PRACTICAL STRESS ANALYSIS™ for DESIGN ENGINEERS

Engineers . . . the Foundation of Modern Technology

PRACTICAL STRESS ANALYSIS ™
for
DESIGN ENGINEERS

Jean-Claude Flabel
Program Director and Professor of Structural Engineering
Engineering Contract Services

Design and Analysis
of
Aerospace Vehicle Structures

Lake City Publishing Company

PRACTICAL STRESS ANALYSIS for DESIGN ENGINEERS

ISBN 0-9647014-0-5

Library of Congress Catalog Card Number: 95-94570

10 9 8 7 6 5

First Edition

Lake City Publishing Company
P.O. Box 2318
Hayden Lake, Idaho 83835
USA

Tel: 1-208-772-7721
Fax: 1-208-762-7466
lakecityusa@mindspring.com

http://www.psa1.com

Printed in the United States of America.

PREFACE

The reason that most aerospace structural design engineers are "underutilized" today is a direct result of the aerospace industries' efforts over the preceding two decades to increase specialization within the structural engineering fields. This prevailing attitude that exists by most companies can however lead to awkward, inefficient, and inadequate structural designs. These designs are often a result of unsatisfactory steps taken during the initial structural analysis effort of the preliminary design concept. To efficiently design an aircraft structure, the structural design engineer must verify his designs by making preliminary and investigative stress analysis computations. To design a structure in synergy with preexisting designs, without the principles of analysis to assist the engineer in arriving at sound conclusions, can severely restrict one's creativity of new and innovative design approaches, and thereby lead to faulty or inadequate structural designs.

Careful planning of a structure comes from a well-disciplined method of attack, and with it the satisfaction of knowing that you have truly done the best job possible. The ability to "visualize and see" structure clearly, and to perceive different relationships from this mental image, will develop into better understanding the behavior of structure. Hence, having a more realistic approach to profound and complex design situations will lead to a greater anticipation and awareness of the consequences of these inherent structural complexities. In the end, one must maintain good judgment in making sound and correct decisions so that the practical use of this technical reference can transcend itself into the engineer's ability to act effectively in different, but yet similar, design situations. Common sense and sound judgment are therefore unique qualities implying diversified training and experience. With these attributes, one can achieve confidence and independence in solving complex design problems.

The material of this book will offer each design engineer a systematic approach to engineering designs based on industry-proven methods of stress analysis. Emphasis will be placed on the solution of actual structural engineering designs so realistic that the engineer can easily relate them to his on-the-job engineering experience. To avoid time-consuming approaches to many designs, wherever possible, shortcuts, approximate methods, and rule-of-thumb methods of analysis will be employed. These approximations will provide convenient and reliable methods of analysis of sufficient accuracy to use in all preliminary and investigative stages of structural design. The simplification of stress analysis methods allows a design engineer a wider latitude of imagination and greater flexibility in expediently solving basic and complex engineering design problems.

This book has a wealth of information about practical engineering problems. But more important than the specific solutions made available to each design engineer is the general attitude of its collections. In other words, interpreting the information collected in a way in which each design engineer can treat effectively alternative forms of structural designs and readily choose the best possible solution. The wise and prudent use of this book will provide the competent design engineer with "many years" of practical stress analysis experience—the same practical experience industry professionals in this field have learned. In summary, the knowledge and experience gained from the study of this material will provide the practicing design engineer with a better understanding relating to the selection of reliable, weight-efficient, and cost-effective aircraft structures. The true *hands-on* engineer will possess the creative and select means to produce "value-added" enhancements for product improvement leading to competitive, end-item hardware—that which is required of truly successful designs. A reduction in the time-consuming, iterative process of developing reliable structure will allow for more attention to be given to other significant design considerations such as maintainability and producibility concurrent with the structural certification process.

This book will serve both as an introduction to the fundamentals of stress analysis for inexperienced design engineers as well as provide a valuable reference for more experienced professionals in this field. The many example problems given throughout this documentary material can be used as standards of comparison against which to check the analysis of other similar and related structural types often encountered in actual engineering designs. The material is presented in such a manner that the subject matter can be easily understood. This book also presents the fundamental principles of stress analysis without requiring the use of advanced mathematics. After these principles have been thoroughly studied and recognized in terms of "practical theory," most of the difficult and complex design problems faced by today's structural design engineer will not seem so confusing nor so complicated. In fact, those of you who will follow through in a diligent study of this material to its conclusion will be better prepared to take on the technological challenges of today—and for years to come.

In closing, this book is a significant attempt to bring new education or re-education to those design engineers who wish to achieve the degree of success their knowledge, background, and experience should promote. It is also envisioned that this critical training will significantly impact a company's bottom line by enhancing the working relationship between design and stress engineering groups. I sincerely wish you mutual success in the challenges ahead and hope this material enables you to accomplish the engineering and professional goals you set out to achieve.

The Author

Hayden Lake, Idaho
January 14, 1997

ACKNOWLEDGMENTS

In the writing of a book there are many people "behind the scenes" who are vital to its success. I would like to express my sincere thanks to my lovely wife, Carroll, for her patience and tolerance during the many difficult years while *Practical Stress Analysis for Design Engineers* was being written, technically illustrated, and produced. Special thanks for her graphics-editing assistance that was required for the multiplicity of scanned images that are used throughout the book. Her effort was truly invaluable.

I would like to express my gratitude to Frank R. Wall, my good friend, for his technical support of the many aircraft designs used throughout the text. His background and experience in aircraft engineering provided me with the key elements necessary to produce this document. It has truly been my privilege to know and work with him.

Also, I would like to give my special thanks to Jim Clark of Wichita, Kansas, who helped edit the original manuscript. His diligence in examining the complete text has contributed substantially to the readability and accuracy of the finished work.

I am also indebted to all of the practicing engineers throughout the aerospace industry who participated in my training program in *Practical Stress Analysis. . . .* Your response in the form of informative, interactive questions over the years has helped to significantly improve the baseline manuscript material. Your encouragement and loyalty has given me the confidence and inspiration of producing this material as an invaluable reference source, and for that I am grateful. Without your expressed support this effort might not have been undertaken.

I also wish to express my sincere appreciation to the following aerospace heritage companies for allowing this critical training to be presented to their engineers at on-site company facilities: Northrop B-2 Division, Lockheed-General Dynamics—Fort Worth Division, NASA—John F. Kennedy Space Center, Lockheed Missiles and Space Company, Boeing Commercial Airplane Group, Bell Helicopter Textron, McDonnell Douglas Corp., Rockwell International—Aircraft and Space Divisions, Sikorsky Aircraft Company, and Douglas Aircraft Company.

Jean-Claude Flabel

TABLE OF CONTENTS

CHAPTER 3. CONNECTION ANALYSIS

CHAPTER 4. SHEARING STRESSES

CHAPTER 5. SHEAR and TENSION CLIP SUPPORTS

CHAPTER 6. CRIPPLING of COMPRESSION MEMBERS

CHAPTER 7. COLUMN MEMBERS

CHAPTER 8. SHEAR-RESISTANT BEAMS

CHAPTER 9. CUTOUTS and HOLE REINFORCEMENTS

LIST OF TABLES

FOREWORD

The structural design engineer's principal job objective is to develop producible hardware that is of high quality, lightweight, and cost-effective. Furthermore, his designs must be functional, and must also be compatible to complement the interfacing structure. All of which must be accomplished within realistic schedules and mandated, budgetary constraints. In order for the design engineer to accomplish this, his work must embody the design philosophies associated with the actual structural behavior of candidate design concepts, with due regards to the analytical methods and approaches of stress analysis.

This book is intended to develop a designer's ability to analyze and study the structural behavior of engineering designs under load. Only through realized confidence and independence can the design engineer provide the leadership required to implement structural designs on major engineering programs. *Practical Stress Analysis (PSA)* will attempt to achieve the creative response to that end.

In this book, the principles and methods of stress analysis are presented to assist and support the design engineer in his selection of the very best alternative structural designs. Only through a comprehensive, practical training program can the engineer hope to fully apply the creativity, intelligence, and imagination required to address the scientific evaluation of reliable and cost-effective aircraft structures. The accomplished design engineer must also rely on his past experience and theoretical ability to arrive at a truly successful, integrated design.

Many detailed stress analysis solutions are incorporated in the material of this book. Only after a thorough study of these solutions, however, can the concepts and ideas of simplified and approximate methods be fully appreciated. The approximate methods of analysis in this book will serve as an invaluable part of the engineer's development and training of his so-called "practical feel" of the structure. The design engineer seldom has the time to completely analyze a structure in detail. Nonetheless, a solid understanding of the basic design process is essential. Therefore, the engineer must first learn to rely on good approximations of complex engineering problems. It is important that the engineer recognize and differentiate between the nature of these approximations and the conditions of more exact methods and approaches of detailed stress analysis. If he is then called upon to take a more active role in the analytical approach, this book will become his guide.

Knowing how to analyze and provide quick, reliable solutions and trade-studies of complex structures *(designer's option)* is what makes the field of structural engineering exciting. If required, structure can be substantiated in detail, only as deemed necessary to validate the design concept. In the real world of engineering, many assumptions and simplifications of a complex structure must be made to achieve a successful engineering design. It takes an engineer many years of practical engineering experience to fully develop the skills necessary to successfully design and analyze actual engineering problems. Engineering is not the substitution of numbers into "magic" equations of stress analysis. The structural design engineer must develop an intuitive "feel" of the structure and know when to recognize and apply simplifications of otherwise *exact solutions*. The design engineer will thereby gain a better understanding behind the philosophy, aesthetics, and economical development of the structural design concept.

In contrast to industry methods, the main focus of attention in most engineering schools is, however, principally directed towards *exact solutions* of hypothetical engineering problems. When an engineering student first attains his degree in engineering, and begins to practice in the industry and apply the teachings of his learned professors, he is shocked to discover that many more years of engineering training must be spent in order to fully complement his new profession. All of the technical training and discipline that he has learned must now be enhanced by directing his energies to the solution of engineering problems using inexact, approximate, and conservative problem-solving techniques. If the graduate engineer is to attain competence in his new professional career, he must acquire these new and sometimes misunderstood methods of analysis.

The bottom line is that this book will provide the necessary training in the specialized concepts involved for the design engineer to further expand his ability to do his own personal stress studies; for example, capable of performing independently in the analysis, design, and investigation of advanced technical systems or concepts. . . . And thereby, gain a greater appreciation of the structural and environmental surroundings of a flight vehicle structure. The creative design engineer who can perform practical stress analysis in the development and application of his ideas has *no limits or bounds* in this competitive industry which demands and rewards perfection. If this book is used consistently by the design engineer, it should serve him well as a guide that is essential to intelligent thinking and independent thought, and as an invaluable reference source.

Frank Reginald Wall

Atlanta, Georgia
February 3, 1996

PRACTICAL STRESS ANALYSIS ™ for DESIGN ENGINEERS

Jean-Claude Flabel

CHAPTER 1

Principles of Statics

1.1 Introduction. It is suggested that the engineer study this chapter carefully, as it will serve as the basis for the fundamental development of stress analysis methods and procedures. Only then can the accomplished design engineer hope to learn and fully understand the assumptions and approaches of subsequent chapters of this book. If the concepts and definitions seem unfamiliar on first reading, do not become discouraged, just continue reading through Sec. 1.4. If, at that time, the theories of these sections have not yet been clearly understood, then the material of the preceding sections should again be thoroughly reviewed.

Previous teaching experience has shown that design engineers who study the fundamentals of stress analysis require some basic review of statics. The equations of static equilibrium are constantly used and applied by structural engineers in the solution of unknown forces and reactions of a structure. Before these fundamental principles are discussed, however, it is necessary to emphasize certain concepts and definitions concerning forces and force systems. These definitions will provide the foundation necessary to develop a thorough and practical working knowledge of stress analysis. Let us now begin these discussions.

A force may be defined as an action which changes the state of motion of a member to which it is applied. The force can be completely described by the following definitions: (1) its point of application, (2) its line of action, and (3) its magnitude. A force is therefore a vector quantity since it specifies both magnitude and direction. The action of one body making direct physical contact with another is an example of an applied force. Although the physical distribution of this force may be rather complex in nature, its idealized representation on the structure can conveniently be described by a concentrated force (more about this in Sec. 1.4).

A moment is defined about an axis through a point as the product of a force times the perpendicular distance from the point to the line of action of the force, or

$$M = Fd. \tag{1-1}$$

To help illustrate the application of Eq. 1-1, consider the diagram of Fig. 1-1. If one end of a string is attached at *A*, considered the pivot axis, and the other end attached perpendicular to the line of action of the vector force *F*, a clockwise rotation is produced by the moment at *A*. In a similar manner, at pivot axis *B*, a counterclockwise rotation is produced by the moment of the vector force *F* at *B*. Using Eq. 1-1, the following mathematical expressions are written for the moments that are calculated at points *A* and *B*:

$$\text{Moment @ } A = M_A = Fd_1 \quad \text{(clockwise rotation)}$$
$$\text{Moment @ } B = M_B = Fd_2 \quad \text{(counterclockwise rotation)}$$

where subscripts *A* and *B* identify the axes perpendicular to the plane of the paper about which moments are calculated, and where the rotations are indicated by the direction specified by the arrowhead of the vector force *F*. The rotations are denoted by the circular arcs (phantom lines) drawn in the figure. If a clockwise rotation is established as a positive quantity and a counterclockwise rotation as a negative, the moment expressions are conveniently rewritten as follows:

$$M_A = Fd_1$$
$$M_B = -Fd_2.$$

Note that if moments are calculated about pivot axis *C*, the perpendicular distance from this axis to the line of action of the vector force *F* is zero, and therefore, the moment M_C based on the definition of Eq. 1-1 is also zero. The importance of a vector force acting through the pivot axis will become clearer as our attention is focused on the calculation of beam reactions in Sec. 1.4.

A free-body diagram is a picture or outline of the structure with all of the applied forces acting and all of the reactions indicated. A free-body diagram is the one most important concept to a successful and dependable stress analysis solution. Most engineering errors can be eliminated by providing a complete and properly oriented free-body diagram of the structure being analyzed. The structure (or body) must be maintained in a state of equilibrium, under the action of a completely balanced set of applied loads and unknown reaction forces. Reactions are identified by the particular type of resistance that a support offers to its beam structure. After

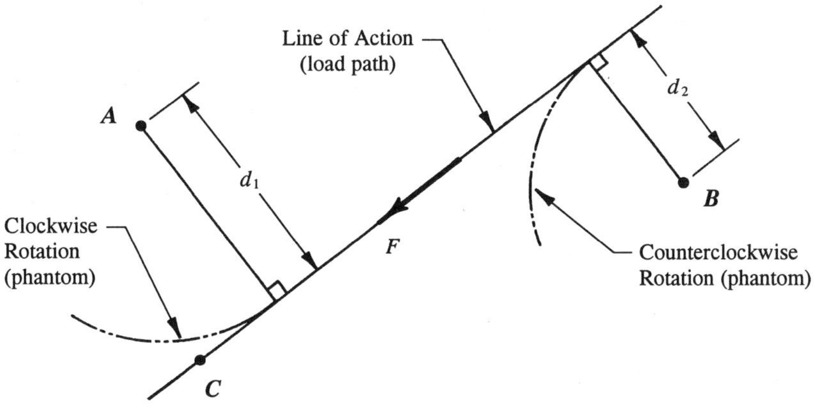

FIGURE 1-1 Illustration of a moment of a force at points A and B.

a free-body diagram has been sketched and all forces applied, unknown reaction forces are then computed. This is accomplished by utilizing the following six equations of static equilibrium:

$$\Sigma F_x = 0 \qquad \Sigma F_y = 0 \qquad \Sigma F_z = 0 \tag{1-2}$$
$$\Sigma M_x = 0 \qquad \Sigma M_y = 0 \qquad \Sigma M_z = 0. \tag{1-3}$$

These equations must be satisfied in their respective x-, y-, and z-directions to maintain a structure in a state of equilibrium; otherwise, a state of unbalance would exist for the structure. Equation 1-2 states that the algebraic sum of all translational forces acting on a structure in the x-, y-, and z-directions must equal zero. Similarly, Eq. 1-3 states that the algebraic sum of the moments of all the translational forces around the x-, y-, and z-axes must also be zero to establish rotational equilibrium of the entire structure. These equations should be somewhat familiar to each engineer. If not, several example problems that follow in Sec. 1.4 should provide all of the review necessary for each engineer to become current in these fundamental principles. Before these examples are presented, however, the different types of supports and conventions of loading a structure that are most common to structural engineering will be defined.

1.2 Conventional Support Types. A beam is one of the most fundamental structural members that is analyzed by the structural design engineer. Most beams are partially or completely restrained from moving freely by their support structure. Even though an infinite number of support types are physically possible, only three conventional types will be presented here: (1) a roller support, (2) a pinned support, and (3) a fixed support. The supports are identified by the kind of resistance they offer to the applied forces. The engineer must keep in mind that many years of engineering experience have correlated these conventional support types with

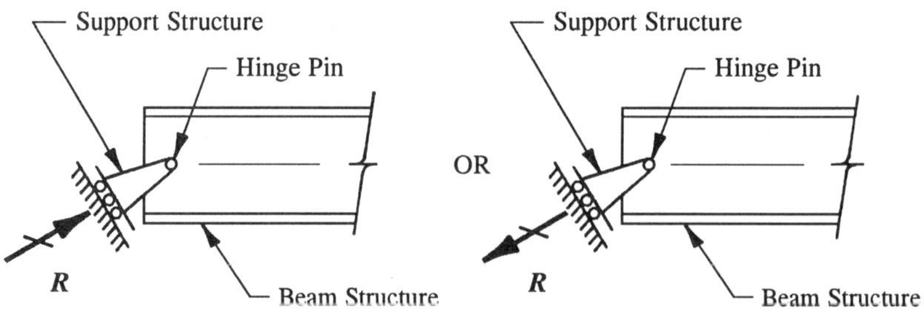

FIGURE 1-2 Roller support. The line of action indicated by the reaction *R*.

the actual behavior of the structure under load. Nevertheless, it is extremely rare for the actual support structure to correspond exactly with the engineer's idealized conception of that structure (more about this in Sec. 1.9). So, in those cases, where the actual degree of restraint of a support may not be known, it is desirable to take a conservative approach to the stress analysis, possibly, using several assumptions or criteria. After a thorough review of these conventional support types have been studied, Sec. 1.9 will treat this condition more specifically.

The first type of structural support arrangement identified is a roller support, as it functions very similar to that of a roller skate, as shown in Fig. 1-2. It is capable of resisting a force acting through the center of its hinge pin either *away* or *toward* the surface on which the rollers roll.[1] By industry convention, the reactive force is usually designated by drawing a line through its force vector, as shown in this figure. Whereas, externally applied forces are not normally indicated in this manner. This is generally a good engineering practice for the design engineer to adopt and use in his study of stress analysis solutions.

At present,[2] we need only concern ourselves with the type of restraint that is offered by these support members; the capability of which is best described by the roller support structure. In Figs. 1-3(a) and (b) are shown two beam structures, the first of which represents an actual beam structure, and the second which depicts the corresponding idealization of the supported structure of that beam. To avoid a weight penalty, a shear clip is principally designed to transfer shear from one structural member to another (vertically as shown in Fig. 1-3). Although shear clips may appear to provide some restraint axially or by rotating, their primary shear load-carrying ability greatly exceeds that of these other forms of resistance. However, if a shear clip is forced to bend or to be pulled in these other failure modes, then, of course, the shear clip must be designed to meet the strength requirements of these additional loading effects. In the final analysis, so long as the design engineer has provided the necessary load paths to carry all of the applied loads efficiently through the structure, the shear clip and its main beam structure should be

[1] This implies that the rollers are trapped between the structures indicated.

[2] Chapter 5 will present a complete detailed analysis of many different types of shear clips: single angle clips, back-to-back angle clips, and tee clips.

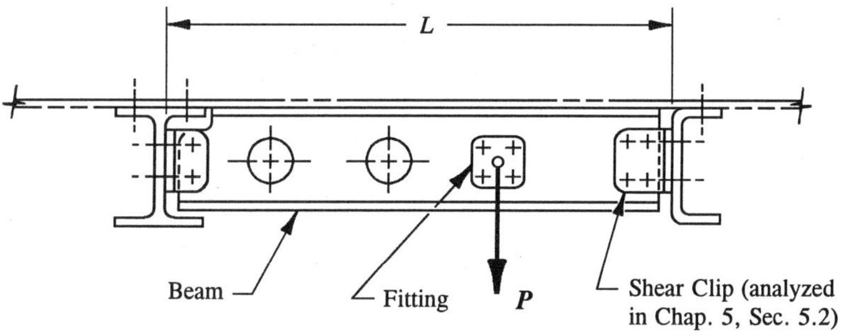

(a) Actual Beam Structure

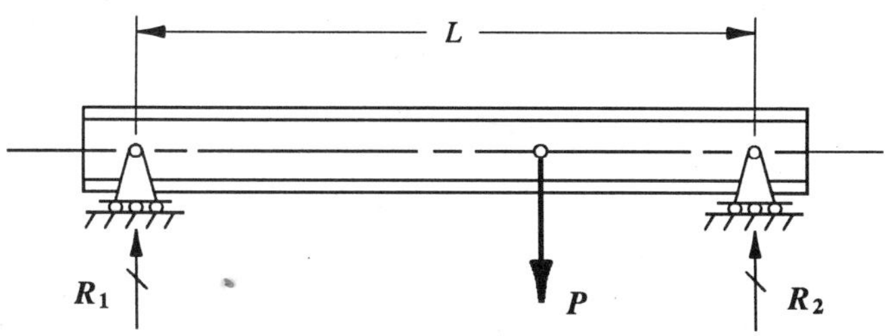

(b) Idealized Beam Structure

FIGURE 1-3 Beam simply-supported at its ends by shear clips.

adequately substantiated. Experience and good engineering judgment are therefore the necessary prerequisites to the determination of reliable shear clip designs.

For critical structures, the analytical approaches and assumptions that are made by the design engineer in his selection of members of adequate strength are eventually verified by actual structural testing. It can be said that no better proof of the true strength and structural integrity of a member can be made than through its physical testing; no matter what results can be shown by rigorous structural analysis. In summary, the main design function of a shear clip is limited to carrying loads in the vertical direction; the horizontal direction simply prevents the overall structure from physically moving or sliding. In addition, this type of support is allowed to freely rotate; thereby producing no appreciable build up of end moment at its support structure. Hence, a shear clip most effectively transmits a reactive shear force at a known point, but the magnitude of which is unknown. The unknown reactive force will be determined in Sec. 1.4 by simultaneously solving the equations of static equilibrium. Although shear clips are depicted by roller supports here, their structural arrangement does in fact prevent the beam from physically moving horizontally under light loading.

The second type of support recognized for a beam is called a pinned support, as shown in Fig. 1-4(a). A pinned support has the capability of resisting a reactive

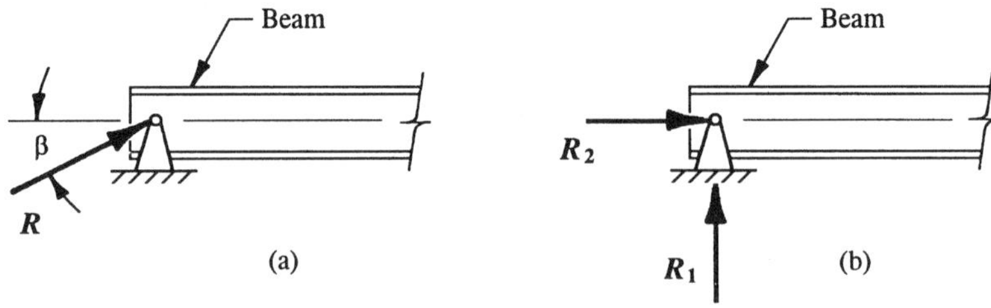

FIGURE 1-4 Pinned support, (a) line of action of the reaction force R, (b) the reaction force R represented by equivalent component forces.

force acting in any direction. In Fig. 1-4(b), such a support is conveniently represented by two equivalent components of force, one acting in a horizontal direction R_2 and the other acting in a vertical direction R_1. The equivalent component forces will exert the same desired physical effects on the structure as the resultant reactive force R. A lug-pin combination such as that of Fig. 1-5 is a good illustration of an actual support structure that can transmit a reactive force in any direction. Since the direction of the resultant force R acting through the hinge pin is not known, it is customary to replace the resultant by its equivalent system of component reactive forces R_1 and R_2, as indicated in Fig. 1-6.

Lastly, in Fig. 1-7, the third type of conventional support is considered for a beam, in which the support structure provides both the capability of resisting a force in any direction and also preventing the end of the beam from rotating. This type of support is illustrated by depicting a beam that is clipped at its supported end and providing continuous upper and lower beam caps. Physically, this support structure could be described by building the end of the beam into a brick wall, or by casting its end into concrete, or by welding its end securely into the attached structure. Such a support is called a fixed support, i.e., where three unknown reactive forces R_1, R_2, and M_R are considered acting, as shown in Fig. 1-8. The splice

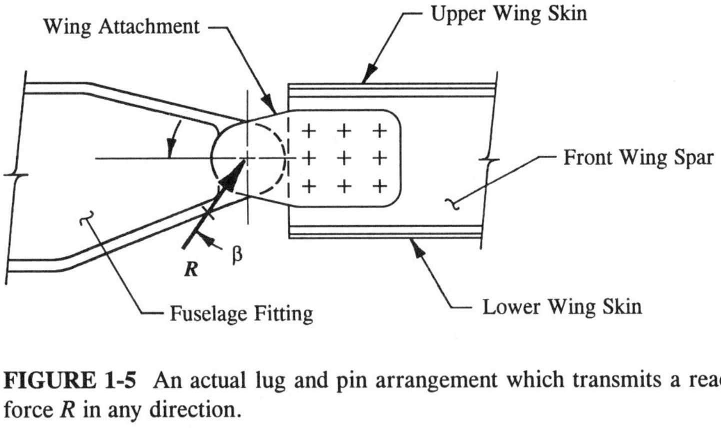

FIGURE 1-5 An actual lug and pin arrangement which transmits a reactive force R in any direction.

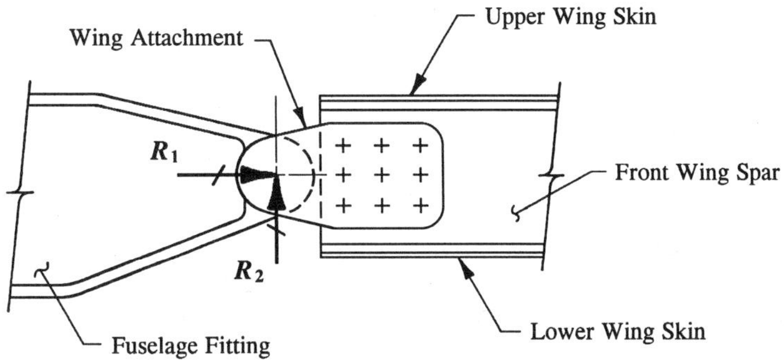

FIGURE 1-6 Resultant force replaced by component forces R_1 and R_2.

plates of the upper and lower beam caps serve two main purposes: each plate can react either tension or compression axial forces, as well as react any bending moment that is developed at the fixed end of the beam. The unknown reactive axial force is designated by the symbol R_1, and the resistance to rotation of the member is described by the reactive moment M_R at the fixed end of the beam. And, as was previously reasoned in this section, a shear clip will provide the vertical reactive shear capability, indicated by the reaction force R_2. As a final note, a complex structure with all of its various structural members possible, i.e., clips, angles, fittings, and all of the many different forms and methods of attaching these

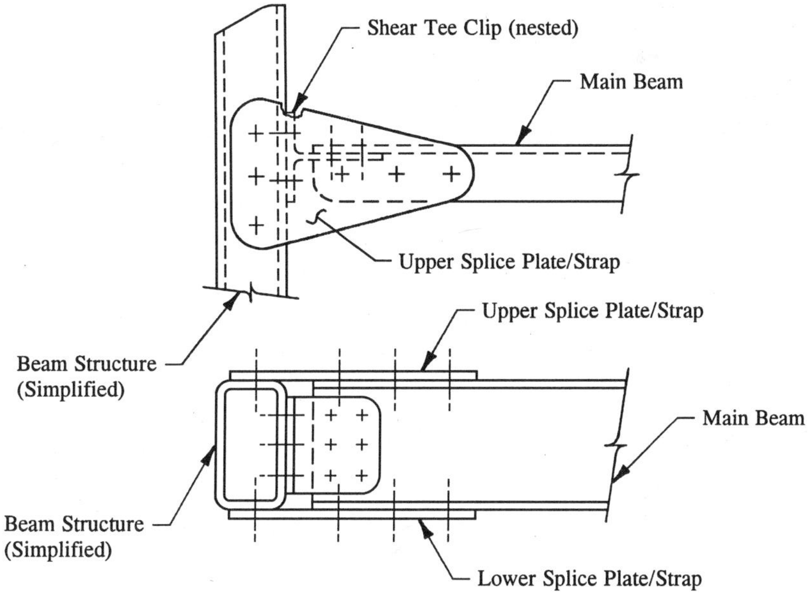

FIGURE 1-7 Fixed support structure represented by actual structure.

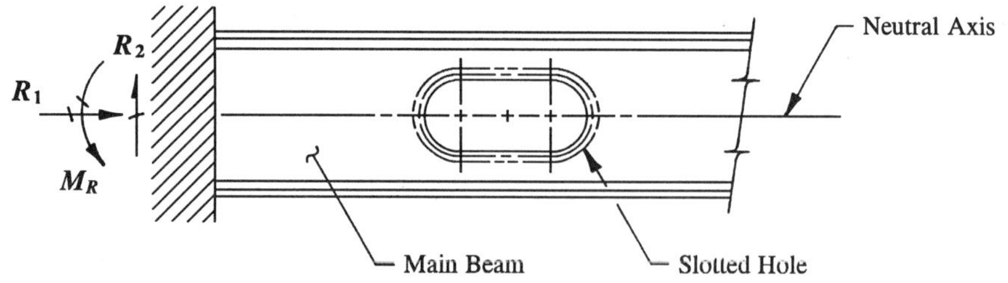

FIGURE 1-8 Idealization of a fixed support structure.

members together, is easily and conveniently simplified by idealizing its component parts in this way. The simplification of the actual support structure outlined here will become more apparent when our discussions proceed to numerical computations of actual structure.

1.3 Conventional Loading Types. In this section, two types of concentrated loads are presented, they are illustrated in Fig. 1-9, where each loading is considered applied at a point; the *concentrated load* and the *concentrated moment.* Realistically, it is physically impossible to apply a concentrated load to a member at a point. The material will begin to yield at the contact point which will tend to spread the load out over some small area. For the purposes of calculating beam reactions (see Sec. 1-4), however, idealizing loads as concentrated at a point is a convenient (also accurate) way of describing externally applied loads.

A multitude of variations of *distributed loads* are possible, i.e., the aerodynamic airloads on an aircraft wing, hydrostatic pressures in a fuel tank, the internal fuselage cabin pressures, to name a few. Under such complex loading conditions, the practicing aerospace engineer will simplify the pressure loading distribution by one or a combination of two commonly known types; the *uniformly distributed load* and the *uniformly varying distributed load*, as shown in Fig. 1-10. As a matter of fact, many hours of detailed stress analysis can be saved by assuming a simplified but yet conservative approach to a complex loading condition. From a design

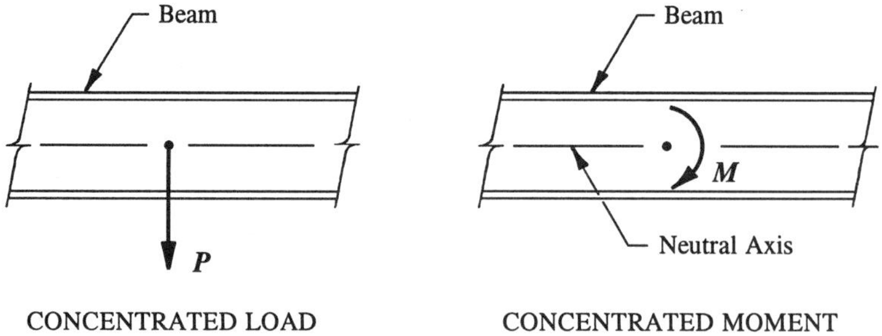

FIGURE 1-9 Idealization of concentrated loading types.

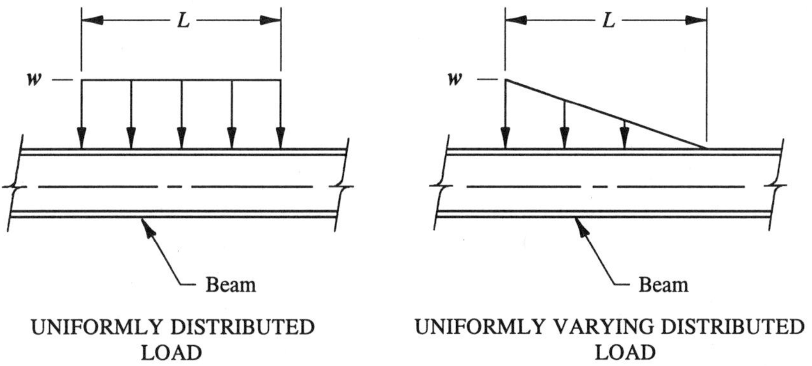

FIGURE 1-10 Representation of distributed loading types.

standpoint, it may be less expensive to overdesign slightly than to save weight by considering time-consuming detailed methods of analysis. Also refer to Table 1-1, Case 3, where the effects of a uniform pressure distribution onto an access door is simplified by the uniformly distributed pressure load carried by the panel stiffener. The engineer is referred to Example 2-1 in Chapter 2 for a specific problem solution depicting this simplified analysis approach.

To explain the meaning of w lb/in for a uniformly distributed load, it is reasoned that for each inch of loading, w lb are applied or introduced into the structure. Until, as we proceed from left to right along the entire length of the beam structure, the total load or wL is represented. Now, if a line is drawn from one corner to the opposite diagonal corner of the uniformly distributed load, the following analogy can be made: if a triangular loading area represents exactly one-half of a rectangular loading area, it then follows directly that the uniformly varying distributed load must represent one-half of the uniformly distributed load or $\frac{1}{2}wL$.

In subsequent sections of this book, it will be found that for the purposes of calculating beam reactions, each distributed loading is conveniently idealized by a concentrated force acting at the center of pressure of the loading area of the particular distribution described, Fig. 1-11. If this procedure is followed, the equations of static equilibrium as given by Eqs. 1-2 and 1-3 (refer back to page 3) can then easily be applied to most any structure. Note that the actual distributions are only idealized by concentrated forces. *At no time have the physical characteristics of the actual loading changed.* Therefore, it would then logically follow that once the reactions have been determined, the original loading distribution that the concentrated force represented be replaced back onto the structure. Much confusion will be avoided by adhering to this principle when our study of internal loads analysis begins. To provide the engineer with some physical meaning to the conventional loading types aforementioned, actual structural members that depict these loadings are summarized and pictured in Table 1-1. Again, as was stated previously, an ample number of example problems will be presented in this chapter for each

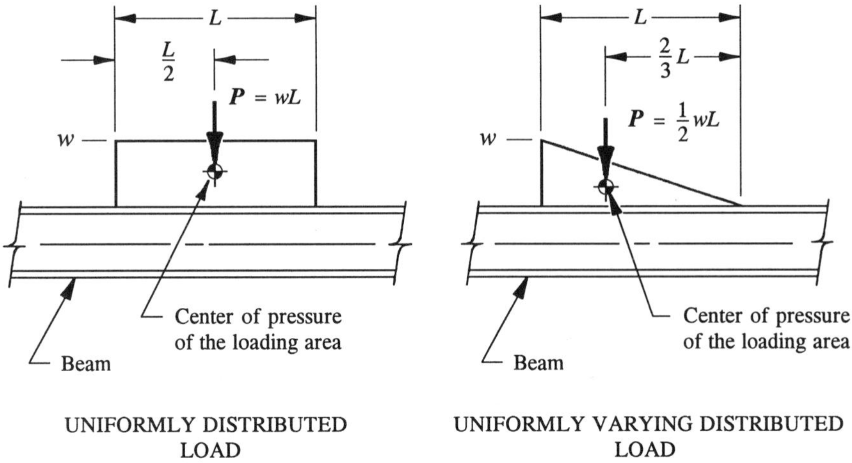

FIGURE 1-11 Idealization of distributed loading types.

engineer to become thoroughly proficient with the new concepts and principles of the preceding sections.

1.4 Calculation of Beam Reactions. The definitions and ideas of the preceding sections are united in this section in an attempt to present the method of calculating beam reactions of a structure. The principles are clear, in order to adequately design a beam to resist the internal stresses which are produced in a structure, it is first necessary to determine "support reactions." To achieve a dependable stress analysis solution for the main structure also requires that the support structure of the beam itself be able to physically withstand the reactions produced there.

A structure is said to be statically determinate if the known reactive forces of the structure can be obtained from the simultaneous solution of the equations of static equilibrium $\Sigma F_x = 0$, $\Sigma F_y = 0$, and $\Sigma M_z = 0$. More specifically, if the number of unknown forces that exist on a structure are the same or fewer than the number of independent equations formulated, the reactions can easily be found by the methods of this section. However, if the structure has more unknown reactive forces than the number of independent equations of statics formulated, no solution can be obtained from statics alone. The particular structure is termed "statically indeterminate" or sometimes referred to as a "redundant structure." The complex mathematics required and advanced nature of indeterminate structures is beyond the main intent and scope of this book. Instead, complete solutions of indeterminate structures, as given by the reference beam formula solutions of Appendix D, page 633, will be used in the solutions of actual stress analysis problems. This basic approach to the analysis of a structure will greatly simplify the overall analysis effort. For the present, all beams analyzed by the methods of this section will be statically determinate. For those engineers who maintain the skills required to

TABLE 1-1 SUMMARY OF CONVENTIONAL LOADING TYPES

Actual Loading Structure	Idealized Loading Structure
Case 1 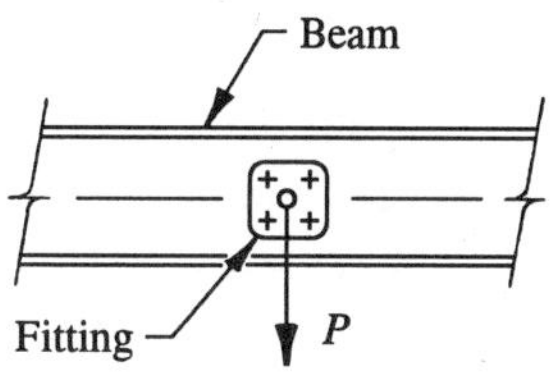	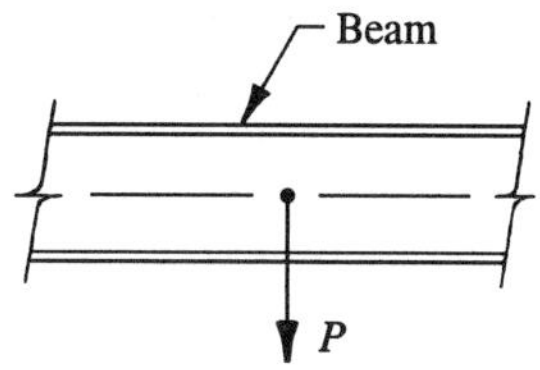 CONCENTRATED LOAD
Case 2 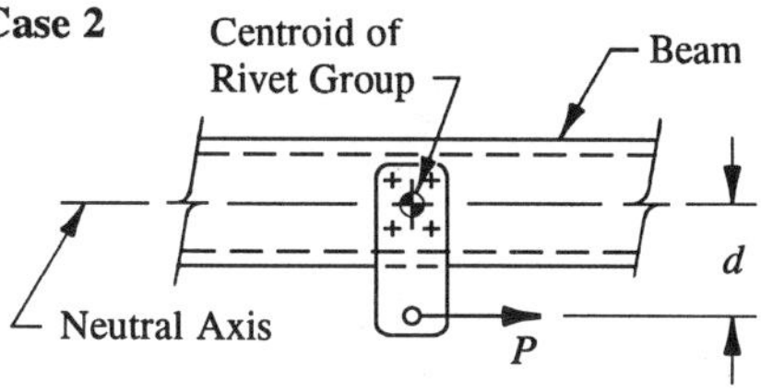	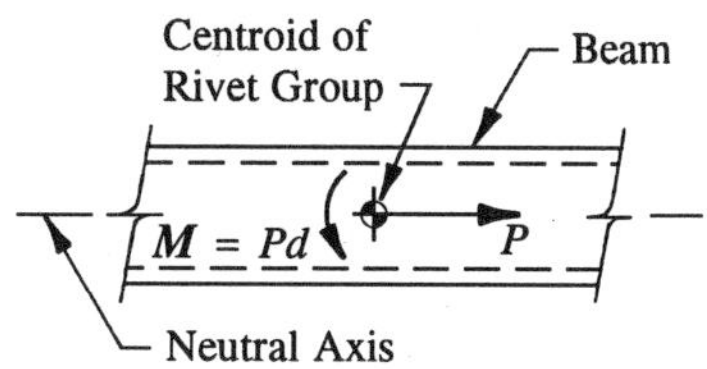 CONCENTRATED MOMENT
Case 3 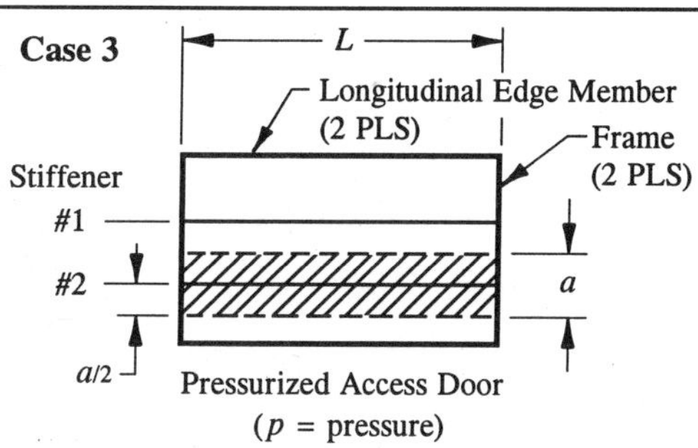 UNIFORM PRESSURE DISTRIBUTION	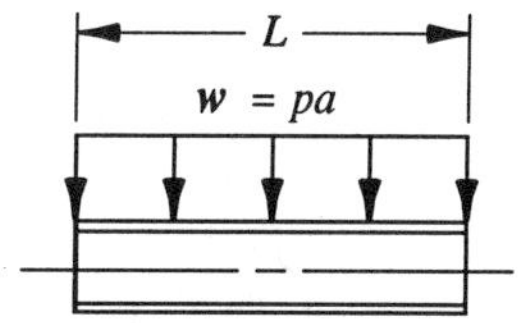 Stiffener UNIFORMLY DISTRIBUTED LOAD (looking at panel in section)
Case 4 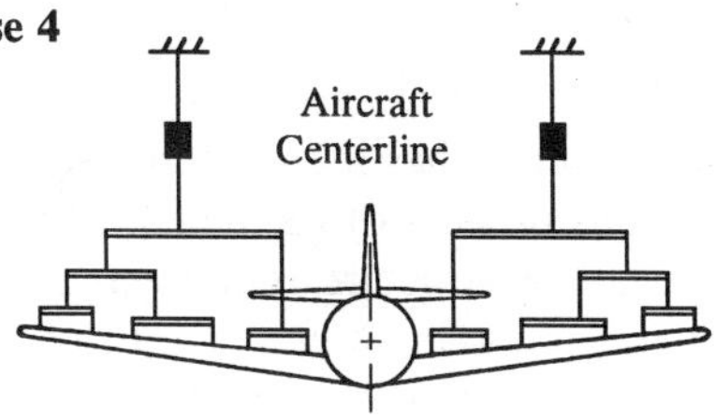 WING UP-BENDING	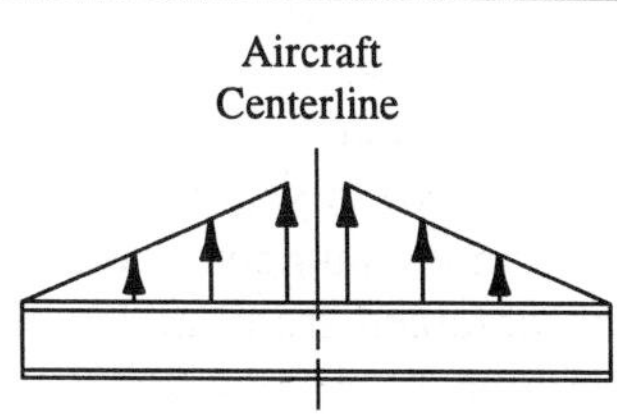 UNIFORMLY VARYING DISTRIBUTED LOAD

successfully apply the equations of statics, proceed ahead to Sec. 1-5. For those who do not, continue to study this section by following the detailed solution of Example 1-1.

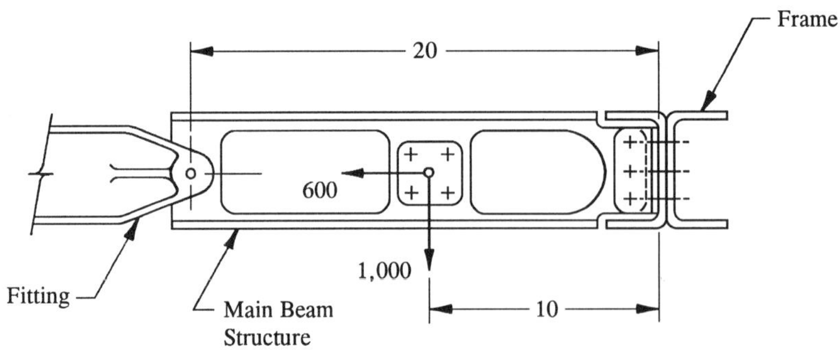

FIGURE 1-12 Beam structure loaded by two concentrated loads.

Example 1-1 For the beam structure of Fig. 1-12, find the magnitude and direction of the beam reactions at the supports. Then, draw a free-body diagram of the structure with the balanced set of applied loads and reaction forces properly indicated.

SOLUTION: The first step in the solution of Example 1-1 is to identify the resistance that each support provides to its main structure. This consists of idealizing the actual supports by one of the three conventional types discussed in the previous sections of this book. The following diagrammatical symbols for these supports are drawn, Fig. 1-13, based on the type of load resistance that each support supplies to the main structure.

To formulate equations from the applied and reactive forces, a rectangular coordinate system is adopted, as shown in the figure. Further, it is assumed that all of the forces (applied or reacted) are arranged on the beam in one plane.[1] From this, the six equations of statics are simplified to three. These are $\Sigma F_x = 0$, $\Sigma F_y = 0$, and $\Sigma M_z = 0$, and are described as follows:

The first of these equations $\Sigma F_x = 0$ requires that all the forces acting in the x-direction be algebraically summed and set equal to zero. Two forces are noted acting horizontally in the figure; R_3 at A and the 600 lb applied force at B. Because the reaction R_3 is acting in the positive x-direction, it is assigned a positive value or $+R_3$, while the 600 lb load applied at B is acting in the negative x-direction, it is assigned a negative value or -600 lb. The two forces are then combined algebraically and set equal to zero.

$$\Sigma F_x = 0, \qquad R_3 - 600 = 0.$$

[1] Even for a single angle shear clip support structure, the out-of-plane loads created by its design configuration are reacted by the shear clip itself. A detailed solution is systematically arrived at by balancing the support structure (shear clip) one plane at a time (for analysis details, see Chapter 5). Hence, for our solution here, no difficulty should be encountered by making this assumption.

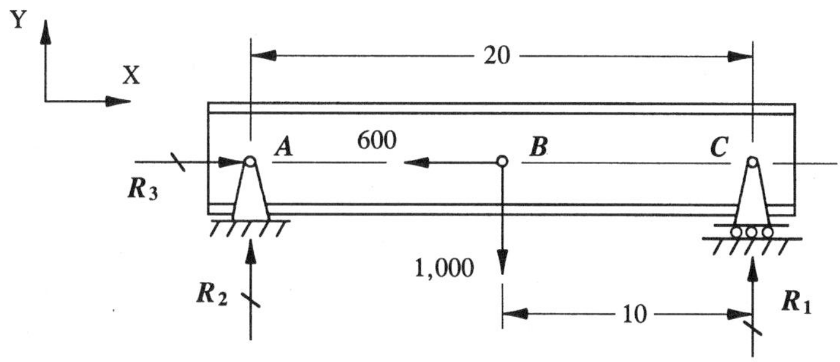

FIGURE 1-13 Free-body diagram of unknown reaction forces.

Then, solving this equation for R_3, we obtain $R_3 = 600$ lb. As expected, an equal and opposite force of 600 lb at *A* was determined to react the 600 lb applied force at *B*.

To apply the second equation of equilibrium $\Sigma F_y = 0$ requires all forces (applied or reacted) acting in the *y*-direction to be algebraically summed and set equal to zero. They are, from left to right, reaction R_2 at *A*, the 1,000 lb applied force at *B*, and the reaction R_1 at *C*. The following signs are indicated for each force: R_2 and R_1 are positive, since each force acts in the positive *y*-direction, the 1,000 lb force is a negative force or $-$ 1,000 lb, since it acts in the negative *y*-direction. Setting the algebraic sum of these forces equal to zero, we obtain:

$$\Sigma F_y = 0, \qquad R_2 + R_1 - 1{,}000 = 0.$$

To arrive at a solution to this equation, one of the two unknown reactive forces must be determined. The third equation of equilibrium $\Sigma M_z = 0$ will be used to establish the moment equation that will provide the solution to the unknown force R_2. Then, with the value of R_2 known, the unknown force R_1 is easily computed. To simplify the moment expression, moments are conveniently calculated at pivot axis *C*, where an unknown force is known to act through this pivot axis. In addition, let us describe these moments by adopting sign conventions for their solutions. For this example, consider all clockwise rotations as positive and all counterclockwise rotations as negative. The force R_2 at *A* and the 1,000 lb load at *B* will produce moments at the pivot axis *C* since these forces have perpendicular distances from their lines of action to this pivot axis. The forces R_3, R_1, and the 600 lb force do not contribute moments to the moment expression since their lines of action pass directly through the pivot axis *C*. The vector force R_2 produces a clockwise rotation, and based on our sign convention for moments, the moment produced by R_2 is positive or $+R_2(20)$. The 1,000 lb applied load produces a counterclockwise rotation and therefore its moment value is negative or $-1{,}000(10)$. Setting these two moments equal to zero has the effect of forcing the

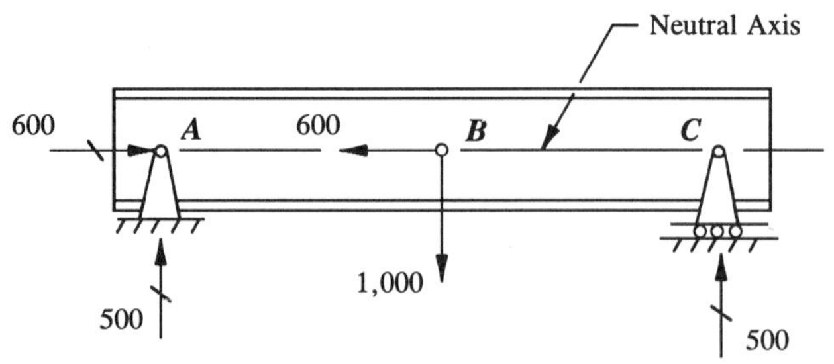

FIGURE 1-14 Beam reactions indicated on a properly drawn diagram of the beam.

beam from physically rotating.

$$(\Sigma M_z)_C = 0, \quad \circlearrowleft + \quad R_2(20) - 1,000(10) = 0.$$

Solving this equation for R_2, we obtain $R_2 = 500$ lb. Now, with the value of R_2 known, we can substitute 500 lb into the second equation of equilibrium that was formulated on the previous page, and solve for R_1. Thus

$$500 + R_1 - 1,000 = 0$$

and hence

$$R_1 = 500 \text{ lb}.$$

Then, with all reaction forces determined, the beam is redrawn with all known loads and reactions properly indicated, as shown in Fig. 1-14.

ALTERNATIVE SOLUTION: To demonstrate how arbitrary the directions of the reaction forces are chosen in the solution of beam reactions, let us reverse the directions of reactions R_3 and R_2 in Fig. 1-15 from those originally assumed, and then again formulate and solve the general equations of static equilibrium. The equations that follow will be presented here without a complete detailed description of how each equation was written:

$$\Sigma F_x = 0, \quad -R_3 - 600 = 0, \quad R_3 = -600 \text{ lb}$$

$$\Sigma F_y = 0, \quad -R_2 - 1,000 + R_1 = 0$$

$$(\Sigma M_z)_C = 0, \quad \circlearrowleft + \quad -R_2(20) - 1,000(10) = 0, \quad R_2 = -500 \text{ lb}.$$

Substituting $R_2 = -500$ lb into the second equation of equilibrium above, we find:

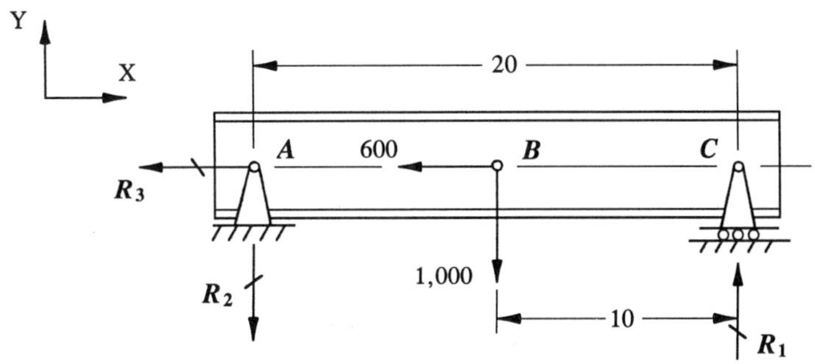

FIGURE 1-15 Free-body diagram of unknown reaction forces.

$$-(-500) - 1,000 + R_1 = 0$$
$$R_1 = 500 \text{ lb}.$$

The alternative solution of beam reactions here reveals that reactions R_3 and R_2 are of the same magnitude but of opposite signs as those values previously calculated by the first method of analysis. The negative signs of R_3 and R_2 simply indicates that the assumed directions of the reactive forces were incorrectly assigned, and should now be correctly indicated on a properly drawn diagram by reversing their directions or simply by circling the arrowheads of these reactive forces, as shown in Fig. 1-16. As before, in the final step, the beam is drawn with all known loads and reactions indicated and the directions of R_3 and R_2 properly oriented, as shown in Fig. 1-17.

In conclusion, when applying the equations of equilibrium, no matter what directions are assumed for the unknown reaction forces, the magnitude of these forces will always be correct. It is their directions that may or may not be properly assigned. However, their directions, as indicated by the sign of their solutions, are easily and conveniently designated on a properly drawn free-body diagram of the structure.

Example 1-2 For the beam loaded as shown in Fig. 1-18, determine the required beam reactions to maintain static equilibrium of this structure. Properly indicate

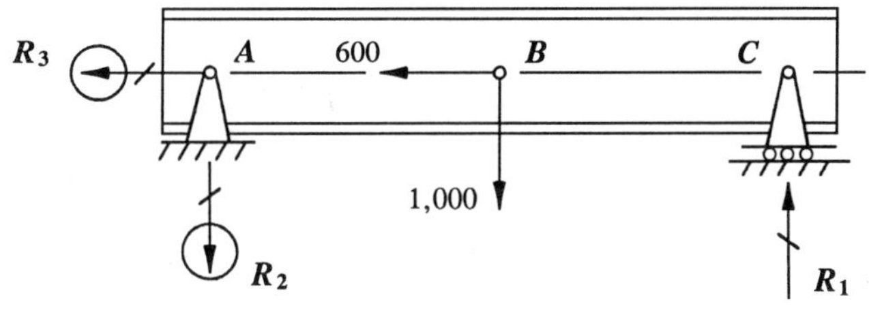

FIGURE 1-16 Alternative free-body diagram of unknown reaction forces.

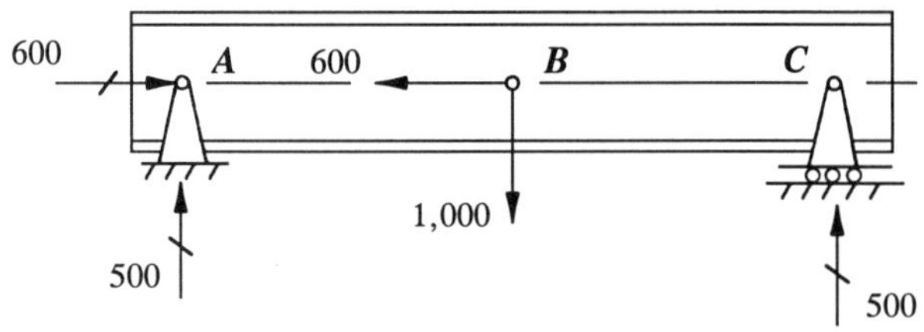

FIGURE 1-17 Beam reactions indicated on a properly drawn diagram of the beam (Repeated).

these reaction forces on a free-body diagram.

SOLUTION: This example problem will clearly demonstrate the solution of beam reactions using the remaining conventional loading types not yet described in this section. As always, the first step in the determination of beam reactions is to replace the support structure of the beam by its corresponding idealized support. This is shown in Fig. 1-19. Secondly, in order to calculate beam reactions using the equations of equilibrium, each distributed load must be replaced by its equivalent concentrated force acting at the centroid of its distribution. The equivalent forces are equal to the sum of all the distributed forces acting along the beam, as was previously shown in Sec. 1.3. To write the three equations of static equilibrium for this structure, proceed as follows:

$$\Sigma F_x = 0, \qquad 0 = 0$$

$$\Sigma F_y = 0, \qquad R_1 - 32 + 13.5 + R_2 = 0, \quad R_1 = -R_2 + 18.5$$

$$\Sigma M_A = 0, \qquad \circlearrowleft + \quad 32(7) + 250 - 13.5(27) - R_2(35) = 0, \quad R_2 = 3.129 \text{ kip}.$$

Now, substituting R_2 into the second equation and simplifying,

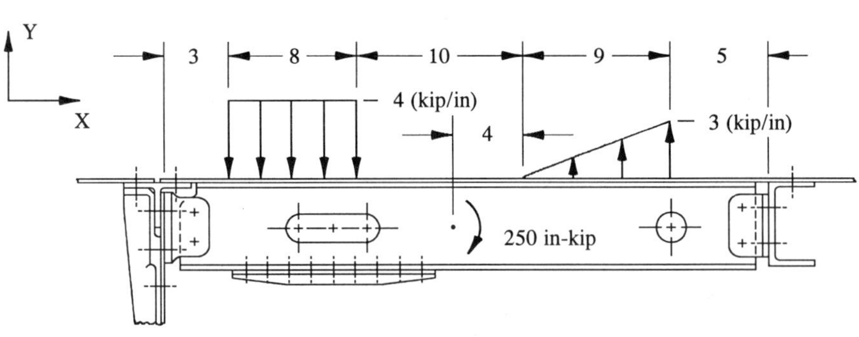

FIGURE 1-18 Beam structure loaded by a concentrated moment and two different distributed loading types.

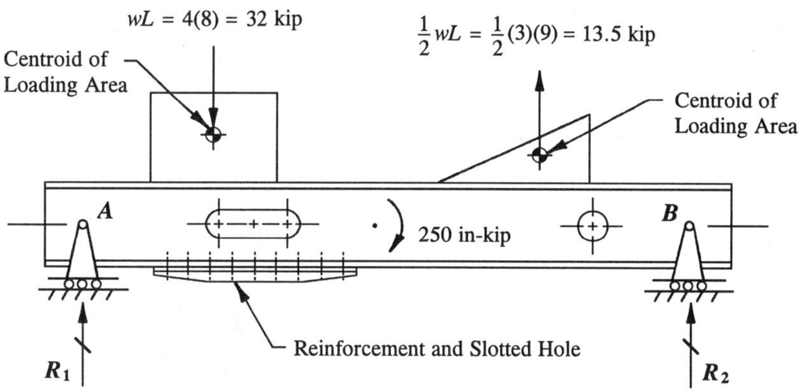

FIGURE 1-19 Idealization of the distributed loading types with unknown reaction forces depicted.

$$R_1 = -(3.129) + 18.5 = 15.371 \text{ kip or } 15{,}371 \text{ lb.}$$

Once the reactions have been computed, the original applied loading distributions are replaced onto the structure. In order to avoid overlooking this principle in design, it is good engineering practice to always show the complete external forces (applied or reacted) in static equilibrium before the internal distributions of stress are made. (The advanced nature of internal stresses in a beam is deferred for discussion until Chapter 2.) The equilibrium of all forces acting on the beam structure is shown in Fig. 1-20.

1.5 Method of Sections Approach to Internal Loads Analysis. The main purpose of this section is to provide a method by which internal forces are determined at any section of a beam. In Chapters 2 and 4, the stresses developed by these internal forces will be computed using conventional stress strength formulas and the results compared to the allowable stresses of the material. The "method of sections approach" is employed here to investigate the internal forces that may exist at any section along the entire length of a beam.

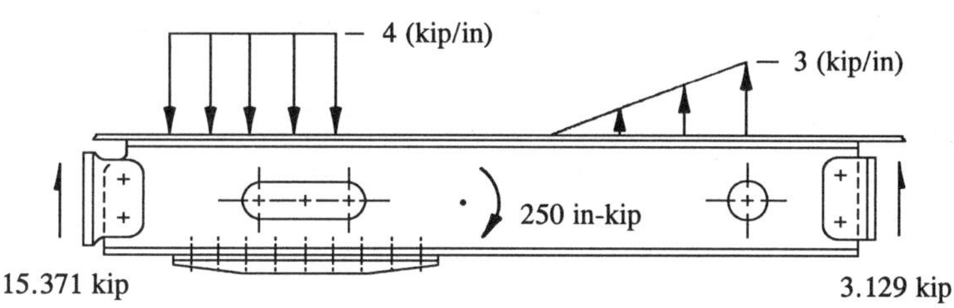

FIGURE 1-20 Free-body diagram of the loaded beam structure.

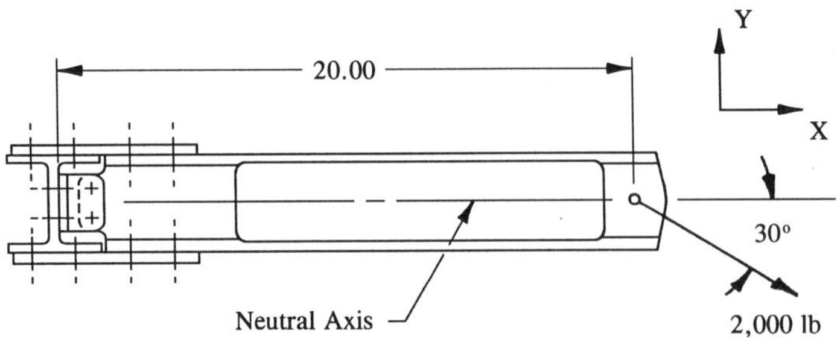

FIGURE 1-21 An actual fixed-supported beam structure.

It is said that if a beam is in equilibrium as a whole, then any isolated part of the beam must also be in equilibrium. To satisfy this condition, it is necessary that there exist a system of internal forces which will establish the isolated part in equilibrium. On each exposed part of the beam, a vertical force *V*, a horizontal force ***P***, and bending moment *M* are the required internal forces to describe the internal state of stress of the beam. The following descriptions are more specifically given to these internal forces:

(1) The internal force *P* acting parallel to the axis of the beam is called the axial force.

(2) The internal force *V* acting perpendicular to the axis of the beam is called the shear force.

(3) The internal force *M* acting in the plane of the beam is called the bending moment.

Each internal force will in turn produce a particular kind of stress on the exposed part of cross-sectional area. It is the internal stresses at a section of a beam that actually determines the ultimate strength of the member—not the internal forces. The internal forces serve as a means of simplifying and idealizing a complex system of stresses that actually creates the physical action of the beam. These stresses will be explained in more detail in the next chapter. To the beam structure shown above, Fig. 1-21, the procedure for computing the internal forces is illustrated.

The reactions necessary to establish equilibrium of this beam as a whole are found before the internal forces at various sections along the beam can be computed. The possible restraining forces offered by such a support are denoted in Fig. 1-22 (see Sec. 1.2, Conventional Support Types). With three unknown reactive forces existing at this support, and three independent equations of equilibrium available for solution, the structure is statically determinate. Having established determinacy of the structure, it then follows that the reaction forces can be computed in the usual manner, using the equations of equilibrium. However, to formulate general expressions from these equations, it is first necessary to arrange the applied load in directions convenient to the established rectangular coordinate

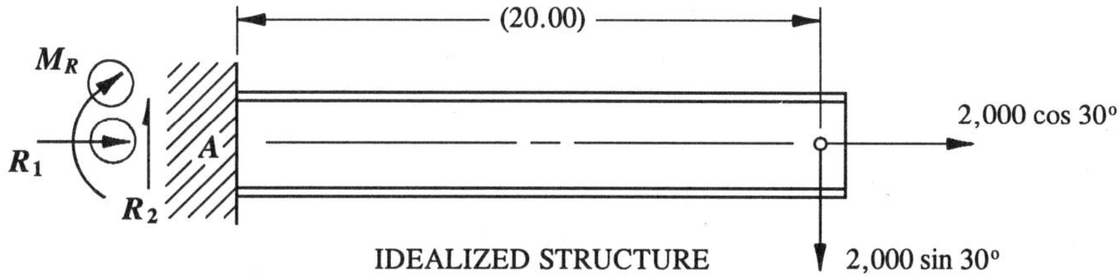

FIGURE 1-22 Idealization of a fixed support structure using unknown reaction forces.

system. This is easily accomplished by the use of trigonometric functions (see Appendix A, Eqs. A-1 and A-2). Hence

$$\Sigma F_x = 0, \quad R_1 + 2,000 \cos 30^\circ = 0, \quad R_1 = -1,732 \text{ lb}$$

$$\Sigma F_y = 0, \quad R_2 - 2,000 \sin 30^\circ = 0, \quad R_2 = 1,000 \text{ lb}$$

$$\Sigma M_A = 0, \quad (+ \quad M_R + 2,000 \sin 30^\circ (20) = 0, \quad M_R = -20,000 \text{ in-lb}.$$

These reaction forces are pictured in Fig. 1-23. To account for the negative signs of R_1 and M_R, the directions of these forces have been reversed. To help illustrate the method of sectıons approach, let us now find the internal forces *V*, *P*, and *M* at a section eight (8) inches from the free end of the beam. An imaginary cut is made there, in which the isolated parts of the beam are separated into two balanced systems of loads. To each of the isolated parts, it is said that a system of internal forces must exist at each section cut to establish the isolated parts in static balance, as indicated in Fig. 1-24.

To determine the magnitude of these internal forces, the equations of equilibrium are applied, but this time, separately to each isolated part. As always, the correct directions of the internal forces will automatically be verified by the signs of the calculated forces. As a convenience, the internal forces are computed using the same coordinate system as was originally adopted for the main structure. When summing moments for each part, the neutral axis of the cross-sectional area is always taken as the pivot axis. The neutral axis is a line of zero stress across a section area subjected to internal bending moments. Strictly speaking, this means that the neutral axis is a function of its internal loading structure, not a function of the

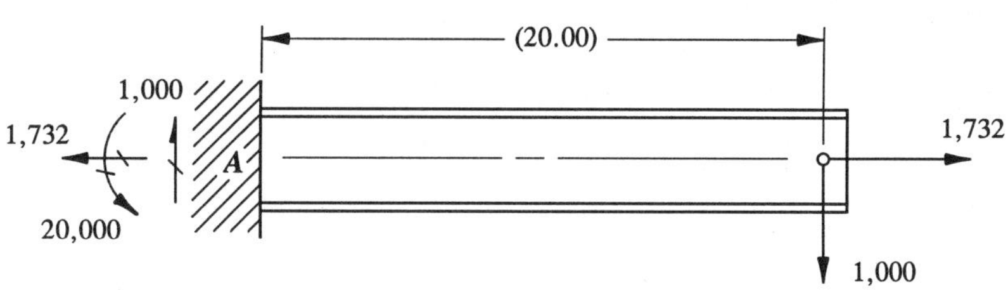

FIGURE 1-23 Magnitude and direction of the reaction forces determined.

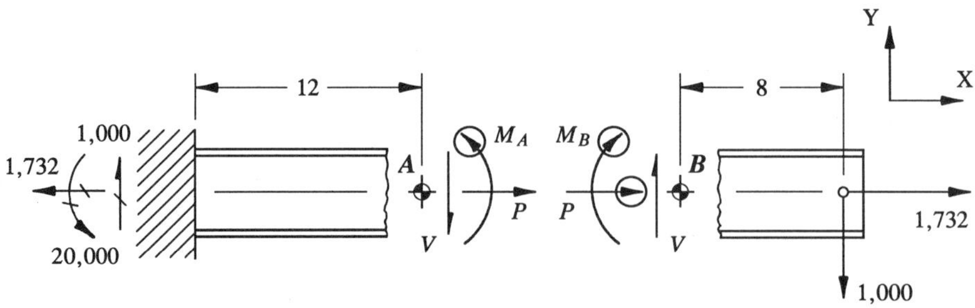

FIGURE 1-24 System of internal forces shown on exposed sections of a beam.

geometry of the section area. In our study of beam solutions in this section, the location of the neutral axis is assumed to be coincidental with the centroidal axis or geometric center of the cross-sectional area. This will be assumed true whether a beam behaves elastically under load or not. A shift in location of the neutral axis when a beam undergoes plastic (or inelastic) deformations is left for discussion to an advanced textbook on this subject.[1]

Equilibrium equations for the left-hand part of the structure:

$$\Sigma F_x = 0, \quad -1{,}732 + P = 0, \quad P = 1{,}732 \text{ lb}$$
$$\Sigma F_y = 0, \quad 1{,}000 - V = 0, \quad V = 1{,}000 \text{ lb}$$
$$\Sigma M_A = 0, \quad (+\circlearrowleft) \quad 1{,}000(12) - 20{,}000 - M_A = 0, \quad M_A = -8{,}000 \text{ in-lb.}$$

Equilibrium equations for the right-hand part of the structure:

$$\Sigma F_x = 0, \quad P + 1{,}732 = 0, \quad P = -1{,}732 \text{ lb}$$
$$\Sigma F_y = 0, \quad V - 1{,}000 = 0, \quad V = 1{,}000 \text{ lb}$$
$$\Sigma M_B = 0, \quad (+\circlearrowleft) \quad 1{,}000(8) + M_B = 0, \quad M_B = -8{,}000 \text{ in-lb.}$$

The correct directions of these forces are then properly drawn for the isolated parts, as shown in Fig. 1-25. Since only one set of internal forces can exist at any one section, it is reassuring to find that the same magnitude of forces are found for each isolated part.

The design engineer's decision as to which of the isolated parts to analyze is principally determined for the part with the fewer number of forces to consider in the analysis. Note the direction of the internal forces at each section cut. The forces that are shown in Fig. 1-25 act in opposite directions on each of the cross-sectional areas of the isolated parts. Actually, this condition is consistent with the physical interpretation of the stresses that these internal loads produce on their exposed

[1] The engineer is also referred to an aerospace company structures manual for the inelastic design and analysis of such beams.

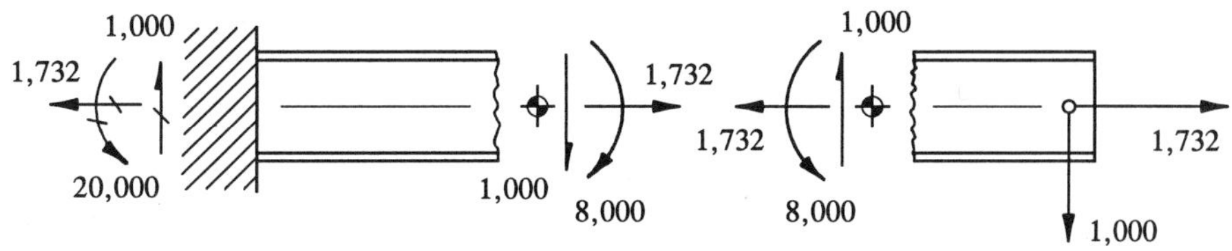

FIGURE 1-25 Magnitude and direction of the internal forces at exposed sections of a beam.

section areas. The axial force is called a tension force if it pulls away from the section and a compression force if it pushes on the section. The axial forces in the diagram are shown pulling away from their exposed section areas and thereby produce the same desired effect on each section area. The bending moments at each section cut are shown acting in opposite rotational directions. This must be so, so that each moment indicated will produce compression in the lower fibers and tension in the upper fibers. Again consistent with the notion that the same physical effects must be produced at the same section cut. The shear is shown acting in opposite directions on the two isolated parts. This is also in agreement with the previously discussed cases of axial loads and bending moments, but is physically more difficult to describe.

In summary, to a completely balanced structure, one simply passes a section cut at a point on the structure where internal loads are sought. To one of the exposed parts, three unknown internal forces are labeled without concern to their correct directions. The unknown forces are easily determined by successfully applying the equations of statics to the isolated part. Additional section cuts are usually made along a beam in order to establish the general loading behavior of its internal structure. In the next section, several section cuts will be made along the entire length of a beam and the computed values plotted on graph paper. The plotted points will establish what are called the axial diagram, shear diagram, and bending moment diagram. The sufficiency of plotted points will be determined by how skillful the engineer is in determining the general trend of the internal loads computed by the methods of this section.

Example 1-3 To the beam structure shown in Fig. 1-26, determine the beam internal forces at a point 9.5 in from support *A* when the upper attached structure reaches its maximum design load of 6,000 lb.

SOLUTION: Since the attached structure is fastened to the main structure over such a short span, it is doubtful that this member will offer any additional stiffness (or bending resistance) to the overall main structure. Therefore, the attached structure should not be treated as part of the main beam for analysis purposes in this region. What this basically means is this: when calculating the stresses produced in

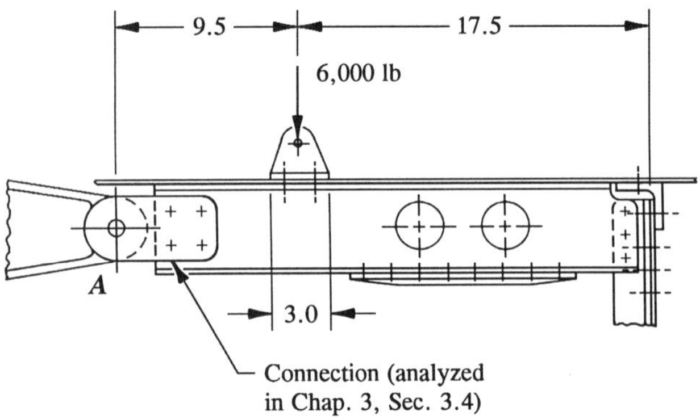

FIGURE 1-26 Beam structure loaded by a concentrated load through its local structure.

the main beam, by the stress methods of Chapter 2, the effective cross-sectional area as a basis for that analysis should not include the area of the attached structure. However, as the attached structure is increased in length, it becomes increasingly probable that this structure will, in fact, act in some capacity in concert with the main structure. The length at which the attached structure can be considered as an effective member of the main beam is strictly based on engineering judgment and, perhaps, verifiable by some form of intermediate structural testing. In the analysis of internal loads, this point must not be overlooked, as the basis of a successful internal loads analysis always considers the position of the neutral axis of the cross-sectional area as the principal location where the internal loads will act if the actual physical stresses of the beam are to be duplicated. This point will become clearer as our attention is focused on calculating stresses in the next chapter.

Another important point: For the purposes of calculating beam reactions, it does not make any difference whether the distribution of load for the attached structure is considered uniform or if a more realistic variable load distribution is represented on the main structure. The reason for this is simple, the true or simplified distribution of bearing stresses, Figures 1-27(a) and (b), respectively, that could be developed by the physical arrangement of the attached structure onto the main structure would be idealized by the same magnitude of equivalent concentrated force, Fig. 1-27(c).

An important concept many times overlooked by the engineer is the static strength of the attached structure to which the applied loads are introduced. The strength of the main beam structure is only as good as the strength of its attached structure. For example, if the strength of the attached structure is not sufficient to introduce the basic applied loads into the main structure, no matter what analytical results are obtained by rigorous analysis, the loads and stresses calculated for the main structure would be physically impossible to attain. Proceeding now with the solution of Example 1-3, the beam reactions necessary to balance the structure of Fig. 1-28 are easily calculated by setting up the equations of equilibrium.

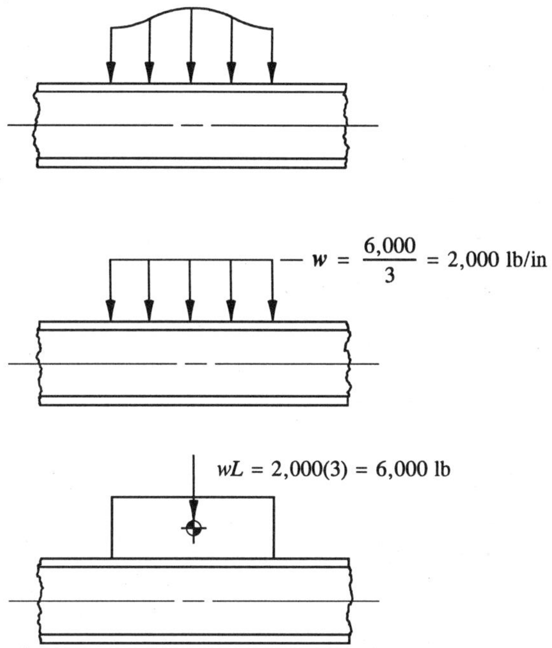

FIGURE 1-27 Distribution of bearing stresses from the physical arrangement of the attaching structure (a) the true bearing stress distribution and (b) the simplified bearing stress distribution. (c) Equivalent concentrated load for the bearing stress distributions depicted in (a) and (b).

Thus

$$\Sigma F_x = 0, \qquad R_3 = 0$$
$$\Sigma F_y = 0, \qquad R_1 - 6{,}000 + R_2 = 0$$
$$\Sigma M_A = 0, \qquad \circlearrowleft\!+ \quad 6{,}000(9.5) - 27R_2 = 0, \quad R_2 = 2{,}111 \text{ lb}.$$

And then substituting back into the second equation gives:

$$R_1 - 6{,}000 + 2{,}111 = 0, \quad R_1 = 3{,}889 \text{ lb}.$$

Before internal loads are calculated, these reactions and the actual bearing distribution in its physically applied form for the attached structure are represented on the completely balanced structure, as shown in Fig. 1-29. To avoid errors in design, it is usually good engineering practice to apply the physical distribution of loading to the main structure when determining or calculating internal loads. This is especially true when internal loads are desired at sections within the physical loading distribution itself. There, caution should be exercised if a reliable and

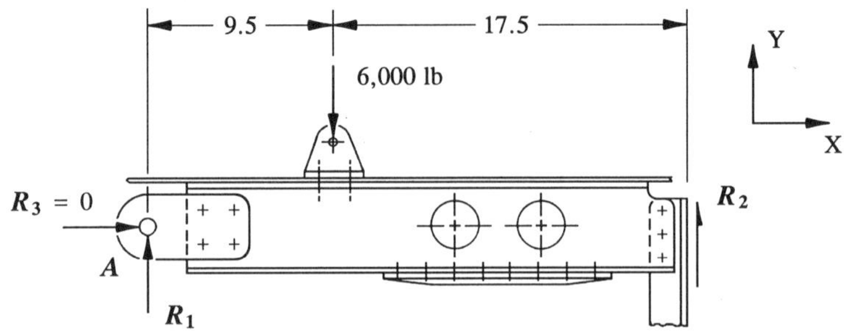

FIGURE 1-28 Unknown beam reactions indicated on a properly drawn diagram of the beam.

intelligent stress analysis solution is to follow. The internal loads for the structure of Fig. 1-29 are found located at point *B* along the neutral axis of the beam in Fig. 1-30, which also corresponds to the desired location of our solution at 9.5 inches from point *A*. By making a section cut through the bearing distribution described at this point, and exposing the left-hand part to the unknown internal forces *V, P,* and *M,* these values are easily computed by the use of the equations of statics. Note, only the portion of loading to the left of the section cut needs to be considered here; as the internal loads on the exposed section to the right of the section cut will produce the same physical loading (compare the physical descriptions of these internal loads to those previously described in Fig. 1-25).

$$\Sigma F_x = 0, \qquad P = 0$$

$$\Sigma F_y = 0, \qquad 3,889 - 3,000 - V = 0, \quad V = 889 \text{ lb}$$

$$\Sigma M_B = 0, \qquad (+ \quad 3,889(9.5) - 3,000\left[\frac{1.5}{2}\right] - M_B = 0$$

$$M_B = 34,695 \text{ in-lb}.$$

To demonstrate the extension of principles to the subject of bearing stresses described previously in this section, consider the structure of Fig. 1-31(a), where

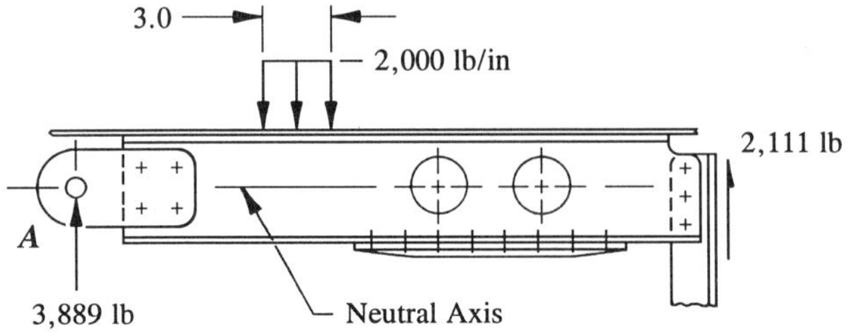

FIGURE 1-29 Balanced structure showing actual bearing distribution of the local structure.

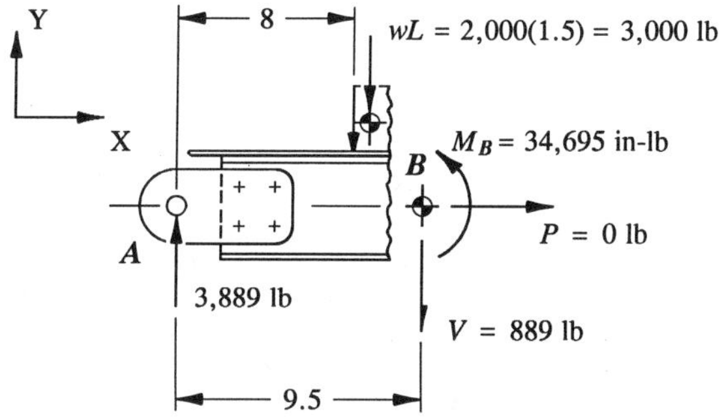

FIGURE 1-30 Internal loads at an exposed section of a beam.

the attached structure is made long enough to be considered effective in bending with the main beam structure. In such a case, if the attached structure is also made sufficiently stiff, the bearing distribution would most likely be described as equally distributed over the entire bearing or contact surface of this member, as shown by the loading structure of Fig. 1-31(b). If, however, the attached structure is made too flexible, a more realistic, conservative approach to the analysis is suggested, as indicated in Fig. 1-31(c) by the effective length L_e used here to represent the

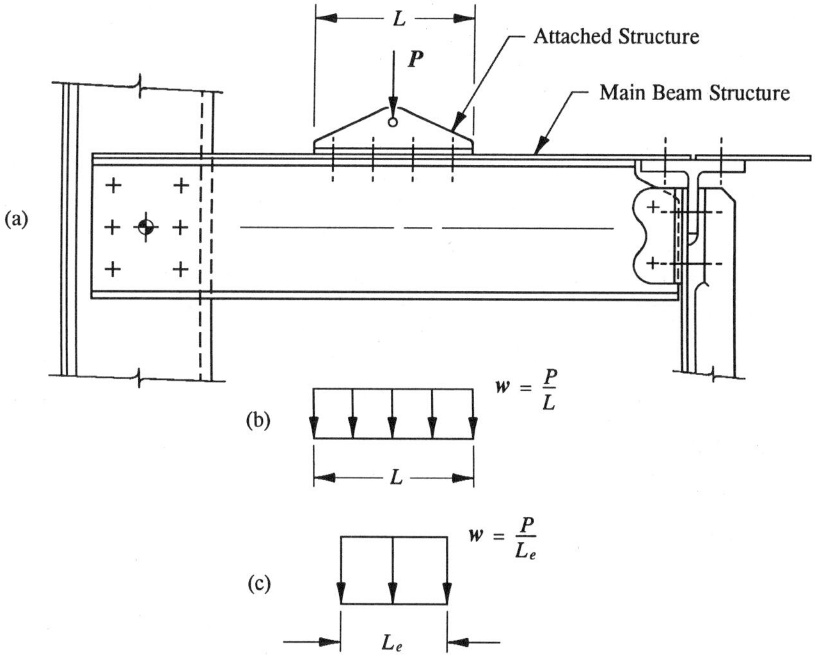

FIGURE 1-31 Effective length of bearing distribution for an attached structure.

assumed bearing stress distribution on the main beam structure of this hypothetical case. This discussion clearly demonstrates a most important principle: that, stiffness of the attached structure governs the distribution of bearing stresses. In conclusion, only good engineering judgment based on an intelligent and rational approach to the basic design concept will dictate the right assumed effective length of bearing stress distribution to use for each particular design problem.

1.6 Axial, Shear, and Bending Moment Diagrams. In this section, the ideas and principles of internal load diagrams are specifically discussed and interpreted. In general, each point along the entire length of a beam has corresponding internal values of axial, shear, and bending moment. The magnitude of the internal forces may easily be computed at any section desired using the method of sections approach of Sec. 1.5. After a series of points have been calculated along the entire length of the beam, the internal forces are plotted for each particular kind of load they represent. These plots are called specifically, the axial diagram, shear diagram, and moment diagram. Most engineering textbooks on this subject will specify a particular sign convention to describe the internal forces of these diagrams. This usually makes a discussion of internal force diagrams only more awkward and confusing, and therefore less practical to use. Instead, this book will place emphasis on the actual physical effect each internal load produces on the structure being analyzed. For example, the axial and bending moment diagrams are labeled by their physical actions on the beam structure; either compression or tension.

The importance of these diagrams cannot be overemphasized. With the assistance of a complete and accurately drawn diagram, the magnitude, direction, and location of the internal loads along the beam can conveniently be obtained. From these diagrams the structural engineer can acquire the desired performance data necessary to support and substantiate his structural design concepts. To illustrate the use of these internal load diagrams, the axial, shear, and bending moment diagrams are constructed for the auxiliary wing spar loaded as shown in Fig. 1-32 (upper and lower skins have been omitted for clarity). The engineer is referred to Appendix C, page 626, for the detailed construction of these diagrams.

The spar caps, physically restrained from moving by the upper and lower wing skins, are considered stabilized and therefore prevented from beam-column action. The secondary bending moments that are normally produced by the axial loads effect of a beam-column will be investigated in Chapter 7, when our study of column instability can more completely and thoroughly be treated.[1]

Now, starting at the left end of the axial diagram, the maximum compression axial load for this beam occurs between points *A* and *C*, while the maximum axial tension load occurs from points *C* to *F*, and zero axial load acting from *F* to *G*. To distinguish between compression and tension axial loads, the axial diagram is conveniently separated by the baseline shown in the figure. What is particularly interesting to note here about this diagram is that even though an applied axial load of

---

[1] In that chapter, it will be shown that when a beam-column undergoes bending, its deflected shape times its axial internal loads will develop secondary bending moments along the beam-column structure.

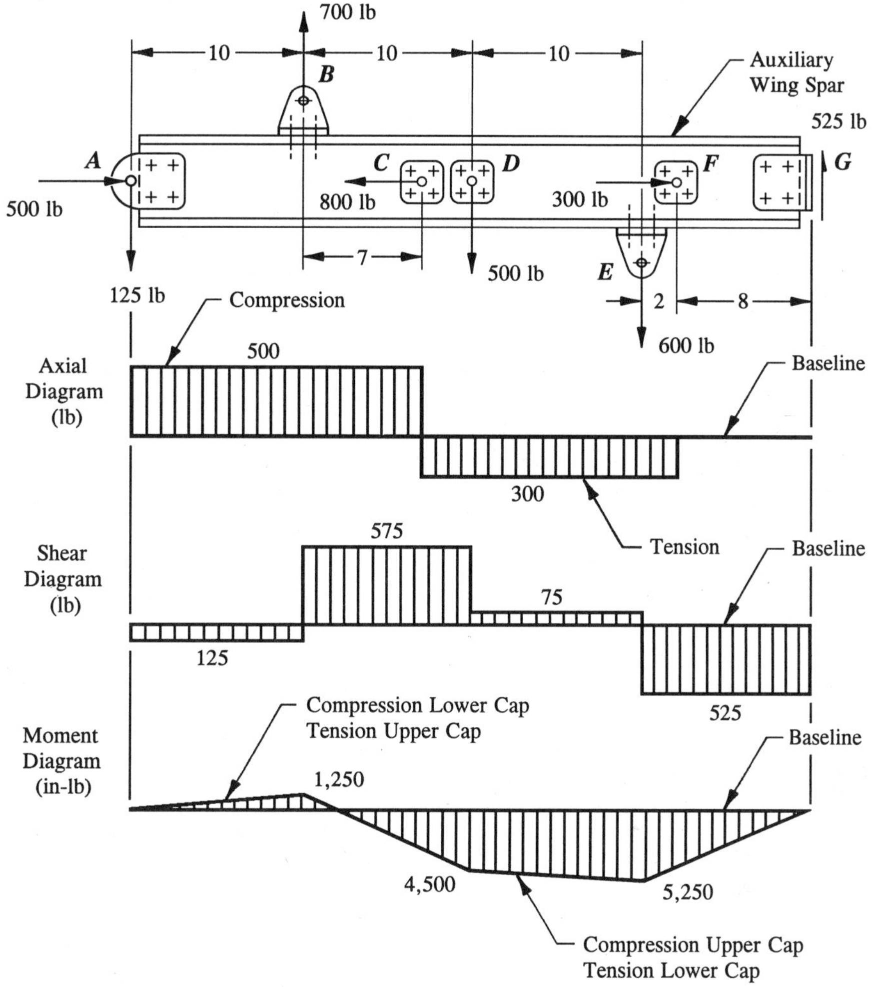

FIGURE 1-32 Auxiliary wing spar with accompanying axial, shear, and bending moment diagrams constructed.

800 lb was externally applied locally to the structure at point *C*, the auxiliary wing spar internally only feels a maximum axial compression load of 500 lb and a maximum axial tension load of 300 lb. This discrepancy that exists between the external loaded structure and its corresponding internal axial diagram clearly demonstrates the importance of a complete and detailed internal loads picture of the loaded structure. Without it, or to do otherwise, would certainly be unacceptable, which would ultimately lead to the overdesign of the basic structure.

In simple terms, one can describe the structural behavior of the loaded structure in the following way: After equilibrium of the auxiliary wing spar has been reached for the applied loads given, the structure is designed for the maximum internal loads indicated by its corresponding axial load diagram. And, since these maximum values are known for this structure, the auxiliary wing spar would then be designed according to the stress analysis methods of Chapter 2. Most importantly, the local structure must be strong enough to support the applied loads introduced into the main structure locally. Here, this refers to adequate strength and proper design of the supporting structures at *A* and *G*, as well as the attached structures at *B*, *C*, *D*, *E*, and *F*. (See Chapter 3 for the analysis and design of connections and Chapter 5 for the analysis and design of shear and tension clips.) Until then, let us assume that these structural components are of sufficient strength to introduce the applied loads and reactions indicated from the balanced structure into the internal loading structure of the auxiliary wing spar. Note that the abrupt changes in loading, vertical lines of the axial and shear diagrams, occur at sections where concentrated loads (or local loads) are either applied or reacted to the structure. Since no applied concentrated moments have been externally applied to the auxiliary wing spar, no such vertical lines are indicated anywhere in the moment diagram.

An analogous interpretation of the shear diagram of the auxiliary wing spar can also be made here. For example, if the spar is of a uniform construction for its entire length, a maximum internal shear of 575 lb will ultimately design the entire length of web structure. Note, in particular, that even though an applied load of 700 lb was externally applied to the structure at *B*, the auxiliary wing spar itself only feels a maximum shear of 575 lb. This again demonstrates the extreme importance of a properly drawn internal loads diagram of the loaded structure. Further, in other designs, where discrete points of a weaker cross-sectional area are located, the weaker sections must also be investigated for static strength, generally, using the corresponding lower values of internal shears at those critical sections. In Chapter 4, the internal shears will also be used in conjunction with the design and analysis of built-up structural beams: members constructed of nested angles, doublers, and straps of similar or dissimilar materials.

Lastly, a maximum moment of 5,250 in-lb is used to design the upper cap of the beam in compression and the lower cap in tension for the entire length of beam corresponding to the region of loading indicated below the baseline of the moment diagram; and design the upper cap of the beam in tension and the lower cap in compression for a maximum moment of 1,250 in-lb for the entire length of beam corresponding to the region of loading indicated above the baseline.

Example 1-4 The main spar of a lightweight cantilevered aircraft is designed to conservatively carry all of the wing aerodynamic lift forces. For the simplified wing up-bending loads given in Fig. 1-33, construct the shear and bending moment diagrams for the main spar.

SOLUTION: Using the methods of Sec. 1.4, the reactions at the wing root (WS 28.0) are computed and their values indicated on a free-body diagram, as shown in

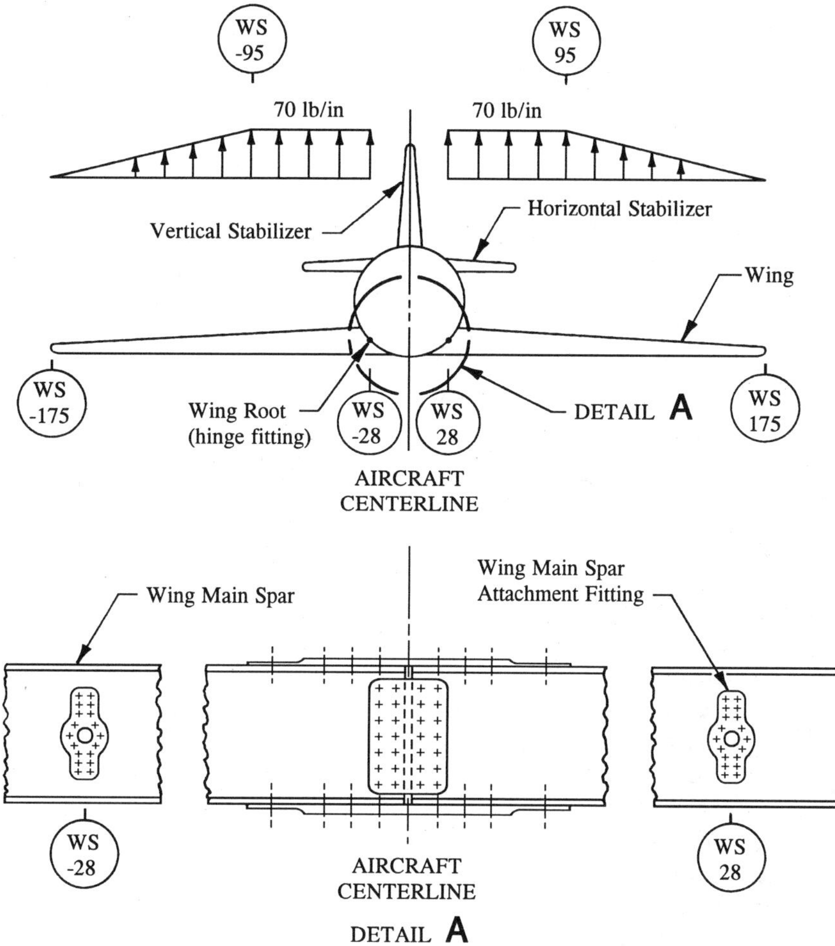

FIGURE 1-33 Simplified aerodynamic wing up-bending loads.

Fig. 1-34. Equivalent concentrated forces for the aerodynamic loading are computed as follows:

$$P_1 = \tfrac{1}{2}wL = \tfrac{1}{2}(70)(175 - 95) = 2,800 \text{ lb}$$

$$P_2 = wL = 70(95 - 28) = 4,690 \text{ lb}.$$

By symmetry of loading, the wing root reactions are determined by inspection. For those who require additional practice in applying the equations of statics, the analytical solution to these reactions follow directly. Essentially, for the wing structure to remain in a state of equilibrium, the following equilibrium equations must be

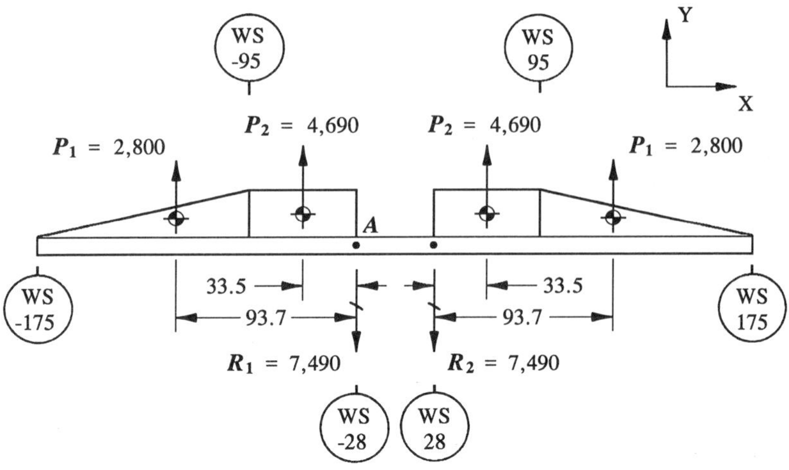

FIGURE 1-34 Wing root reactions indicated on a free-body diagram of the main spar.

satisfied:

$$\Sigma F_y = 0 \quad \text{and} \quad \Sigma M_z = 0.$$

In the example considered, this gives:

$$\Sigma F_y = 0, \qquad P_1 + P_2 - R_1 - R_2 + P_2 + P_1 = 0.$$

Substituting for P_1 and P_2,

$$2,800 + 4,690 - R_1 - R_2 + 4,690 + 2,800 = 0$$
$$-R_1 - R_2 = -14,980.$$

From $\Sigma M_z = 0$ at point A, R_2 is obtained directly:

$$\Sigma M_A = 0, \quad (+) \quad 4,690(33.5) + 2,800(93.7) + R_2(56.0)$$
$$-4,690(89.5) - 2,800(149.7) = 0$$
$$R_2 = 7,490 \text{ lb.}$$

Hence, from $\Sigma F_y = 0$, R_1 is

$$-R_1 - 7,490 = -14,980$$
$$R_1 = 7,490 \text{ lb.}$$

Now, with a completely balanced structure, Fig. 1-35, the internal forces V and M at points a and b are computed, and their values plotted on shear and

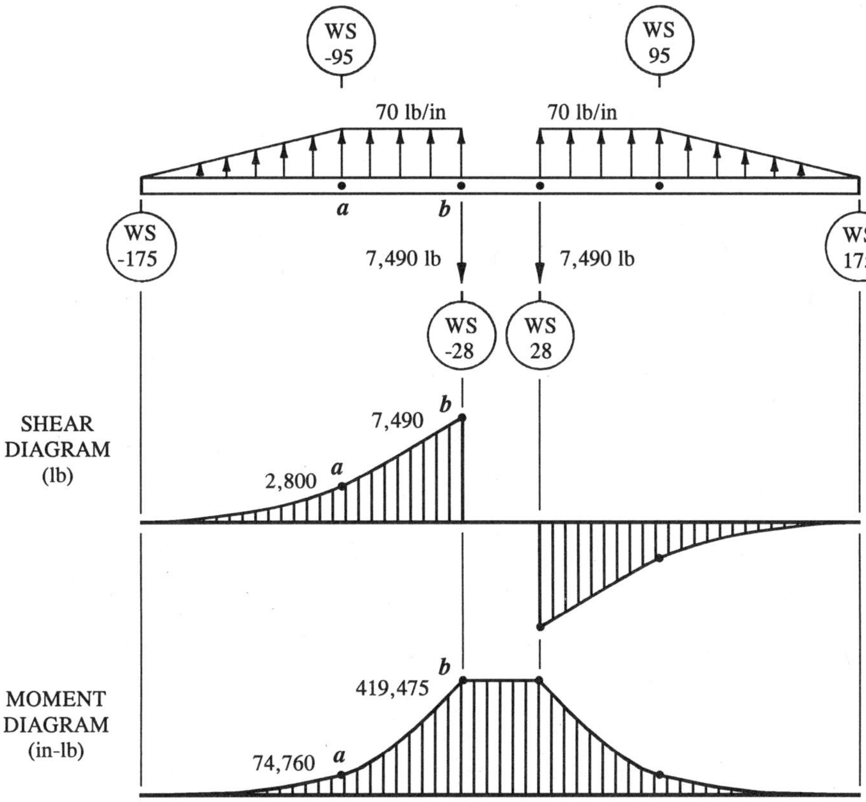

FIGURE 1-35 Completely balanced main spar, (a) shear diagram, (b) bending moment diagram.

bending moment diagrams, respectively.

Internal loads at point *a*, Fig. 1-36:

$$\Sigma F_x = 0, \qquad P = 0$$

$$\Sigma F_y = 0, \qquad 2,800 - V = 0, \quad V = 2,800 \text{ lb}$$

$$\Sigma M_a = 0, \qquad (+ \quad 2,800(26.7) - M_a = 0, \quad M_a = 74,760 \text{ in-lb.}$$

Internal loads at point *b*, Fig. 1-37:

$$\Sigma F_x = 0, \qquad P = 0$$

$$\Sigma F_y = 0, \qquad 2,800 + 4,690 - V = 0, \quad V = 7,490 \text{ lb}$$

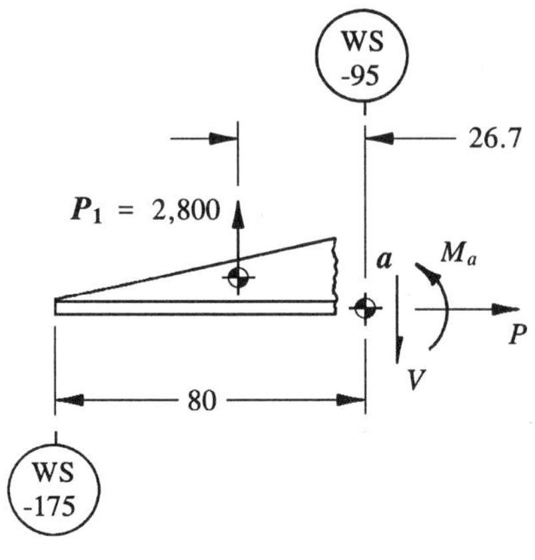

FIGURE 1-36 Internal loads at an exposed section of beam at point *a*.

$$\Sigma M_b = 0, \quad \circlearrowleft + \quad 2,800(93.7) + 4,690(33.5) - M_b = 0$$
$$M_b = 419,475 \text{ in-lb.}$$

From this point on, the construction of these diagrams is straightforward. Using a little ingenuity and symmetry of loading, these diagrams are easily figured out. Of course, if necessary, intermediate points along the beam may be taken to deduce the general behavior or trend of the loaded wing structure.

In summary, the completeness of a free-body diagram is generally what makes an accurate and reliable solution of shear and bending moment diagrams possible. When the engineer has fully mastered the basic techniques outlined in this and other sections of this book, he may then wish to take intermediate steps or

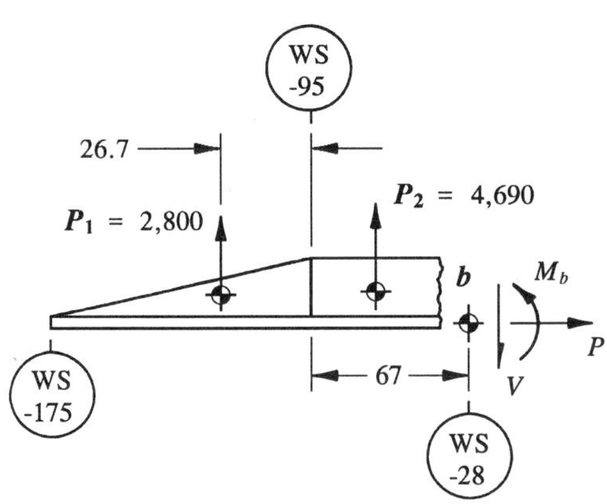

FIGURE 1-37 Internal loads at an exposed section of beam at point *b*.

short cuts to arrive at quicker methods of constructing these diagrams. Until the engineer acquires these skills, and learns to apply them correctly, it is advisable that he maintain a systematic approach to their construction. Clearly, the construction of these diagrams is tedious and can easily become the time-consuming part of the structural analysis effort. In most cases, the engineer's ability to pinpoint the location of maximum internal loads along a structural member will usually dictate whether or not he should construct detailed shear and bending moment diagrams.

1.7 Principle of Superposition. The principle of superposition states that the resultant effect of several applied forces on a structure is the algebraic sum of those effects when the applied forces are acting separately. In other words, the effect of each force acting separately is superimposed algebraically to obtain the total effect of all the forces acting simultaneously on the structure. Specifically, the superimposed effects can be internal loads, reactions, elastic stresses, strains, and small deflections of a structure.[1]

The principle of superposition is very important in the solution of complex loading. In particular, its real power lies with its ability to resolve the complex loading using known or standard beam solutions of determinate and indeterminate beam structures (see ahead to Sec. 1.8, Example 1-6). Specifically, it enables the engineer to simplify a complex system of loads into several simpler ones. However, the principle is not valid in cases where deflections of the structure are not directly proportional to the applied loads. This condition occurs for a member that is stressed above the proportional limit of the material. In this higher range of stresses, the material is said to behave inelastically, or sometimes referred to as the plastic or inelastic range of a stress-strain curve of the material (see Appendix E, Fig. A-14). Elastic or inelastic behavior of a structure depends upon its response to the application of externally applied forces. For instance, if a structure returns to its original design configuration after all applied forces have been removed from it, the structure is said to behave elastically. Otherwise, if permanent set or deformation of the structure is prevalent, this condition would be characteristic of inelastic stress behavior, and the methods of handling such designs are more aptly treated in an advanced textbook (see also Appendix J, "Inelastic Bending," for the specific treatment of rectangular-shaped sections in bending). Careful review of a stress-strain diagram for each particular material used in a design will determine whether the existing region of stress is elastic or not.

Let us now apply the principle of superposition to the reaction forces of the proposed system of loads in Fig. 1-38(a). The following procedural set up is devised: the forces P_1 and P_2 are separately applied to the beam structure, as shown by System II and System III loads of Figs. 1-38(b) and (c), respectively. The

---

[1] A beam-column is a structural member where the principle of superposition is not valid, not even below the proportional limit of the material, because the transverse loads of such a member produce deflections which in turn induce additional bending moments by the axial applied loading times the deflected shape of the beam. Fortunately, a beam-column is easily perceived, and the basis of its analysis more conveniently treated in an advanced textbook on this subject.

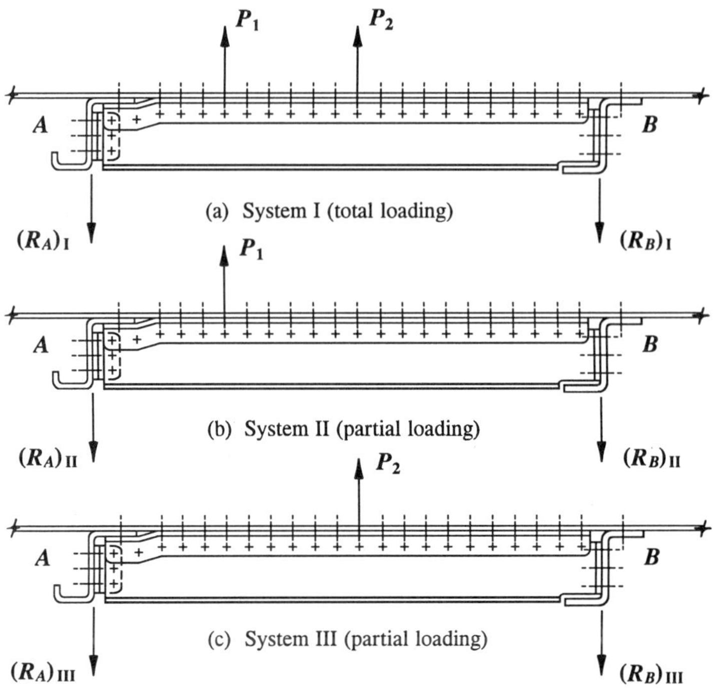

FIGURE 1-38 Principle of superposition of reaction forces.

following mathematical expression is formulated:

System I = System II + System III.

This expression can be further generalized to include n loading systems:

$$\text{System I} = \text{System II} + \text{System III} + \ldots + \text{System } n \tag{1-4}$$

where: n = number of loading systems.

If we now apply this general expression to the solution of reactions at supports A and B of System I above, we obtain:

$$(R_A)_{\text{I}} = (R_A)_{\text{II}} + (R_A)_{\text{III}}$$
$$(R_B)_{\text{I}} = (R_B)_{\text{II}} + (R_B)_{\text{III}}\,.$$

Now, to fully illustrate the power of this method and its applications, the following example is presented, and will focus on the superposition of (1) applied loads, (2) reactions, and (3) internal loads of a determinate beam structure:

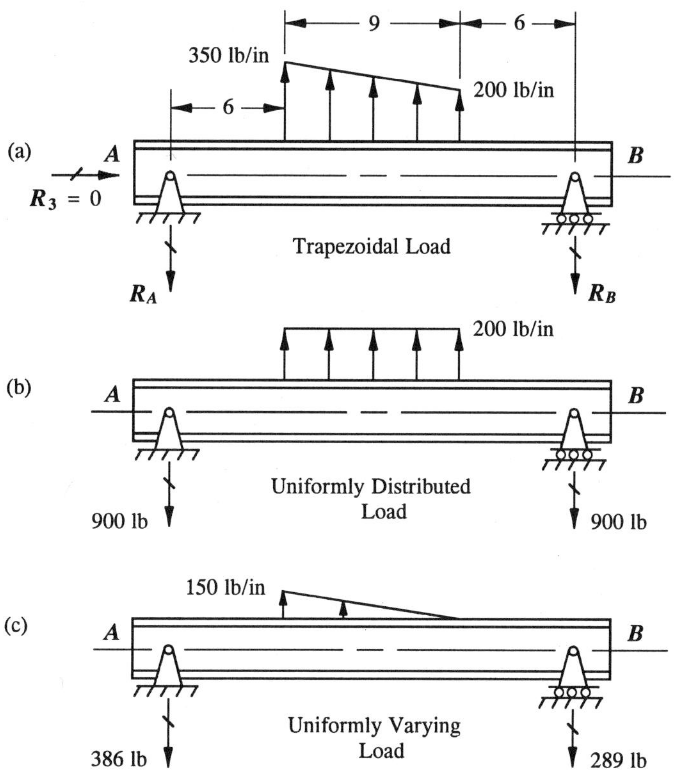

FIGURE 1-39 (a) Trapezoidal loaded beam. Separation of the trapezoidal loading into two separate loading types: (b) the uniformly distributed load and (c) the uniformly distributed varying load.

Example 1-5 To the beam structure shown in Fig. 1-39, find the internal forces 5.0 in from the support at *A* for the trapezoidal loading given. Then, properly orient these forces on the beam segments to each side of the proposed section cut.

SOLUTION: The simplest way to solve this problem is to separate the trapezoidal loading for this beam into two convenient conventional loading types: that is, the uniformly distributed load and the uniformly distributed varying load, as shown in Figs. 1-39(b) and (c). To each of these loading types, individual solutions are obtained using standard methods of analysis; namely, the equations of equilibrium are applied to each separate loading system to determine beam reactions. The reactions at points *A* and *B* for each loading are given without analytical substantiation or proof. If desired, the engineer is encouraged to verify the magnitude of these reactions by using or reviewing the methods of Sec. 1.4. For the most part, no difficulty should be encountered if a logical and systematic approach to their solutions are used. Now, by applying the concept of superposition of reactions, Eq. 1-4, the reactions at A and B are easily determined by algebraically combining the reactions of each separate system.

System I = System II + System III (formulated from Eq. 1-4).

Hence,

$$R_A = 900 + 386 = 1,286 \text{ lb}$$

and

$$R_B = 900 + 289 = 1,189 \text{ lb}.$$

In a similar manner, the internal loads V, P, and M at each proposed section cut of the two separate loading systems can be found using in this case the concept of superposition of internal loads. That is, using the methods of Sec. 1.5, section cuts are passed 5.0 inches from the beam supports at A for each separate loading system. And, from this, the isolated parts either to the left or right of each section cut are free-bodied and the internal loads determined. To simplify this solution somewhat, the left-hand parts are chosen for the actual calculation of these quantities. These diagrams are shown in Figs. 1-40(a) and (b), where from statics the internal loads are determined. Next, the two separate solutions are algebraically combined into one, thereby obtaining the total solution to the original problem, as shown in Fig. 1-41.

In an analogous manner, the internal forces on the right-hand segment of the proposed section cut can be calculated using the same techniques of analysis that were applied to the left-hand segment. Or, the astute engineer will recognize the

(a)

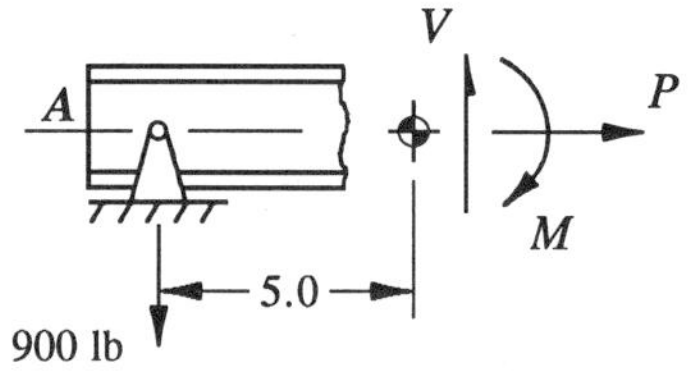

From statics:

$V = 900$ lb
$P = 0$ lb
$M = 900(5.0) = 4{,}500$ in-lb.

(b)

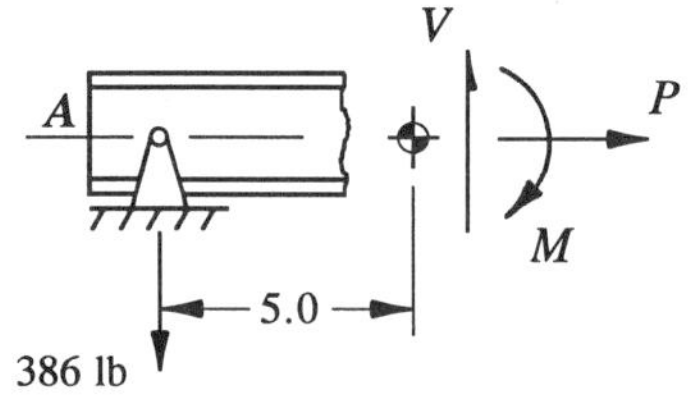

From statics:

$V = 386$ lb
$P = 0$ lb
$M = 386(5.0) = 1{,}930$ in-lb.

FIGURE 1-40 Internal loads at exposed sections of beam: (a) for the uniformly distributed load and (b) for the uniformly distributed varying load.

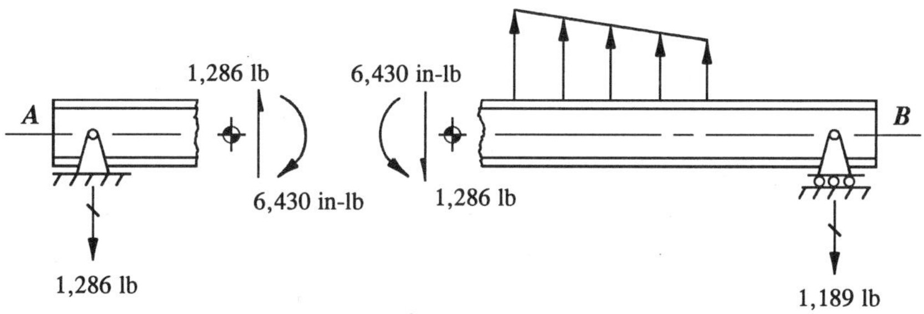

FIGURE 1-41 Final system of loads for the two separate loading types.

compatibility of internal loads that exist at a section cut, as they were described in Sec. 1.5, and make by intuitive reasoning the proper orientation of these internal loads on that segment. However, if the basic methods of determining reactions and internal loads are not as yet clearly understood, it is suggested that to achieve a better understanding and working knowledge of their solutions, the methods of Secs. 1.4 and 1.5 should again be reviewed. The extra effort spent now to learn these fundamentals correctly will help to promote a better understanding of more advanced concepts later in our study of more complex structures. Of course, those of you who feel confident in their applications should instead just proceed ahead to Sec. 1.8.

1.8 Reference Beam Formula Solutions. In the solution of most structural engineering designs, the engineer is required to make simplifications of a complex structure. For the most part, these simplifications often lead to the same types of idealized structures being analyzed. To take full advantage of these repetitive cases, a tabulation of their solutions expressed in general formula form are presented in Appendix D, Table A-1. These formula solutions are tabulated and indicate the support reactions, internal shears and bending moments at any point along the entire span of a beam for many different typical loading cases. Of course, any combination of these solutions can be combined algebraically by employing the principle of superposition of forces, as was demonstrated in the previous section of this book. The tabulation of these solutions are described into two general classifications: the first lists the formulas of statically determinate beams and the second for statically indeterminate beams. The engineer is referred to Sec. 1.4 for definitions of these structural terms. Also included are shear and bending moment diagrams for each specific type of beam. These internal load diagrams will provide the design engineer with a better perspective and general feel of the structural behavior of a beam under different loading conditions. The engineer should become thoroughly familiar with the general usage of these formulas and the physical interpretation of these diagrams. The example that follows will specifically demonstrate the use of these tables.

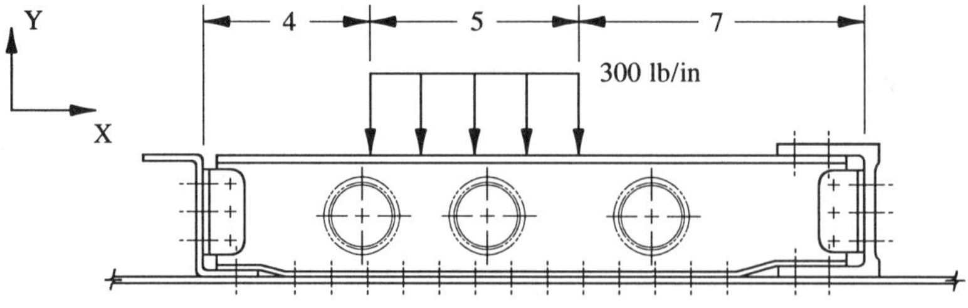

FIGURE 1-42 Intercostal loaded by a uniformly distributed load.

Example 1-6 If the intercostal shown in Fig. 1-42 is loaded by a uniformly distributed load of 300 lb/in, determine the support reactions using the appropriate beam formula solution provided in Appendix D, Table A-1, for this structure. Also, indicate the maximum shears and bending moments on properly drawn shear and bending moment diagrams, respectively.

SOLUTION: The symbolic representation of the real supports of this beam is shown in Fig. 1-43. The structure is indeterminate because more unknown reaction forces (R_A, R_D, and M_D) exist than independent equations of statics. Remember, since no horizontal loads are applied to the beam, $\Sigma F_x = 0$ is a singular solution. Hence, the following equations of equilibrium are available for solution: $\Sigma F_y = 0$ and $\Sigma M_z = 0$. The reactions for this structure are determined from the equations given in Appendix D (Table A-1, Reference Beam Formula Solutions, Case 18):

$$(1)\quad R_A = \frac{1}{8}\frac{wc}{L^3}\left[4L(a^2 + ab + b^2) - a^3 - ab^2 - a^2b - b^3\right]$$

$$(2)\quad R_D = wc - R_A$$

$$(3)\quad M_D = \frac{wc}{2}(c + 2a) - R_AL.$$

Substituting $a = 7$, $b = 12$, $c = 5$, $d = 4$, $L = 16$, and $w = 300$ into the first equation for R_A, we obtain $R_A = 644$ lb. With the value of R_A known, the second and third equations are solved for R_D and M_D, respectively. This gives:

$$R_D = 856 \text{ lb}$$

$$M_D = 3,946 \text{ in-lb}.$$

Since all calculated reactions are positive quantities, their indicated directions are correct and compatible with those designated in Fig. 1-43.

When using the beam formula solutions given in Appendix D, be sure to reverse the direction of any reaction that is calculated negative, or simply circle its

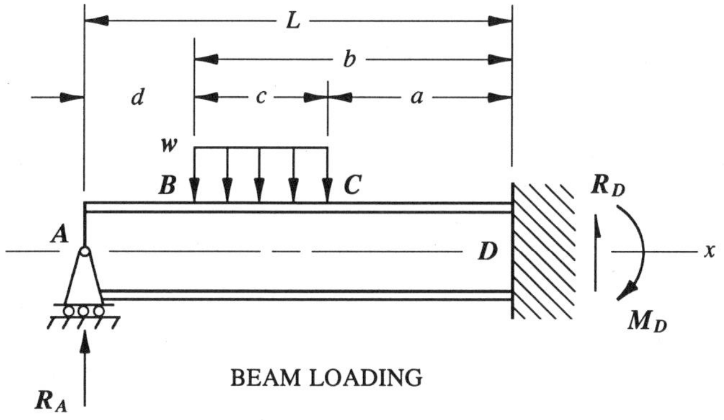

FIGURE 1-43 Unknown beam reactions indicated on the idealized beam structure.

arrowhead as a reminder of its true intended direction on the structure. But, always remember to use the actual calculated value in all subsequent calculations, even if the value is negative; thereby maintaining a consistent relationship with the original orientation of applied and reacted loads. Also, for any particular loading case, if the applied loading is opposite to that indicated by the beam loading solutions given in this appendix, simply use a negative value for this loading in each expression given.

The maximum bending moment that occurs for this beam between B and C, at a distance x from point A, is given by the following equation:

$$x = d + \frac{R_A}{w} = 6.15 \text{ in.}$$

Now, substituting x into the moment expression corresponding to this region of maximum bending gives:

$$M = -R_A x + \frac{w}{2}(x - d)^2 = -3{,}267 \text{ in-lb.}$$

Shear and bending moment diagrams are conveniently drawn in Fig. 1-44.

1.9 Partial Degree of Restraint of Support Types. It was shown in preceding sections of this chapter that the degree of restraint that a support provides to its beam structure must first be determined before the beam itself can be properly designed. Our discussions of support conditions thus far have concentrated on the following three specific types: (1) a roller support, (2) a pinned support, and (3) a fixed support. In many engineering designs, however, the actual degree of restraint of a support may not be precisely known nor easily determined by analysis. At his discretion, the structural engineer may elect to account for the unknowns that exist

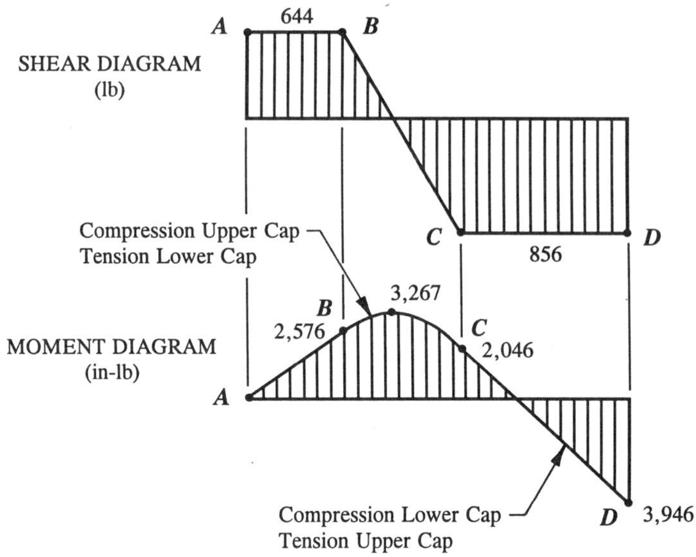

FIGURE 1-44 Shear and bending moment diagrams.

at such a support by making some conservative assumptions. For example, one could actually modify the analysis of a structure by making what is sometimes referred to as "overlapping assumptions." That is, the analysis of the structure would be performed twice based on two different assumptions or criteria; thereby overlapping a wider range of possible design solutions. To do otherwise would require initiating some sort of structural test effort to substantiate the support. As a general rule, though, even for major aircraft companies, structural testing of the simplest structural forms would be too cost prohibitive. Therefore, in the absence of reliable data to aid the engineer in making his preliminary evaluations and assumptions, a conservative approach to the design of supports is recommended.

A simply-supported beam is principally designed to transfer shearing forces from one structure to another in one specified direction at its supported ends (see Sec. 1.2, Fig. 1-3). In effect, this type of beam is allowed to freely rotate its supported ends without causing any appreciable build up of end moments, no matter how stiff the actual beam structure is made. Also, keep in mind that the rigidity of the backup structure to which a simply-supported beam is attached can also influence the degree of restraint provided by the support structure itself. In general, though, if a backup structure is made relatively thin and flexible, for instance, a beam web, the amount of additional restraint that the support structure would actually provide would be negligible. In fact, even if the backup structure were made relatively stiff, and the beam allowed to freely rotate, the support structure would still remain effectively flexible (or simply-supported).

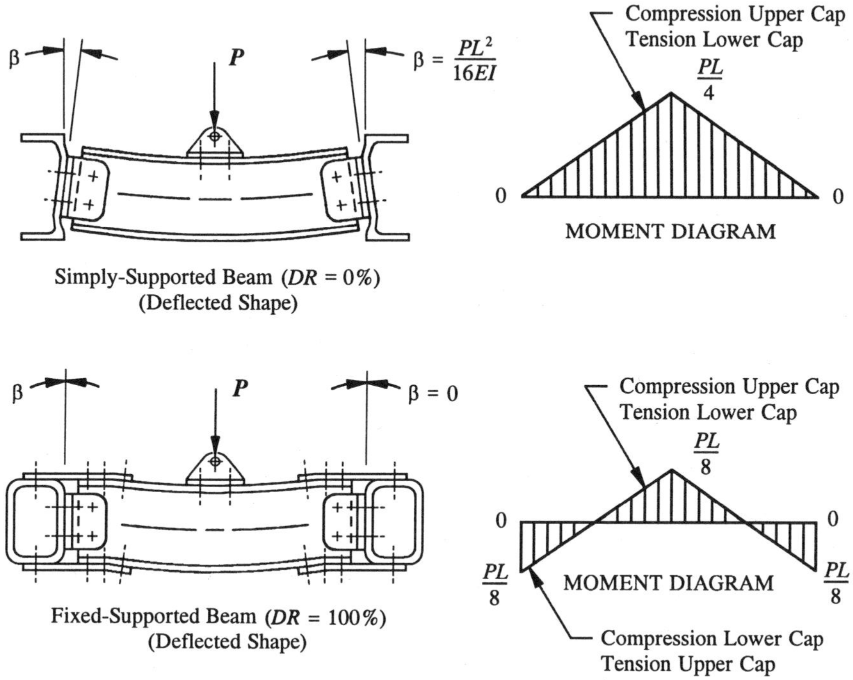

FIGURE 1-45 Supported beams and their deflected shapes.

For a fixed beam, the support structure, specifically, the web and flange members of the main beam structure, must be securely attached to prevent any rotation of the supported ends of the beam. These two types of supported beams and their deflected shapes are shown in Fig. 1-45. The engineer should compare the two bending moment diagrams that are provided in this figure. It should be observed from these diagrams that by increasing the amount of restraint that is offered by the simply-supported beam to that of the fully fixed beam, the center moment will decrease from a maximum value of $M = PL/4$ to a maximum value of $M = PL/8$, at center span, while the end-fixity moments will increase from $M = 0$ to their maximum values of $M = PL/8$, at the supported ends. For a beam of homogeneous construction, i.e., a beam of a constant cross-sectional area, the fully fixed beam would be designed for a maximum moment or $M = PL/8$ throughout its entire length or span. The simply-supported beam is clearly at a disadvantage here, even less weight-efficient, over its counterpart the fixed-supported beam since its entire length must be designed for twice this value or a maximum moment of $M = PL/4$, which is clearly indicated by its peak value at midspan.

Let us now look at the partial degrees of restraint offered by the beams supported as shown in Figs. 1-46(a) and (b). It will be most desirable and exceedingly beneficial to a better understanding of partial support structures if we describe

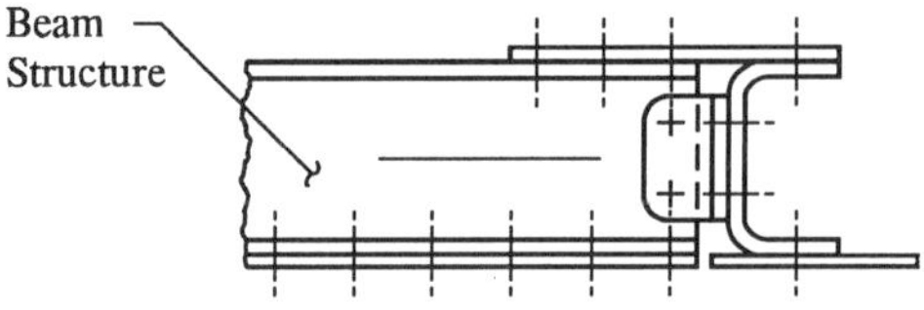

(a) Support provides greater than 0% fixity.

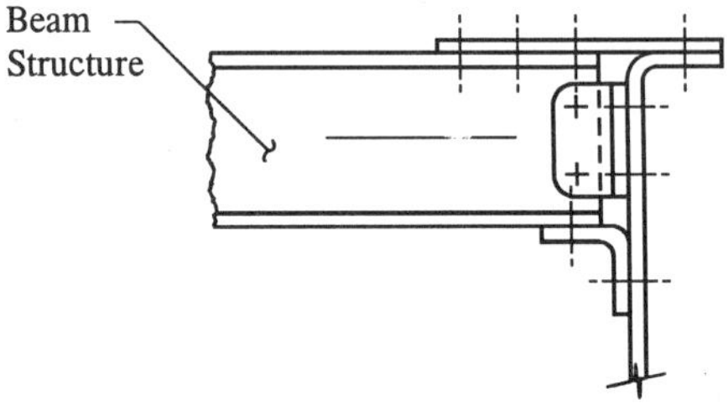

(b) Support provides less than 100% fixity.

FIGURE 1-46 Partial degree of restraint of support types.

these supports mathematically. To do this, let us measure the degree of restraint of a typical support by the ratio of the actual moment of the support to that of a moment that would be realized if that same support structure had instead been theoretically designed fully fixed, or

$$\text{Degree of Restraint}, DR = \frac{\text{actual support moment}}{\text{fixed support moment}}(100). \tag{1-5}$$

Of course only through structural testing can the actual degree of restraint of a support structure be known. Even so, it can still be rather helpful, if only for engineering discourse, to describe the support structure in terms of Eq. 1-5. For now, let us consider the simplest, yet the most conservative approach to the analysis of partial restraints that we can possibly make. That is, to design a beam for the maximum moment that would occur at the midspan of a simply-supported beam or $M = PL/4$ ($DR = 0\%$); and to design its support structures for the end moments that would occur if the beam were then considered fully fixed or $M = PL/8$ ($DR = 100\%$). This rather conservative approach based on overlapping assumptions may however produce too severe a weight penalty for the overall structure. Consequently, their solutions may be entirely unacceptable. The alternative approach to a more efficient design of these members (which is sometimes recommended by experienced engineers) is to consider a 50 percent partial degree of restraint for their designs. However, even this assumption can lead to faulty designs. For instance, if the actual degree of restraint, realized from structural testing, should prove to be slightly more rigid than the 50 percent design value assumed, the end moments would increase to more than what the supports were originally designed to. Or, if the actual degree of restraint should prove to be more flexible than the 50 percent design value, the center moment would instead increase. This would make the design of the structure in either case structurally understrength and potentially unsafe. Therefore, to avoid the possibility of premature failure of unknown support types, some latitude or overlapping in the analysis process of these members must be considered. The degree of overlapping or conservatism that is acceptable for each particular design is of course a function of many different design variables. Consider the following questions as your answers relate to the amount of conservatism required for each particular design case:

(1) How reliable are the applied loads?
(2) How important is the structure to the overall safety of the aircraft?
(3) How much of a weight penalty is acceptable for the structure?
(4) How many man-hours could be saved by simplifying the analysis?
(5) How would the performance characteristics of the aircraft change?

After a careful evaluation of each support structure has been made, in some cases their values possibly correlated from existing test results or analysis, it is recommended that the beam and its supports be substantiated for the higher of the loads resulting from either a 15 percent increase or decrease in the analyst's prediction of the support structure. This therefore establishes our overlapping approach to the design of partial support structures. Of course, no matter what conservative approaches are taken to the analysis, in no case should the design of a support be greater than the minimum values known.

Thus far, from our discussion of this section, it should be apparent that the structural behavior of a beam is greatly influenced by its support structure. For example, it was previously observed in this section that as the degree of restraint of a support structure is increased, the bending moment at center span decreases, and the bending moments at the ends will increase. The analysis of a complex structure is simple and usually straightforward, it is the simplification of that structure which often leads to difficulty. It is the engineer's prerogative, therefore, to modify his analysis according to the best of alternative designs based on past experience and existing conditions.

During structural testing many critical areas of an aircraft structure are monitored by the engineer. Using strain gauges and load-cell indicators, the true behavior of the structure under load can be accurately described. These instruments of structural testing are strategically placed throughout the aircraft in locations where the engineer intends to correlate test values with those computed from analysis. Strain gauges are used to measure surface strains that occur from calibrated electrical resistance changes in the gauge. The strain values are then converted to actual stresses using transformation equations. If test values are found to be higher than those predicted by analysis, the analyst must re-examine his original approaches and assumptions to the basic solution of that particular design. If he does not, and

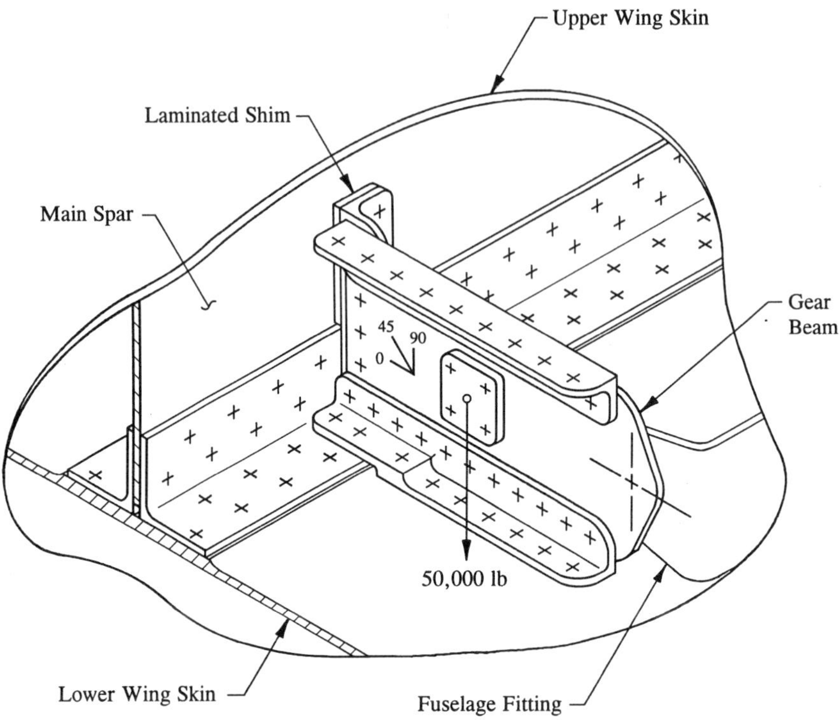

FIGURE 1-47 Vertical shear in a gear beam measured with a rectangular strain rosette.

the test is continued to ultimate load, premature failure of the structure is possible. Which would indeed be extremely embarrassing for those engineers principally involved in support of the basic structural design. Aerospace companies spend millions of dollars in engineering salaries to prevent such failures; the engineer must avoid their occurrences at all costs.

Example 1-7 The main landing gear was loaded to 110% of limit load. With the aid of a rectangular strain rosette, as shown in Fig. 1-47, the electrical resistance of the web was measured and its value converted to a vertical shear of 36,000 lb at the location indicated in the figure. Determine the actual degree of restraint that is offered by this support structure. If the gear beam was preliminarily designed to an acceptable design range of 40 to 60 percent degree of restraint, should testing of this structure be continued to 150% limit load?

SOLUTION: When the 50,000 lb load is physically applied to the gear beam web, part of this load will shear into the right side of the beam and be reacted at the fuselage; the rest will shear into the left side and be reacted at the main spar. The

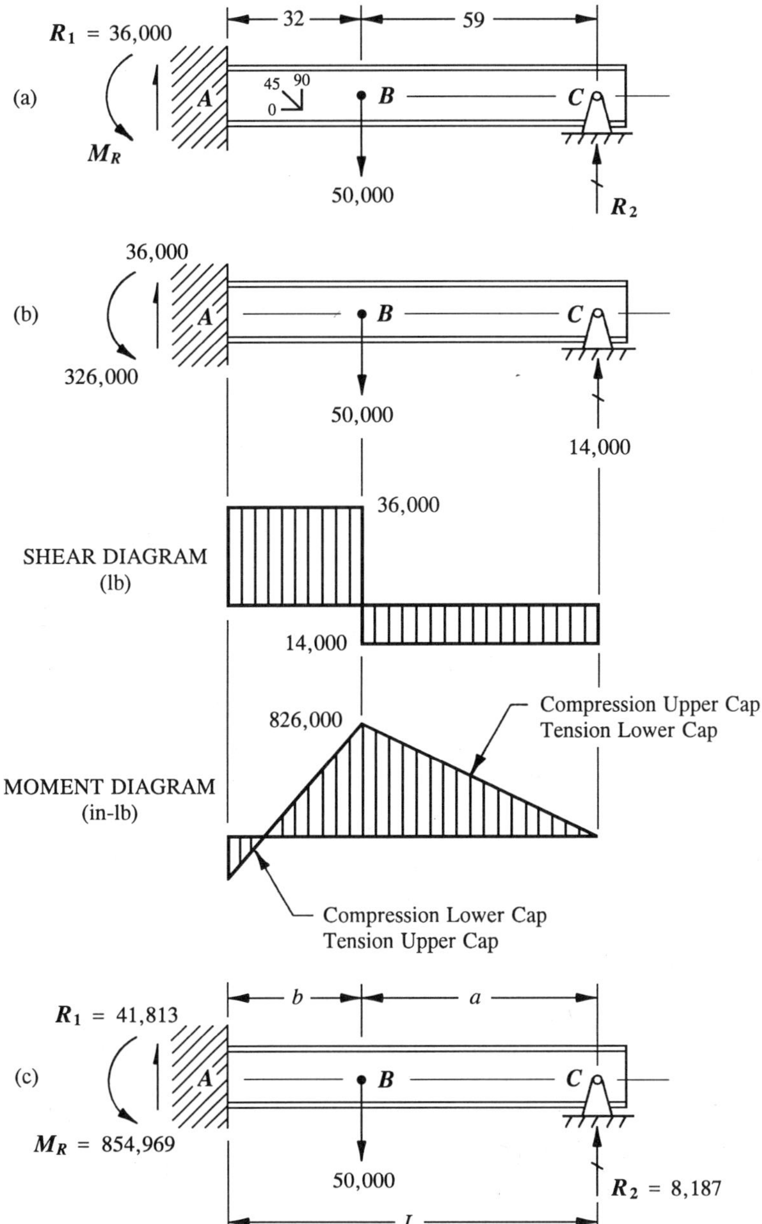

FIGURE 1-48 (a) Actual fixity of the support structure from test. (b) Free-body diagram of the actual tested structure and corresponding shear and bending moment diagrams. (c) Balanced structure for a theoretically fixed support.

magnitude of each shear force will correspond to the magnitude of the beam reactions. This structure is shown free-bodied in Fig. 1-48(a). For the gear beam, intuitively, it is observed that the shear force between A and B is constant. As such, the reaction at A must also be 36,000 lb, as given by the transformation value of the test strain gauge. The shear diagram in Appendix D, Case 16 (page 640), can be used to help the engineer better understand the internal loads picture of the structure, i.e., the internal shears that exist along the entire length of the gear beam. With the value of R_1 known, R_2 is directly obtained from the second equation of equilibrium, or

$$\Sigma F_y = 0, \qquad R_1 - 50,000 + R_2 = 0 .$$

Substituting for R_1,

$$36,000 - 50,000 + R_2 = 0.$$

Hence, this gives:

$$R_2 = 14,000 \text{ lb}.$$

To obtain the moment at end A, the third equation of statics is applied at point A, or

$$\Sigma M_A = 0, \quad \circlearrowleft + \quad -14,000(91) + 50,000(32) - M_R = 0$$
$$M_R = 326,000 \text{ in-lb}.$$

With the actual loading having been determined, as shown in Fig. 1-48(b), the entire structure is now accurately described. This is shown by the shear and moment diagrams just below the loaded structure in this figure.

Now, to complete our discussion of this problem, let us investigate the loads that would result if the gear beam was considered fully fixed at A. With the aid of the reference beam formula solutions available in Appendix D, Case 16, the following balanced structure, Fig. 1-48(c), is arrived at:

$$R_2 = \frac{1}{2}\frac{P}{L^3}(3b^2L - b^3) = 8,187 \text{ lb}$$
$$R_1 = P - R_2 = 41,813 \text{ lb}$$
$$M_R = \frac{1}{2}\frac{P}{L^2}(b^3 + 2bL^2 - 3b^2L) = 854,969 \text{ in-lb}.$$

The actual degree of restraint DR as measured by Eq. 1-5 is now written for the support at A as follows:

$$DR = \frac{\text{actual support moment}}{\text{fixed support moment}}(100) = \frac{326,000}{854,969}(100) = 38.1\%.$$

Hence, the actual degree of restraint of the main landing gear beam does not lie within the acceptable design range of 40 to 60 percent degree of restraint. Whether testing of this structure should be continued to 150% limit load or not will entirely depend upon the test stresses developed for this structure at higher loads, not on its preliminary design factors. The reason being, at higher loads some redistribution of peak loads can occur in areas actually unsubstantiated by analysis. This condition is undesirable, but its occurrence is realistic behavior of structure. That is to say, specifically, outside this design range when the applied loads are continued to increase, some regions of the structure will begin to yield, sustaining their loads, while other areas of the structure will accept the ever-increasing load. In effect, the structure changes its structural characteristics during actual testing. In retrospect, there is no more reliable substitute than the careful monitoring of stresses during structural testing, no matter what calculated or projected stresses are indicated at higher loads by analysis.

A final note to this problem: If structural testing is resumed and the main landing gear beam is substantiated at 150% limit load, the results of this test can then be fully utilized to more efficiently optimize this structure for subsequent production model aircraft. This time, of course, with the confidence and assurance gained from our test study of this problem, and without having to make conservative overlapping assumptions, the actual degree of restraint or $DR = 38.1\%$ is used to redesign the structure.

Test data can also be obtained from strain-gauge studies of an aircraft under actual flight and landing conditions. This is accomplished by using an aircraft that is heavily instrumented so that the structural loads throughout the aircraft can be measured and transmitted real-time to an automated telemetry tracking station. Engineers monitor these loads and determine whether they are acceptable or not. This automatic telemetry system will record the test data in real-time, enabling engineers to analyze the resulting stresses on the aircraft as the maneuver is being performed, and report to the pilot immediately with an evaluation of the results.

Today, the design engineer is a thoroughly integrated member of the design and developmental team. Along with other engineers, he understands the theory beyond the design objectives and the safe operational limits of the aircraft. Flight testing involves a highly discrete incremental testing procedure that will start with simulation trials on the ground of all test regimes before ultimately taking the aircraft to first flight. The intent of a flight test program is therefore to increase the maneuvering envelope over that which the aircraft was originally designed. The engineer's experience and ability to do the job of flight and structural testing of the aircraft and its derivatives are critical to the success of the production aircraft.

1.10 Method of Joints Approach to Internal Loads Analysis. The method of joints approach to internal loads analysis is a technique used by engineers to

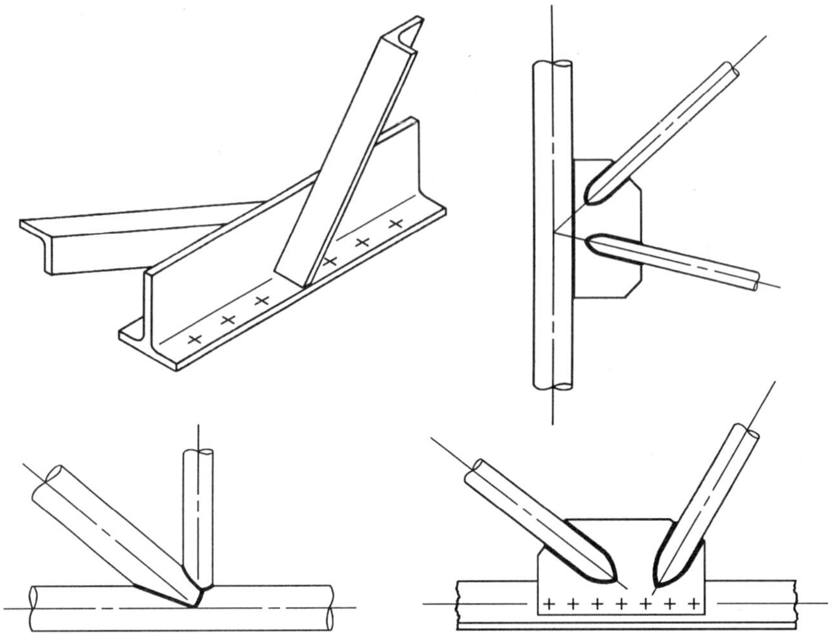

FIGURE 1-49 Welding and riveting of members to a common joint of a truss framework.

determine the internal axial forces (tension or compression) that may exist in the bar members of a truss framework. The procedure for calculating the internal axial forces of a truss is the same whether studying a beam (Method of Sections Approach to Internal Loads Analysis, Sec. 1.5) or for any other type of structure. In most actual truss systems, the joints connecting all members are seldom completely free of shearing forces and bending moments. For all practical purposes, however, the axial internal forces of an idealized truss are usually sufficient to describe the stress intensities that an actual truss system would produce, even if shearing forces and bending moments do slightly occur.

If a joint of a truss is arranged so that no significant amounts of shear and bending moment can be carried across the joint to other axial members, the joint can be considered pinned and frictionless. To accomplish this in actual design, the centroid of the bar members must coincide with the centroid of the joint or connection. Since all forces would then pass through the center of the joint, little or no shear force or bending moment would be produced. Most joints of an actual truss are fabricated by welding or riveting its members to the joint (see Fig. 1-49). Even so, if the joints have been properly designed to eliminate or minimize the eccentricities that may occur, the idealized truss should provide an invaluable source of information to satisfactorily design an actual truss framework.

The method of joints approach to the analysis of a truss will be explained by a specific example. The simple truss in Fig. 1-50(a) is isolated without regard to the

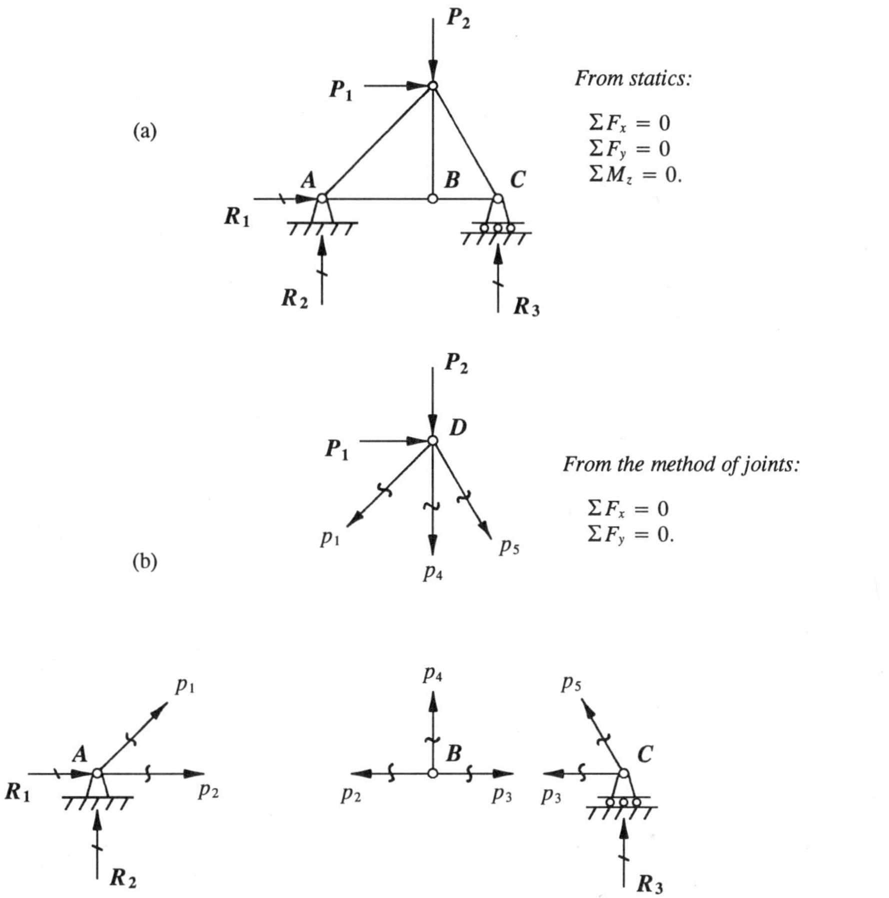

FIGURE 1-50 Truss framework, (a) free-body diagram of the external system of equilibrium forces, (b) unknown internal axial bar forces of the truss framework.

interior makeup of the truss, and reactions determined from statics, $\Sigma F_x = 0$, $\Sigma F_y = 0$, and $\Sigma M_z = 0$ to establish overall equilibrium. Then, imaginary cuts are conveniently made through all of the bar members of the truss that completely isolate a particular joint, as shown in Fig. 1-50(b). Since no moment can exist for a concurrent system of forces at a joint, only two independent equations are available for solution at each isolated joint. Assuming that the axial forces are tension for these members, equilibrium of forces is established if the equations $\Sigma F_x = 0$ and $\Sigma F_y = 0$ are both satisfied. If, however, more than two unknown bar forces exist at a joint, the unknown bar axial forces cannot immediately be found from these two equations. The extra unknown bar force or forces may however be found from the computations of other isolated joints. These extra forces then become

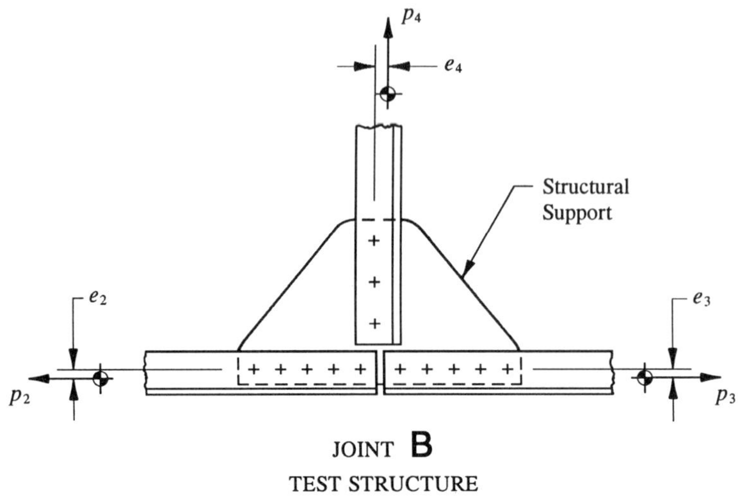

FIGURE 1-51 Joint eccentricity of a truss framework.

known values acting on subsequent isolated joints being analyzed. Applying these two equilibrium force equations at each joint, the magnitude and proper direction of the bar axial forces will be determined. If the sign of an unknown bar force is computed and found to be positive, the indicated direction is therefore correct and the bar force remains tension; however, if the sign is found to be negative, this would indicate that the assumed direction was chosen incorrectly and the bar axial force must be reversed (i.e., compression). The strength of a member is then measured by comparing the calculated tension stresses (Chapter 2, Eq. 2-2) to the corresponding allowable tension stress of the material. The compression axial bar members are designed as Euler or Johnson-Euler columns (see Chapter 7, Secs. 7.4 and 7.5, respectively).

To design a joint efficiently requires that the eccentricity of the bar axial forces also be investigated in detail at each joint. For example, if the neutral axis of

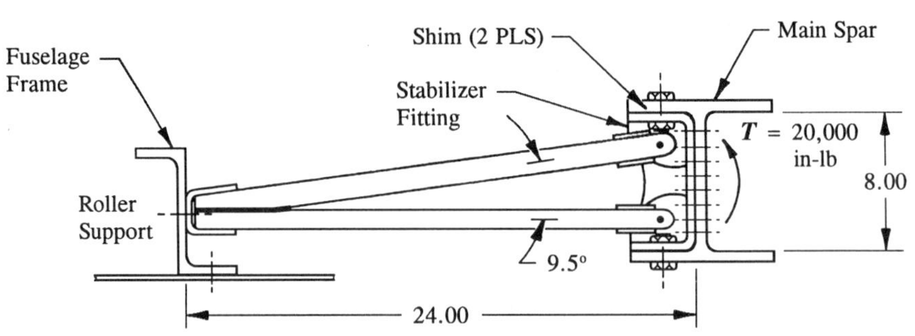

FIGURE 1-52 Stabilizer truss arrangement of tubular members.

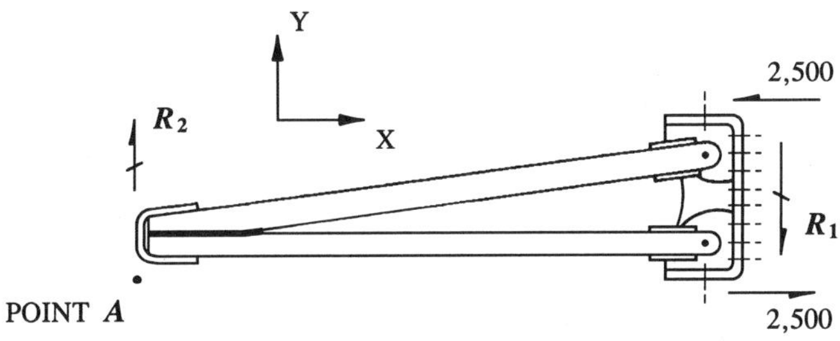

FIGURE 1-53 Equilibrium of forces acting on the truss framework.

the cross-sectional area of a bar member does not line up with the centroid of its rivet pattern, a twisting of the member will result. From Fig. 1-50, a detail of joint *B* depicting these eccentricities is shown in Fig. 1-51. The effects of twisting on a riveted connection will be treated in Chapter 3 when our attention is focused on the analysis of eccentrically loaded connections.

Example 1-8 To stabilize (prevent twisting) of the main spar, a simple truss arrangement of tubular members is proposed, as shown in Fig. 1-52. If the main spar carries a maximum torque of 20,000 in-lb, what are the axial forces in the stabilizer tubes? Where would strain gauges be strategically placed on the stabilizer truss to monitor the actual behavior of this structure under load?

SOLUTION: The torque T is physically introduced into the truss system as an equivalent horizontal couple[1] of magnitude 2,500 lb through the upper and lower fitting bolts, as shown in Fig. 1-53.

$$P_{\text{couple}} = \frac{M}{H} = \frac{20,000}{8} = 2,500 \text{ lb}.$$

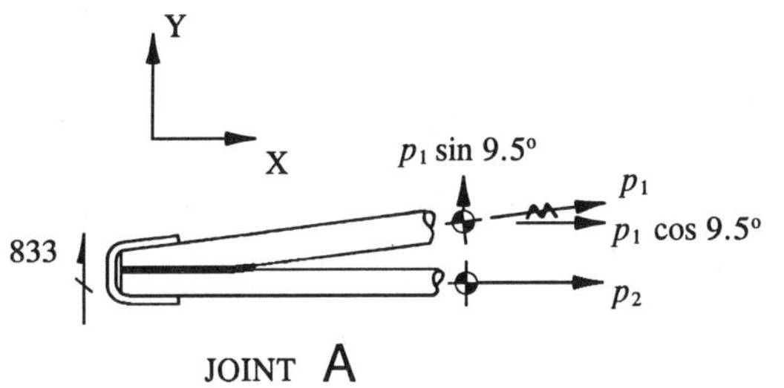

FIGURE 1-54 Internal bar forces at an isolated joint.

[1] It is shown in Appendix B that a moment M is equivalent to a couple of magnitude M/H.

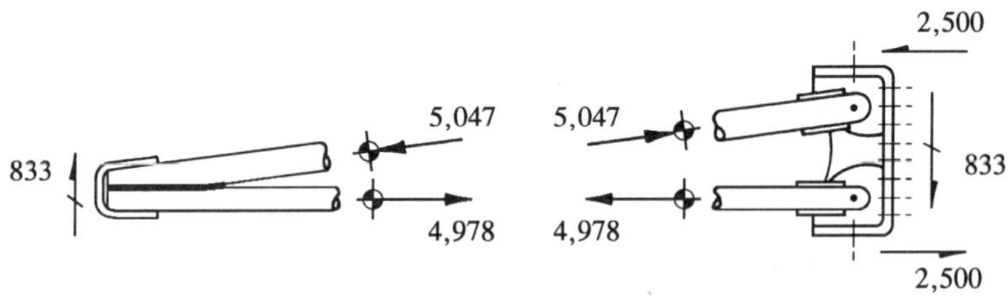

FIGURE 1-55 Internal axial bar forces indicated for the truss framework.

Since the method of attaching the stabilizer to the fuselage frame web allows the joint to freely rotate, no build up of moment is possible at this joint. Additionally, the web cannot provide significant out-of-plane loads and the basic frame section cannot provide much torsional restraint. Hence, joint A is assumed to be simply-supported, and the roller support with its vertical shear capability describes this joint tendency. From earlier discussions, the joint is said to be pinned and frictionless since shearing forces and bending moments have been minimized.

Next, consider the equilibrium of all the forces acting on the truss framework, and take moments of all these forces about point A (see Fig. 1-53), we obtain:

$$\Sigma M_A = 0, \quad \circlearrowleft{+} \quad -2,500(8) + R_1(24) = 0, \quad R_1 = 833 \text{ lb}.$$

From $\Sigma F_y = 0$, $\quad R_2 - R_1 = 0$

$$R_2 = R_1 = 833 \text{ lb}.$$

Imaginary cuts are now made through the diagonal and horizontal tubular members of the truss with the intent of isolating the joint at A. The internal axial bar forces are labeled p_1 and p_2 in Fig. 1-54. Applying the following two equations of equilibrium at joint A will establish their values.

$$\Sigma F_x = 0, \quad p_1 \cos 9.5^\circ + p_2 = 0$$

$$\Sigma F_y = 0, \quad 833 + p_1 \sin 9.5^\circ = 0$$

$$p_1 = -\frac{833}{\sin 9.5^\circ} = -5,047 \text{ lb}.$$

And then substituting p_1 back into the first equation gives:

$$-5,047 \cos 9.5^\circ + p_2 = 0$$

$$p_2 = 4,978 \text{ lb}.$$

The internal axial bar forces determined are then properly drawn on the isolated joint, as shown in Fig. 1-55.

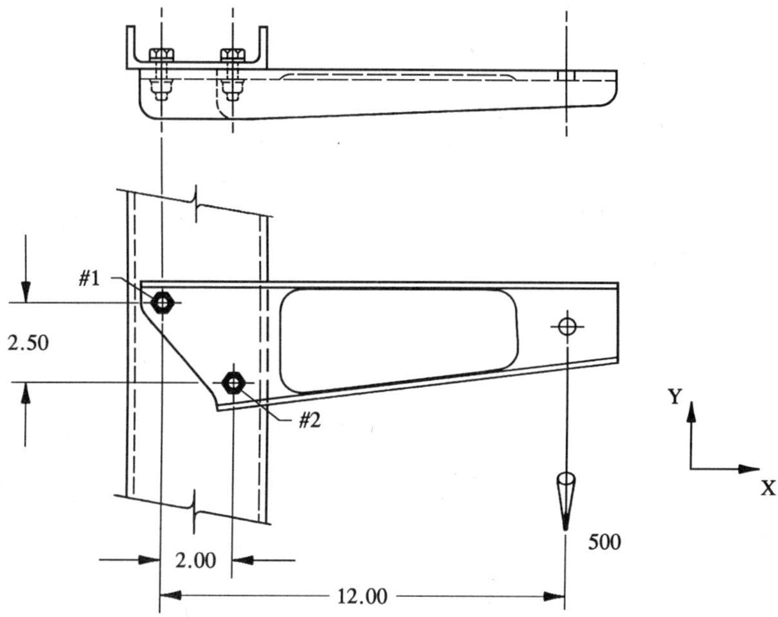

FIGURE 1-56 Cantilever beam support structure.

1.11 Problem for Solution. The cantilever support beam shown in Fig. 1-56 is subjected to a vertical load of 500 lb. (a) Locate the center of resistance of the fastener pattern and then find the resultant shearing force on each fastener. Assume that both fasteners are the same size and type. (*Hint:* Balance the beam with reactive loads at the center of resistance of the fastener pattern and then distribute these forces separately to each fastener.) (b) Indicate these forces on a properly drawn free-body diagram of the beam. Also state whether the forces indicated represent plate or fastener forces.

CHAPTER 2

Axial and Bending Members

2.1 Introduction. Stress is an internal force exerted on the interior parts of a structure that was acted upon by externally applied forces at the surface of the structure. The intensity of force or stress is measured by the ability of the member to resist the internal forces at critical interior sections of the structure. In Fig. 2-1, each member of the control system mechanism is labeled by the particular type of internal forces it is subjected to. It is therefore the objective of this book to determine the internal stress distributions of these internal forces through the application and proper usage of conventional stress analysis formulas. In our study of stresses in this chapter, only the effects of axial and bending stresses either combined or acting separately at a particular exposed section of a structure are investigated. A complete study of shearing stresses will be deferred until Chapter 4, where our attention will be specifically focused there on how to relate the internal shears in a beam to shearing stresses that they produce.

In all phases of stress analysis, the following questions must be answered to achieve a complete and dependable structural design solution: (1) What magnitude of force can be applied to the structure or to its component parts before failure occurs? (2) How much deformation is acceptable under prescribed loading conditions? and (3) What is the most efficient size member required for the structure to withstand these forces? The material of this chapter will attempt to answer these and many other related questions to their solutions.

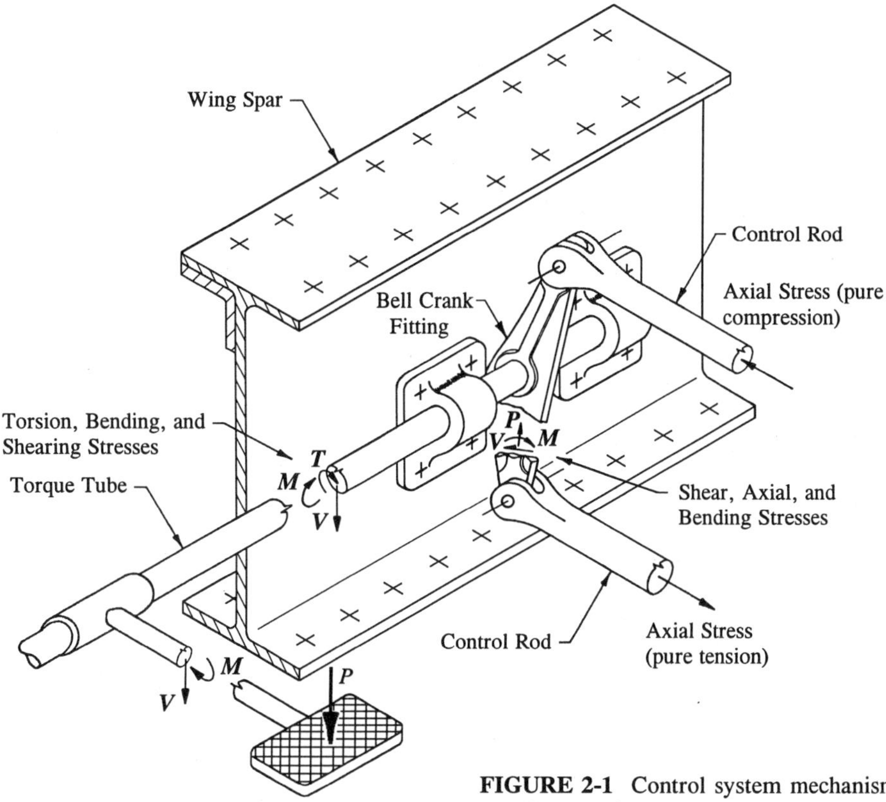

FIGURE 2-1 Control system mechanism showing the internal loads members are subjected to.

Using the method of sections approach to internal loads analysis of Sec. 1.5, the internal forces at any section, identified by the symbols *V*, *P*, and *M*, along a member can directly be computed. In general, the internal forces are resolved into perpendicular and parallel component forces to a section being examined. The component force is called "normal" if it represents the force perpendicular to the section. In particular, when the normal force is directed toward the section (or push) it is called axial compression. Whereas, if it is directed away from the section (or pull) it is called axial tension. The other internal component force *V* acting parallel to the exposed section of the member being investigated is called "shear." The internal forces (*V*, *P*, and *M*) will then in turn produce corresponding stresses on the cross-sectional area of the member based upon the appropriate stress formulas applied for each particular kind of load. The stress formulas necessary to apply to these members for the loading types indicated are listed in Table 2-1. For easy reference, also included in this table are those equations described in other chapters of this book where, for example, shearing and crippling stresses are also prevalent in the loaded structure.

TABLE 2-1 STRESS FORMULAS

Type of Stress	Formula	Ref.
Normal Stress, Eq. 2-2	$f_n = \pm \frac{P}{A}$	Chapter 2, p. 57
Bending Stress, Eq. 2-5	$f_b = \pm \frac{Mc}{I_{na}}$	Chapter 2, p. 63
Shear Stress, Eq. 4-2	$f_s = \frac{VQ}{I_{na}\,t}$	Chapter 4, p. 227
Crippling Stress, Eq. 6-16	$F_{cc} = \frac{C_e \sqrt{F_{cy} E_c}}{(b'/t)^{3/4}}$	Chapter 6, p. 387

By themselves, the solutions to these equations (or stresses) have no real meaning unless their calculated values can be directly compared to laboratory test results for each material being used for design. Fortunately, allowable values are easily determined from physical testing of different materials and are readily available from most aerospace company material manuals and various government publications. In this book, all design mechanical and physical properties as they pertain to specific problem solutions will be taken from the Military Standardization Handbook, *Metallic Materials and Elements for Aerospace Vehicle Structures* or MIL-HDBK-5F. This handbook is maintained with the latest available information from aerospace industry sources and in joint operation with the Department of Defense and Federal Aviation Administration to establish its currency. Engineers who are not thoroughly familiar with the general usage of this document are encouraged to review the material of Appendix E of this book for more information. In this appendix the mechanical-property tables available, not continually maintained or updated by this author or its editors, should only be used for general guidelines or instructional purposes: unless of course, each table is specifically verified beforehand from the most current edition of MIL-HDBK-5. Then, the values given here (in this appendix) can be used for design.

The basic jargon or terminology used by structural engineers to measure the degree of reliability that a structure can withstand or realize above or below its minimum guaranteed requirements is called "margin of safety." Its numerical value provides a means by which the engineer can communicate to his associates and others of his analytical findings relating to his predictions of structural failure as a result of some prescribed physical characteristic of the structure, such as ultimate failure stresses, fatigue considerations, instability requirements, deformation criteria, etc. Specifically, the applied or calculated design stress of a member is compared to the allowable stress of the material used for that member. From this, the following mathematical expression is formulated:

$$\text{Margin of Safety} = \text{M.S.} = \frac{\text{allowable stress}}{\text{applied stress}} - 1. \tag{2-1}$$

Where possible, the engineer should strive to optimize his designs by maintaining "zero" margins of safety. Or, at least, to avoid premature failure, he must realize slightly "positive" values for each of his calculated predictions or margins of safety.

The number of stress formulas necessary to effectively analyze and design most structures are surprisingly few in number. Success in stress analysis will depend on a well-disciplined method of attack in the treatment of real engineering problems. It is the methods and approaches to the solution of these problems on a rational and intelligent basis which the engineer must develop to fully understand the internal stress distributions of a complex structure. Past teaching experience has proved that a logical sequence of study of stresses is to introduce axial and bending stresses in one chapter (Chapter 2), and to postpone a discussion of shearing and crippling stresses into separate chapters of their own (Chapters 4 and 6, respectively).

2.2 Axial Compression and Tension Stresses. The general expression used to calculate axial compression and tension normal stresses is

$$f_n = \pm \frac{P}{A} \tag{2-2}$$

where: P = internal axial force acting perpendicular (or normal) to a section and passing through the centroid of the cross-sectional area of a beam

A = effective cross-sectional area (see specific applications using gross and net areas, Eqs. 2-3 and 2-4).

Two types of normal or axial forces are considered in this section: an axial compression force and an axial tension force. Furthermore, if we adopt the industry convention for stresses, a + sign will be used when the stress is indicated as tension (or pulling), and a – sign when the stress is compression (or pushing). From these, and the application of Eq. 2-1, the following predictions of tension and compression failures of the material are written:

Ultimate Tension Failure:

$$\text{Margin of Safety} = \text{M.S.} = \frac{F_{tu}}{f_t} - 1$$

where: F_{tu} = ultimate tension stress allowable of the material

f_t = applied ultimate axial tension stress (from Eq. 2-2).

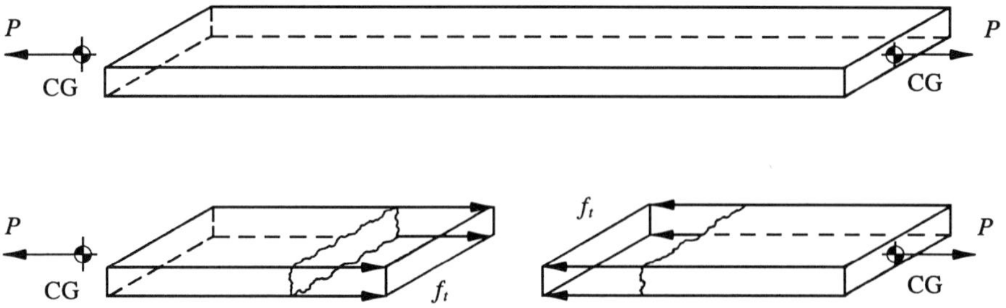

(a) Axial tension force.

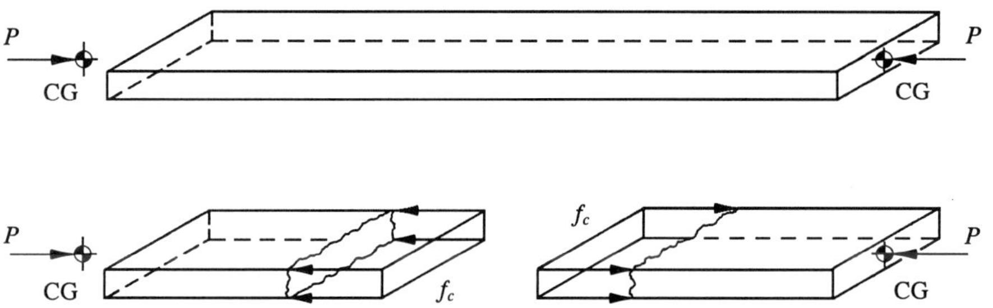

(b) Axial compression force.

FIGURE 2-2 (a) Internal axial tension stress distribution. (b) Internal axial compression stress distribution.

Yield Compression Failure:[1]

$$\text{Margin of Safety} = \text{M.S.} = \frac{F_{cy}}{f_c} - 1$$

where: F_{cy} = yield compression stress allowable of the material
f_c = applied ultimate axial compression stress (from Eq. 2-2).

The axial forces that are represented internally at a section must also pass through the centroid of area (center of gravity of the cross-sectional area) to develop an internal stress distribution across the section area which is nearly uniform. Refer to the isometric views drawn in Figs. 2-2(a) and (b). The axial tension and compression stresses that are developed in those figures are shown uniformly

[1] The margin of safety expression for yield compression failure assumes that compression instability or local crippling failure of the section is not critical (see Chapter 6, "Crippling of Compression Members," for this particular structural requirement).

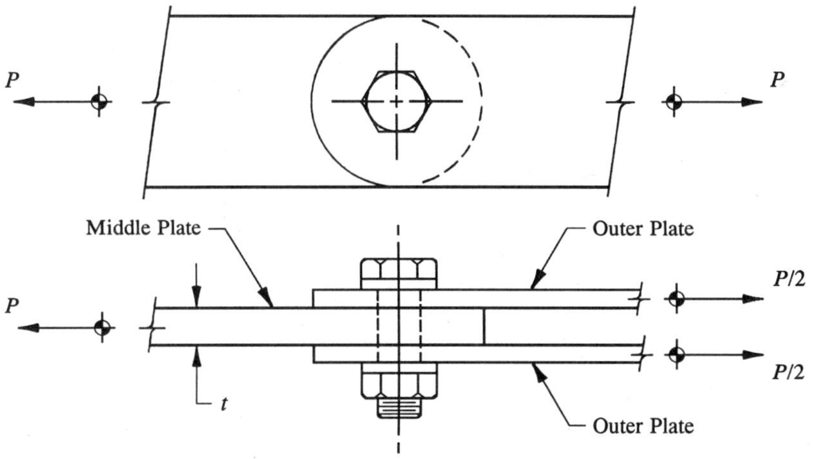

FIGURE 2-3 Double-shear lap joint loaded by a tension load *P*.

distributed across their exposed sections. If the centroids of different sections along a structural member are known, the line formed by joining these points together will establish the centroidal axis of the member. Sometimes confused with the neutral axis, the centroidal axis is described as a function of the geometric shape of a member and therefore is a constant for any particular shaped area. The neutral axis is used in conjunction with the solution of bending stresses (elastic or inelastic), and is established by the equilibrium of internal forces that exist at a section being investigated.[1]

In another case, see ahead to Fig. 2-14, an internal axial force is shown correctly diagrammed at the center of gravity of the member. But, the force does not line up with the externally applied force system. In such a case, the resulting eccentricity of force will induce secondary internal bending stresses across the section area of that member. The nonuniform distribution of bending stresses caused by this condition of loading will be covered in Sec. 2.5, where a discussion of combined axial and bending stresses can more suitably be treated.

Whenever fasteners are used to attach members in a tension joint, the joint is weakened by the fastener holes existing in each of the attached members. The reason for this is simple, a tension load transfers its maximum value across the centerline of a fastener where the minimum cross-sectional area of the member exists. The tension stresses produced in such a joint are calculated using the net area of each member. To illustrate the principle further, the double-shear lap joint loaded by the tension load *P* shown in Fig. 2-3 will be used to help describe the concept of net tension stresses across the hole.

---

[1] For a complete discussion of this topic, the engineer is referred to E.F. Bruhn, *Analysis and Design of Flight Vehicle Structures*, Chap. C3, "Yield and Ultimate Strength in Bending," Tri-State Offset Company, Cincinnati, Ohio, 1965.

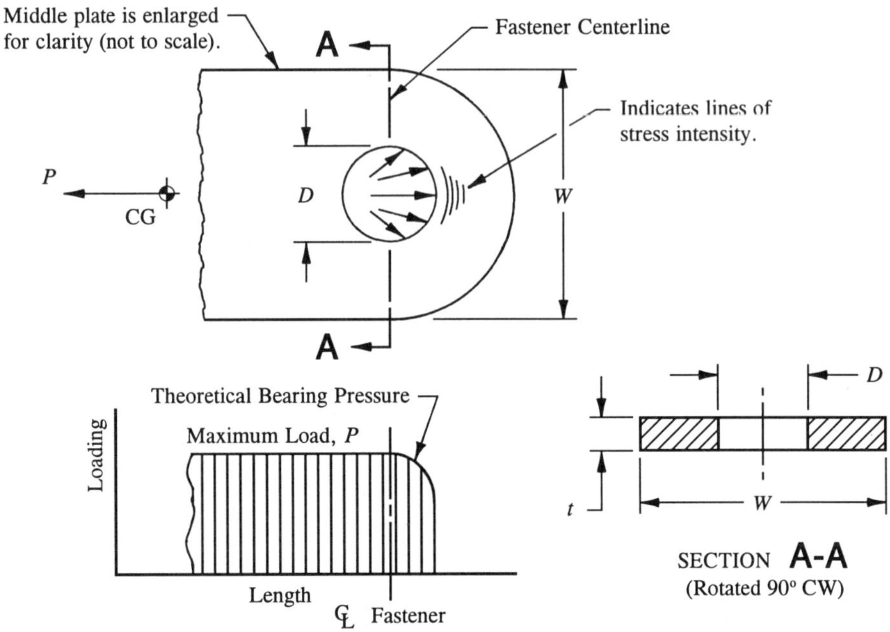

FIGURE 2-4 Axial tension diagram of the middle plate.

If the middle plate of this joint is isolated, Fig. 2-4, it is observed from the axial diagram of this plate that a maximum load *P* exists across the fastener centerline where the plate area at Section A-A is a minimum. This combination of maximum load and minimum plate area will produce the highest level of stress intensity at any point along the middle plate when Eq. 2-2 is applied. The same basic analogy can be shown to exist for the outer plate members. Except, in these cases, only ½ the applied load *P* would be used to describe their structural behavior. Note that the bearing stress distribution used to construct the axial diagram of the middle plate is entirely theoretical. The complexity of bearing failures of most ductile metals makes it physically impossible to measure this quantity accurately. For this reason, in most practical applications, it is common practice to conservatively base the theoretical bearing stress distribution of a member on a uniform stress distribution across the centerline of the hole. This assumption is completely justified since published allowable bearing stresses are customarily determined from structural testing anyway using the projected area of the fastener onto the plate. That is, the yield and ultimate bearing stresses of a material used in the analysis of structural designs are usually established by dividing the actual test load of a fastener by its projected bearing area (i.e., the product of the fastener diameter[1] and the plate thickness). Additional comments on this subject will be presented and made

[1] For a hole-filling fastener (rivet) the nominal hole diameter is used; for a nonhole-filling fastener (such as a bolt or screw) the nominal pin or shank diameter is used.

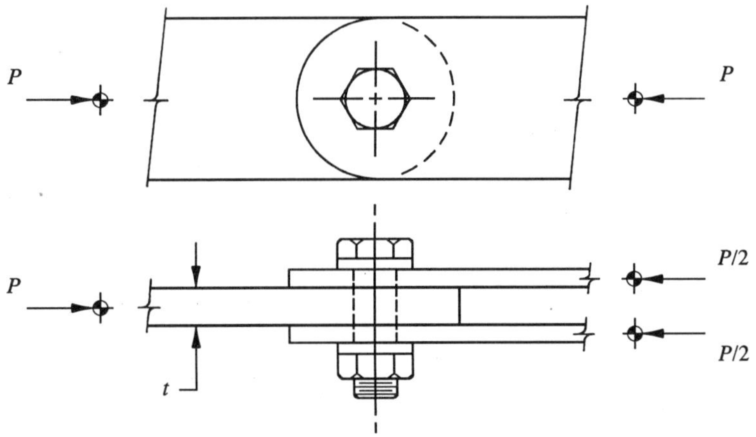

FIGURE 2-5 Double-shear lap joint loaded by a compression load *P*.

clearer in Chapter 3, where a more thorough treatment of bearing failure of plate and fastener designs will be considered. From Eq. 2-2, the maximum net tension stress is written for the middle plate:

$$f_t = +\frac{P}{A_{\text{net}}} = +\frac{P}{(W-D)t} \tag{2-3}$$

where: P = internal axial tension force
W = width of the plate
D = actual hole diameter[1]
t = thickness of the plate.

For the compression-loaded, double-shear lap joint in Fig. 2-5, no reduction in cross-sectional area is made. The fastener in this case transfers the load *P* from the middle plate to each of the outer plates before reaching the minimum plate area at the fastener centerline. This is why the net section area of a compression-loaded joint is not used in the analysis of such members. The fastener is said to "fill the hole." With the aid of the axial diagram drawn in Fig. 2-6, the transfer of load for the middle plate of this compression joint can clearly be seen. The same analogy can also be drawn for the outer plate members, but in these cases only ½ of the applied load *P* would be considered for their load transfers. From Eq. 2-2, the maximum compression stress for the middle plate in terms of its gross cross-sectional area is written:

$$f_c = -\frac{P}{A_{\text{gross}}} = -\frac{P}{Wt} \tag{2-4}$$

[1] See footnote p. 60.

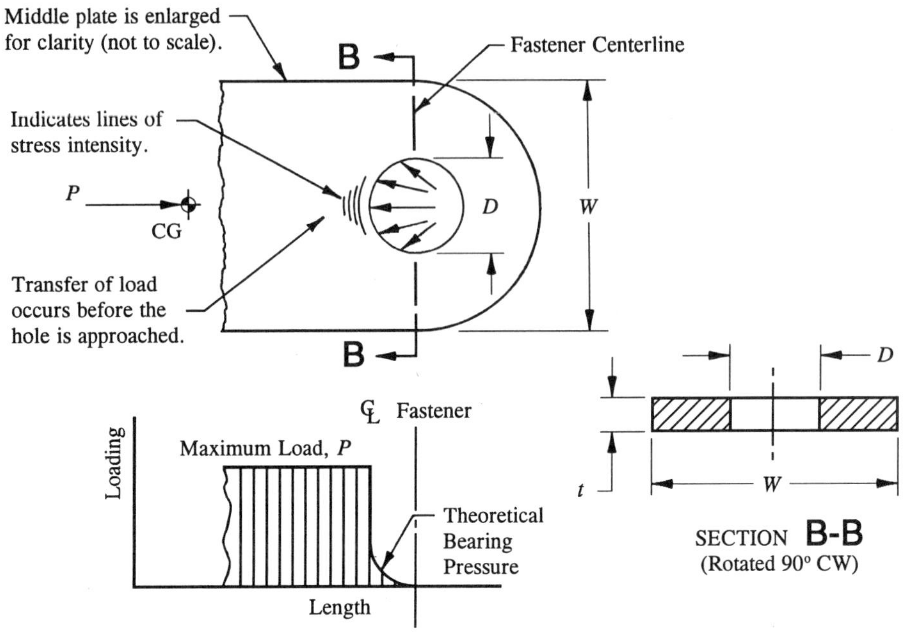

FIGURE 2-6 Axial compression diagram of the middle plate.

where: P = internal axial compression force
W = width of the plate
t = thickness of the plate.

A final note: The load-carrying capacity of a compression joint is also governed by its resistance to bearing stresses (see Chapter 3, Eqs. 3-2 and 3-3, for specific application and theory).

2.3 Bending of Beams in One Plane. The flexure formula is one of the most fundamental equations used in the design and analysis of structural engineering problems. Its formulation is used to determine stresses in straight, homogeneous beams[1] caused by internal bending moments in the elastic range of a stress-strain curve of a material. The general expression to compute the internal elastic bending stresses is

---

[1] For all practical purposes, most curved beams used in conventional aircraft structures can be analyzed by straight beam theory. For example, the circular frames supporting the fuselage shell are regarded as straight beam members. For an excellent method of calculating actual stresses in curved beams, the engineer is referred to Raymond J. Roark, *Formulas for Stress and Strain,* Table VII, "Formulas for Curved Beams," p. 164, McGraw-Hill Book Company, New York, 1965, Fourth Edition.

$$f_b = \pm \frac{Mc}{I_{na}} \tag{2-5}$$

where: M = internal bending moment around the neutral axis passing through the geometric center (or centroid) of the cross-sectional area

c = distance measured perpendicular from the neutral axis to any point on the cross-sectional area

I_{na} = moment of inertia around the neutral axis of the entire cross-sectional area (see Appendix F for detail calculations).

The following predictions of elastic bending failure of the material in tension and compression are written:

Ultimate Tension Failure:

$$\text{Margin of Safety} = \text{M.S.} = \frac{F_{tu}}{f_t} - 1$$

where: F_{tu} = ultimate tension stress allowable of the material

f_t = tension ultimate bending stress (from Eq. 2-5).

Yield Compression Failure:[1]

$$\text{Margin of Safety} = \text{M.S.} = \frac{F_{cy}}{f_c} - 1$$

where: F_{cy} = yield compression stress allowable of the material

f_c = compression ultimate bending stress (from Eq. 2-5).

In this section, we will limit our discussions to cross-sectional areas having at least a horizontal or vertical axis of symmetry. Such an axis will always coincide with one of the principal bending axes[2] of the cross-sectional area. This can be seen from the cross-sections depicted in Fig. 2-7. For example, if a cross-sectional area has an axis of symmetry, the maximum and minimum principal bending axes are easily ascertained by simply inspecting the design configuration of the section area. Conversely, if a cross-sectional area has no axis of symmetry, the principal bending axes are such as to make their determinations less obvious. In fact, the proper orientation of these axes must be mathematically computed (for explicit

---

[1] The margin of safety expression for yield compression failure assumes that compression instability or local crippling failure of the section is not critical (see Chapter 6, "Crippling of Compression Members," for this particular limitation or requirement of the structure).

[2] Principal bending axes are mutually perpendicular axes about which the maximum and minimum moments of inertia of a cross-sectional area are computed. These axes are also closely related to the neutral axis of the section area.

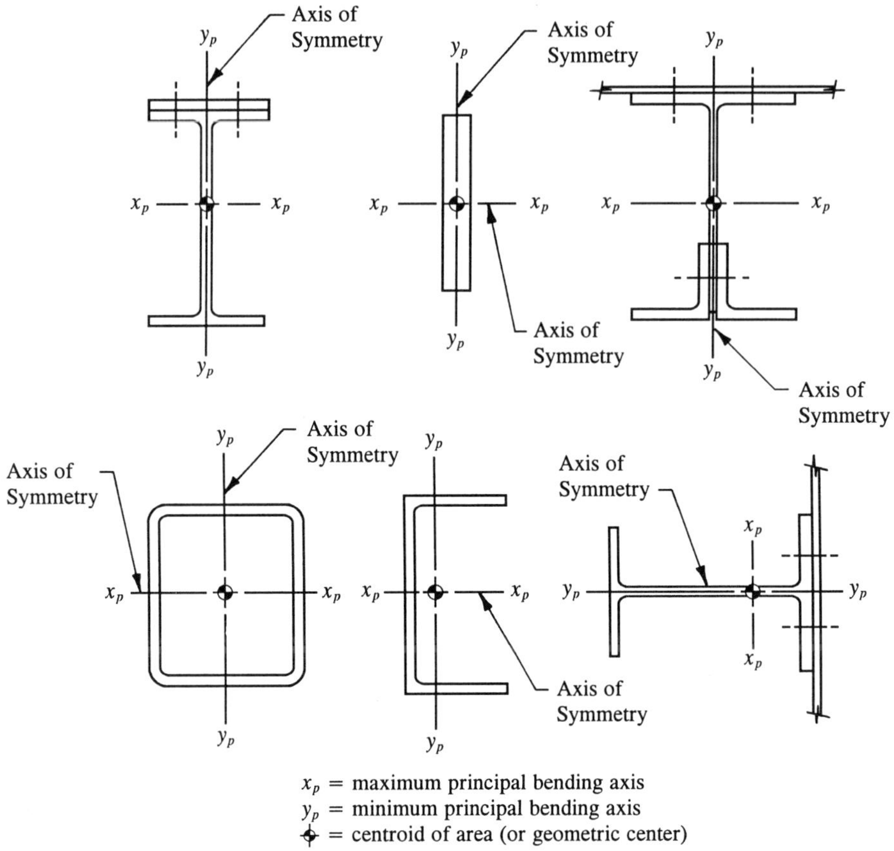

FIGURE 2-7 Beam cross-sections with at least one axis of symmetry. This establishes the maximum and minimum principal bending axes of the beam.

details, see Appendix G, "Calculation of Principal Moments of Inertia").

When a beam is subjected to bending, its physical action on the structure will cause bending around one of the principal axes of the cross-sectional area, unless of course the structure is physically constrained from doing so by other external forces. Such a force can be supplied by the attached skin of the fuselage outer shell or by the structural shear panels of the wing and empennage structures. In these cases, bending is forced to act in planes either parallel or perpendicular to the skin surfaces, not as might be presumed around the principal axes of bending of the cross-section. Such a structural arrangement is shown in Fig. 2-8.

A further limitation is imposed in this section, that is, the internal bending moments are restricted in planes which are coincident with the principal axes. In this way, the bending stress formula of this section can be correctly applied. This is done by resolving the internal moments into components which then coincide with

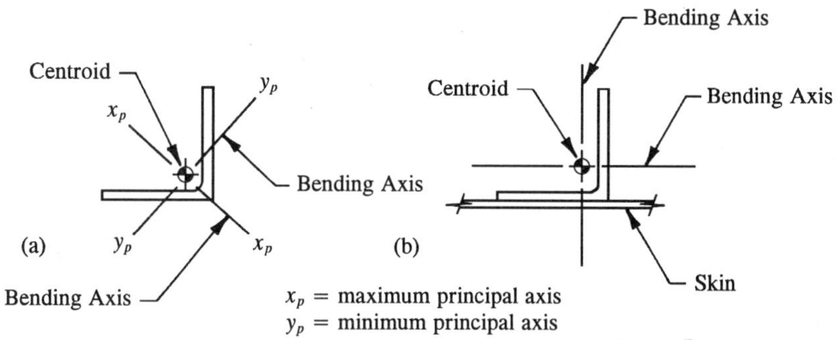

FIGURE 2-8 (a) Principal bending axes of a section area. (b) Skin forces bending to occur in planes either parallel or perpendicular to its surfaces.

the principal bending axes. The resolution of these moments are specifically treated in Sec. 2.9, "Axial and Bending Stresses of Beams That Bend in Two Different Planes." In that section, the internal bending moments considered will not be confined to the planes containing the principal bending axes, nor will the cross-sectional areas be limited to those having an axis of symmetry.

Although the flexure formula is restricted to the special case of bending stresses in the elastic range, its application to problems of inelastic stress design will nevertheless provide a basis for a conservative approach to their solutions. In all cases, calculated stresses using the flexure formula will provide nearly exact to slightly higher values than the true inelastic stresses that would otherwise occur if the methods of inelastic stress design were instead employed. Hence, the engineer should have no difficulty applying Eq. 2-5 to inelastic beam designs. To apply these ideas early in our study of bending stresses would only cause considerable confusion in this only an introductory discussion of this subject.

The amount of conservatism realized by the application of Eq. 2-5 to most inelastic stress designs will depend strictly on the material characteristics and the geometric shape of the structural members involved. Whether a member is or is not stressed to ultimate failure as prescribed by its inelastic behavior might entirely depend upon other design considerations or circumstances, such as fatigue requirements, distortion criteria, permanent deformations, etc. In addition to these limitations, the flexure formula is used only where a force is applied by steady loading without impact or shock. Also, all beams are assumed to remain stable (nonbuckled) under the action of externally applied forces. After a better understanding of basic stress fundamentals and techniques has been developed, the theory of stability as it applies to compression members will be studied (see Chapter 7, "Column Members").

The internal elastic bending stress distribution across a typical section of beam caused by an internal bending moment M is shown in Fig. 2-9. The bending moment occurs in a plane parallel to the x-y rectangular coordinate axes and bends the beam around its neutral axis. Its equivalent internal bending stresses are zero at

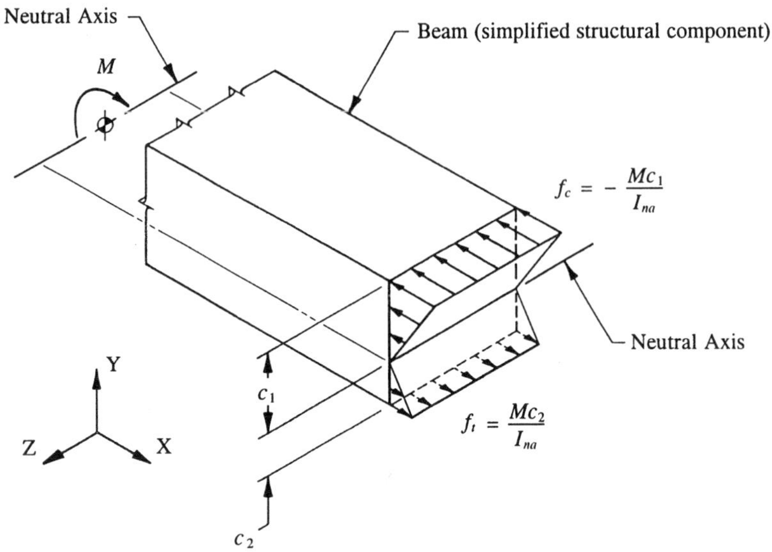

FIGURE 2-9 Elastic bending stress distribution.

the neutral axis, and will vary linearly to maximum values at the most distant points c_1 and c_2 of the section being examined. The linearity of bending stresses at a section will greatly simplify the application relating to the solution of Eq. 2-5. In that expression, the distance c to the most extreme points of the cross-sectional area of the beam are taken to either side of the neutral axis. In this way, the maximum compression and tension stresses along the surfaces of the cross-sectional area of the beam can be found. From a textbook on mechanics of materials, it is recalled, in designing a member for static strength, the maximum extreme fiber stresses are the most significant, as they will cause the ultimate failure of the material. These stresses when used in conjunction with prescribed allowable stresses of the material are sufficient to efficiently design the member in bending. From the couple-force relationship of moments derived in Appendix B ($P_{\text{couple}} = M/H$), the direction of these calculated stresses across the entire section can easily be figured out. In other words, inasmuch as a moment can be thought of as a couple, as such, a push (or compression force) must exist on the upper part of the beam while a pull (or tension force) must exist on the lower part for the moment M indicated in this figure.

The neutral axis, as the name might imply, is an axis of neutrality or a line of zero stress across the cross-sectional area of a beam subjected to bending. So long as the physical properties of the material behave elastically, and the compression and tension stress-strain curves are identical, the neutral axis remains coincident with the centroidal axis of the beam. Or, quite simply, the neutral axis passes through the centroid of the cross-sectional area. After a complete and practical study of elastic bending stresses has been presented, the particular complexities of inelastic or plastic bending of beams will become clearer (see Appendix J, "Inelastic Bending," for an introduction to the inelastic bending of rectangular-shaped sections[1]). Until then, let us assume that the location of the neutral axis is identical with the established location of the centroidal axis. Using the tabular methods employed in Appendix F, the centroidal axis, located a distance Y_{cg} from an arbitrary established reference axis, is systematically determined. The following example problem will help to illustrate the principles just outlined in this section while also focusing and expanding on ideas of similar or related subjects of previous discussions.

Example 2-1 To provide additional stiffness to the engine air-inlet duct skin, it is proposed that four (4) typical stiffeners equally spaced between Frame Stations 495.0 and 535.0 be used. Such an arrangement is shown in Fig. 2-10, where, based on the duct geometry given, the stiffeners are of unequal lengths. If the combined pressure of the internal cabin pressure and external air pressure on the surface of the duct is 39.3 psi ultimate acting outward from the center of the fuselage, what are the maximum fiber stresses for the most critical stiffener? To simplify the solution, neglect the distribution of pressure loading that is carried by the longitudinal edge members. Assume that the air-inlet duct skin rivets are .159 inch in diameter.

SOLUTION: The first step in the solution of this problem is to determine the amount of pressure loading that is carried by each stiffener. This is done conveniently by proportioning one-half (½) of the pressure loading acting in each of the air-inlet duct bays to each of the adjacent transverse structural members: the stiffeners and frames, as shown in Fig. 2-11(a), provide this function. To accomplish this mathematically, the pressure loading is idealized as a distributed load w (lb/in) acting along the length of each stiffener or frame, and their numerical values are computed by taking the product of the pressure p and the effective width b of loading considered, or

$$w = pb \quad \text{(see Table 1-1, Case 3 in Sec. 1.3, p. 11)}$$
$$w = 39.3(8.0) = 314.4 \text{ lb/in ultimate.}$$

Since the proposed stiffeners are evenly spaced, they will each carry the same distribution of load w. In Fig. 2-11(b), a typical stiffener is shown completely isolated from its main structure, and its free-body diagram drawn.

In Chapter 5, a method of isolating and analyzing shear clips will be presented. For the time being, let us assume that the stiffener shear clips are of adequate strength to transfer the shear reactions R_1 and R_2 indicated in the figure. The maximum bending moment for any stiffener occurs at midspan, and is represented

[1] The advanced nature of inelastic bending stresses for complex shapes is left for further investigation by the engineer.

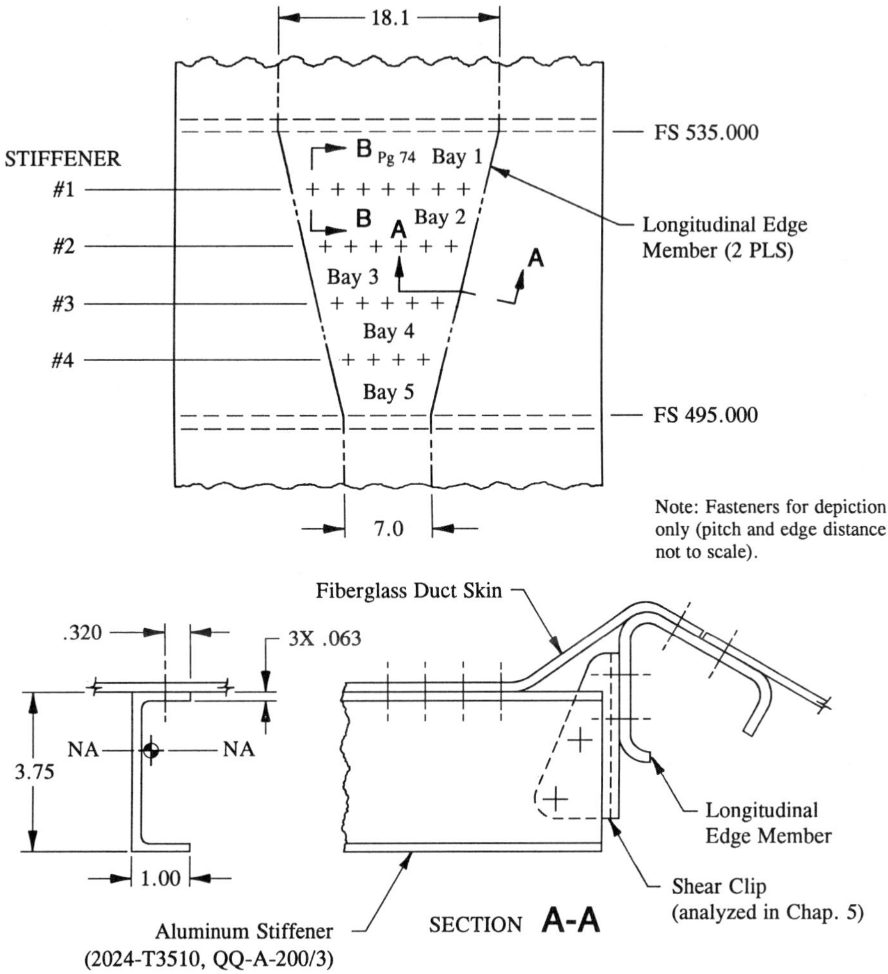

FIGURE 2-10 Engine air-inlet duct shown with typical stiffeners equally spaced.

by the following equation: $M = wL^2/8$ (see Reference Beam Formula Solutions, Case 11, Appendix D). This expression is formulated from a statics analysis of an isolated stiffener, and can easily be verified by the usual methods and techniques of internal loads analysis of Chapter 1, Sec. 1.5. As a brief review of that section, it is recalled that where a maximum internal bending moment is thought to occur along a member, a perpendicular section cut to the longitudinal axis of the beam is made. The maximum internal bending moment is then idealized on either of the isolated parts, and its value is calculated from the equations of statics. As an expedient, however, the magnitude of M will be computed using the beam formula solution already provided here. Hence, solving for M in this equation, we find:

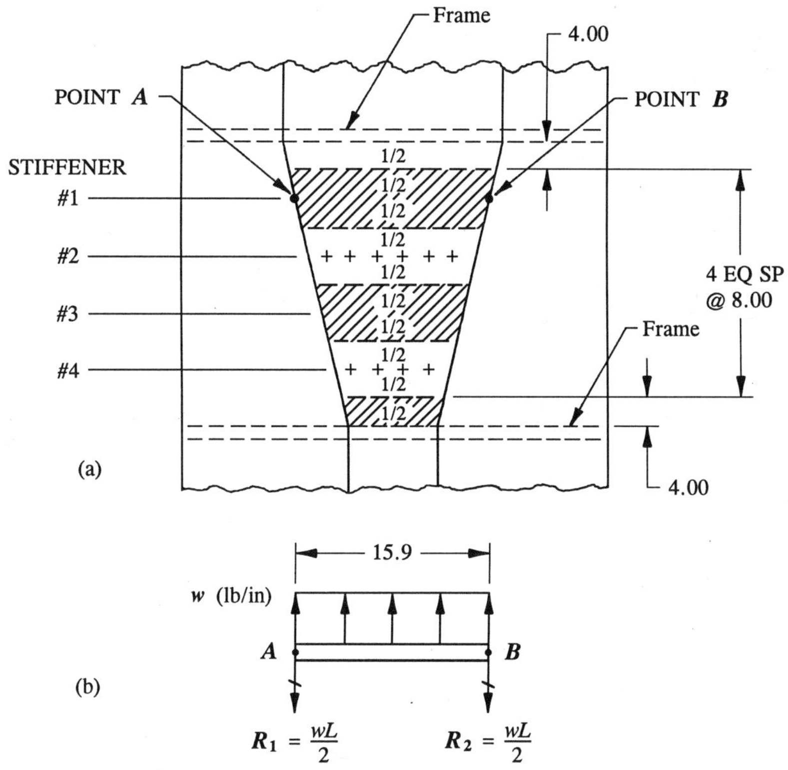

FIGURE 2-11 (a) Pressure loading on the engine air-inlet duct is idealized by conveniently distributing the loading to adjacent structural members. (b) Stiffener #1 is isolated from the main structure and free-bodied.

$$M = \frac{wL^2}{8} = \frac{314.4(15.9)^2}{8} = 9,935 \text{ in-lb ultimate}$$

where from the geometry given in this problem, the length of stiffener #1 from A to B is 15.9 in. Based upon principles previously learned in Chapter 1, the direction of this moment is easily figured out: tension on the outer flange (skin side) and compression on the inner flange side.

Those of you who are unable to determine the correct direction of this maximum moment should carefully review the moment diagram provided in Appendix D for this loading case. From the proportionality of terms in this expression, it is clear that the longer stiffener is more critical. This is true because the ultimate strength of a member is usually based on its maximum design moment, which, in this case, occurs at center span for the longer stiffener.

In order to apply the flexure formula ($f_b = \pm Mc/I_{na}$), the moment of inertia I_{na} around the neutral axis of the cross-sectional area of the stiffener must be computed. This computation will also establish the maximum c distances measured from the neutral axis to the location on the surface where the maximum compression and tension stresses occur. Since fiberglass is structurally many times weaker than aluminum, the fiberglass duct skin will not be considered as an effective member in providing any appreciable bending resistance with the attached stiffener. The duct skin does however provide the physical restraint to prevent the stiffener from twisting out-of-plane. The skin actually forces bending to occur about an axis parallel to its skin line. Of course, this axis must also pass through the neutral axis of the effective stiffener area. Note, in particular, that if the fiberglass duct skin was not present to stabilize the stiffener, bending would then occur around the principal axes of the cross-sectional area. With no axis of symmetry, the principal axes of the section would have to be computed (see Appendix G, "Calculation of Principal Moments of Inertia"). And then the flexure formula would apply around these axes.

To account for the loss of bending stiffness of the outer flange of the stiffener when a hole is present, the net area through the hole must be considered. This is shown in Fig. 2-12, where the rivet hole (element #4) is shown shaded-in. The computation of moment of inertia of the unshaded portions of the stiffener area is now performed by the tabulation method of Appendix F.

MOMENT OF INERTIA

Element	b	h	y	A	Ay	Ay^2	I_o
1	1.000	0.063	0.031	0.063	0.002	0.000	0.000
2	0.063	3.624	1.875	0.228	0.428	0.803	0.250
3	1.000	0.063	3.718	0.063	0.234	0.871	0.000
4	0.159*	0.063	3.718	- 0.010	- 0.037	- 0.138	- 0.000
			Total	0.344	0.627	1.536	0.250

* Nominal hole diameter for rivets (see specific values given in Table 3-1, p. 146).

Then, from Eqs. A-10 and A-11, we find the centroid location and moment of inertia to be

$$Y_{cg} = \frac{\Sigma\, Ay}{\Sigma\, A} = \frac{.627}{.344} = 1.823 \text{ in}$$

$$I_{cg} = \Sigma\, I_o + \Sigma\, Ay^2 - Y_{cg}\,(\Sigma\, Ay)$$

$$I_{cg} = .250 + 1.536 - 1.823(.627) = .643 \text{ in}^4 .$$

If the bending stresses calculated by Eq. 2-5 are elastic, the neutral axis is coincident with the center of gravity of the cross-sectional area, and it would

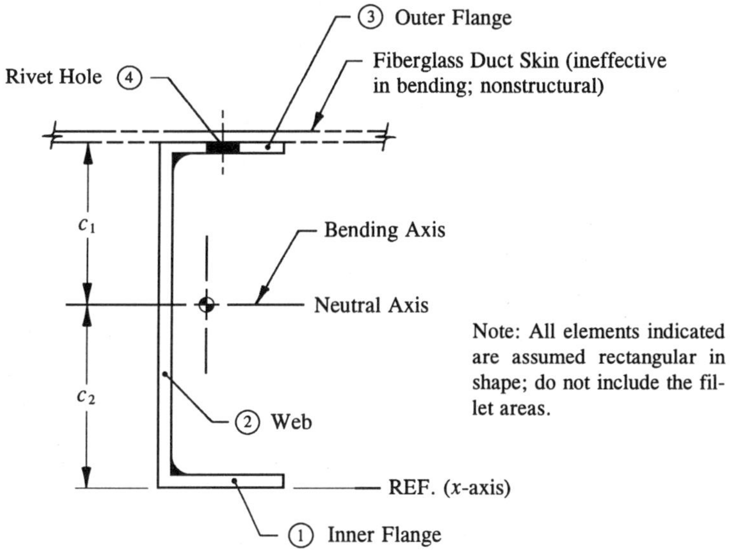

FIGURE 2-12 Stiffener net cross-sectional area through the hole. (Dimensions pertinent to the analysis are shown on page 68.)

follow directly from this assumption that

$$Y_{na} = Y_{cg} = 1.823 \text{ in}$$

and

$$I_{na} = I_{cg} = .643 \text{ in}^4.$$

On the basis of this assumption, the extreme fiber stresses are computed for the critical stiffener:

$$f_t = +\frac{Mc_1}{I_{na}}$$

$$f_t = \frac{9,935(3.75 - 1.823)}{.643} = 29,774 \text{ psi ult} \quad \text{(tension skin side)}$$

$$f_c = -\frac{Mc_2}{I_{na}}$$

$$f_c = -\frac{9,935(1.823)}{.643} = -28,167 \text{ psi ult} \quad \text{(compression inner flange)}.$$

The final step in the solution of this problem is to compare each calculated stress with its corresponding allowable stress, as given by Table A-2 of Appendix

E for 2024-T3510 aluminum alloy extrusion (QQ-A-200/3). Using the A-basis values in the longitudinal direction and a sheet thickness of .063 of an inch, we find: $F_{tu} = 57$ ksi, $F_{ty} = 42$ ksi, and $F_{cy} = 34$ ksi. Since the computed stresses are well below the tension and compression yield values of the material, our original assumption of elasticity is confirmed. Hence, the following margins of safety are written:

Ultimate tension failure of the outer flange:

$$\text{M.S.} = \frac{F_{tu}}{f_t} - 1 = \frac{57,000}{29,774} - 1 = +0.91 \text{ or } 91\%.$$

Yield compression failure of the inner flange:

$$\text{M.S.} = \frac{F_{cy}}{f_c} - 1 = \frac{34,000}{28,167} - 1 = +0.21 \text{ or } 21\%.$$

This solution has purposely omitted the consideration of the effects of crippling failure of the inner flange of the critical stiffener. Crippling is a condition of buckling whereby a member under compression loading can fail by virtue of its instability at a compression stress level which may be lower than the indicated yield compression value of the material F_{cy}. To avoid the possibility of this type of failure occurring unexpectedly or prematurely, the crippling allowable F_{cc} of a compression member must be investigated, and its value compared to the calculated compression stress f_c. Mathematically, this says that if $F_{cc} < F_{cy}$, the condition of instability is more critical and therefore governs the compression strength criterion of its design. Using Eq. 2-1, the following expression would then be formulated for crippling failure:

$$\text{M.S.} = \frac{F_{cc}}{f_c} - 1.$$

In Chapter 6, this condition will be treated more specifically.

In consideration of possible weight savings for this structure, it might be very cost-effective to evaluate other design alternatives to the solution of this problem. Actually, many different solutions are possible here depending on how efficiently one wishes to optimize the structure. For instance, instead of spacing the stiffeners equally between frame stations, they could be respaced according to some graduated scale. In this way, the shorter stiffeners which carry considerably less load in their present positions would be moved to positions of higher load intensity where a more proportionate distribution of pressure loading would be achieved. Some trial and error must of course be used to relocate each new stiffener position. Ingenuity and patience are the prime ingredients for the complete optimization of this alternative structural arrangement.

2.4 Method of Approximations Approach to the Analysis of Bending Members. The structural designer in the performance of his professional engineering duties is constantly called upon to estimate and approximate solutions to structural engineering designs. Approximation methods of analysis can provide the proficient design engineer with a means of quickly eliminating inefficient or totally unacceptable design concepts, as well as provide a reliable method of appraising those of existing ones. Quick and reliable methods based on approximation techniques of stress analysis are an indispensable part of a design engineer's forte. The competent engineer must learn these simple techniques if he is to become competitive with other highly skilled aerospace engineers in this field.

The material of this section will establish a method of approximation to the analysis of members subjected to bending. Before we start our discussion, however, the engineer is referred to the couple-force relationship of a moment as it applies to a beam section, described mathematically in Appendix B by Eq. A-7 ($P_{\text{couple}} = M/H$). As a brief review of these principles, it was previously shown that the internal bending moment M that exists across a beam section can conveniently be replaced by an equivalent couple-force, P_{couple}, each acting in opposite directions and separated by a distance H between them. From this relationship, not only is the physical action of the beam mentally comprehended but by the use of Eq. 2-2 ($f_n = \pm P/A$), as it applies to each separate cap area, the following equations in terms of tension and compression stresses can be written:

Tension stress:

$$f_t = +\frac{P_{\text{couple}}}{A_{\text{net}}} \tag{2-6}$$

where: $P_{\text{couple}} = M/H$

A_{net} = net cross-sectional area of the tension cap.

Compression stress:

$$f_c = -\frac{P_{\text{couple}}}{A_{\text{gross}}} \tag{2-7}$$

where: $P_{\text{couple}} = M/H$

A_{gross} = total cross-sectional area of the compression cap.

Once the application of these equations has been thoroughly learned, bending stress calculations, normally performed laboriously by using the flexure formula ($f_b = \pm Mc/I_{na}$), can now be alternatively done with rapidity and with a remarkable degree of accuracy. The reason this method is so quick, is that the bending stresses as defined by Eqs. 2-6 and 2-7 are entirely derived independent of moment

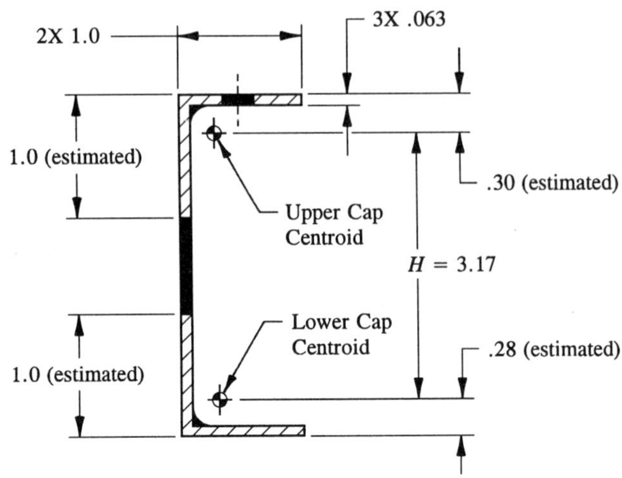

FIGURE 2-13 Distance between the upper and lower cap centroids is estimated for Section B-B.

of inertia calculations. The most time-consuming and boring part of a stress analysis solution of bending members is usually the calculation of this term.

Having applied the flexure formula to the solution of Example 2-1, page 67, let us now compare the results of that solution to the approximation method of this section. First, the distance H between cap centroids is estimated for Section B-B, as pictured in Fig. 2-13. The effective cap areas (shown cross-hatched) are written as follows:

$$A_{\text{upper cap}} = (1.0 + 1.0 - .159 - .063)(.063) = .112 \text{ in}^2$$

$$A_{\text{lower cap}} = (1.0 + 1.0 - .063)(.063) = .122 \text{ in}^2.$$

Since our solution is intended to be approximate in nature, just guess at the distance H between cap centroids of the cross-sectional area. From the sketch, it is apparent that

$$H = 3.75 - .300 - .280 = 3.17 \text{ in}.$$

The moment M is then replaced by an equivalent couple-force between the cap centroids of Section B-B using Eq. A-7 of Appendix B. Thus, in the example considered, this gives:

$$P_{\text{couple}} = \frac{M}{H} = \frac{9,935}{3.17} = 3,134 \text{ lb}.$$

Next, Eqs. 2-6 and 2-7 are applied to each designated cap area.

$$f_t = +\frac{P_{\text{couple}}}{A_{\text{net}}} = \frac{3,134}{.112} = 27,982 \text{ psi} \quad \text{(tension outer flange)}$$

$$f_c = -\frac{P_{\text{couple}}}{A_{\text{gross}}} = -\frac{3,134}{.122} = -25,689 \text{ psi} \quad \text{(compression inner flange)}.$$

The stress results obtained from the approximation method here and the flexure formula (Example 2-1) are summarized below:

Member	Approximation Method (M/H)	Flexure Formula (Mc/I_{na})	% Deviation
Outer Flange	27,982	29,774	6.0
Inner Flange	- 25,689	- 28,167	8.8

It should be clear from the comparison made above that the approximation method is sufficiently accurate to use for investigative stages of structural design. To develop a better feel for the approximation method of analysis presented here, the engineer is encouraged to change the estimated values of the centroid locations slightly of Section B-B, and observe the sensitivity of the resulting bending stresses. In this way, the engineer can develop the confidence to make good estimations in his own preliminary design work.

In the next section, Example 2-2, a method will be devised whereby the internal axial forces that sometimes occur simultaneously with internal bending moments can also be approximated—the axial forces are distributed to each designated cap by a ratio of their individual cap areas to the total area of the section considered. The final results are obtained when these values are superimposed with the bending loads of this section. This gives the combined effects desired. Using the following expression, the magnitude of force of each cap can be found:[1]

$$P_{\text{cap}} = P\left[\frac{A_{\text{cap}}}{A_{\text{total}}}\right] \tag{2-8}$$

where: P = internal axial force (from statics)

A_{cap} = individual cap area

A_{total} = total beam cross-sectional area.

2.5 Axial and Bending Stresses of Beams That Bend in One Plane. In this section, we shall focus our attention on the ideas and concepts of earlier sections and

[1] This equation is derived from axial stiffness considerations.

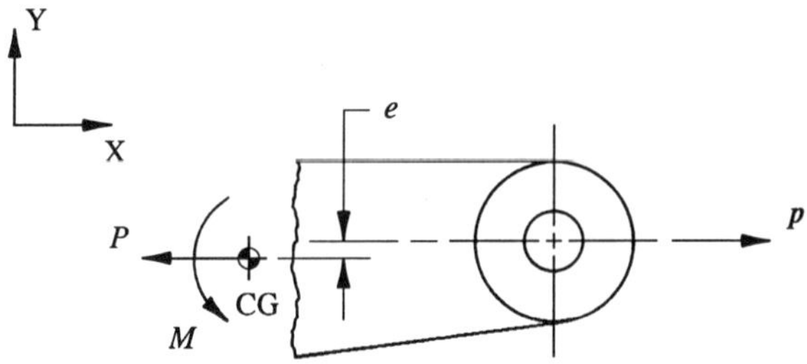

FIGURE 2-14 Internal bending moment is developed across the section area due to an eccentrically applied axial force.

bring together these principles as they relate to axial and bending stresses of stable[1] beams. The limitations imposed in Sec. 2.3 for beams subjected to bending will again be used and restricted to the beams of this section. Among the types of stable beams that will be considered in this section are the following: beams axially loaded in tension and to very short axial members in compression, each of which are simultaneously subjected to bending loads. The resulting stress system can be combined using the principles of superposition so long as the structure to which these stresses are applied behaves elastically (for a brief review of these principles, see Sec. 1.7, "Principle of Superposition").

For illustrative purposes, when an externally applied axial force does not act through the centroidal axis of the cross-sectional area of a beam, as shown in Fig. 2-14, the eccentricity of force e will cause a bending stress distribution by virtue of the internal bending moment M which is developed across the section area. As a good design practice, to limit the increase in overall structural weight of a final design, all member eccentricities should be avoided or at least minimized, and a deliberate and careful consideration made to eliminate their occurrences. To find the internal forces at this section, an imaginary section cut is made through the member and the equations of statics applied by the usual methods of internal loads analysis.

$$\Sigma F_x = 0, \qquad P = p$$

$$\Sigma M_{cg} = 0, \qquad (+\!\!\curvearrowleft) \quad pe - M = 0, \quad M = pe.$$

Physically, to produce the actual stresses on the cross-sectional area, the internal force P must be represented at the centroid of the cross-sectional area of the member, while the bending moment M establishes its stress distribution with respect to the neutral axis of the section area. Then, the appropriate stress formulas

[1] That is, where the stability and buckling characteristics of such beams, terms often used synonymously with members loaded in compression, are not primary design considerations in the overall evaluation of their designs. A comprehensive and thorough treatment of these specific topics will be better served when our study of columns (see Chapter 7, "Column Members") is fully treated.

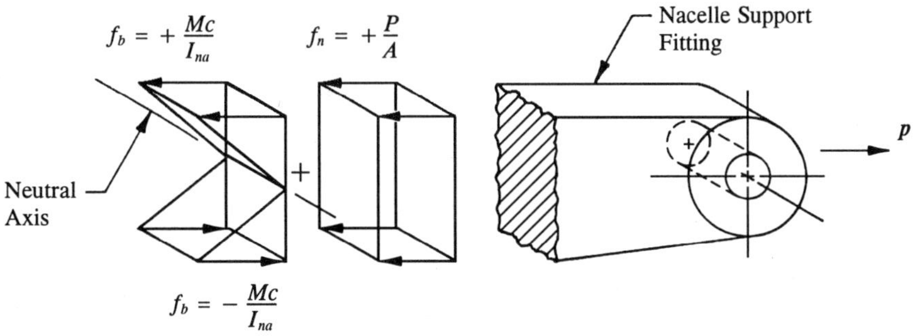

FIGURE 2-15 Axial and bending stresses produce similar stresses normal to the plane of the section area.

are each applied separately to determine the internal stresses which are caused by these internal forces, as shown in Fig. 2-15.

Since the axial and bending stresses each produce stresses of the same particular kind, normal to the exposed section, the principle of superposition as it applies to elastic structures is valid. The equivalent stress distributions are combined and are indicated in Fig. 2-16. Mathematically, the axial and bending stresses, as defined by Eqs. 2-2 and 2-5, respectively, are combined into one representative equation of stress. Namely,

$$f = \pm\frac{P}{A} \pm \frac{Mc}{I_{na}}. \tag{2-9}$$

Whenever making this or any other stress calculations, be sure to carefully review a stress-strain diagram to make sure the values calculated are associated with the elastic region of the material being used (see Appendix E, Fig. A-14, page 651, for a typical stress-strain diagram).

If the existence of shear at a section produces stresses simultaneously with other known stresses (axial or bending stresses), the shearing stresses that occur are

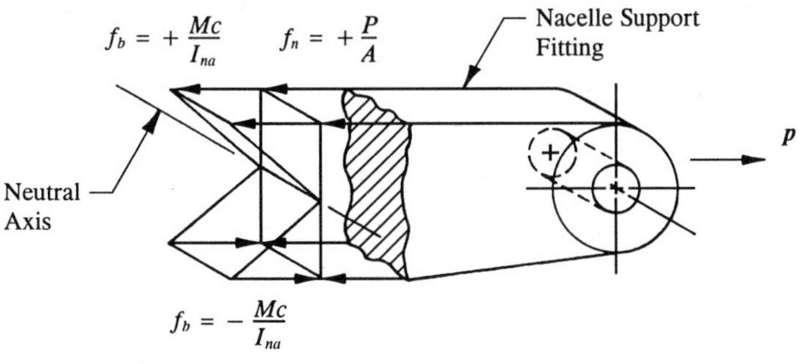

FIGURE 2-16 Axial and bending stresses combined into an equivalent stress distribution.

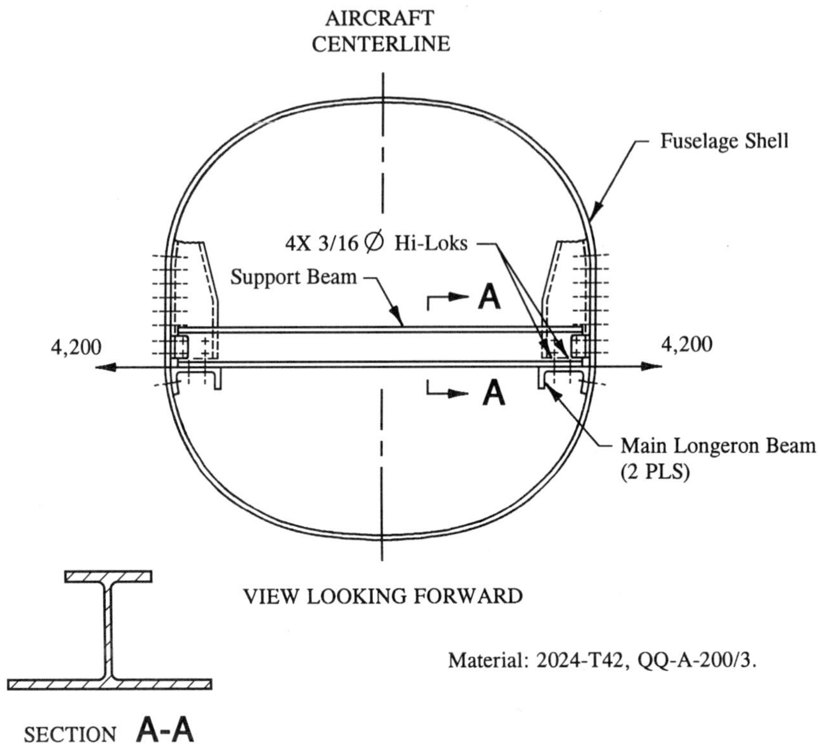

FIGURE 2-17 Support beam spanning the fuselage shell.

of such a kind that they can not be directly combined with these other known stresses. For members subjected to bending, the shearing stresses developed present no real complications: since maximum internal bending stresses will occur at points of zero internal shearing stresses across a section area. But axial stresses do occur at points of maximum internal shearing stresses at the neutral axis, and if proper selection of a member is to be made, their combined effects must be considered.[1] The generalization of these concepts will be made clearer by the methods of Chapter 4, when a more detailed study of the nature of shearing stresses can more specifically be treated.

Example 2-2 Instead of redesigning the main longeron beams of an increased-gross-weight model aircraft, it was proposed to provide an additional support for these members by spanning a support beam completely across the fuselage shell, as shown in Fig. 2-17. The additional support will have the desired effect of decreasing the peak internal loads for the longerons. (a) If the support beam reacts

[1] The "interaction equation method" is used to design structures for stability and strength requirements under combined loading conditions.

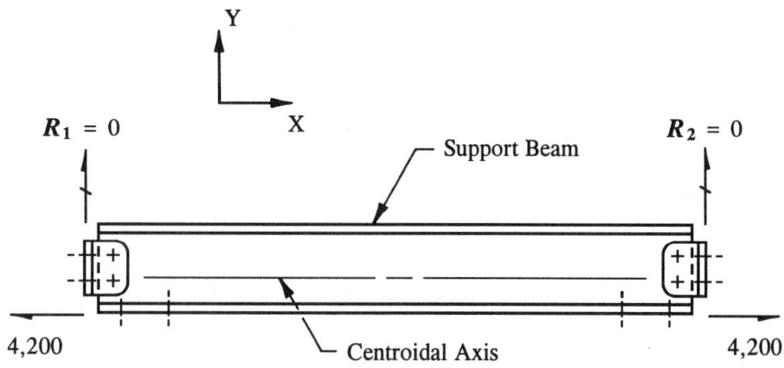

FIGURE 2-18 Support beam is isolated from the fuselage shell and free-bodied.

4,200 lb ultimate load through its lower flanges, what maximum extreme fiber stresses will occur for this member? (b) Write the margins of safety in compression and tension.

SOLUTION: Since the applied loads do not lie in the same plane with the centroidal axis of the beam, it should be clear that this effect will produce an eccentricity of load e which in turn will induce a constant internal bending moment $M = 4,200(e)$ along the entire length of the support beam. Once the eccentricity is found, the magnitude of this moment can be computed. To determine these unknown quantities, the usual methods of analysis are employed: the support beam is completely isolated from the fuselage shell and the corresponding structure free-bodied. This is shown in Fig. 2-18.

Inasmuch as there are no applied forces acting vertically, the support reactions R_1 and R_2 are not necessarily required to maintain vertical equilibrium of the structure. Consequently, their values equal zero. This condition should not be misconstrued as an indication that the shear clips of the support beam serve no real purpose, and therefore, as a potential weight savings, should be removed from the structure. Although this notion might at first seem to be a reasonable one to make, the engineer must also consider other loading conditions that may exist for an aircraft which might necessarily obviate this misconception. The point is that an

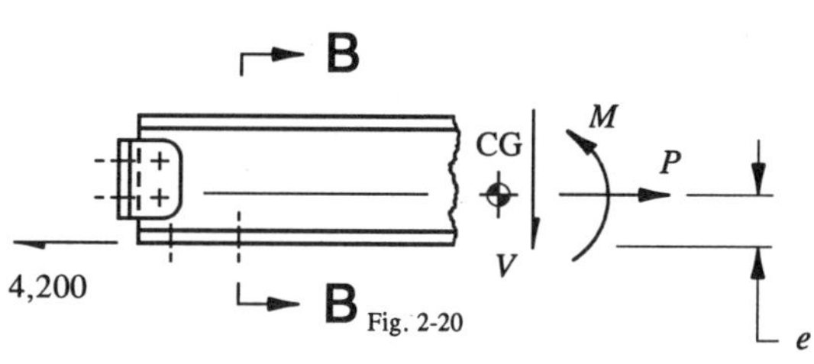

FIGURE 2-19 Internal loads represented on an exposed section of beam.

aircraft undergoes many different loading conditions, and to design all components of the structure effectively from these conditions requires that all parameters of design be fully considered. This includes all flight and landing conditions that an aircraft generally encounters. The engineer is referred to Chapter 5 for a complete study and design of support shear clips.

Next, the magnitude of the internal loads are investigated at arbitrary points along the entire length of the support beam, see Fig. 2-19 for the representation of these loads on an exposed section of beam. If we apply the method of sections approach to internal loads analysis at this section, we obtain the following values for *V, P,* and *M:*

$$\Sigma F_y = 0, \qquad V = 0$$

$$\Sigma F_x = 0, \qquad P - 4,200 = 0, \quad P = 4,200 \text{ lb ult}$$

$$\Sigma M_{cg} = 0, \qquad \circlearrowleft + \quad 4,200(e) - M = 0, \quad M = 4,200(e) \text{ in-lb ult.}$$

From these equations, it can be seen that the internal loads *P* and *M* are constant anywhere between the supported ends of the beam, but not specifically including the joints themselves. A complete and practical approach to the analyses of joint and connection designs will be deferred until Chapter 3. For the reasons described in Sec. 2.2, fastener holes are considered open (or ineffective in resisting tension) in a tension-loaded joint. On this basis, the support beam is critical at Section B-B, where the axial tension and bending loads across the net area of the support beam will produce the highest combination of stress intensity. Using the structural methods of analysis of Appendix F, the following section properties are computed for the unshaded areas of Section B-B, Fig. 2-20.

MOMENT OF INERTIA

Element	b	h	y	A	Ay	Ay^2	I_o
1	2.300	0.080	0.040	0.184	0.007	0.000	0.000
2	0.080	1.200	0.680	0.096	0.065	0.044	0.012
3	0.190*	0.080	0.040	- 0.015	- 0.001	- 0.000	- 0.000
4	0.190*	0.080	0.040	- 0.015	- 0.001	- 0.000	- 0.000
5	0.500	0.080	1.320	0.040	0.053	0.070	0.000
			Total	0.290	0.123	0.114	0.012

* The nominal pin or shank diameter is normally used for bolts in a tension joint (see specific values given in Table 8.1.5.2(n) of MIL-HDBK-5F for this fastener).

$$Y_{cg} = \frac{\Sigma Ay}{\Sigma A} = \frac{.123}{.290} = .424 \text{ in}$$

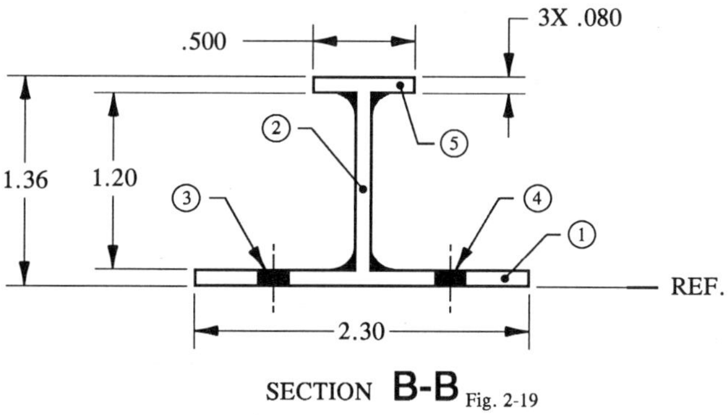

FIGURE 2-20 Support beam cross-sectional area. Neglect the fillet areas of the extruded I-beam.

$$I_{cg} = \Sigma I_o + \Sigma Ay^2 - Y_{cg}(\Sigma Ay) = .012 + .114 - .424(.123) = .074 \text{ in}^4.$$

The eccentricity of force e corresponds to the value Y_{cg} above, or

$$e = Y_{cg} = .424 \text{ in}$$

and, from $M = 4,200(e)$, we now obtain:

$$M = 4,200(.424) = 1,781 \text{ in-lb ult}.$$

And if we assume that calculated stresses from Eq. 2-9 will be elastic, this presumption further implies the following:

$$Y_{na} = Y_{cg}$$

and

$$I_{na} = I_{cg}.$$

Thus, the elastic stresses at the extreme fibers caused by the combination of axial force P and bending moment M are determined:

Ultimate tension stress of the lower flange:

$$f_t = \pm\frac{P}{A} \pm \frac{Mc}{I_{na}}$$

$$f_t = +\frac{4,200}{.290} + \frac{1,781(.424)}{.074} = 14,483 + 10,205 = +24,688 \text{ psi}.$$

Ultimate compression stress of the upper flange:

$$f_c = \pm \frac{P}{A} \pm \frac{Mc}{I_{na}}$$

$$f_c = +\frac{4,200}{.290} - \frac{1,781(1.36 - .424)}{.074} = 14,483 - 22,527 = -8,044 \text{ psi}.$$

The mechanical properties of 2024-T42 aluminum alloy extrusion (QQ-A-200/3) in the longitudinal direction are as follows: $F_{tu} = 57$ ksi, $F_{ty} = 38$ ksi, and $F_{cy} = 38$ ksi (see mechanical-property table for this material in MIL-HDBK-5F). If we compare these allowable values with those stresses calculated, clearly, we find that tension and compression stresses are well below yield allowable values. And this necessary condition therefore confirms or validates our original assumption of elastic stress behavior of the support beam. The margins of safety are then computed as follows:

Ultimate tension failure of the lower flange:

$$\text{M.S.} = \frac{F_{tu}}{f_t} - 1 = \frac{57,000}{24,688} - 1 = +1.31 \text{ or } 131\%.$$

Yield compression failure of the upper flange:

$$\text{M.S.} = \frac{F_{cy}}{f_c} - 1 = \frac{38,000}{8,044} - 1 = +\text{HIGH!!}$$

As is quite often done by practicing engineers, let us now focus our attention on how to verify this solution using an alternative method of analysis. Preferably, let this method be approximate in nature which will produce results which are quick, reasonably consistent and, hopefully, reliable with its corresponding detailed solution. Essentially, whenever bending is present in an axially loaded member, an approximate solution to the problem is accomplished by superimposing axial and equivalent bending loads directly. When combining these loads, care must also be taken to superimpose their correct physical effects on the structure, such as compression or tension, which these loads may produce.

The procedure for replacing a bending moment with an equivalent couple-force was explained earlier in Sec. 2.4. Again, as we did before, the distance between cap centroids is first approximated at Section B-B. This is shown in Fig. 2-21 where the effective cap areas for this section are shown cross-hatched. From the estimated values chosen in this figure,

$$H = 1.36 - .070 - .060 = 1.23 \text{ in}.$$

The upper and lower cap areas are written as follows:

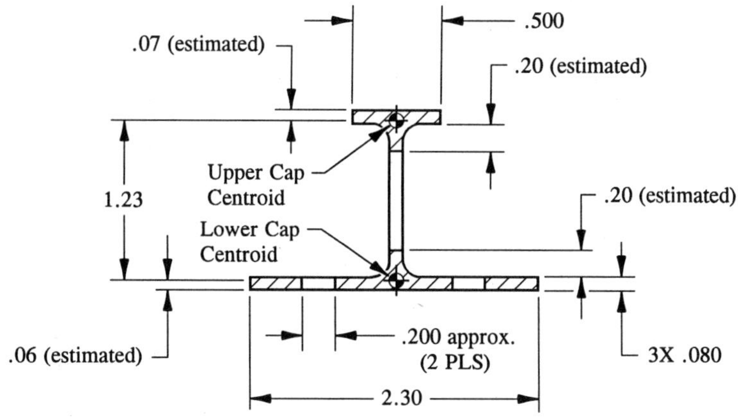

FIGURE 2-21 Effective cap areas shown cross-hatched for the beam section.

$$A_{\text{upper}} = (.500)(.080) + (.20)(.080) = .056 \text{ in}^2$$

$$A_{\text{lower}} = (2.30 - .200 - .200)(.080) + (.20)(.080) = .168 \text{ in}^2.$$

The total cross-sectional area of the support beam is

$$A_{\text{total}} = (.500 + 1.20 + 2.30 - .200 - .200)(.080) = .288 \text{ in}^2.$$

Now, using Eq. A-7 of Appendix B, the equivalent couple-force is computed:

$$P_{\text{couple}} = \frac{M}{H} = \frac{1,781}{1.23} = 1,448 \text{ lb ult}.$$

The physical action of this loading on the cross-sectional area is to produce compression on the upper cap and tension on the lower cap.

If we now consider the internal axial load P (from page 80) proportionately distributed between the upper and lower cap areas, the following axial cap loads are determined (see Eq. 2-8, page 75):

Axial load of the upper cap:

$$P_{\text{cap}} = P\left[\frac{A_{\text{cap}}}{A_{\text{total}}}\right] = P\left[\frac{A_{\text{upper}}}{A_{\text{total}}}\right]$$

$$P_{\text{cap}} = 4,200\left[\frac{.056}{.288}\right] = 817 \text{ lb ult} \quad \text{(tension)}.$$

Axial load of the lower cap:

$$P_{cap} = P\left[\frac{A_{cap}}{A_{total}}\right] = P\left[\frac{A_{lower}}{A_{total}}\right]$$

$$P_{cap} = 4,200\left[\frac{.168}{.288}\right] = 2,450 \text{ lb ult} \quad \text{(tension)}.$$

The axial loads of the upper and lower caps are now combined with the corresponding couple-force. That is,

$$P_{upper} = P_{couple} + P_{cap} = -\,1,448 + 817 = -\,631 \text{ lb ult} \quad \text{(compression)}$$

$$P_{lower} = P_{couple} + P_{cap} = +\,1,448 + 2,450 = 3,898 \text{ lb ult} \quad \text{(tension)}.$$

From Eq. 2-2 ($f_n = \pm P/A$), as it applies to each effective cap area, the following uniform cap stresses are obtained:

$$f_c = -\frac{P_{upper}}{A_{gross}} = -\frac{631}{.056} = -\,11,268 \text{ psi ult} \quad \text{(compression)}$$

$$f_t = +\frac{P_{lower}}{A_{net}} = \frac{3,898}{.168} = 23,202 \text{ psi ult} \quad \text{(tension)}.$$

These stresses compare very well with those values previously calculated. Approximation methods of analysis are the most important first steps necessary for a design engineer to master in his search for alternative forms of good designs. The engineer is encouraged to memorize this and any other similar techniques of analysis which can afford such considerable time-savings.

Example 2-3 The internal loads acting at designated node points around the fuselage frame structure of Fig. 2-22 were obtained from a finite-element computer model analysis[1] of that structure. After a careful review of all flight and landing conditions around this frame, the following locations were found to have critical loading combinations:

Critical Node Points	*P* (lb)	*V** (lb)	*M* (in-lb)
32	8,000	2,000	10,000
29	- 9,500	1,000	- 11,000
25	- 4,500	4,000	- 3,700

* The shearing force *V* developed around this frame will be treated by the methods and techniques of analysis in Chapter 4, "Shearing Stresses."

[1] The following books are recommended for additional information: (1) Harold C. Martin and Graham F. Carey, *Introduction to Finite-Element Analysis,* McGraw-Hill, New York, 1973 and (2) O.C. Ziendiewicz, *The Finite-Element Method,* 3d ed., McGraw-Hill, New York, 1977.

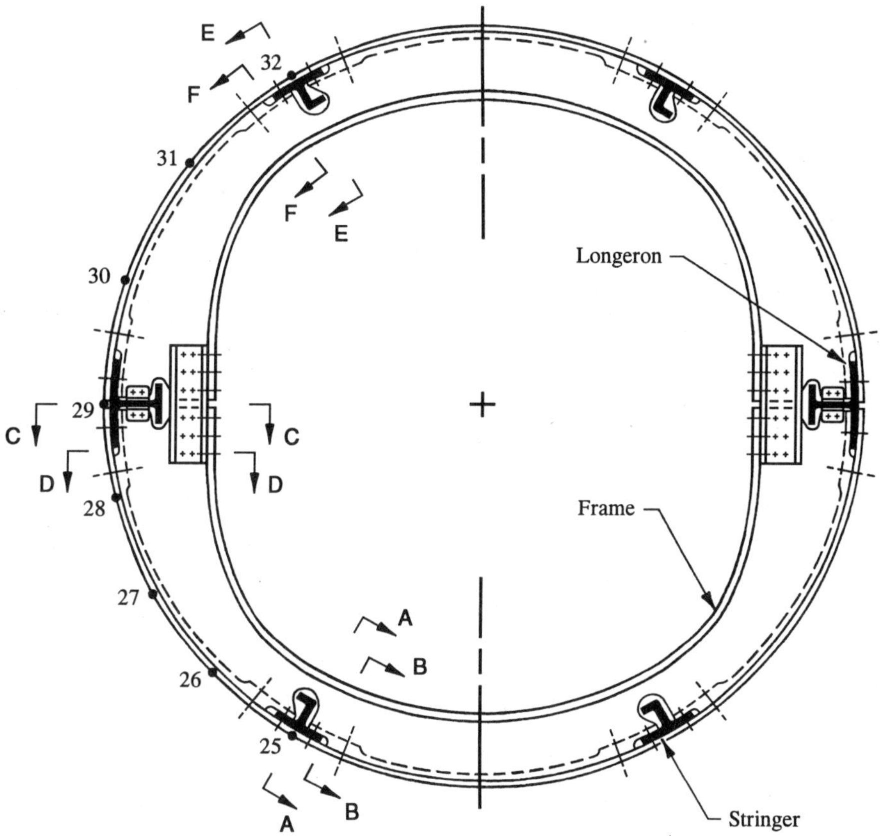

FIGURE 2-22 Designated node points around a fuselage frame structure.

Critical loads are those combinations of axial and bending internal loads that will produce the highest levels of compression and tension stresses across a section area. Calculate the combined axial and bending stresses at these locations using the computer internal loads given.

General Discussion of Fuselage Frame Design: Before the solution to this example problem is fully developed in detail, several comments and general observations essential to fuselage frame design will be made. The fuselage is most simply described in terms of two simple beams which are cantilevered off both sides of its wing box assembly structure. Composed of skin, stringers, and longerons, fuselage frames vary in size from very light to a much heavier construction depending on whether the structure must absorb or transmit large concentrated loads. In aircraft design, frames are primarily used to support or reinforce the shell of the fuselage while simultaneously supporting or distributing many different types of flight and landing conditions under load. Among the most important of these load types are

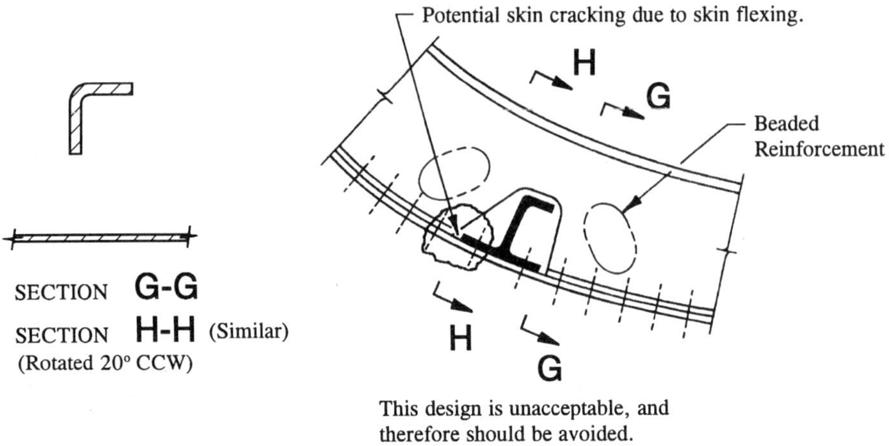

FIGURE 2-23 Stringer cutout in a fuselage frame depicting weakened cross-sectional area across the cutout region.

the following: (1) surface airloads, (2) landing gear reactions, (3) wing pivot reactions, and (4) floor beam reactions. Fuselage frames are designed to resist these loads while still maintaining the general design shape or configuration of the fuselage shell.

Longerons and stringers are riveted to the fuselage outer shell (or skin) longitudinally to meet general aviation strength and bending stiffness requirements of the fuselage. It is customary to allow these longitudinal members to pass directly through the fuselage frame structure. To accomplish this, the basic frame structure is cut out, and the outer flanges of the stringers and longerons passing through these cutouts are attached to the outer flanges of the frame. This will insure continuity of the structure and thus provide a continuous load path necessary to carry the internal frame loads across the cutout region. A similar analogy can be made at Section C-C, Fig. 2-22, where a splice channel is used to insure a continuous load path for the inner cap of the frame structure at this location.

Hypothetically, let us say, if a fuselage frame is cut out, but is not joggled and fastened over the outer flanges of its stringers or longerons, such a joint arrangement can be seen in Fig. 2-23, the weaker cross-sectional area as shown across the frame structure at G-G and H-H will severely weight penalize the frame design—an obvious impractical and unacceptable design choice to make. Bear in mind that the initial load that was carried by the frame cap before it was cut away, in effect, must now theoretically transfer through the skin. The additional increase in load by the skin, particularly in compression, will severely buckle the skin at low stress levels. This situation is undesirable and should be avoided if potential weight reduction and cost-savings of any consequence are to be realized for the structure.

An important consideration many times overlooked in frame design is the influence that curvature has on the internal stress distribution of the structure. In principle, if the radius of a fuselage frame is relatively small, the neutral axis will be pulled significantly toward the center of the fuselage by the higher stresses which are developed on the inner cap of the frame structure. To account for this increase in stress, a curved beam analysis is typically done. The theory and relative importance of curvature as it relates to frame or beam design can be found in most strength of material textbooks on this subject.[1] From a design standpoint, suffice it to say that the curvature and the relative size of most frames of conventional aircraft fuselages of commercial or military types are such as to cause a negligible effect on the final system of stresses. Therefore, this condition is usually ignored in their design.

The many discontinuities that exist when cutouts, shear-ties, and splice members are used further complicate frame design. For all practical purposes, however, these particular design areas are considered as local aberrations whose distinctive physical loading effects on the main frame structure are quickly dissipated. This means that each fuselage frame can be idealized with externally applied loads without specific regards to the local effects of the discontinuities on the loaded structure. Of course, once the internal frame loads have been obtained, each particular discontinuity must be individually treated and investigated for stiffness and structural strength.

In most practical frame designs, calculated frame stresses are sufficiently low to satisfy the condition of elastic stress design (see Appendix E, Fig. A-14, for the elastic range of a stress-strain curve of a material). The reason that this is so, is that in most applications of frame design, other design criteria are imposed on the skin to limit operating stress levels. For instance, the skin is prevented from reaching inelastic stress levels when the basic frame cap is designed to its compression crippling allowable F_{cc} (see Chapter 6, "Crippling of Compression Members"), or when the frame cap is designed to a value not to exceed the inter-rivet buckling stress allowable F_{ir} (see Sec. 6.2 of Chapter 6, "Inter-Rivet Buckling of Compression Members"). The effect of inter-rivet buckling can dramatically change the panel edge-restraint conditions that are used to design skin panels—causing the panels to buckle at stress levels which are unacceptably low. Inter-rivet buckling is not considered a failure of the skin but rather a structural design limitation; the skin can only maintain the compression load which created its buckled state. A better design is achieved when this condition is prevented from occurring at operating stress levels.

SOLUTION: In most cases, the internal loads acting around a fuselage frame are given at different sections along the centroidal axis of area of the frame. If this is true, then the analysis is rather simple, Eq. 2-9 is applied at these sections for the combined effects of axial and bending loads. Further, to simplify the entire analysis process, only the most critical sections of the frame structure will require

[1] One such source is the book *Formulas for Stress and Strain* by Raymond J. Roark (see Table VII, "Formulas for Curved Beams").

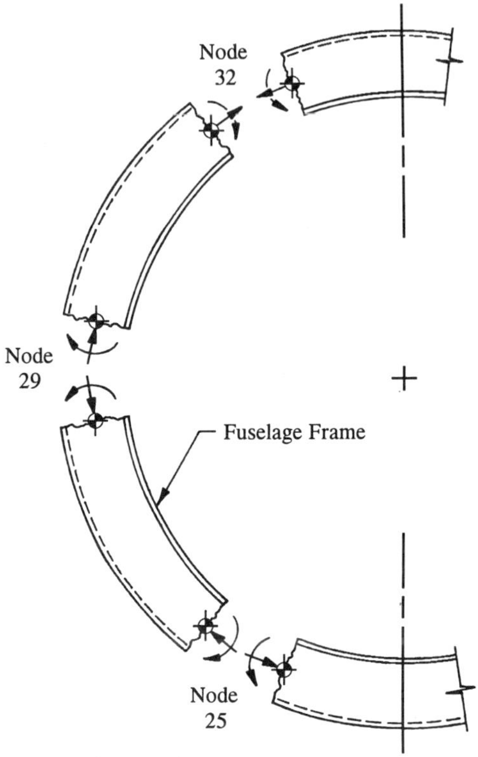

FIGURE 2-24 Orientation of internal loads on a fuselage frame structure.

investigation. Specifically, if sections of maximum stress are shown to be of adequate structural strength, then all other areas of lower stress intensity will consequently be substantiated. There is no need to spend extra engineering time analyzing areas that can easily be verified by other simpler methods of analysis. To avoid repetitious calculations, the process of elimination can serve as a most reliable expedient to fundamental frame design verification. In some cases, when areas of maximum stress are too difficult to locate by simple visual inspection, it is suggested that the engineer construct axial, shear, and bending moment diagrams in a circular fashion around the fuselage frame structure. It is the highly skilled, competent aerospace engineer who can effectively economize his time and still safeguard the structural reliability and integrity of his structural designs.

Before attempting to use computer program loads in any technical analysis, two basic questions must be answered: (1) What sign convention is specified for the internal loads? (2) Where along the structural model are the internal loads actually idealized? To answer the first question, simply review the following sign conventions adopted and then select one system as a basis for internal loads interpretation:

(1) P is a compression load if its value is positive (negative).

(2) P is a tension load if its value is negative (positive).

(3) M produces compression on the skin side and tension on the inner frame cap side if its value is positive (negative).

(4) M produces tension on the skin side and compression on the inner frame cap side if its value is negative (positive).

Remember, a computer can only indicate either a positive or a negative value for its internal loads output. It is the user who must be able to properly orient these loads in accordance with their true physical effect on the structure. Inasmuch as no two program solutions are ever exactly alike, one must always establish the appropriate sign convention for the load output before attempting a stress analysis solution. For the purposes of illustration, let us define the internal loads of our particular example by the sign convention specified in parentheses above. The correct orientation of these loads on the actual frame structure are shown in the schematic of Fig. 2-24.

Simply stated, the answer to the second question is: A computer-generated solution should represent its internal loads at the centroidal axis of its structural model.[1] From this, the appropriate stress formulas can be applied and used to physically represent the true structural behavior of the actual structure under load. Otherwise, the loads designated at points other than at the centroid must be transferred there in order to correctly duplicate the true loading effects of the structure. The engineer is referred to Example 3-4, page 204, for a complete discussion of this subject. To simplify the analysis of our example problem, let us assume for now that the loads given here do in fact act at the centroid of each frame section. In so doing, these loads can then be substituted directly into Eq. 2.5.

A complete and thorough analysis of combined axial and bending stresses at the frame cutouts must also include separate analysis checks of those sections nearest to either side of the stringer cutouts but far enough away from the local aberrations of the joint. The engineer should now study the frame sections making up the effective cross-sectional areas of Fig. 2-25. Refer to Table 2-2 for the section properties of these frame sections. Notice, in particular, which members of each section have been chosen as effective in carrying loads. Also, note that to either side of the fuselage frame, the skin, doublers, and outer flanges of the stringers and longerons extend indefinitely. In Chapter 6, a method of analysis will be devised whereby the structural effectivity of a member as a flat sheet under compression loading for indefinite (continuous) members will be determined. In theory, even a sheet of paper can effectively resist tension loads when pulled; but that same sheet in compression, if pushed, buckles under very light loading. Until this numerical value is calculated for indefinite members, just accept the premise that some limitation must be imposed on the amount of effective material that can be used with each cross-sectional area.

---

[1] In most cases, however, this is usually a matter of convenience or personal preference dictated by engineers of the initiating group.

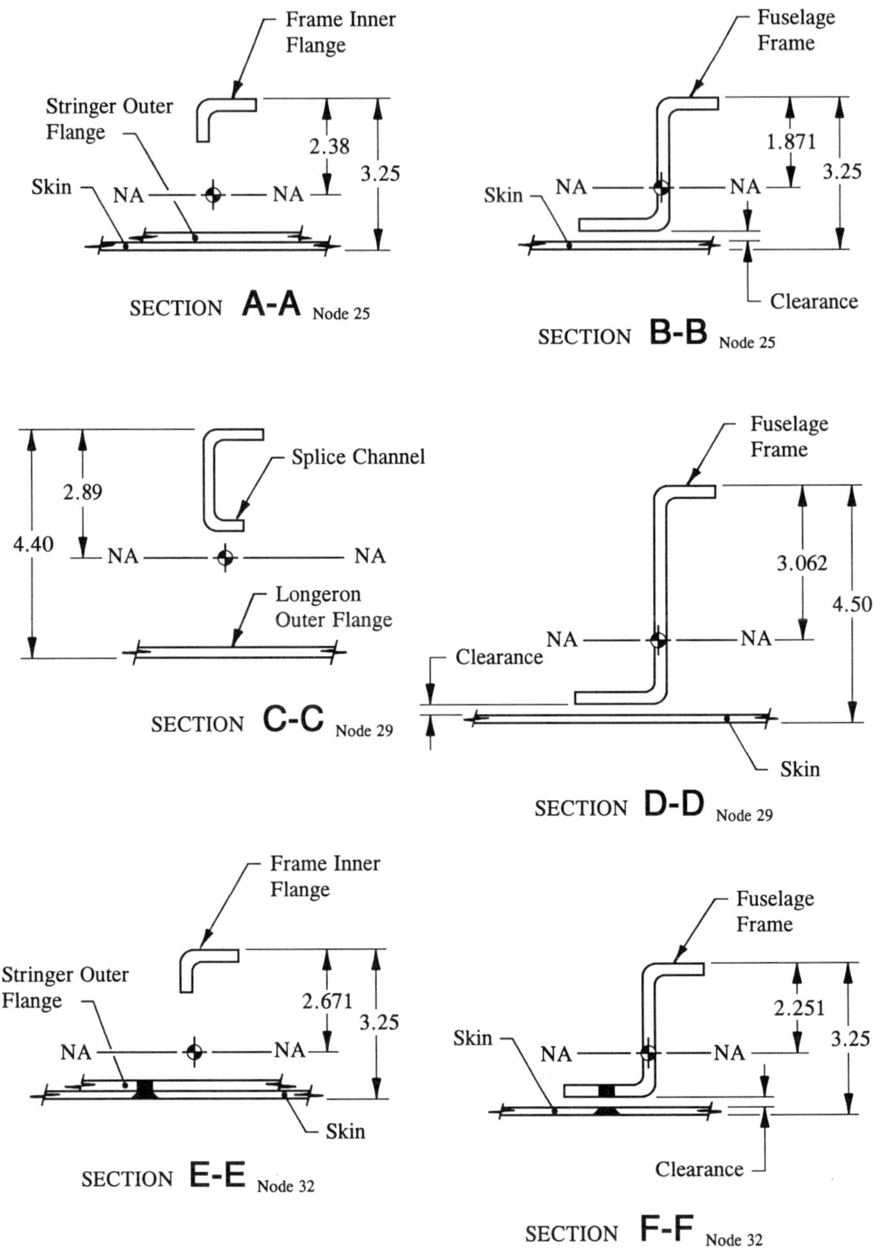

FIGURE 2-25 Fuselage frame effective cross-sectional areas.

TABLE 2-2 SECTION PROPERTIES

Section	Area* A, in^2	Moment of Inertia I_{na}, in^4
A-A	.529	.830
B-B	.388	.601
C-C	.863	2.575
D-D	.650	1.740
E-E	.829	.955
F-F	.538	.795

* Areas include effective width of skin.

The easiest way to visualize the load effectivity of members across discontinuities of a frame cutout is to imagine an axial load being carried around the frame through each joint. Those members that can transfer part of the imaginary axial load across the joint by the most direct load paths are considered effective; while those members that require special or ingenious manipulations or considerations of their load directions are not. The justification for this concept is founded on the general principle that axial and bending stresses are typically of the normal loading type anyway. And, as such, their combined stress distributions can be represented by an equivalent system of axial forces. It will be shown in Sec. 2.6, "Member Forces," how the stress distributions across the section area of a beam can be replaced by equivalent internal axial forces.

The internal loads at Node 32 produce combined tension and bending stresses on the skin side of Sections E-E and F-F, and in accordance with previous discussions of hole-filling fasteners in a tension stress field (Sec. 2.2), their shaded areas are considered ineffective (refer again to Fig. 2-25). Pay particular attention to the skin and stringer outer flange which extend indefinitely to either side of the frame at those sections. It is the judgment of the engineer who will establish the most realistic design cutoffs for these members in tension. However, do not extend these members beyond what can be reasonably expected to occur in the local proximity of the actual structural design. The analyst must take into account the influence of adjacent structures which may also consider these indefinite members as effective components for their designs. In simple words, do not use indefinite members in two separate analyses unless their effects on the structure can be successfully mediated.

With all values of internal loads properly described and all section properties clearly defined and calculated, the axial and bending stresses across each particular section area are computed. Their combined stress distributions are obtained from Eq. 2-9, and the results of those solutions conveniently itemized as follows:

$$f = \pm \frac{P}{A} \pm \frac{Mc}{I_{na}}$$ (see page 77 for definition of terms).

SECTION A-A (Node 25)

Inner Flange:

$$f_t = -\frac{4,500}{.529} + \frac{3,700(2.38)}{.830} = 2,103 \text{ psi.}$$

Skin:

$$f_c = -\frac{4,500}{.529} - \frac{3,700(3.25 - 2.38)}{.830} = -12,385 \text{ psi.}$$

SECTION B-B (Node 25)

Inner Flange:

$$f_c = -\frac{4,500}{.388} + \frac{3,700(1.871)}{.601} = -79 \text{ psi.}$$

Skin:

$$f_c = -\frac{4,500}{.388} - \frac{3,700(3.25 - 1.871)}{.601} = -20,088 \text{ psi.}$$

SECTION C-C (Node 29)

Inner Flange:

$$f_t = -\frac{9,500}{.863} + \frac{11,000(2.89)}{2.575} = 1,338 \text{ psi.}$$

Skin:

$$f_c = -\frac{9,500}{.863} - \frac{11,000(4.40 - 2.89)}{2.575} = -17,458 \text{ psi.}$$

SECTION E-E (Node 32)

Inner Flange:

$$f_c = +\frac{8,000}{.829} - \frac{10,000(2.671)}{.955} = -18,318 \text{ psi.}$$

Skin:

$$f_t = +\frac{8,000}{.829} + \frac{10,000(3.25 - 2.671)}{.955} = 15,713 \text{ psi.}$$

SECTION F-F (Node 32)

Inner Flange:

$$f_c = +\frac{8,000}{.538} - \frac{10,000(2.251)}{.795} = -13,445 \text{ psi.}$$

Skin:

$$f_t = +\frac{8,000}{.538} + \frac{10,000(3.25 - 2.251)}{.795} = 27,436 \text{ psi.}$$

SECTION D-D (Node 29)

Inner Flange:

$$f_t = -\frac{9,500}{.650} + \frac{11,000(3.062)}{1.740} = 4,742 \text{ psi.}$$

Skin:

$$f_c = -\frac{9,500}{.650} - \frac{11,000(4.50 - 3.062)}{1.740} = -23,706 \text{ psi.}$$

A final note: The aerodynamic forces on a fuselage can cause longitudinal (fore-and-aft) stresses to develop in its stringers and main longeron members. Therefore, where applicable, particularly at frame cutouts, these stresses must interact, combine with the circumferential frame stresses obtained here in this solution. The method of combining these stresses together, sometimes called the "interaction equation method," is however postponed for future presentation and study until a better, more detailed understanding of stress theory in general (concepts in this chapter) has been learned.[1]

In retrospect, it is hoped that the discussions presented thus far have not been too confusing nor too difficult to understand. Each particular aspect of this solution that was not explained in detail will be more appropriately described in other chapters. After these chapters have been carefully read, the engineer is encouraged to reread this example so that a clear and intelligible understanding of its design peculiarities can better be appreciated. The numerical solution to this example problem is very simple, it is the simplification and theoretical considerations which require diligent observation if confidence and a high degree of reliability of its solutions are to be achieved.

2.6 Member Forces. It is the subject of this section to evaluate the member forces that are carried by the element areas[2] that make up the cross-sectional area of a beam. And then, by a logical and rational approach to splice-joint analysis, determine the shearing forces that must pass through the fasteners of a typical stringer cutout. To perform the actual stress analysis solution, both axial and bending stress distributions that are normally present across an exposed cross-sectional area of a beam are replaced by equivalent member forces designated at specific element areas. Mathematically, this is accomplished by multiplying the average stress level of an element by its corresponding element area, or

---

[1] Interaction equations are used to design structures for stability and strength requirements under combined loading conditions. The engineer is referred specifically to Example 5-6 for a brief introduction to this method of analysis.

[2] Here, element area refers to the term used in moment of inertia calculations (see Appendix F).

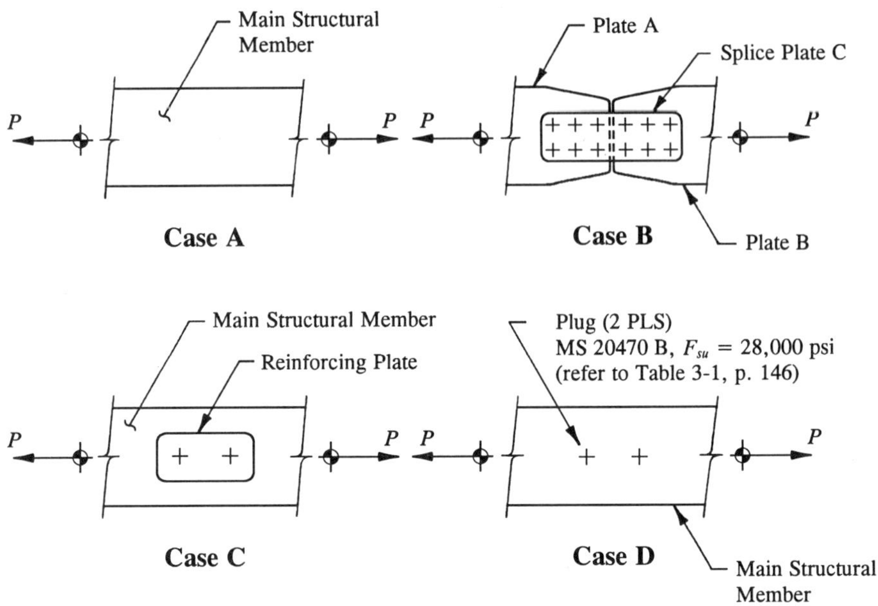

FIGURE 2-26 Diagrams are used to show concepts and theory of load transfers through various joints.

$$P = fA \tag{2-10}$$

where: f = average stress level of an element area (if present, include both axial and bending stresses)

A = element area.

This equation is by definition a derivative of the basic equation for normal or axial stresses ($f_n = \pm P/A$). The following sign convention for stresses will be adopted in this section: a + sign is used when the stress is tension (or pulling), and a − sign when the stress is compression (or pushing). Before Eq. 2-10 is applied to a specific engineering problem, a brief discussion pertaining to concepts and fundamentals of splice-joint analysis will be illustrated.

Consider the plates diagrammed in Fig. 2-26. If the plate member of Case A is cut into two parts, some type of splicing member would be needed to transfer the force P from one plate to the other. This is accomplished as shown in Case B, where the transfer of force from plate A to plate B is achieved through each group of fasteners of splice plate C. Or, to say it another way, the load P that the plates carried before they were cut must now be transferred by each group of fasteners of plates A and B across the discontinuity through splice plate C.

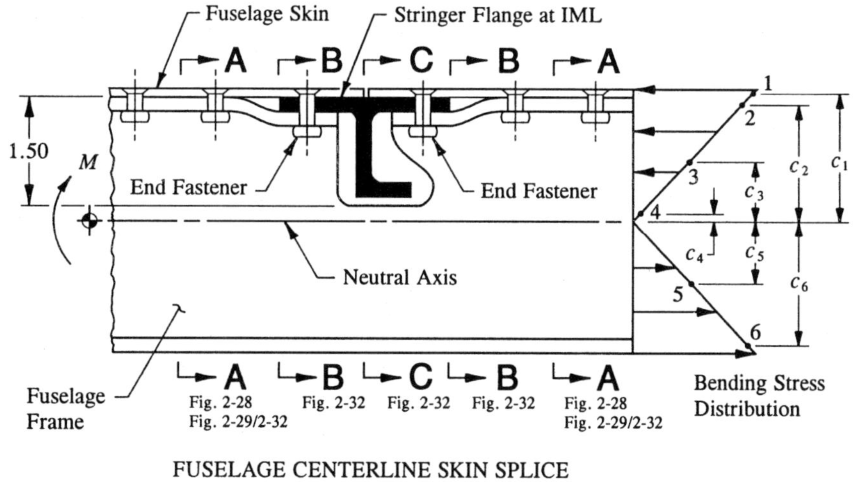

LOADS: $M = 3{,}000$ in-lb (compression skin side)
$P = 0$
$V = 0$.
MATERIAL: Aluminum 2024-T3 Clad
2024 Aluminum Alloy (Extrusion).

FIGURE 2-27 Stringer cutout in pure bending.

If, however, a reinforcing plate is riveted to a continuous structural member, as shown in Case C, the transfer of load through the reinforcing plate would then be entirely dependent upon the strains (or stretching) of the main structural member. For example, if the main structure was strained very little, the transfer of force would be small. Practically speaking, no transfer of force would occur through this member or its fasteners. But, if that same plate was strained much more, the transfer of force would be larger. In either case, the reinforcing plate would be considered as a local aberration and its effectivity as a primary load-carrying member conservatively neglected. The main structural member is said to be of sufficient strength by itself to efficiently sustain the load *P*.

In Case D, no transfer of force would take place; the rivets would however weaken the structural member across the net area through the holes (see Eq. 2-3, page 61, $f_t = +P/A_{\text{net}}$). The two main points of this discussion are summarized below:

(1) Continuous members across a splice-joint provide a continuous load path to sustain their internal forces across the joint.

(2) Discontinuous members across a splice-joint must transfer their internal forces through other structural members that can provide a continuous load path across the joint.

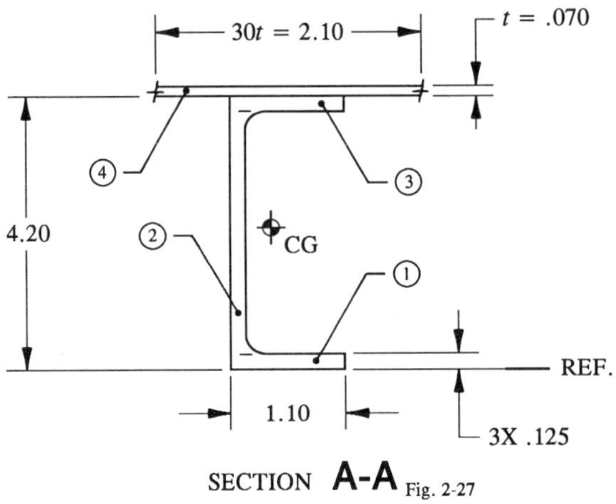

FIGURE 2-28 Fuselage frame cross-sectional area. All fillet radii neglected.

Now, with the benefit of these discussions, the stringer cutout arrangement depicted in Fig. 2-27 will be analyzed in pure bending. To achieve such a configuration, the outer flange and web of the basic frame structure must be cut away to allow the stringer through clearance. The engineer is again referred to Fig. 2-22 where an actual design of a typical aircraft fuselage frame is drawn. Note how the stringers and longerons are allowed to pass through the fuselage frame structure in this figure. By a similar analogy here, the transfer of internal member forces across the joint of the stringer cutout are easily seen by directly relating each structural member to the simple splice-joint concepts depicted earlier in this section. The internal forces that are carried by the skin, outer frame flange, and part of the web that was cut away must now transfer across the joint through the end fasteners of the stringer flange. The stringer flange, in effect, provides a continuous load path for these members. All members that are discontinuous at a splice-joint must transfer their internal forces through other members that can provide a continuous load path across the joint. If the load each member carried before it was cut away can be found, one can then logically reason out the internal member forces that must transfer through the end fasteners of the stringer flange. The elastic bending stress distribution corresponding to pure bending across the frame section is also depicted in this figure (see Sec. 2.3, "Bending of Beams in One Plane").

To form the basis for a reliable and dependable stress analysis solution of member forces, it is essential that the most typical cross-sectional area of frame structure in this region be used to calculate bending stresses. Since many different cross-sectional areas are possible along the frame structure, the section area which best typifies the most typical bending stress distribution of the basic frame structure is chosen for our investigation of these loads. Without a question, this occurs on either side of the splice-joint, at Section A-A in Fig. 2-27, where the internal forces of these members will clearly represent a better internal stress distribution away from the local discontinuities and member irregularities that exist at the joint center. In accordance with the tabulation method of Appendix F, the following section properties are computed for Section A-A (see Fig. 2-28):

MOMENT OF INERTIA

Element	b	h	y	A	Ay	Ay^2	I_o
1	1.100	0.125	0.062	0.137	0.009	0.001	0.000
2	0.125	3.950	2.100	0.494	1.037	2.177	0.642
3	1.100	0.125	4.137	0.137	0.569	2.353	0.000
4	2.100*	0.070	4.235	0.147	0.623	2.636	0.000
			Total	0.915	2.238	7.167	0.642

* The effective area of skin in compression for aluminum alloy 2024-T3 clad is approximated by the formula $30t$ (30 times the material thickness t). The formulation of this expression is specifically derived empirically (for other materials, the engineer is referred to Chapter 6).

$$Y_{cg} = \frac{\Sigma\, Ay}{\Sigma\, A} = \frac{2.238}{.915} = 2.446 \text{ in}$$

$$I_{cg} = \Sigma\, I_o + \Sigma\, Ay^2 - Y_{cg}\,(\Sigma\, Ay)$$
$$I_{cg} = .642 + 7.167 - 2.446(2.238) = 2.335 \text{ in}^4.$$

If we assume that calculated bending stresses will occur in the elastic range of stresses, then from Eqs. A-12 and A-13, the neutral axis is coincident with the centroidal axis, or

$$Y_{na} = Y_{cg} = 2.446 \text{ in}$$

and

$$I_{na} = I_{cg} = 2.335 \text{ in}^4.$$

Now, refer to Section A-A of Fig. 2-29. The element areas in this figure are chosen as a function of the internal member forces desired for our particular splice-joint configuration. To find the internal member forces of these element areas, use will be made of Eq. 2-10, where the average bending stress across each element of the section is multiplied by its corresponding element area. This can be done most conveniently in tabular form, as shown in Table 2-3.

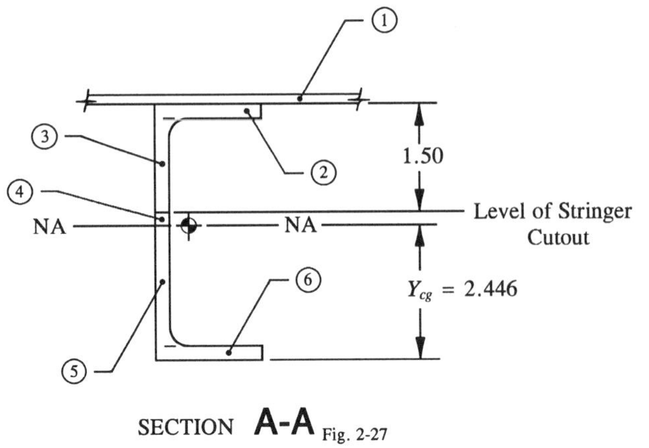

FIGURE 2-29 Fuselage frame element areas used to determine internal member forces.

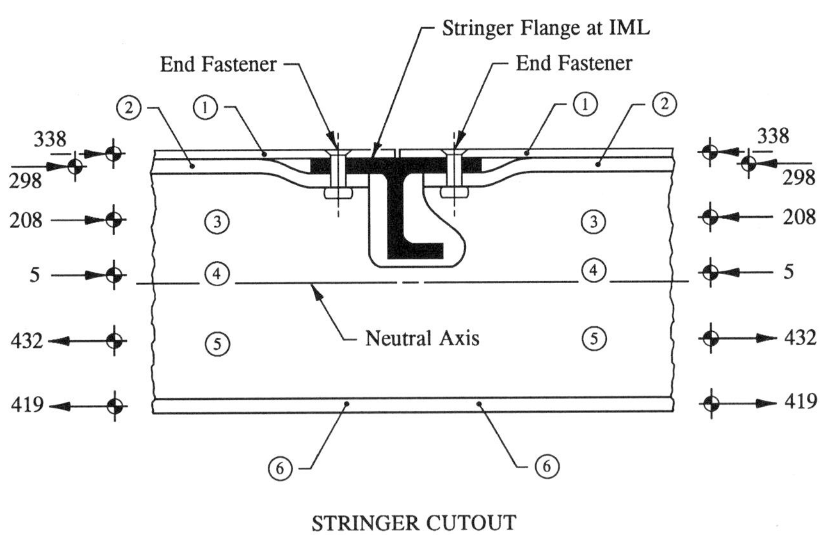

FIGURE 2-30 Fuselage frame internal member forces.

TABLE 2-3 MEMBER FORCES

Element	Member	b	h	A	c	f^*	$P^\dagger$
1	skin	2.100	0.070	0.147	1.789	- 2,299	- 338
2	outer frame flange	1.100	0.125	0.137	1.691	- 2,173	- 298
3	portion of web (cutout)	0.125	1.375	0.172	0.941	- 1,209	- 208
4	web above the neutral axis	0.125	0.254	0.032	0.127	- 163	- 5
5	web below the neutral axis	0.125	2.321	0.290	1.160	1,490	432
6	inner frame flange	1.100	0.125	0.137	2.383	3,062	419

* $f = f_b = \pm Mc/I_{na}$ (refer to Eq. 2-5).

† $P = fA$ (refer to Eq. 2-10).

In this table, the average stresses f at the midpoints of designated element areas are indicated by the distances c from the neutral axis of the bending stress distribution (see Fig. 2-27). The internal member forces P are shown conveniently drawn in Fig. 2-30. The ideas of this section may now be fully utilized here most efficiently in describing the transfer of these forces across the stringer cutout. These ideas, as they relate to the internal forces which are carried by members that can provide continuous load paths across the joint, will show that elements #4, #5, and #6 will not necessarily transfer their internal member forces to other structural members of the joint. Instead, these members will sustain their loads and thereby maintain a fairly constant stress level across the joint. By taking an intelligent and logical approach to the analysis of discontinuous members, it can be reasoned out that the loads of elements #1, #2, and #3 must transfer through the end fasteners of the stringer flange. Also, it is interesting to note that the load carried by element #3 could conceivably redistribute (disperse) some of its load to the inner frame cap side of the fuselage frame. The percentage of redistribution will depend upon the magnitude of the inner frame stresses. If the inner frame stresses are high, very little additional load would be expected to actually redistribute to the inner frame cap (elements #4, #5, and #6). In problems where the inner frame cap stresses are relatively low, the engineer must decide, hopefully, conservatively, how much of this load will actually distribute to the inner frame cap. Realistically, however, only a strain-gauge survey of this joint during flight or structural testing will accurately establish the actual load distribution. Keeping this point in mind then, the most direct approach to a conservative stress analysis solution of the end fasteners would be to completely force the entire load of element #3 or 208 lb through each

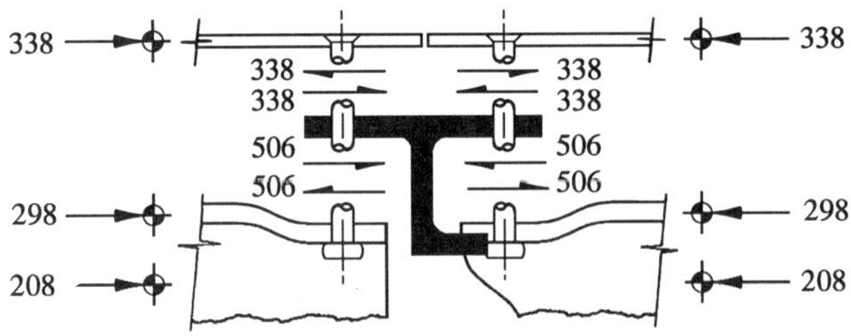

FIGURE 2-31 Transfer of shear forces across the frame cutout.

end fastener.

According to the results given in Table 2-3, and discussions pertaining there to, the transfer of shear forces across the frame cutout by the end fasteners of this joint are diagrammed as shown in Fig. 2-31. Since these forces were derived from the circumferential frame loads of the fuselage, they must also be algebraically

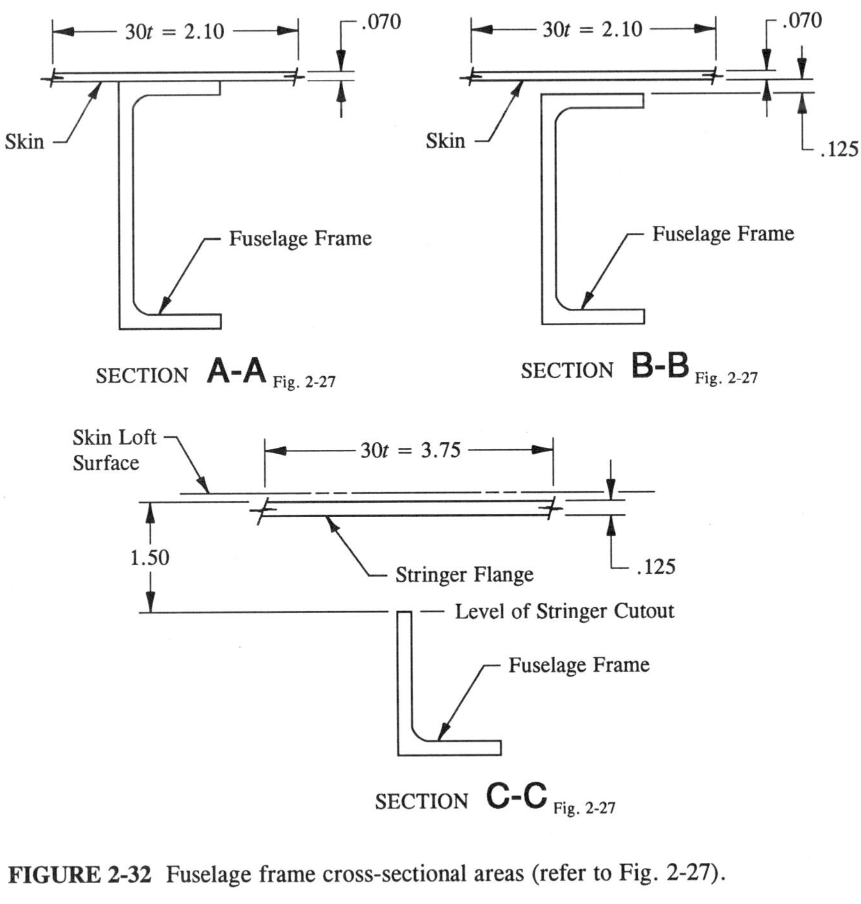

FIGURE 2-32 Fuselage frame cross-sectional areas (refer to Fig. 2-27).

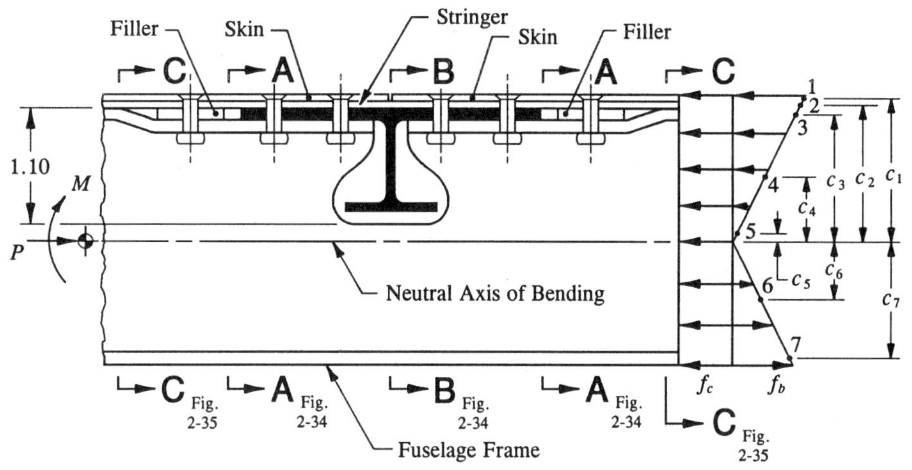

FIGURE 2-33 Stringer cutout subjected to an axial force and a bending moment.

combined with longitudinal fuselage skin shears (those forces perpendicular to the plane of the frame). Here, the shear forces in both planes of the frame cutout are resolved into a single resultant fastener shear force. This is computed mathematically from the Pythagorean theorem, or using Eq. A-6 of Appendix A, $P = (p_x^2 + p_y^2)^{1/2}$. The higher magnitude of shear existing at these fasteners is generally the reason why fasteners common to both stringer and frame are of a higher shear strength (usually of the same size diameter) than those fasteners used between frames or between stringers. In Chapter 3, a method of analyzing a fastener for the transfer of shear will be fully treated. There, fasteners of a multi-riveted connection are sized based on established shear allowables, and the attached members designed from prescribed allowable bearing stresses.

The rest of this solution, as it pertains to fundamental frame design, is to determine the bending stresses that occur along the most critical sections of the fuselage frame structure (if necessary, see Example 2-3, page 84, for a review of actual calculations of a typical frame structure). *All members offering effective means of load transfer, or providing the most direct load paths across the splice-joint, are used in the calculation of basic section properties.* As a brief review of those principles here, conventional stress analysis methods require a complete investigation of the basic frame structure at Sections A-A, B-B, and C-C. These sections are shown in Fig. 2-32. Note, in particular, that the stringer flange (Fig. 2-30) provides an effective load path for the frame outer cap. For this reason, this member becomes part of the effective cross-sectional area of Section C-C. After the section properties of these sections are calculated, the extreme fiber stresses are computed using the flexure formula, Eq. 2-5 ($f_b = \pm Mc/I_{na}$). Further, it will be recalled that the fuselage structure is basically a simple beam, and the longitudinal stresses which it develops from the aerodynamic loads on its structure must also interact

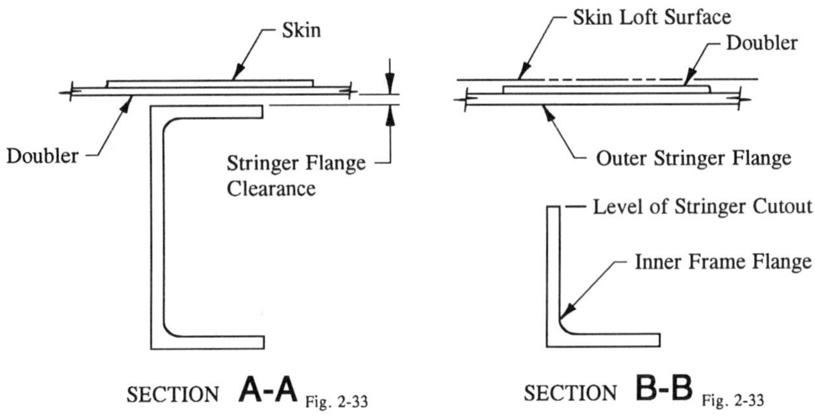

FIGURE 2-34 Fuselage frame cross-sectional areas.

with these stresses (more about this in subsequent chapters when our study of biaxial stresses will focus on their combined solutions using interaction equations[1]).

The material outlined in this section has been presented here as a means of broadening the design engineer's conceptual perception of the actual design problem. Hopefully, we have accomplished this endeavor. However, if the discussions of this section have not been clearly understood, it is suggested that the engineer again review the basic concepts and fundamentals of previous sections of this book as they pertain to the material of this section. In the example which directly follows, the combined effects of axial and bending stresses will be considered across a slightly different but similar stringer cutout arrangement.

When all of the underlying fundamentals of splice-joint analysis have been thoroughly studied and their applications completely understood, the engineer is encouraged to proceed ahead with the solution to Example 2-4. In this example, the principles of splice-joint analysis are again used but in this case the solution is applied to a slightly different configuration of members than was previously used in Example 2-3.

Example 2-4 The stringer cutout arrangement in Fig. 2-33 is subjected to an axial force P of 2,000 lb (compression) and a bending moment M of 4,000 in-lb (compression skin side) across its joint. The corresponding axial and bending stress distributions are indicated as shown. From these distributions, determine the internal member forces, and using these values describe the shear transfer forces of the end fasteners of the stringer flange on a properly drawn exploded view of the joint. Material: fuselage frame and stringer, 2024 aluminum alloy extrusion; skin, clad 2024-T3 aluminum alloy.

[1] Interaction equations are used to design structures for stability and strength requirements under combined loading conditions. The procedure for handling these loads, however, will be covered on an individual problem basis.

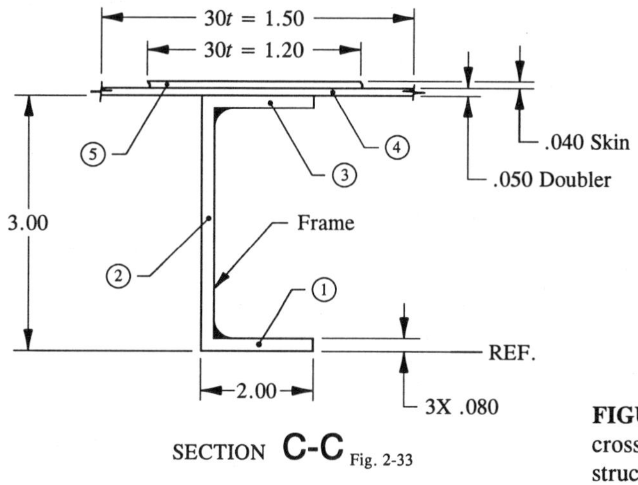

FIGURE 2-35 Representative cross-section of fuselage frame structure. All fillet areas neglected.

SOLUTION: Before performing the actual stress analysis, it is recommended that the engineer formulate in his mind a mental picture of the particular design parameters of the structure and the associated phases of analysis to its analytical substantiation. Most well-designed aircraft structures are a direct result of well-trained, competent design engineers who can maintain the flexibility to correlate their scientific findings of one particular design solution to those of other similar design types. For this problem, the following steps have been collectively accumulated and should now be reviewed in advance of performing the actual stress analysis:

(1) The basic frame structure is analyzed by conventional stress analysis methods at Sections A-A and B-B, Fig. 2-34, for the combined effects of axial and bending stresses at the extreme fibers. The stress values are then compared to the prescribed mechanical properties of the material and in some cases to more stringent design limitations or requirements that may have been imposed on the structure for fuselage frame design, such as inter-rivet buckling, crippling, fatigue, deformations, etc. Use only those structural members of a section area which can most efficiently carry the primary design loads of the basic frame structure.

(2) After the frame structure is sized and is found to be of adequate structural strength, use Section C-C, Fig. 2-35, as a basis for a typical frame section and find the internal member forces of designated element areas of that section area. To approximate the amount of effective width of aluminum skin and doubler in compression use 30t (30 times the individual material thickness t).

(3) Indicate the structural members that can provide the most direct load paths for the internal member forces of discontinuous members across the joint. Then, transfer these forces across the joint through the end fasteners of these structural members.

(4) To complete the analysis, the shear forces and stresses across the joint are

combined with the longitudinal shear forces and stresses of the main fuselage shell, respectively. The transfer of shear forces in both circumferential and longitudinal directions are algebraically combined into a single resultant shear force using Eq. A-6 of Appendix A. Whereas, the combined effects of biaxial stresses are specifically treated using interaction equations to design for stability and strength requirements under combined loading conditions.

The efficient and productive use of engineering time in the performance of the actual stress analysis can better be achieved when a clear and precise understanding of the entire analysis process has been mentally formulated. After all the mental gymnastics of this design have been contemplated, the concepts and fundamentals as they relate to specific analysis solutions of this example can then be performed with a sense of confidence and acquired independence.

In the vicinity of the stringer cutout, Section C-C is taken as the most representative cross-section of frame structure, where the local discontinuities and member irregularities of the joint have been avoided. In fact, even the filler material (see Fig. 2-33) is omitted from the section properties. Basically, this member is not long enough to be considered effective in carrying the basic internal frame loads; consequently, it simply serves as a nonstructural member. However, if the filler had been considerably longer, possibly spanning from stringer to adjacent stringer, its load capacity would then have been utilized. Using the tabulation method of Appendix F, the following table is set up to compute the section properties of Section C-C:

MOMENT OF INERTIA

Element	b	h	y	A	Ay	Ay^2	I_o
1	2.000	0.080	0.040	0.160	0.006	0.000	0.000
2	0.080	2.840	1.500	0.227	0.341	0.511	0.153
3	2.000	0.080	2.960	0.160	0.474	1.402	0.000
4	1.500	0.050	3.025	0.075	0.227	0.686	0.000
5	1.200	0.040	3.070	0.048	0.147	0.452	0.000
			Total	0.670	1.195	3.051	0.153

$$Y_{cg} = \frac{\Sigma\, Ay}{\Sigma\, A} = \frac{1.195}{.670} = 1.784 \text{ in}$$

$$I_{cg} = \Sigma\, I_o + \Sigma\, Ay^2 - Y_{cg}\,(\Sigma\, Ay)$$
$$I_{cg} = .153 + 3.051 - 1.784(1.195) = 1.072 \text{ in}^4.$$

If the combined bending and axial stresses are calculated to values within the elastic range of a stress-strain curve of a material, the neutral axis will remain coincident with the centroidal axis. In most common frame designs where frame stresses are deliberately kept low, this condition should be true. And so, it follows directly that

$$Y_{na} = Y_{cg} = 1.784 \text{ in}$$

and

$$I_{na} = I_{cg} = 1.072 \text{ in}^4.$$

With all of the section properties known, the axial and bending elastic stress distributions which are represented across the frame area in Fig. 2-33 can now be replaced by equivalent internal forces designated at specific element areas. To accomplish this, the average stress levels at the midpoints of designated element areas, Fig. 2-36, are computed using Eq. 2-9 ($f = \pm P/A \pm Mc/I_{na}$). With these values determined, the equivalent internal member forces are found by multiplying this average stress by the corresponding element areas of the frame section (see Eq. 2-10, $p = fA$). A summary of these calculated quantities are presented in Table 2.4.

TABLE 2-4 MEMBER FORCES

Elem.	Member	b	h	A	c	f_n	f_b	f^*	$p^†$
1	skin	1.200	0.040	0.048	1.286	- 2,985	- 4,799	- 7,784	- 374
2	doubler	1.500	0.050	0.075	1.241	- 2,985	- 4,631	- 7,616	- 571
3	outer frame flange	2.000	0.080	0.160	1.176	- 2,985	- 4,388	- 7,373	- 1,180
4	portion of web (cutout)	0.080	1.020	0.082	0.626	- 2,985	- 2,336	- 5,321	- 436
5	web above the neutral axis	0.080	0.116	0.009	0.058	- 2,985	- 216	- 3,201	- 29
6	web below the neutral axis	0.080	1.704	0.136	0.852	- 2,985	3,179	194	26
7	inner frame flange	2.000	0.080	0.160	1.744	- 2,985	6,507	3,522	564

* $f = f_n + f_b$ where: $f_n = \pm P/A$ (see Eq. 2-2)
$f_b = \pm Mc/I_{na}$ (see Eq. 2-5).

† $p = fA$ (see Eq. 2-10).

To help illustrate the transfer of forces across the stringer cutout, all internal member forces are conveniently drawn at the centroids of their corresponding

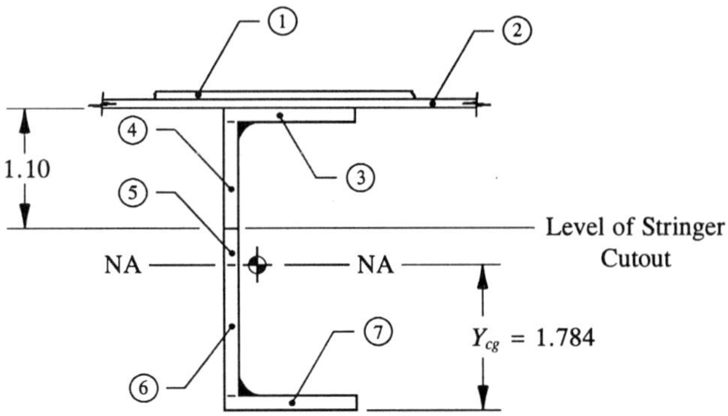

FIGURE 2-36 Fuselage frame element areas used to determine member forces.

element areas, as shown in Fig. 2-37. From our previous discussions of splice-joint analysis, it is observed here that the skin, web, and outer frame flange members that were cut away will transfer their internal member forces through each of the two end fasteners of the stringer flange. The doubler in this case will provide a continuous load path across the joint. As such, this member will not transfer its internal force to other adjacent structural members. Instead, it will be a recipient of the internal skin forces.

It is conservatively assumed here that all of the internal member force that is carried by the cut web (element #4) will transfer through the two end fasteners of the stringer flange. The reason that this is so, is that since fuselage design stresses are normally kept relatively low, most of the load carried by this member will likely transfer through the end fasteners of the stringer flange. Moreover, after all

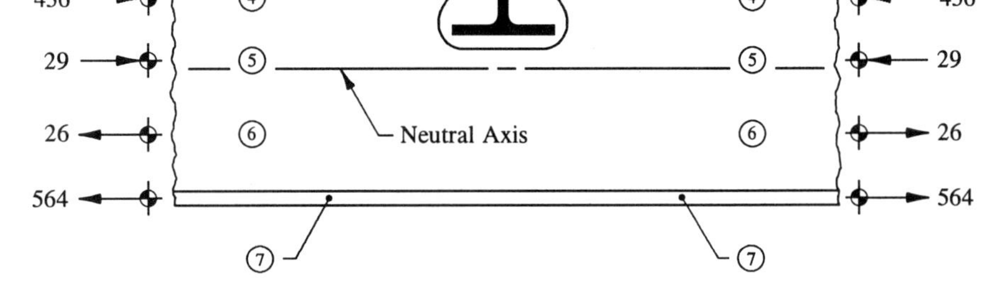

FIGURE 2-37 Fuselage frame internal member forces.

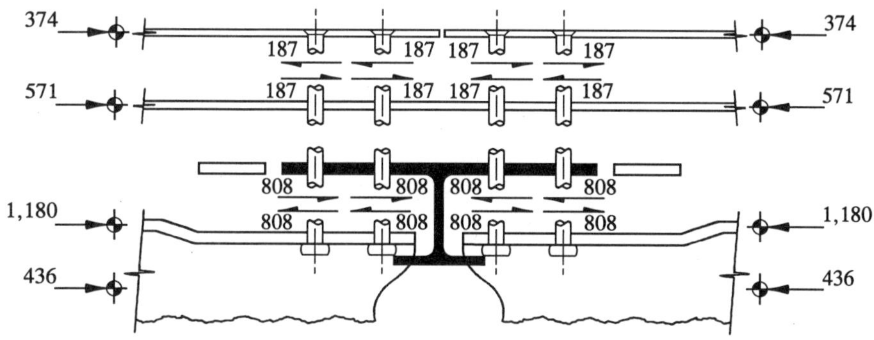

FIGURE 2-38 Transfer of shear through the end fasteners of the stringer cutout.

joint frictional effects have been overcome, it is generally accepted engineering practice to equally divide the total member force between end fasteners of equal strength (see multi-riveted connection analysis in Chapter 3). This is shown in Fig. 2-38 for each of the two fasteners of the stringer flange. In the final step, the shear transfer forces of each fastener are logically reasoned out and their values described diagrammatically in this figure. Although many other variations of a stringer cutout are physically possible, the approaches and techniques to their analyses remain very similar.

2.7 Method of Transformations Approach to Bending of Beams of Dissimilar Materials. So far in our study of stress analysis, the beams analyzed in this book have been constructed of similar (homogeneous) materials. Beams composed of dissimilar (heterogeneous) materials are also commonly used in aircraft structural designs. In this section, the methods and ideologies of beams constructed of different materials are specifically treated. Following these discussions, the importance and practical considerations of their designs will be additionally emphasized using several illustrative examples of actual engineering hardware.

In general aircraft design, beams constructed of dissimilar materials usually produce rather inefficient structures; and therefore, their use in production model aircraft designs should be avoided. However, if their designs are nonetheless contemplated, each particular design case should be thoroughly reviewed and evaluated before employing them in actual design practice. The effects of galvanic action between members of dissimilar materials can sometimes produce a slight weakening of their material properties. An additional consequence of their poor designs is that the allowables of their materials will not be reached simultaneously during structural loading. Hence, when several members of different materials are loaded together jointly, while one material begins to reach its allowable stress the others are stressed below their maximum allowable values. This inconsistency in their designs is inferior to designs of similar materials because they (beams of dissimilar materials) do not fully utilize their available strengths. However, in some structural design applications, i.e., repairs, structural testing and modifications, their practicability can be most important to the success of the total design effort. Their utility and general purpose in practical design cases will be further elaborated upon in later parts of this section.

Now, the method of transformations approach of beams of dissimilar materials in bending is presented. If a built-up beam is constructed of several different materials, to account for the difference in the material stiffnesses of its members, the dissimilar members of the section are transformed into equivalent areas of one base material. This is done by selecting one of the dissimilar materials of the actual built-up section. The section area is then conformed and suitable to use in the bending stress equation (see Sec. 2-3, Eq. 2-5, $f_b = \pm Mc/I_{na}$).

To accomplish the actual transformation, the bending stiffnesses[1] of the dissimilar materials are each separately equated in terms of the bending stiffness of the selected base material. Or, simply

$$(EI)_{\text{base material}} = (EI)_{\text{dissimilar material}}$$
$$E_B I_B = E_D I_D.$$

Solving for I_B,

$$I_B = I_D \left[\frac{E_D}{E_B} \right] \tag{2-11}$$

where: E = modulus of elasticity (use E_c and E_t when stresses are compression and tension, respectively)

I = moment of inertia of a member around its own axis of bending

B = subscript used to designate the base material

D = subscript used to designate the dissimilar material.

It will be observed from this equation that by a simple ratio of elastic moduli E_D/E_B each dissimilar material may be transformed into its equivalent base material. Conditionally, however, the location of the internal member force acting at the centroid of the transformed area must also correspond to the same centroid location on the original dissimilar area. If the location of these forces on both cross-sectional areas remains the same, the same internal resisting moment M across the whole cross-sectional area will be developed. Consequently, this condition makes the transformed area compatible with the original design area by virtue of their equivalent applied moments.

Before members of dissimilar materials are transformed into members of equivalent base material, it will be convenient to represent their geometric shapes into combinations of known or standard shaped areas. Since most cross-sectional

[1] Bending stiffness is measured by the product of the modulus of elasticity E of the material and the moment of inertia I around the neutral axis of bending of the cross-sectional area.

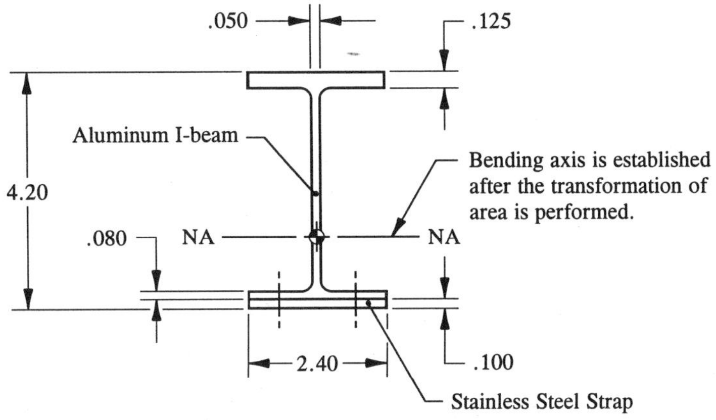

FIGURE 2-39 Cross-sectional area of a beam made up of dissimilar materials.

areas of a typical aircraft structure are composed of structural members made up of rectangular-shaped areas, this particular shape will be utilized as a special case to illustrate the application of Eq. 2-11. In most cases, the actual calculation of moment of inertia I is performed by the simple tabulation method of Appendix F. From this appendix, the moment of inertia for a rectangular-shaped area about its own axis of bending is $I = bh^3/12$. Substituting this value into Eq. 2-11 gives:

$$\frac{b_B h_B^3}{12} = \left[\frac{b_D h_D^3}{12}\right]\left[\frac{E_D}{E_B}\right].$$

It will be recalled that the axis of bending is what firmly establishes the dimensions b and h when calculating moment of inertia by our tabular method. In Appendix F, the b dimension is always selected parallel to the axis of bending; the h dimension is then established perpendicular to that axis. As a required condition to the actual material transformation, the h dimensions of each material are set equal to each other. That is, if $h_B = h_D$, the location of the internal member force of the original dissimilar material is fixed at the centroid of the equivalent base material. In this way, the same original resisting moment M is developed across the transformed section area. It then remains to simplify this equation and solve for b_B, we obtain:

$$b_B = b_D\left[\frac{E_D}{E_B}\right] \quad \textbf{(2-12)}$$

$$h_B = h_D. \quad \textbf{(2-13)}$$

The following example will help to illustrate the simple techniques of transformation using these equations. As shown in Fig. 2-39, a stainless steel strap or

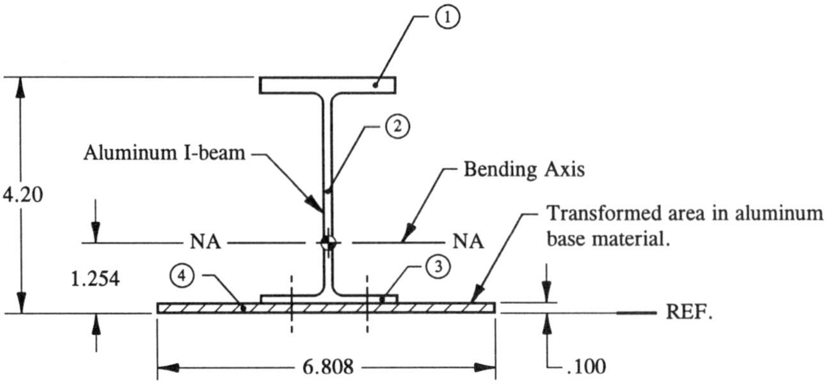

FIGURE 2-40 Cross-sectional area showing stainless steel reinforcement represented in equivalent aluminum base material.

reinforcement of a different material several times stiffer than that of the aluminum I-beam is used. From the mechanical-property tables in MIL-HDBK-5F, use values of $(E_c)_{\text{aluminum}} = 10.4 \times 10^6$ psi for the aluminum I-beam and $(E_c)_{\text{steel}} = 29.5 \times 10^6$ psi for the stainless steel strap. Consider an internal maximum moment of 22,000 in-lb across the total section area (compression strap side). The smaller gage of the steel reinforcement is used to facilitate fabrication and thereby avoid a costly redesign effort of the original design. If the reinforcement is not to be a permanent part of the actual structure, its strength characteristics should be patterned to a weaker section area than that of the actual production model structure. If the weaker section proves to be of adequate structural strength during all particular phases of structural testing, then the higher strength characteristics of the production model structure will be substantiated.

The steel reinforcement in its present design configuration does not conform to the implied rules of conventional stress analysis; therefore, it cannot be used in the application of the flexure formula. Instead, a transformation of the steel reinforcement material into its equivalent aluminum base material is required. The steel reinforcement was selected instead of the aluminum I-beam for the obvious reason that, for the actual transformation fewer transformations would be required for this individual member. (Compare the number of transformations that would be required in equivalent steel base material.) After the engineer has studied the remaining procedure to the analysis of dissimilar materials, it is suggested that he then go back and again use the method of transformations approach to the solution of this example, but this time, perform them in equivalent steel base material. Surprisingly, the final stresses he determines will be the same. Now, let us continue, utilizing Eqs. 2-12 and 2-13, the steel strap is transformed into equivalent aluminum base material:

$$b_B = b_D\left[\frac{E_D}{E_B}\right] = 2.40\left[\frac{29.5 \text{ x } 10^6}{10.4 \text{ x } 10^6}\right] = 6.808 \text{ in}$$

$$h_B = h_D = .100 \text{ in.}$$

The steel reinforcement in equivalent aluminum base material is redrawn in Fig. 2-40. In this form, the moment of inertia of the entire cross-sectional area is calculated, as tabulated in Table 2-5.

TABLE 2-5 MOMENT OF INERTIA IN EQUIVALENT ALUMINUM BASE MATERIAL

Element	b	h	y	A	Ay	Ay^2	I_o
1	2.400	0.125	4.137	0.300	1.241	5.134	0.000
2	0.050	3.895	2.127	0.195	0.414	0.881	0.246
3	2.400	0.080	0.140	0.192	0.027	0.004	0.000
4	6.808	0.100	0.050	0.681	0.034	0.002	0.001
			Total	1.368	1.716	6.021	0.247

$$Y_{cg} = \frac{\Sigma\, Ay}{\Sigma\, A} = \frac{1.716}{1.368} = 1.254 \text{ in}$$

$$I_{cg} = \Sigma\, I_o + \Sigma\, Ay^2 - Y_{cg}\,(\Sigma\, Ay)$$
$$I_{cg} = .247 + 6.021 - 1.254(1.716) = 4.116 \text{ in}^4.$$

Next, if we assume calculated bending stresses will occur in the elastic range, then the flexure formula is applicable for our solution in aluminum base material. And, if this assumption proves correct, then the following is also true:

$$Y_{na} = Y_{cg} = 1.254 \text{ in}$$

and

$$I_{na} = I_{cg} = 4.116 \text{ in}^4.$$

Now, the bending stresses at the extreme fibers of our equivalent section are calculated below:

$$f_b = \pm\frac{Mc}{I_{na}}$$

$$(f_t)_{\text{aluminum}} = \frac{22,000(4.20 - 1.254)}{4.116} = 15,746 \text{ psi} \quad \text{(true stress)}$$

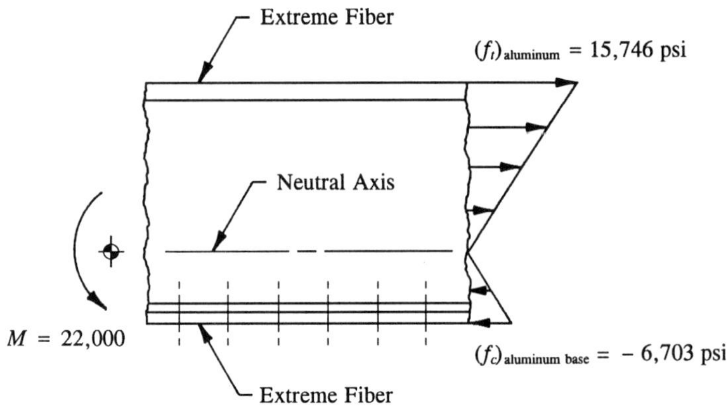

FIGURE 2-41 Elastic bending stress distribution across a beam section.

$$(f_c)_{\text{aluminum base}} = -\frac{22,000(1.254)}{4.116} = -6,703 \text{ psi}.$$

The stress distribution across this section is established as shown in Fig. 2-41.

Question: Are the bending stresses calculated in the transformed aluminum base material true stresses? To answer this question, the stresses at the interface of the dissimilar materials must be investigated. There, when the beam undergoes bending, the strains (or stretching) that occur between the surfaces of contact of these different members must be the same. Using this knowledge, the true stress distribution caused by the bending moment M can be found by relating the linear strains of each member to Hooke's Law (see Appendix E, $f_n = \varepsilon E$). Note from this expression that if the strains of each member are the same, and their elastic moduli E are different, the elastic stresses f_n of their materials must also be of different magnitudes. To show these principles clearly, the compatibility requirements of their strains are mathematically equated at the surfaces of contact of their materials. Thus from Hooke's law:

$$\varepsilon_{\text{steel}} = \frac{f_{\text{steel}}}{E_{\text{steel}}} \quad \text{and} \quad \varepsilon_{\text{aluminum}} = \frac{f_{\text{aluminum}}}{E_{\text{aluminum}}}.$$

The equations are then equated like this:

$$\varepsilon_{\text{steel}} = \varepsilon_{\text{aluminum}}.$$

Substituting their corresponding material strains into this equation gives:

$$\frac{f_{\text{steel}}}{E_{\text{steel}}} = \frac{f_{\text{aluminum}}}{E_{\text{aluminum}}}. \tag{2-14}$$

The true elastic stress in the steel material in terms of the aluminum base material can now be written:

$$f_{\text{steel}} = f_{\text{aluminum base}} \left[\frac{E_{\text{steel}}}{E_{\text{aluminum}}} \right]. \tag{2-15}$$

Hence, the true elastic stress of the steel reinforcement is found by multiplying the stress of the aluminum base material by the ratio of $E_{\text{steel}}/E_{\text{aluminum}}$. It should also be observed from this expression that, because of compatibility of strains, the stiffer steel material must actually operate at a higher stress level than the aluminum material. This observation is of course consistent with the notion that the transformed steel material does not behave nor physically exist as an equivalent aluminum material, but rather only as steel. And that calculated stresses in its equivalent aluminum form must therefore, that is, for compatibility sake, undergo a transformation back to the stresses that should actually have been developed in its original steel form. If the transformation had instead been performed in equivalent steel, the true stress in the actual aluminum material would have been found by ratioing down the stress level in the equivalent steel material by $E_{\text{aluminum}}/E_{\text{steel}}$. That is, solving for f_{aluminum} in Eq. 2-14, we obtain a slightly different mathematical expression for this alternative transformation:

$$f_{\text{aluminum}} = f_{\text{steel base}} \left[\frac{E_{\text{aluminum}}}{E_{\text{steel}}} \right]. \tag{2-16}$$

This then meets the strain compatibility requirements at the interface of the dissimilar materials. For our particular example, Eq. 2-15 is used for the transformation back to the true stress levels that would exist in the actual steel material. At the interface, the stresses in the aluminum and steel materials are determined:

$$f_b = \pm \frac{Mc}{I_{na}}$$

$$(f_c)_{\text{aluminum}} = (f_c)_{\text{aluminum base}} = -\frac{22,000(1.254 - .100)}{4.116} = -6,168 \text{ psi}$$

$$(f_c)_{\text{steel}} = (f_c)_{\text{aluminum base}} \left[\frac{E_{\text{steel}}}{E_{\text{aluminum}}} \right] = -6,168 \left[\frac{29.5 \text{ x } 10^6}{10.4 \text{ x } 10^6} \right]$$

$$(f_c)_{\text{steel}} = -17,496 \text{ psi}.$$

Now, at the lower extreme fibers of the composite beam section, the true stress in the steel reinforcement is found:

$$(f_c)_{\text{steel}} = (f_c)_{\text{aluminum base}} \left[\frac{E_{\text{steel}}}{E_{\text{aluminum}}} \right], \text{ from Eq. 2-15}$$

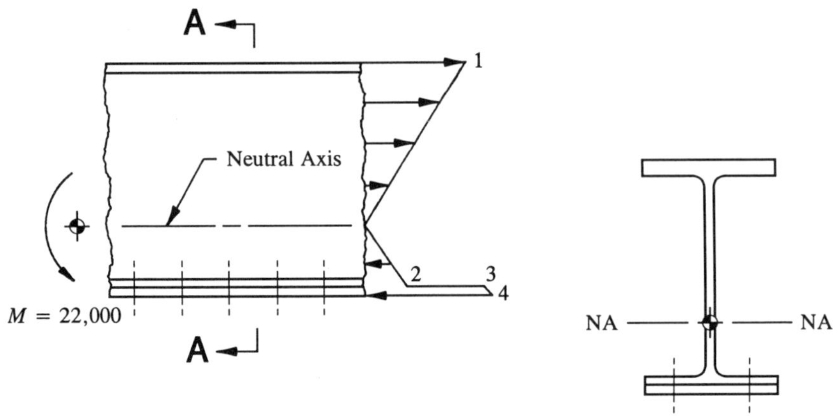

Point	Material	Stress (psi)
1	aluminum	15,746
2	aluminum	- 6,168
3	steel	- 17,496
4	steel	- 19,013

SECTION **A-A**

FIGURE 2-42 True stress distribution across a beam made up of dissimilar materials.

$$(f_c)_{\text{steel}} = -6,703\left[\frac{29.5 \text{ x } 10^6}{10.4 \text{ x } 10^6}\right] = -19,013 \text{ psi} \quad \text{(true stress)}$$

$$(f_t)_{\text{aluminum}} = 15,746 \text{ psi} \quad \text{(duplicated here from page 111)}$$

$$(f_c)_{\text{aluminum base}} = -6,703 \text{ psi} \quad \text{(from page 112)}.$$

The true stress distribution across this beam is detailed in Fig. 2-42.

To more clearly emphasize the method of transformations approach to the solution of dissimilar materials outlined in this section, the following procedural steps are summarized below:

(1) First, decide which of the dissimilar materials of the cross-sectional area are to be transformed into equivalent base material.

(2) Transform each of the dissimilar materials chosen in step 1 into equivalent base material using Eqs. 2-12 and 2-13. Remember that the b and h dimensions of a transformed area must be compatible with the axis of bending of that section area.

(3) Next, calculate the moment of inertia of the entire transformed cross-sectional area by the tabulation method of Appendix F (this method will also locate the centroidal axis of the entire transformed section area).

(4) Using Eq. 2-5 ($f_b = \pm Mc/I_{na}$), determine bending stresses at critical points of the transformed section area.[1]

[1] It will be demonstrated in Sec. 2.8 that for combined axial and bending loads the general expression for their combined stress effects is used, or $f = \pm P/A \pm Mc/I_{na}$.

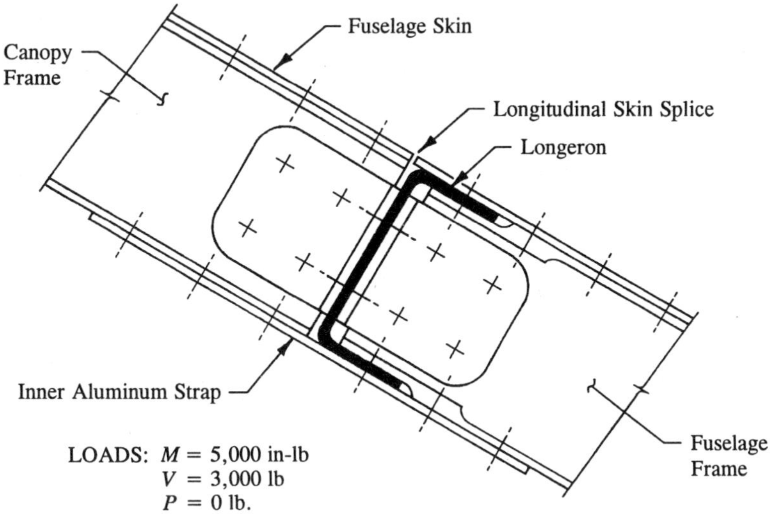

FIGURE 2-43 Structural arrangement of members attached together at a common joint intersection.

(5) Lastly, the true elastic stresses developed in the dissimilar materials are found by the application of Eq. 2-15 or 2-16; no modification of elastic stresses is required for those members that exist in the selected base material.

Example 2-5 Several main structural members are attached together at a joint intersection to form the structural arrangement of members shown in Fig. 2-43. To increase the clarity of the intersecting members in this view, only the fuselage frame, longeron, and canopy frame structures are drawn. Entirely overlooked by the structures group, it is now proposed as a temporary repair of the structure to add a stainless steel strap .016 in thick and 2.50 in wide underneath the fuselage skin so it straddles across the longitudinal skin splice. The strap provides an effective load path for both the fuselage and canopy frame structures on the skin side of the longitudinal splice. Its proper position under the fuselage skin is drawn as shown in Fig. 2-44. If the maximum bending moment M across the joint is 5,000 in-lb (compression on the inner flange side as given by a computer solution of this structure), what are the maximum bending stresses across this joint? (Note: Unless the frame and canopy structures are again remodeled by the computer analysis group for the effects of a partial degree of restraint[1], the existing design must carry the original bending moment M. Material: aluminum strap, $E_{\text{aluminum}} = 10.5 \times 10^6$ psi; stainless steel strap, $E_{\text{steel}} = 30.0 \times 10^6$ psi.

[1] The engineer is referred to Chapter 1, Sec. 1.9, for a discussion of partial degree of restraint of support types.

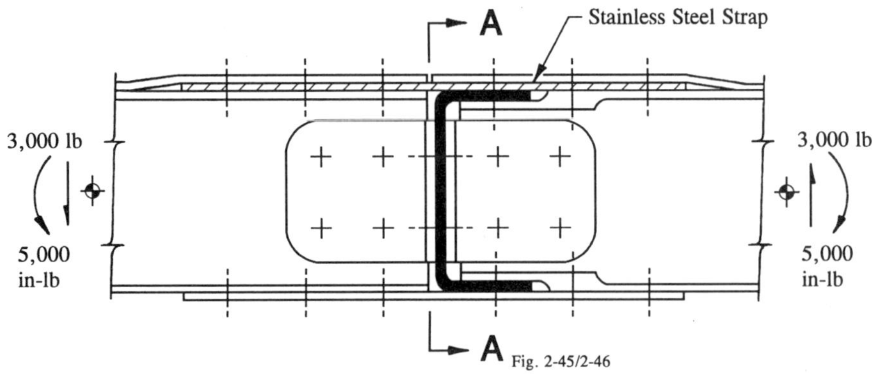

FIGURE 2-44 Reinforcement strap (shown cross-hatched) is used to provide a continuous load path for the outer frame cap.

General Discussion of This Design: In the course of an engineer's career many unusual design configurations will cross the engineer's desk, including, perhaps, even some faulty ones like this. Such an oversight is of particular interest to us at this time as it specifically relates to the subject matter of this section. Its particular details are subsequently discussed here. During the investigative design phases of this particular joint intersection, all intersecting structural members should have been carefully examined for continuity of load paths. Through a closer examination of these members now, it can be seen that no load path is provided for the fuselage and canopy frame structures across the longitudinal skin splice. However, if these frame members were originally designed to have a continuous load path, and if their structural configurations were computer modeled for this specification, then the maximum bending moment M produced from a computer solution of the joint intersection would still have to be carried by the original design. In essence, this means that no matter what deliberate changes or redesign efforts have been initiated to correct the existing structure, the same computer bending moment would have to be accounted for. In light of the partial degree of restraint capability of this joint, this would be a considerable undertaking, not at all consistent with acceptable frame designs of this type.

The load path discontinuity which exists across this joint is better perceived when the maximum bending moment M is represented as an equivalent couple-force system (see Appendix B, Eq. A-7, $P_{couple} = M/H$). In this alternative loading form, the load, P_{couple}, on the outer frame cap, now viewed as a simple axial compression load, will not be able to transfer its value across the longitudinal skin splice by the most direct or efficient load path possible. Instead, the frame shear clips must now provide the load path continuity that the original design concept neglected to do. Even for temporary structural design situations, e.g., those that might be expected when used in static verification tests, this design flaw would prove impractical. It is ill-advised to force additional loads through the shear clips when a better, more direct load path can be achieved through the outer frame cap. Conversely, if no moment exists at this joint, the shear-ties offered by the shear clips will be sufficient by themselves to carry the internal shear across the longitudinal skin splice. Here, the internal shear V of magnitude 3,000 lb will then be effectively carried across the joint by these structural members, and their static strengths can be assured in accordance with the methods of analysis of Chapter 5.

An undesirable consequence of this poorly designed structure is the severe weight penalty that must be realized by the existing structure. Additionally, it will be extremely difficult to substantiate the production model aircraft structure by simple means of comparative analysis if the existing structure is designed with different load paths than what the actual structure uses in production. In all structural verification tests using temporary reinforcements, the test structure is usually made of a weaker strength than the actual structure of the production model aircraft. If the test structure proves to be of adequate structural strength, by simple deductive reasoning the higher strength characteristics of the production model aircraft structure is also substantiated. On the basis of these discussions, then, it is recommended that a corrosion-resistant metal reinforcement (or strap) be added across the longitudinal skin splice. Of course, the skin must be partially de-skinned to allow the reinforcement to slide between the skin and flanges of the fuselage and canopy members. To accomplish this, the strap should be thin enough to pick up the existing holes when these members are reassembled. The best choice to achieve this structural arrangement is to use a stainless steel reinforcement .016 in thick.

In today's aircraft markets, commercial airline companies, the U.S. Military Armed Forces and many other non-Communist governments will be sending their most capable and competent engineering representatives to carefully inspect and review pertinent performance data of the static test article. These same representatives will be submitting their acceptance or rejection buy recommendations back to their parent companies for approval. The catch phrase, "What looks good, is good," has a subtle implied connotation to "good aircraft designs," whether or not the actual aircraft is in fact a truly good design. Therefore, based on this human emotion, it is the well-disciplined engineer who will strive to avoid awkward, unusual looking structures even for the most structural worthiness of aircraft designs. For most structural design applications, a temporary strap on the outside of the fuselage shell, even for the test article, could considerably detract from the basic aesthetics of the aircraft.

SOLUTION: To solve this problem by the methods of analysis of this section, the proposed stainless steel reinforcement is transformed into equivalent aluminum base material, and using its equivalent section properties the moment of inertia I_{na} around the neutral axis of the total section is determined. However, before this member is transformed into equivalent aluminum base material, the bending axis of the beam must first be established. This axis is clearly viewed in Fig. 2-45. Inasmuch as the beam is known to physically bend about a horizontal axis, the horizontal dimension b of the steel reinforcement area is changed; the vertical

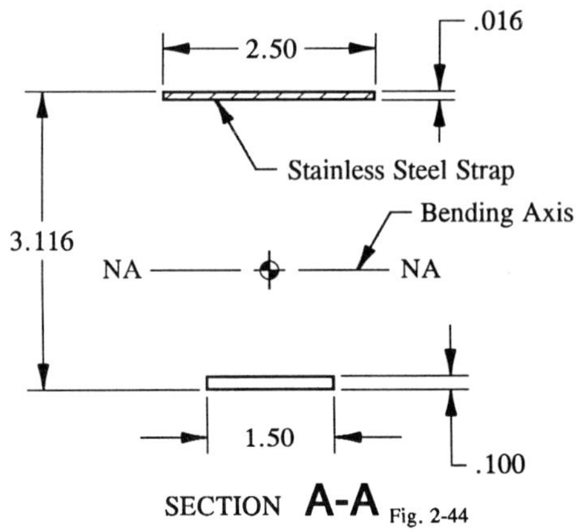

FIGURE 2-45 Cross-sectional area depicting dissimilar materials.

dimension h remains the same. The actual transformation is accomplished using Eqs. 2-12 and 2-13. Thus, the following dimensions are transformed:

$$b_B = b_D\left[\frac{E_D}{E_B}\right] = 2.5\left[\frac{30.0 \times 10^6}{10.5 \times 10^6}\right] = 7.143 \text{ in}$$

$$h_B = h_D = .016 \text{ in.}$$

The stainless steel strap in equivalent aluminum base material is shown in Fig. 2-46. Now, the moment of inertia I_{na} of the total section area is computed in the usual convenient tabular way, as shown in Table 2-6.

TABLE 2-6 MOMENT OF INERTIA OF THE TOTAL SECTION AREA

Element	b	h	y	A	Ay	Ay^2	I_o
1	7.143	0.016	3.108	0.114	0.355	1.104	0.000
2	1.500	0.100	0.050	0.150	0.007	0.000	0.000
			Total	0.264	0.362	1.104	0.000

$$Y_{cg} = \frac{\Sigma Ay}{\Sigma A} = \frac{.362}{.264} = 1.371 \text{ in}$$

$$I_{cg} = \Sigma I_o + \Sigma Ay^2 - Y_{cg}(\Sigma Ay)$$

$$I_{cg} = 0 + 1.104 - 1.371(.362) = .608 \text{ in}^4.$$

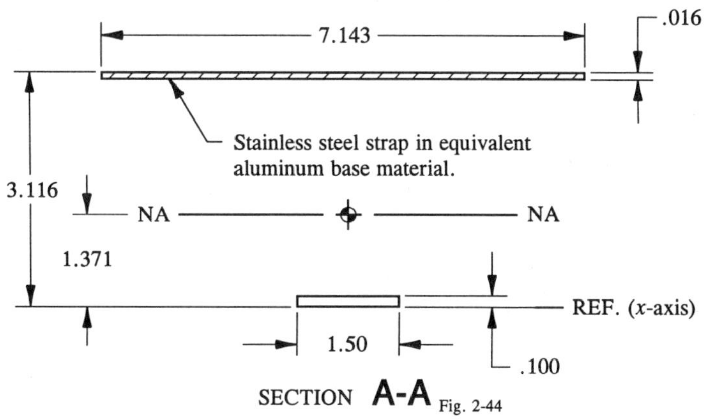

FIGURE 2-46 Cross-sectional area showing stainless steel reinforcement represented in equivalent aluminum base material.

If we assume elastic stress design, then

$$Y_{na} = Y_{cg}$$

and

$$I_{na} = I_{cg}.$$

The true extreme fiber stresses are now computed using the flexure formula ($f_b = \pm Mc/I_{na}$):

$$(f_c)_{\text{aluminum}} = -\frac{Mc}{I_{na}} = -\frac{5,000(1.371)}{.608} = -11,275 \text{ psi} \quad \text{(true stress)}$$

$$(f_t)_{\text{aluminum base}} = +\frac{Mc}{I_{na}} = \frac{5,000(3.116 - 1.371)}{.608}$$

$$(f_t)_{\text{aluminum base}} = 14,350 \text{ psi} \quad \text{(fictitious stress)}.$$

Using Eq. 2-15, the fictitious stress of the aluminum base material is transformed into the true stress that exists in the steel material.

$$(f_t)_{\text{steel}} = (f_t)_{\text{aluminum base}}\left[\frac{E_{\text{steel}}}{E_{\text{aluminum}}}\right] = 14,350\left[\frac{30.0 \times 10^6}{10.5 \times 10^6}\right]$$

$$(f_t)_{\text{steel}} = 41,001 \text{ psi} \quad \text{(true stress)}.$$

The internal member forces which transfer through the cap fasteners of the outer and inner straps across the joint intersection are found according to the

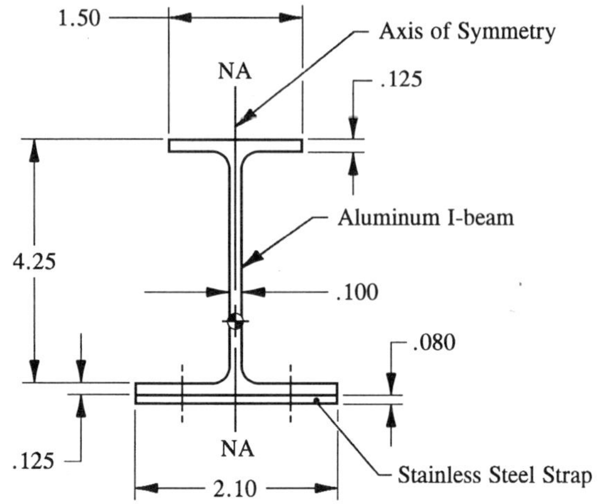

FIGURE 2-47 Cross-sectional area of a beam made up of dissimilar materials.

methods of stress distribution of Sec. 2.6, "Member Forces." To remain relatively current in the analysis methods of that section, it is recommended that each design engineer mentally prepare a step-by-step solution of those principles here. Remember, one should not attempt the numerical computations of a design problem before all the basic steps to its fundamental solution have been clearly formulated.

2.8 Method of Transformations Approach to Combined Axial and Bending of Beams of Dissimilar Materials. To complete our investigation of dissimilar materials, the following discussion will present the methods of analysis to the solution of combined axial and bending of beams. To illustrate these principles, let us turn our attention to the cross-sectional area shown in Fig. 2-47. If an axial load was applied to this section, what method of transformation would be proposed for the stainless steel strap? The actual transformation is performed using the analogous procedure derived in the preceding section for bending of beams of dissimilar materials. For axially loaded members, however, the transformation of steel material into its equivalent aluminum base material is achieved by simple correlation of axial stiffnesses of their materials. The transformed area is then compatible with the base material of the whole cross-sectional area. As was previously developed in Sec. 2.7, our basic approach here is typically the same. The axial stiffness of the proposed or selected base material is equated to the axial stiffness of the dissimilar material. This equality is formulated below:

$$(AE)_{\text{base material}} = (AE)_{\text{dissimilar material}}$$

$$A_B E_B = A_D E_D .$$

Solving for the area A_B in equivalent base material, we find that

$$A_B = A_D\left[\frac{E_D}{E_B}\right] \tag{2-17}$$

where: E = modulus of elasticity (use E_c and E_t when stresses are compression and tension, respectively)
A = cross-sectional area of a member
B = subscript used to designate the base material
D = subscript used to designate the dissimilar material.

The actual transformation of area of the dissimilar material into its equivalent base material is accomplished by a simple ratio of elastic moduli E_D/E_B. Further, the location of the internal member force of the original dissimilar material must correspond to the same location in equivalent base material. Or, simply, the centroid of areas of each material must be coincident (having the same original position). Here, the condition that satisfies this requirement for a rectangular-shaped area is such that $h_B = h_D$. If the area of a rectangle ($A = bh$) is now substituted into Eq. 2-17, we obtain:

$$b_B h_B = b_D h_D\left[\frac{E_D}{E_B}\right].$$

And, since $h_B = h_D$, this equation reduces further to:

$$b_B = b_D\left[\frac{E_D}{E_B}\right] \tag{2-18}$$

$$h_B = h_D. \tag{2-19}$$

Let us now compare these equations with those from Sec. 2.7 (refer specifically to Eqs. 2-12 and 2-13). Clearly, this comparison demonstrates that the actual transformation of area for axial members is accomplished using the same identical set of transformation equations as was previously developed for bending members in that section.

This conclusion makes the solution of beams with combined axial and bending stresses of dissimilar materials in this section very convenient to solve. That is, only one actual transformation of material is required even when axial and bending loads are simultaneously applied. An additional point of convenience of this result is that Eqs. 2-15 and 2-16 (page 113) of the previous section are also applicable here in this section to the fictitious stress system obtained for an axial member in equivalent base material. Specifically, Eqs. 2-15 and 2-16 lend themselves directly to the solution of true combined stresses in the steel material from strain compatibility requirements at the interface of the dissimilar materials (i.e.,

$\varepsilon_{steel} = \varepsilon_{aluminum}$). For easy reference, these equations are again written below:

$$f_{steel} = f_{aluminum\ base}\left[\frac{E_{steel}}{E_{aluminum}}\right]$$, see Eq. 2-15, p. 113

$$f_{aluminum} = f_{steel\ base}\left[\frac{E_{aluminum}}{E_{steel}}\right]$$, see Eq. 2-16, also from p. 113.

To study the application of this method to combined axial and bending of dissimilar materials, the following example is formulated to illustrate the procedure in detail.

Example 2-6 A stainless steel strap reinforcement (301 ½ hard) is mounted to the base of an aluminum I-beam (once again refer to Fig. 2-47). Given the following design internal loads, what are the maximum operating stresses for the different materials used for this structural member?

$P = -\ 17,000$ lb (compression)

$V = 8,000$ lb (see Chapter 4 for details pertaining to the design and analysis of beams subjected to shearing stresses)

$M = 2,000$ in-lb (this bending moment will produce compression on the right side of the vertical axis of bending of the section).

For stainless steel $E_c = 26.0 \times 10^6$ psi; for aluminum $E_c = 10.4 \times 10^6$ psi. Neglect the fillet areas of the extruded I-beam.

SOLUTION: There is essentially very little difference in the method of attack here compared with that of Example 2-5 of Sec. 2.7 (page 115). Using the method of transformations approach to solve this problem, the stainless steel reinforcement is transformed into equivalent aluminum base material. Only then can the geometric properties of the transformed section area be applied to the fundamental stress equations developed in this and previous sections of this chapter. In this example problem, inasmuch as the basic beam section bends about a vertical axis, the vertical dimension b of the steel reinforcement is transformed; however, the horizontal dimension h is not. This condition is required so that the original resisting moment of 2,000 in-lb will be appropriately duplicated across the entire cross-sectional area now containing the transformed steel material. Using Eqs. 2-18 and 2-19, the actual transformation of steel material into equivalent aluminum base material is performed. Here, the following equivalent dimensions are obtained:

$$b_B = b_D\left[\frac{E_D}{E_B}\right] = .080\left[\frac{26.0 \times 10^6}{10.4 \times 10^6}\right] = .200 \text{ in}$$

$$h_B = h_D = 2.10 \text{ in.}$$

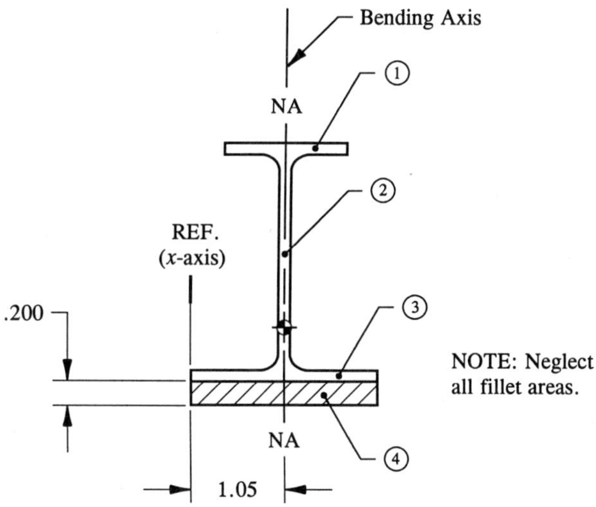

FIGURE 2-48 Cross-sectional area showing stainless steel reinforcement represented in equivalent aluminum base material.

From our earlier discussions of strain compatibility in this section, these values are also in agreement with axial compatibility requirements. Therefore, as such, no additional transformation of these dimensions is necessary. The transformed stainless steel reinforcement is shown cross-hatched in Fig. 2-48. In this form, the moment of inertia of the total cross-sectional area is computed (see Table 2-7 below).

TABLE 2-7 MOMENT OF INERTIA OF THE TOTAL CROSS-SECTIONAL AREA

Element	b	h	y	A	Ay	Ay^2	I_o
1	0.125	1.500	1.050	0.187	0.197	0.207	0.035
2	4.125	0.100	1.050	0.412	0.433	0.455	0.000
3	0.125	2.100	1.050	0.262	0.276	0.289	0.096
4	0.200	2.100	1.050	0.420	0.441	0.463	0.154
			Total	1.281	1.347	1.414	0.285

$$Y_{cg} = \frac{\Sigma\, Ay}{\Sigma\, A} = \frac{1.347}{1.281} = 1.052 \text{ in}$$

$$I_{cg} = \Sigma\, I_o + \Sigma\, Ay^2 - Y_{cg}\,(\Sigma\, Ay)$$

$$I_{cg} = .285 + 1.414 - 1.052(1.347) = .282 \text{ in}^4.$$

As is commonly acknowledged for elastic stress design,

$$Y_{na} = Y_{cg}$$

and therefore

$$I_{na} = I_{cg}.$$

These properties may now be substituted into Eq. 2-9 ($f = \pm P/A \pm Mc/I_{na}$) and the maximum combined axial and bending stresses of the entire cross-sectional area computed. Thus, we obtain:

Extreme fiber stresses on the left side of the bending axis of the beam:

$$f = \pm \frac{P}{A} \pm \frac{Mc}{I_{na}}$$

$$f_c = -\frac{17,000}{1.281} + \frac{2,000(1.052)}{.282} = -13,271 + 7,461$$

$$f_c = -5,810 \text{ psi} \quad \text{(true stress in the aluminum material)}.$$

Extreme fiber stresses on the right side of the bending axis of the beam:

$$f = \pm \frac{P}{A} \pm \frac{Mc}{I_{na}}$$

$$f_c = -\frac{17,000}{1.281} - \frac{2,000(2.10 - 1.052)}{.282} = -13,271 - 7,433$$

$$f_c = -20,704 \text{ psi} \quad \text{(true stress in the aluminum material)}.$$

These stresses are true stresses in the aluminum material but imaginary or fictitious stress values in the equivalent aluminum base material. To obtain the true stresses in the actual stainless steel material, Eq. 2-15 is applied. For easy reference, this equation is rewritten here below:

$$f_{\text{steel}} = f_{\text{aluminum base}} \left[\frac{E_{\text{steel}}}{E_{\text{aluminum}}} \right].$$

The formulation of this expression was derived in Section 2.7 of this book from strain compatibility requirements at the interface of dissimilar materials. Applying this equation here, the true stresses in the stainless steel reinforcement are found:

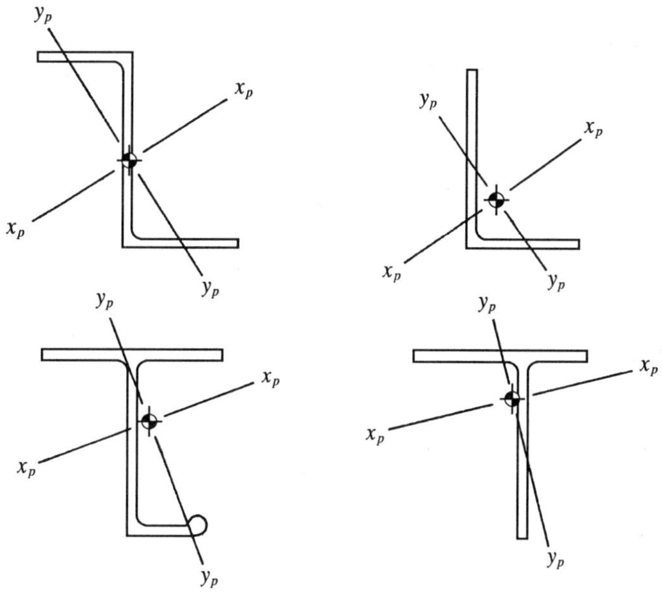

x_p = maximum principal moment of inertia
y_p = minimum principal moment of inertia
⌖ = centroid of area (or geometric center)

FIGURE 2-49 Principal bending axes of beam sections having no definite axes of symmetry.

Extreme fiber stresses on the left side of the bending axis of the beam:

$$f_c = -5{,}810\left[\frac{26.0 \text{ x } 10^6}{10.4 \text{ x } 10^6}\right]$$

$$f_c = -14{,}525 \text{ psi} \quad \text{(true stress in the steel material).}$$

Extreme fiber stresses on the right side of the bending axis of the beam:

$$f_c = -20{,}704\left[\frac{26.0 \text{ x } 10^6}{10.4 \text{ x } 10^6}\right]$$

$$f_c = -51{,}760 \text{ psi} \quad \text{(true stress in the steel material).}$$

This result completes the basic requirements and conditions of this problem: that of making stress computations. In the final analysis, though, the true stresses in the aluminum and steel materials are each compared to their respective yield compression stress allowables, unless, of course, a more critical design condition actually supersedes or prevents their use.

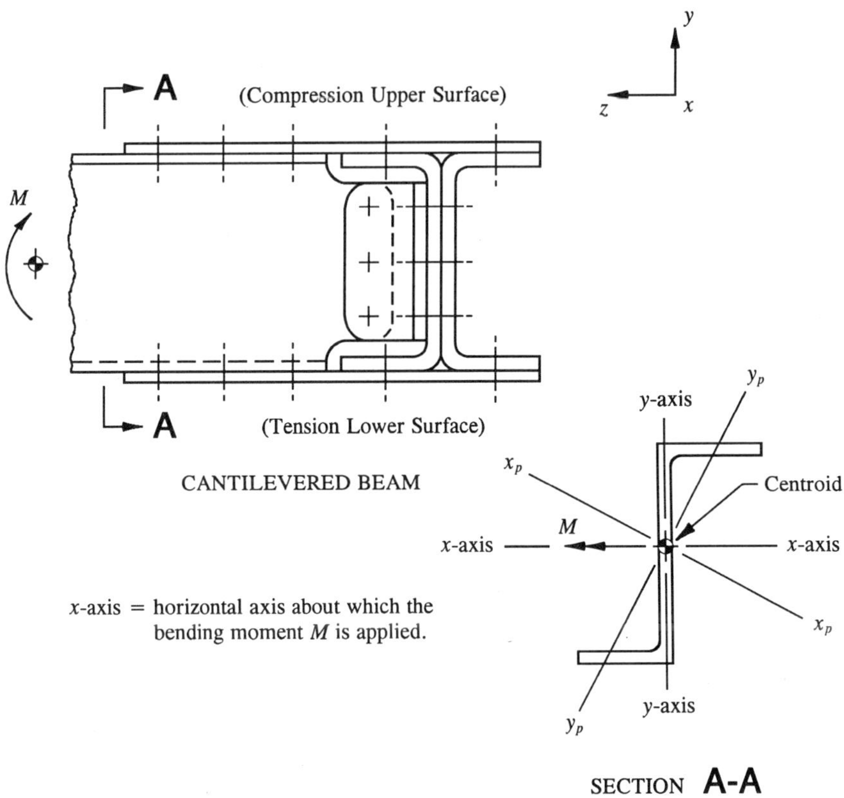

FIGURE 2-50 Section area of a cantilevered beam showing its principal axes of bending.

2.9 Axial and Bending Stresses of Beams That Bend in Two Different Planes. The limitations imposed thus far in the preceding sections of this book have been restricted to beam cross-sectional areas with at least one axis of symmetry (see complete details in Sec. 2.3, "Bending of Beams in One Plane"). While these limitations have been useful in the elementary discussions of bending fundamentals up to now, they are too restrictive and impractical to use in a wider range of beam design selections that are available for general aircraft usage. In order to expand on the concepts and principles of compound bending (beams that bend in two planes), these restrictions will be completely relaxed. The beam structure that will be illustrated in the example problem in this section will consider the more general case of a cross-sectional area having no definite axes of symmetry. Several cross-sectional areas that fit this general category are presented in Fig. 2-49.

It will therefore be the main emphasis of this section to determine the bending stresses that develop when beams having such cross-sectional areas are subjected to bending moments which do not lie in the planes of either of the principal

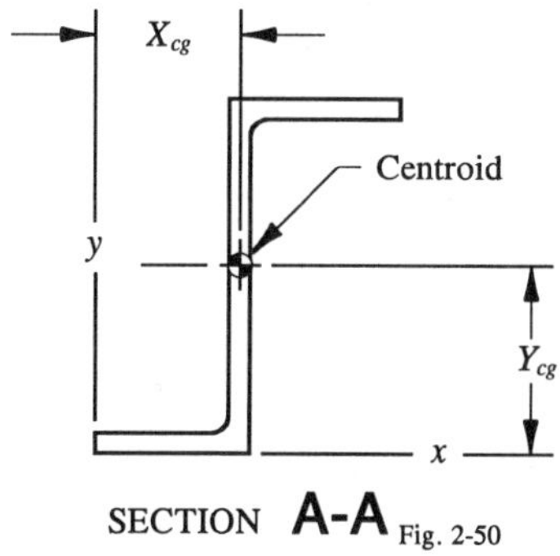

FIGURE 2-51 Cross-sectional area of a beam showing the location of the centroid.

bending axes[1]. The method of solution is rather straightforward, each bending moment is resolved into components that act in planes which contain the principal bending axes of the cross-sectional area. In this way, the well-known flexure formula ($f_b = \pm Mc/I_{na}$) as it applies to elastic stress design of beams can be fully utilized as a separate problem around each axis of bending. To illustrate this type of compound or multi-bending system, the cantilevered beam structure depicted in Fig. 2-50 is used. Note particularly that the cross-sectional area of the beam

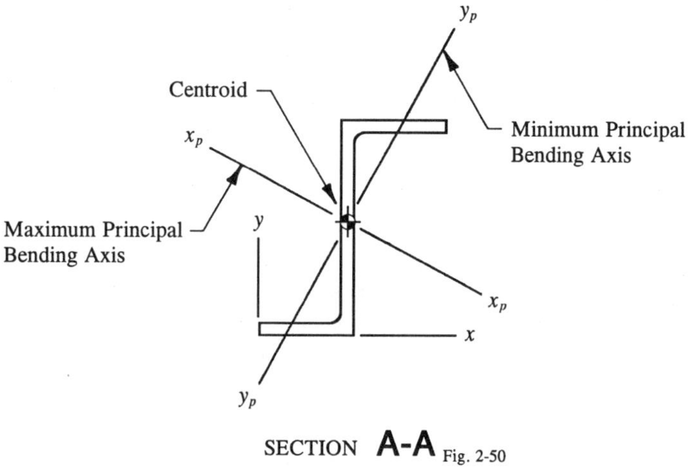

FIGURE 2-52 Cross-sectional area of a beam showing its principal axes of bending.

[1] Principal bending axes are those axes about which the maximum and minimum moments of inertia of a cross-sectional area are computed. Such axes are always mutually perpendicular. And, of course, these axes must also pass through the centroid of area of the member if the true bending stress distribution caused by these bending moments are to be accurately described for the structure.

(Section A-A in this figure) does not have an axis of symmetry. Nor does the applied bending moment M lie in planes coincident with the principal bending axes of the section. Instead, the bending moment is applied around the horizontal x-axis of the beam. To establish the true internal state of stress that will develop for such a member, the following step-by-step procedure is proposed and summarized below:

(1) Locate the center of gravity (centroid) of the cross-sectional area around an arbitrary chosen set of horizontal and vertical reference axes x and y, as shown in Fig. 2-51. This is most easily done using Eq. A-10 of Appendix F ($Y_{cg} = \Sigma Ay/\Sigma A$).

(2) Locate the principal bending axes x_p and y_p through the centroid of the cross-sectional area. Then calculate the principal moments of inertia I_{x_p} and I_{y_p} around these axes (see Appendix G, "Calculation of Principal Moments of Inertia," for explicit details of these computations). The principal bending axes are shown in Fig. 2-52.

(3) Resolve the applied bending moment M into equivalent component moments, $M_{x_p} = M \cos \beta$ and $M_{y_p} = M \sin \beta$, in planes coincident with the principal bending axes that pass through the centroid of area of the section. This can be viewed in Fig. 2-53, where the resolution of this bending moment is done in the same way as when a force is resolved into an equivalent system of component forces (Eqs. A-4 and A-5 in Appendix A, "Resolution of Forces," are used for this computation).

(4) In Fig. 2-54, the bending stress distributions across the entire section area for each component of bending are computed around the principal bending axes x_p and y_p using the flexure formula ($f_b = \pm Mc/I_{na}$) developed in Sec. 2.3. Each

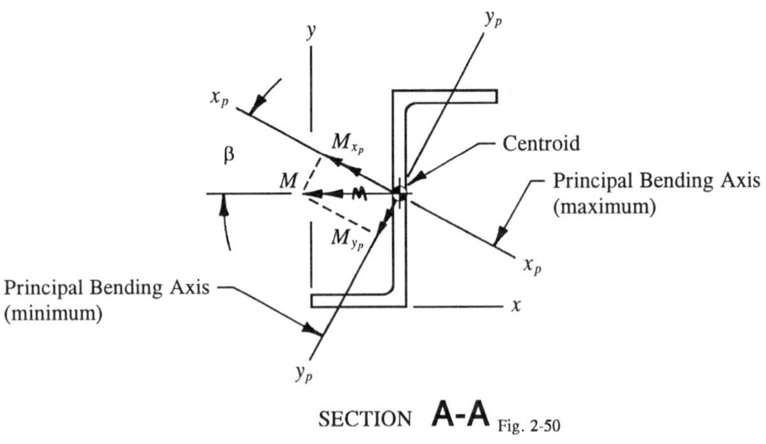

FIGURE 2-53 The moment M resolved into equivalent component moments acting in planes containing the principal bending axes.

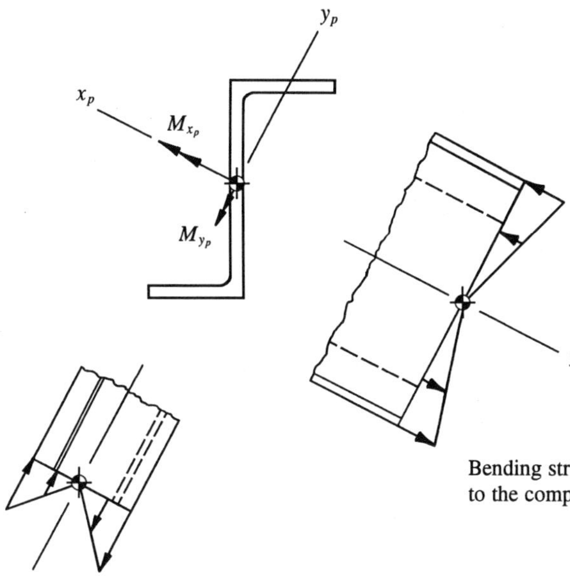

Bending stress distribution due to the component moment M_{x_p}.

Bending stress distribution due to the component moment M_{y_p}.

FIGURE 2-54 Bending stress distributions for the equivalent component moments.

separate stress calculation is then algebraically combined using the Principle of Superposition[1] as it relates to the design of elastic structural members. Thus, the following general expression is written for a compound bending system described in two different planes of bending:

$$f_b = \pm \frac{M_{x_p} c_{y_p}}{I_{x_p}} \pm \frac{M_{y_p} c_{x_p}}{I_{y_p}} \tag{2-20}$$

where: M_{x_p} and M_{y_p} = bending moments around the principal bending axes x_p and y_p, respectively

c_{x_p} and c_{y_p} = distances measured perpendicular from the principal bending axes x_p and y_p, respectively, to any point on the cross-sectional area being examined

I_{x_p} and I_{y_p} = moments of inertia around the principal bending axes x_p and y_p, respectively, passing through the centroid of area of the cross-sectional area.

---

[1] The justification for this principle asserts that the total stress of an elastic system due to several applied bending moments is the algebraic sum of their individual stresses when caused by each of the bending moments acting alone (see discussion in Chapter 1, Sec. 1.7, "Principle of Superposition").

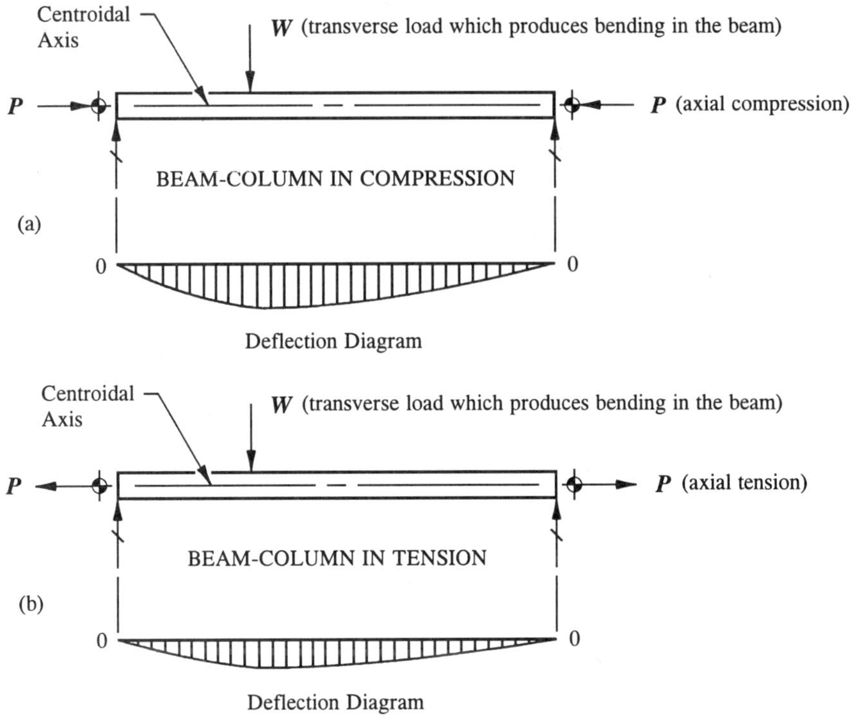

FIGURE 2-55 Beam-columns and their deflected shapes: (a) in compression and (b) in tension.

Next, the foregoing principles of compound bending are expanded to include the simultaneous application of axial normal stresses. The axial tension or compression stresses which they produce must be linearly related to the applied axial forces which caused these particular stresses. If such a system is to achieve elastic stress design implications, this condition must be met. All prior limitations, if applicable, must also be presumed.

Consider the beam-columns described in Fig. 2-55. In general, when such members are simultaneously subjected to axial tension or compression forces with bending loads, superposition of their separate effects, such as reactions, elastic stresses, deflections, etc., does not as a general rule or consequence necessarily apply. However, if the beam is laterally restrained from sidewise motion, then the effects from these loads acting separately on the structure can be superimposed. Theoretically, axial loads that are applied to the deflected shape of a laterally unsupported beam will induce additional (secondary) bending moments internally along the centroidal axis of the deflected structure. Mathematically, this is equivalent to the axial load P times the deflected shape of the beam. The secondary internal bending moments will then produce secondary deflections which in turn will produce more internal moments from the applied axial forces times the new deflected shape of the beam. This structural member is commonly referred to as a "beam-column," and all details pertaining to its design solution will be deferred to an advanced textbook on this subject.

In the remaining few paragraphs of this section, the limitations imposed on the use of "short" beam-column members will be specifically treated. Simply put, axial tension loads will tend to straighten a beam subjected to bending, and, as such, will cause a decrease in the internal bending moments that normally exist along that structural member. Conversely though, axial compression loads will have the opposite effect of producing higher values of internal bending moments while considerably increasing the deflected shape of the member. This latter occurrence is usually a more substantial loading condition for aircraft structures of this particular type. In any case, their suitability to production design hardware should be thoroughly perceived before such members are seriously contemplated in actual design use. In all cases, a severe weight penalty is usually the outcome if beam-column members are nevertheless decided upon for use in structural design situations.

If, however, certain restrictions pertaining to relatively "short members" are strictly enforced, their applications to aircraft structural designs can be routinely followed. That is, once the principles of superposition are appraised, and deemed permissible to use, the nature of short beam-column designs of the compression kind can be clearly administered, and their designs accurately evaluated by the generalized equations of this section. Conditionally, however, these compression members are judged in a manner which is consistent with the stability of their designs. Typically, such members must exhibit stability and nonbuckling characteristics under load. From the foregoing discussions, a more general expression may be formulated where axial normal stresses are simultaneously applied with compound bending stresses. This combination equation should yield adequate stress results for most short beam-column members of the compression or tension kind.

$$f = \pm \frac{P}{A} \pm \frac{M_{x_p} c_{y_p}}{I_{x_p}} \pm \frac{M_{y_p} c_{x_p}}{I_{y_p}}. \tag{2-21}$$

Collectively, they constitute the final stress picture. Notice the obvious similarities between this equation and Eq. 2-20.

It is important for the design engineer to understand all aspects of compound stress behavior so that he can relate and blend this knowledge into practical theories that can be useful in the study of other structural designs. One of the best ways to develop such a practical feel for the methods and principles of compound bending is by implementing these new ideas on an actual engineering structural design (see ahead to Example 2-7). Such a design will help to demonstrate the procedures and techniques outlined in this section while providing a good working model for industry-related problems. Whether or not the actual numerical calculations of this example or of any other similar types are necessarily performed in detail by the design engineer is irrelevant. What is important is knowing that the acquired skills and techniques to perform the detailed computations are learned and readily

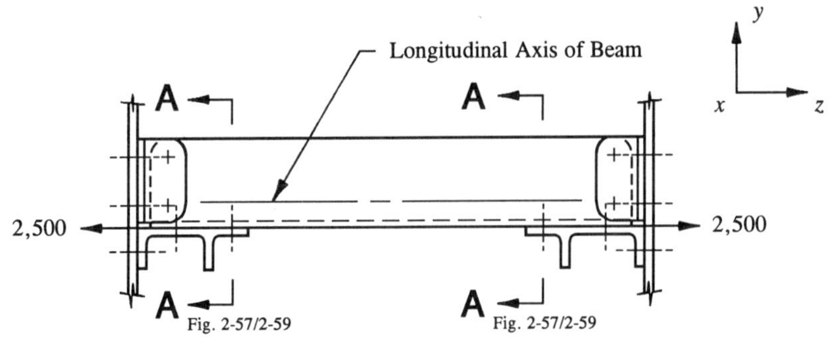

FIGURE 2-56 Eccentrically loaded beam. Axial tension force applied through the lower flanges of the beam.

available to use if the engineer is ever called upon to take a more active role in the analysis effort. The added difficulties which are encountered in the technical analysis of compound bending will probably contribute to some extent to the reevaluation of the final designed structure; unless that structure and its relation to the principles of this section are thoroughly understood.

Example 2-7 Consider the homogeneous beam structure in Fig. 2-56 in which an axial tension force of 2,500 lb is applied through the lower flanges of the beam. For this eccentrically loaded member, determine the critical combinations of tension and compression stresses as computed by Eq. 2-21. The rectangular coordinate system adopted for this beam is based on the principles of right-hand rule. Using these principles, the indicated direction of the x-axis can be properly designated by the index finger of the right-hand which goes into the plane of this page. And it is further assumed that stability and buckling are not primary influences in the overall design integrity of this member. Therefore, the member is not to be considered a beam-column, at least for this analysis.

SOLUTION: In general, wherever possible, the effects of eccentricities in actual design situations should be completely controlled by avoiding or at least minimizing their occurrences. This design practice should be considered foremost in the engineer's overall evaluation and selection of his design choices. If sheer avoidance is somewhat impractical or impossible to negotiate in certain design cases, the adverse effects realized from the additional bending loads that these eccentricities produce must be fully considered on their designs. Essentially, in our example problem here, since the axial tension force is not applied in line with the centroidal axis of the beam structure, an offset or eccentricity of load e will develop. The eccentricity is viewed on the surface of the cross-sectional area in Fig. 2-57. Its numerical value is measured from the centroid of the cross-sectional area to the point of application of the applied tension force. Only after the location of the centroid of area of the beam has been precisely defined can the magnitude of this

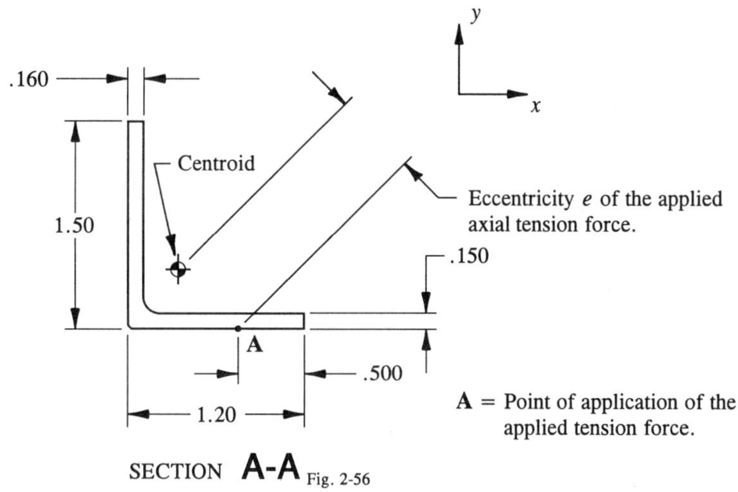

FIGURE 2-57 Eccentricity measured from the centroid of the cross-sectional area to the point of application of the applied tension force.

eccentricity be accurately measured. Until then, all computations will be performed in terms of this unknown value.

The usual conventional methods of internal loads analysis are employed in the solution of this example problem.[1] A section cut is passed through the cross-sectional area of the beam at Section A-A (Fig. 2-56) perpendicular to the longitudinal axis of the member. The isolated beam segments to either side of the section cut are then separated and the internal forces *V, P,* and *M* required to establish equilibrium are determined. This is shown in Fig. 2-58. For this example, the left-hand segment is chosen for the actual computation of these quantities. The proper orientation of these same loads on the right-hand segment will follow directly from the basic definitions of compatibility of internal loads at this section.

Now, utilizing the equations of static equilibrium, the internal forces necessary to balance the left-hand segment of this beam are computed:

$$\Sigma F_y = 0, \qquad V = 0$$

$$\Sigma F_z = 0, \qquad -2,500 + P = 0, \quad P = 2,500 \text{ lb}$$

$$\Sigma M_{cg} = 0, \qquad \circlearrowleft\!+ \; 2,500(e) - M = 0, \quad M = 2,500(e) \text{ in-lb.}^2$$

From this result, and considering the homogeneous construction of this beam, it is evident that the internal loads *V, P,* and *M* are constant values along the entire

[1] For a review of these principles, the engineer is referred to Chapter 1, Sec. 1.5, "Method of Sections Approach to Internal Loads Analysis."

[2] Note how similar the moment expression here resembles that of the basic definition used to define a bending moment (see Chapter 1, Eq. 1-1, $M = Fd$).

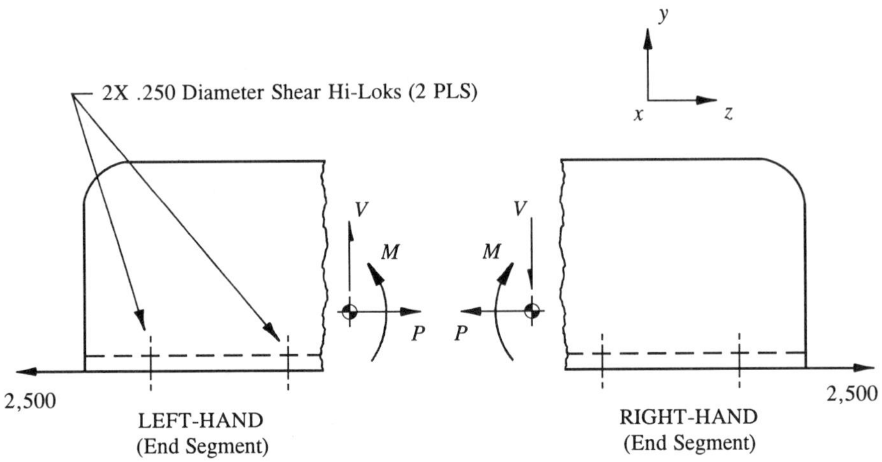

FIGURE 2-58 System of internal forces shown on exposed sections of the beam.

length of the beam structure. To verify this generalization, the same internal loads analysis can be performed, but this time, at several other sections along the beam structure. Looking ahead to Fig. 2-60, it can be seen that this moment will act in a plane indicated by the moment vector M. Also shown in that same figure are the equivalent component moments M_{x_p} and M_{y_p} which must appropriately act around the principal bending axes x_p and y_p of the cross-sectional area, respectively. Clearly, the application of the equations of static equilibrium has demonstrated how an eccentrically applied tension force can effectively be carried (across any section) by the structural member itself. Before the magnitude of this moment can be evaluated, however, the eccentricity $\boldsymbol{e}$ must first be found. To accomplish this, the tabulation method of Appendix F is employed using the unshaded areas of Section A-A. The element areas assigned for this section are shown in Fig. 2-59. The actual computations are performed in Tables 2-8 and 2-9.

TABLE 2-8 MOMENT OF INERTIA I_x AROUND THE $\bar{x}$-AXIS

Element	b	h	y	A	Ay	Ay^2	I_o
1	0.160	1.350	0.825	0.216	0.178	0.147	0.033
2	0.825	0.150	0.075	0.124	0.009	0.001	0.000
3	0.250	0.150	0.075	- 0.037	- 0.003	- 0.000	- 0.000
4	0.375	0.150	0.075	0.056	0.004	0.000	0.000
			Total	0.359	0.188	0.148	0.033

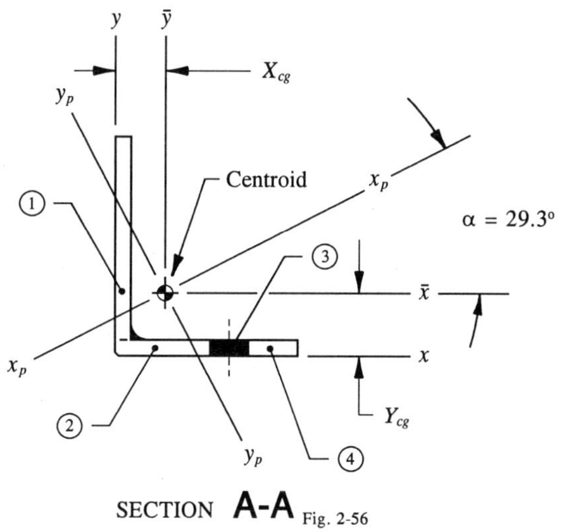

FIGURE 2-59 Beam section area. Shaded areas (fillet and fastener hole) are assumed ineffective.

$$Y_{cg} = \frac{\Sigma Ay}{\Sigma A} = \frac{.188}{.359} = .524 \text{ in}$$

$$I_x = I_{cg} = \Sigma I_o + \Sigma Ay^2 - Y_{cg}(\Sigma Ay)$$
$$I_x = .033 + .148 - .524(.188) = .082 \text{ in}^4.$$

TABLE 2-9 MOMENT OF INERTIA I_y AROUND THE $\bar{y}$-AXIS

Element	b	h	x	A	Ax	Ax^2	I_o
1	1.350	0.160	0.080	0.216	0.017	0.001	0.000
2	0.150	0.825	0.412	0.124	0.051	0.021	0.007
3	0.150	0.250	0.700	- 0.037	- 0.026	- 0.018	- 0.000
4	0.150	0.375	1.012	0.056	0.057	0.058	0.001
			Total	0.359	0.099	0.062	0.008

$$X_{cg} = \frac{\Sigma Ax}{\Sigma A} = \frac{.099}{.359} = .276 \text{ in}$$

$$I_y = I_{cg} = \Sigma I_o + \Sigma Ax^2 - X_{cg}(\Sigma Ax)$$
$$I_y = .008 + .062 - .276(.099) = .043 \text{ in}^4.$$

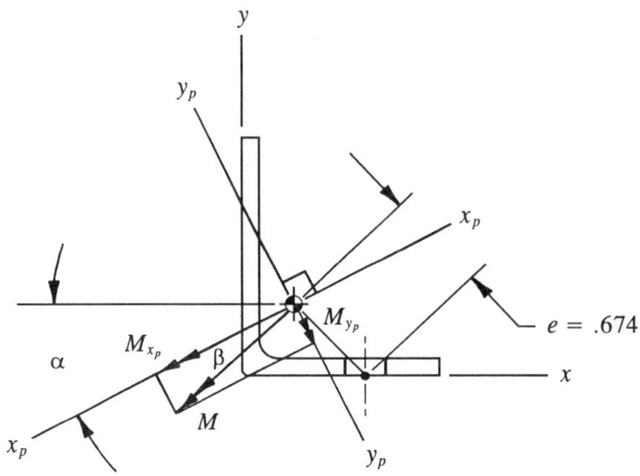

FIGURE 2-60 The moment M resolved into equivalent component moments acting in planes containing the principal bending axes.

The basic theory of holes in a tension stress field, as described in Sec. 2.2, asserts that whenever fasteners are used in a tension joint application, the holes they introduce into the basic structure are ineffective in resisting the applied tension forces. The higher stresses caused by the slight weakening effect of the structure by these holes are determined by using the net cross-sectional area of the beam. This condition will govern the structural adequacy of our particular design example at Section A-A. Note that at all other locations along the beam structure, the combination of computed stresses should be slightly below these apparent critical values. Precluding instability and buckling effects, this beam is designed by the most critical combinations of either maximum compression stresses or maximum tension stresses, or both. This occurs at the most critical section areas of the member.

Now, having located the centroid of this section area, the eccentricity e of the applied tension force can be determined. The numerical details of this computation, however, are left as an exercise for the engineer to complete. The predetermined value of e is .674 in. With this value, the magnitude of the internal bending moment M may also be computed. This gives:

$$M = 2,500(e) = 2,500(.674) = 1,685 \text{ in-lb}.$$

This moment is now resolved into two equivalent components M_{x_p} and M_{y_p} which act in planes containing the principal bending axes x_p and y_p, respectively:

$$M_{x_p} = M \cos \beta$$
$$M_{y_p} = M \sin \beta.$$

This corresponds to Fig. 2-60. The proper orientation of the principal bending axes and their corresponding principal moments of inertia are computed using Eqs. A-10 through A-13 of Appendix G as follows:

$$
\begin{aligned}
(1)\quad I_{xy} &= \Sigma Axy - AX_{cg}Y_{cg} \\
&= .216(.080)(.825) + .124(.412)(.075) - .037(.700)(.075) \\
&\quad + .056(1.012)(.075) - .359(.276)(.524) \\
&= .014 + .004 - .002 + .004 - .052 \\
I_{xy} &= -\ .032 \text{ in}^4.
\end{aligned}
$$

$$
\begin{aligned}
(2)\quad \tan 2\alpha &= \frac{2I_{xy}}{I_y - I_x} = \frac{2(-.032)}{.043 - .082} = 1.641 \\
2\alpha &= \tan^{-1} 1.641 = 58.6^\circ \\
\alpha &= 29.3^\circ.
\end{aligned}
$$

$$
\begin{aligned}
(3)\quad I_{x_p} &= I_x \cos^2\alpha + I_y \sin^2\alpha - I_{xy}\sin 2\alpha \\
&= .082(.872)^2 + .043(.489)^2 - (-.032)(.854) \\
&= .062 + .010 + .027 \\
I_{x_p} &= .099 \text{ in}^4 \quad \text{(maximum principal moment of inertia)}.
\end{aligned}
$$

$$
\begin{aligned}
(4)\quad I_{y_p} &= I_x \sin^2\alpha + I_y \cos^2\alpha + I_{xy}\sin 2\alpha \\
&= .082(.489)^2 + .043(.872)^2 + (-.032)(.854) \\
&= .020 + .033 - .027 \\
I_{y_p} &= .026 \text{ in}^4 \quad \text{(minimum principal moment of inertia)}.
\end{aligned}
$$

With the basic dimensions of this cross-sectional area properly described, and the value of α known,[1] the angle β is found to be 9.7°. The actual proof of this is left for the engineer's own verification. Substituting the angle β into the two expressions for component moments gives:

$$
\begin{aligned}
M_{x_p} &= M\cos\beta = 1,685 \cos 9.7^\circ = 1,661 \text{ in-lb} \\
M_{y_p} &= M\sin\beta = 1,685 \sin 9.7^\circ = 284 \text{ in-lb}.
\end{aligned}
$$

The remaining solution is essentially divided into two separate bending solutions using the component moments around each of their respective principal bending axes of the cross-sectional area. According to Eq. 2-21, the computed stresses of each solution are then superimposed together with the corresponding axial stresses. For easy reference, this equation is rewritten as follows:

[1] A positive angle for this quantity is measured counterclockwise between the centroidal and principal axes.

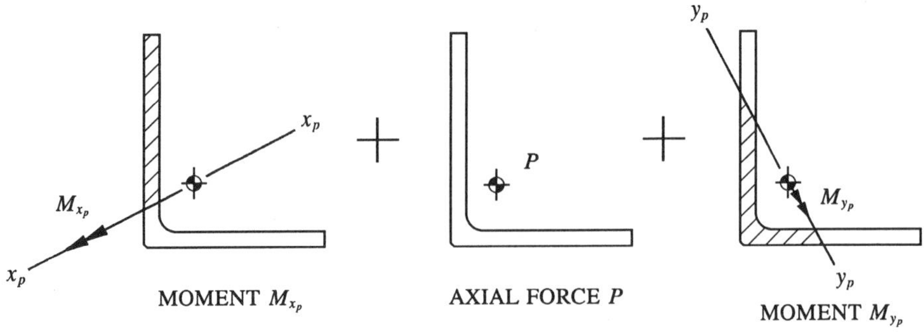

FIGURE 2-61 Diagram shows stresses that are produced on the surface of a cross-sectional area for different loading types. Compression stresses are shown cross-hatched, while areas in tension are not.

$$f = \pm \frac{P}{A} \pm \frac{M_{x_p} c_{y_p}}{I_{x_p}} \pm \frac{M_{y_p} c_{x_p}}{I_{y_p}}.$$

The proper sense of each computed stress, + for tension and – for compression, is determined by the particular effect each stress will produce on the surface of the cross-sectional area. This is observed in Fig. 2-61 for each separate loading case. The compression stresses are shown cross-hatched on the cross-sectional area, while areas in tension are not. The final state of stress is accurately described by algebraically combining the individual stresses at different points on the cross-sectional area. The process of finding the maximum compression and tension stresses is an extremely tedious one; determination is usually accomplished by trial and error.

It is hoped that from this relatively straightforward approach to the solution of this problem will emerge a better understanding and knowledge of the theoretical concepts of compound bending. From the general theories, direct implementation of basic concepts and principles to the structural behavior of similar or related members can directly be made. Of course, it is particularly prudent for each design engineer to mentally review in advance all of the different aspects and assumptions required of a particular design before initiating the actual detailed analysis effort.

Once the basic techniques of compound bending and the particular details of its application to the solution of this example are clearly understood, it should then be quite easy to extend these principles to the analysis of other compound bending solutions. Before doing so, however, all the design factors associated with their implementation should be accurately perceived and explored by taking certain initial design steps to simplify their construction. If we have some idea of at least the approximate level of behavior of the structure under load, we can avoid some of the more serious ambiguities associated with their solutions.

Realistically, compound bending solutions are perhaps too long for the practicing design engineer to perform as a normal daily routine. Nevertheless, the processes of understanding what is "perceived" is certainly useful to our basic understanding of more complicated problems. In most cases, the amount of original thinking you acquire is a function of previously learned skills. Therefore, it is exceedingly important to be able to generalize by logic and inferences if careful observations of factual data to conclusions are not to be ultimately confused.

2.10 Problem for Solution. Perform a complete stress analysis solution for the beam loaded as shown in Fig. 2-62. The analysis should include: (1) a complete free-body diagram of the structure, (2) shear and bending moment diagrams, (3) calculation of maximum bending stresses using Eq. 2-5, (4) margins of safety in tension and compression, (5) a list of assumptions and approaches to the solution

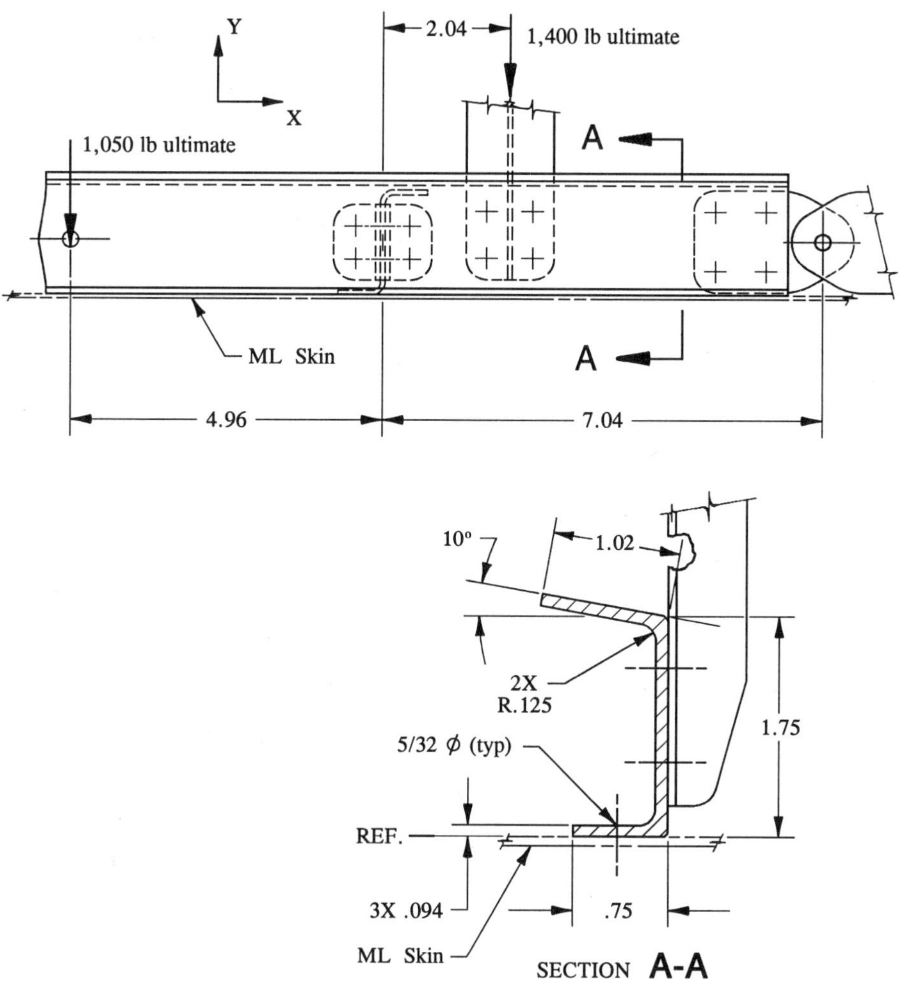

FIGURE 2-62 Spanner beam and sectional area detail.

of this problem, (6) calculation of moment of inertia by approximation—neglecting the 10-degree slope of the upper flange, and (7) calculation of maximum bending stresses by approximation. (*Hint:* Again calculate maximum bending stresses, but this time, use Eq. A-7, page 623, with each effective chord cross-sectional area.) Consider the extruded member made of 2024-T3 aluminum alloy material (QQ-A-200/3) and a design load factor of 1.5. Assume the skin is nonstructural.

CHAPTER 3

Connection Analysis

3.1 Introduction. In this chapter, the structural methods of analysis of mechanically fastened connections are studied. Their practical applications to aircraft design are many, particularly where a load is transferred from one structural member to another. There are two basic joint arrangements that make up a connection design: the single-shear lap joint and the double-shear lap joint, as shown in Figs. 3-1 and 3-2, respectively. From these, a multitude of other design configurations are possible to construct for general aircraft usage: such as shear clips, brackets, web splices, support fittings, backup fittings, and various types of reinforcement members that are used in conjunction with the repair and modification of in-service flight vehicle structures.

It is the subject of this chapter therefore to examine these and other similar types of configurations as they relate specifically to the structural design behavior of commonly used aircraft joint designs. The standard method of analysis that is predominantly used by the aerospace industry in the solution of connection designs will be the preferred method of analysis of this chapter. The application of this method to industry-related aircraft designs is fully discussed and illustrated in the many example problems contained within this chapter. The structural methods and approaches used to solve these problems should provide the design engineer with a step-by-step procedure to a dependable solution of most related or similar joint designs encountered in actual aircraft structure. Each solution is optimized according to the required number and size of fasteners and the proper selection of sheet or plate material for its particular design configuration.

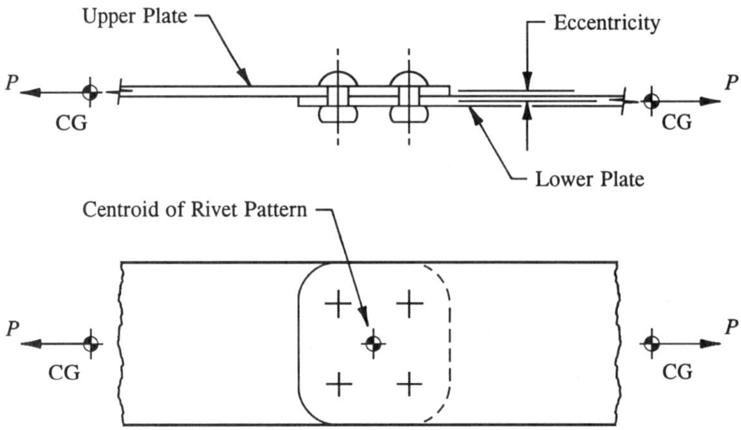

FIGURE 3-1 Single-shear lap joint.

Since double-shear lap joints are composed of three or more plate-like members, they are usually of a heavier type of construction than the lighter weight two-plate lap joint varieties. But since lap joints develop eccentricities of their load paths from the overlapping nature of their design configurations, the double-shear lap joint is the preferred design alternative of the two basic joint arrangements described. This condition can be clearly seen from the side view drawn of the lap joint arrangement shown in Fig. 3-1. The inherent eccentricity or offset that exists for this joint is measured (perpendicularly) between the lines of action of the plate forces. For most commercial and military aircraft, such irregularities in joint

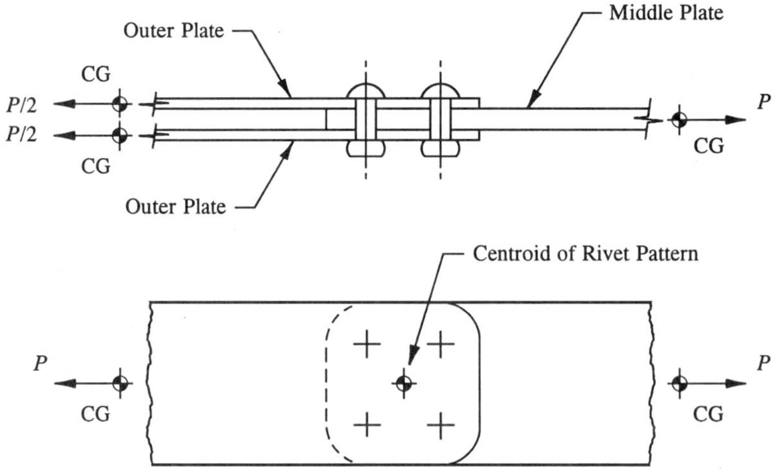

FIGURE 3-2 Double-shear lap joint.

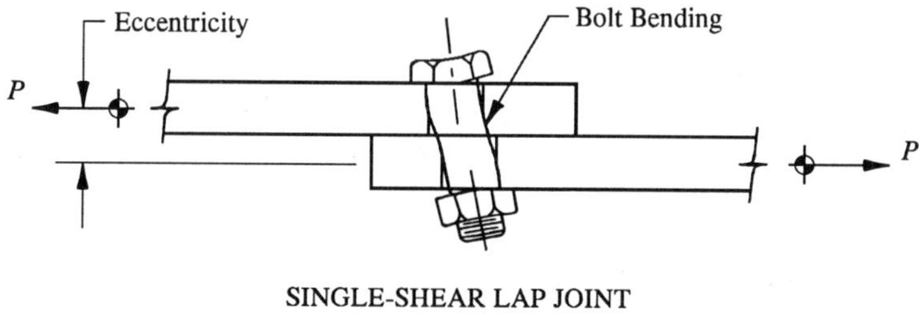

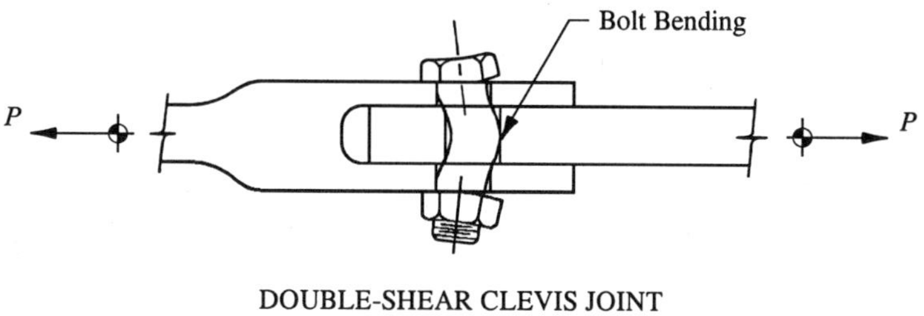

FIGURE 3-3 Bolt bending: (a) in a single-shear lap joint and (b) in a double-shear clevis joint.

designs are fully deliberated and taken into account by applying a prescribed fitting factor.

In general, if relatively thin plate-like members of either the single-shear lap or double-shear lap joint varieties are used, the local bending effect on the joint fasteners arising from the eccentricities and anomalies of their designs can be completely ignored, and therefore, disregarded from analytical consideration. Careful deliberation of thick plate-like members, however, reveals that, although a fitting factor may be applied, bending of the joint fasteners in these cases cannot be neglected. Their damaging effects must be fully considered if the effects of binding and jamming of fasteners in their holes are to be prevented. The undesirable consequences of such a design, commonly referred to as "bolt bending," should be avoided under normal operating flight and landing conditions.[1] See Fig. 3-3 for an actual detailed description of this joint tendency. Equilibrium forces for the bolts are determined from the deflected shape of the bolts under load.

Static tests of single bolt fittings have shown that joint failures are principally due to failure of the lugs. However, it is bolt bending which causes the peak bearing stresses to develop on the lugs that precipitates the lugs to fail. Additionally, it is important to provide sufficient bending strength for the bolt to prevent permanent bending deformation of the bolt at limit load. In this way, the bolts can easily be removed from the structure during routine maintenance operations.

[1] For specific details of their solutions, the engineer is referred to M.A. Melcon and F.M. Hoblit, *Product Engineering*, "Developments in the Analysis of Lugs and Shear Pins," 1953, pp. 160-170.

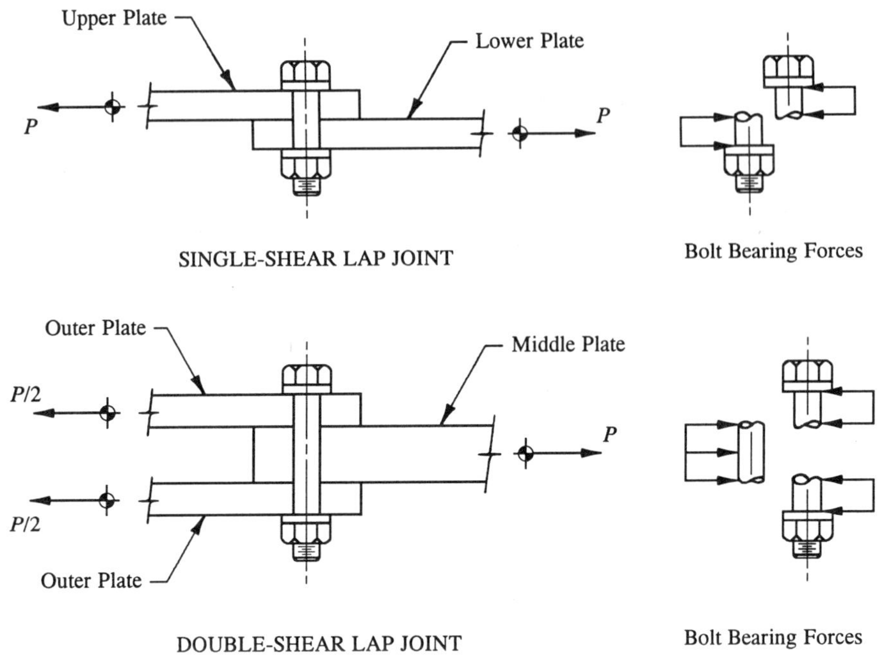

FIGURE 3-4 Joint shear failures: (a) in a single-shear lap joint and (b) in a double-shear lap joint.

3.2 Strength Criteria for Mechanically Fastened Connections. The strength of a mechanically fastened joint is governed by a complement of ultimate joint failures which can occur by shearing and tension failures of the fastener, tension and compression failures of the plate, and bearing, shearing and tearing failures of the sheet or plate material. Each possible mode of failure must be carefully reviewed and investigated by the analyst to assure the structural reliability and integrity of the joint design. Before the structural methods of analysis of Secs. 3.3 and 3.4 are presented, the following strength criteria established for the design of a mechanically fastened connection are defined:

Ultimate Allowable Shearing Strength P_{su} of a Solid, Protruding-Head Rivet:

The shearing failure that occurs for fasteners of both the single-shear lap joint and double-shear lap joint configurations are shown in Fig. 3-4. In either case, the bearing pressures that are developed by the plate forces bearing up against the fastener are assumed to be uniformly distributed along the fastener. Since most metals used in aircraft joint designs will exhibit some ductile behavior of their materials, this simplified distribution is completely justified, and should prove sufficiently accurate to use in the analysis of mechanically fastened connections at ultimate flight and landing conditions. Such is the case when stresses occur above the elastic limit of the material.

A riveted or bolted connection is primarily designed to transfer shear through its joint fasteners from one structural member to another. It is therefore the "transfer of force" that is resisted by the shear area or areas of a fastener. For a single-shear lap joint, only one shear area or A_{shr} is provided by each fastener to overcome this transfer of force. In the case of a double-shear lap joint, however, two shear areas or 2 A_{shr} are resisted by each joint fastener. In effect, it can be said that the fastener of a double-shear joint has approximately twice the strength or capacity of that same fastener if used in a single-shear joint application.

To identify the plate and fastener internal forces of a single-shear lap or double-shear lap joint, it is helpful to recognize and understand the transfer of forces that occur within the actual joint arrangement. For purposes of illustration, therefore, Fig. 3-4 will again be used, but this time, to physically describe the internal transfer forces that occur for individual members that make up both lap joint designs. In the case of a single-shear lap joint, the internal force P of one plate is transferred directly to the fastener by bearing pressure from the plate onto the fastener. The bearing pressure is then transferred along the fastener to bearing pressure resisted by the other plate. The same basic line of reasoning can be explained for a double-shear lap joint configuration. Here, the internal force P of the middle plate is also transferred to the fastener by bearing pressure from the plate onto the fastener. But, then, the bearing pressure divides along the fastener to bearing pressures on the outer plates. If identical outer plates are used, the bearing pressure of the middle plate will divide equally between the outer plates or ½P, as viewed in this figure.[1]

The ultimate allowable shearing strength of a solid, protruding-head rivet in either a single-shear or double-shear joint application, expressed in pounds (lb), is defined by the following expression:

$$P_{su} = F_{su} A_{shr} C_r \tag{3-1}$$

where: $A_{shr} = \frac{\pi}{4} D^2$ for single-shear joints; and $2A_{shr}$ for double-shear joints

F_{su} = ultimate shear stress of the rivet material (see Table 3-1 for conventional rivet types)

D = nominal hole diameter (see Table 3-1 for standard values based on the drill size of a rivet)

C_r = shear strength correction factor (see Table 3-2 for appropriate tabulated values for single-shear and double-shear joints).

---

[1] If the outer plates are of different thicknesses, distribution of plate forces is achieved from axial stiffness considerations. Here, this simply means that the bearing pressure will divide in proportion to the plate cross-sectional areas.

TABLE 3-1 ULTIMATE ALLOWABLE SHEAR STRENGTH P_{su} OF SOLID, PROTRUDING-HEAD RIVETS*

Diameter of Rivet				1/16	3/32	1/8	5/32	3/16	1/4	5/16	3/8
Drill Number				51	41	30	21	11	F	P	W
Nominal Hole Diameter				0.067	0.096	0.1285	0.159	0.191	0.257	0.323	0.386
Rivet Standard	Rivet Code	Rivet Material	Rivet Ultimate Shear Stress (psi)	Shear Strength, P_{su} (lb)†							
MS 20470 B		5056-H321	28,000	99	203	363	556	802	1450	2295	3275
MS 20470 AD	BJ	2117-T3	30,000	106	217	388	596	862	1555	2460	3510
		2017-T31	34,000	120	247	442	675	977	1765	2785	3980
MS 20470 D		2017-T3	38,000	134	275	494	755	1090	1970	3115	4445
MS 20470 DD	CX	2024-T31	41,000	145	296	531	814	1175	2125	3360	4800
		7050-T731	43,000	152	311	558	854	1230	2230	3525	5030
MS 20615 M	LN	Monel	49,000	173	355	635	973	1405	2540	4015	5735
		Ti-45Cb	53,000	187	384	687	1050	1520	2750	4340	6200
NAS 1198	MM	A-286	90,000	317	651	1170	1790	2580	4670	7370	10500

* Reference MIL-HDBK-5F, Tables 8.1.2(a) and 8.1.2(b).

† Shear strength values are based on shear areas of rivets computed using the nominal hole diameters specified above ($A_{shr} = \pi D^2/4$, where D = nominal hole diameter).

TABLE 3-2 SHEAR STRENGTH CORRECTION FACTORS C_r FOR SOLID, PROTRUDING-HEAD RIVETS*

Diameter of Rivet (in)	1/16	3/32	1/8	5/32	3/16	1/4	5/16	3/8
	Single-Shear Strength Correction Factors							
Sheet Thickness† (in)								
0.016	0.964							
0.018	0.981	0.912						
0.020	0.995	0.933				unacceptable regions		
0.025	1.000	0.970	0.920			of design		
0.032		1.000	0.964	0.925				
0.036			0.981	0.946	0.912			
0.040			0.995	0.964	0.933			
0.045			1.000	0.981	0.953			
0.050				0.995	0.970	0.920		
0.063				1.000	1.000	0.961	0.922	
0.071						0.979	0.944	0.909
0.080						0.995	0.964	0.933
0.090						1.000	0.981	0.953
0.100							0.995	0.972
0.125							1.000	1.000
	Double-Shear Strength Correction Factors							
0.016	0.687							
0.018	0.744	0.518						
0.020	0.789	0.585				unacceptable regions		
0.025	0.870	0.708	0.545			of design		
0.032	0.941	0.814	0.687	0.560				
0.036	0.969	0.857	0.744	0.630	0.518			
0.040	0.992	0.891	0.789	0.687	0.585			
0.045	1.000	0.924	0.834	0.744	0.653			
0.050		0.951	0.870	0.789	0.708	0.545		
0.063		1.000	0.937	0.872	0.808	0.679	0.550	
0.071			0.966	0.909	0.852	0.737	0.622	0.508
0.080			0.992	0.941	0.891	0.789	0.687	0.585
0.090			1.000	0.969	0.924	0.834	0.744	0.653
0.100				0.992	0.951	0.870	0.789	0.708
0.125				1.000	1.000	0.935	0.870	0.805
0.160						0.992	0.941	0.891
0.190						1.000	0.981	0.939
0.250							1.000	1.000

Note: Linear or graphical interpolation of shear strength correction factors between sheet thicknesses not given in Table 3-2 is entirely permissible. However, in no case should extrapolated values be taken above D/t values of 5.5, where D = rivet diameter and t = sheet thickness.

* Reference MIL-HDBK-5F, Table 8.1.2.1(b).

† Sheet thickness is that of the thinner sheet in single-shear lap joints and the middle sheet in double-shear lap joints. All values are based on tests of aluminum rivets.

Shearing failure is then predicted by making the following load comparison:

$$\text{Margin of Safety} = \text{M.S.} = \frac{P_{su}}{p_s k} - 1$$

where p_s = ultimate shearing force of a fastener due to the applied force P (use the full load or $p_s = P$ when analyzing a fastener in either a single-shear lap joint or a double-shear lap joint) and k = fitting factor[1] for joint design (use 1.15 for commercial and military flight vehicles).

For a multi-riveted connection, however, fastener shearing force distributions are expressed in accordance with the structural methods and techniques developed in Sec. 3.3, "Concentrically Loaded Connections" (see ahead to Eqs. 3-9, 3-10, and 3-11 of that section for explicit details of joint fastener load distributions). Whenever protruding-head rivet shear strengths are used, their values must be computed by multiplying the shear strength of the rivet given in Table 3-1 by the correction factors listed in Table 3-2. This accounts for the reduction of rivet shear strength resulting from high bearing stresses that develop from the knife-edge effect of thin sheet thicknesses on solid, protruding-head rivet shanks.[2] Also, the effective shear and bearing areas of hole-filling fasteners (or rivets) should be based on the nominal hole diameter of the rivets, as prescribed by MIL-HDBK-5. This is usually a standard value for rivets based on drill size (see values listed in Table 3-1).

Equation 3-1 is valid only for solid, protruding-head rivets. For all other types of fasteners, which include countersunk rivets, lockbolts, jo-bolts, screws, hi-loks, etc., joint fastener allowables P_{su} are based on prescribed company and government agency specifications. These publications list the allowables of many preferred fasteners in various alloy materials in terms of their static joint strengths. The reason for confirmatory test data to substantiate fastener joint strength allowables is that sometimes, especially in thin members, fasteners will not develop their full shear strength allowables in the materials in which they are installed. For this reason, to determine the true strength of a mechanically fastened joint, the allowable joint strength properties of a fastener must be established when that fastener is in its installed condition. The engineer is referred specifically to MIL-HDBK-5, Sec. 8, for the static joint strength allowables of fasteners when installed in various thicknesses of different materials. Many more joint fastener allowables are also available and documented by aerospace and military standards (i.e., MS, NAS, AN), and by certain manufacturers which establish proprietary fastener specifications.

Rivets under primary tension loads should not be used in structural design applications; however, secondary tension loads on rivets, if they occur, are

---

[1] A fitting factor may not be required for commercial and military aircraft when static testing is used to substantiate the basic structure.

[2] This corresponds to the established criteria in MIL-HDBK-5 for D/t values greater than 3 for single-shear joints and 1.5 for double-shear joints, where D is the nominal hole diameter and t is the sheet thickness.

permissible if their effects are fully considered. For example, secondary rivet tension loads are most prevalent in "diagonal-tension webs" where the web or sheet panel under load is allowed to buckle. The buckled state of the web, in effect, induces tension loads into the rivets supporting the panel that fasten together the panel and its boundary of support members.

Inter-rivet buckling between rivets is also another condition where rivet tension is considered incidental to the main shear load-carrying ability of the rivets (see Sec. 6.2, "Inter-Rivet Buckling of Compression Members"). If secondary tension loads on rivets do occur, the following rule-of-thumb criteria are recommended for their ultimate design:

FOR SOLID, PROTRUDING-HEAD RIVETS:

$$P_{tu} = \tfrac{2}{3} P_{su}$$

where: P_{tu} = ultimate allowable tensile strength
P_{su} = ultimate allowable shear strength (from Eq. 3-1).

FOR COUNTERSUNK, SOLID-HEAD RIVETS:

$$P_{tu} = \tfrac{1}{2} P_{su}$$

where: P_{tu} = ultimate allowable tensile strength
P_{su} = ultimate allowable shear strength (from MIL-HDBK-5, MS, NAS, AN, etc.).

A final note should also be mentioned about mechanically fastened joints consisting of a mixed pattern of attachments, such as rivets and bolts, rivets and screws, etc. In few words, they should be avoided in the same common joints or connections. Rivets are hole-filling fasteners and therefore should provide a better fit in the holes than bolts. In theory, the rivets load up first, even yield, until they have deflected enough to cause the clearance between the bolts and the bolt holes to diminish and thus begin loading the bolts. Because of this, a mixed fastener pattern of rivets and bolts tends to overload the rivets before the bolts have begun to load. In some cases, the rivets may even fail prematurely. To minimize this occurrence, close tolerance bolts should be contemplated in mixed fastener patterns.

Ultimate Allowable Bearing Strength P_{bru} of a Plate or Fastener:

Failure of a connection can occur in bearing when a fastener crushes or deforms the material of the plate caused by the bearing pressures that build up between the fastener and the plate. This type of failure is viewed in Fig. 3-5. Conversely, though, if the fastener is made of a weaker material (that is, of a lower

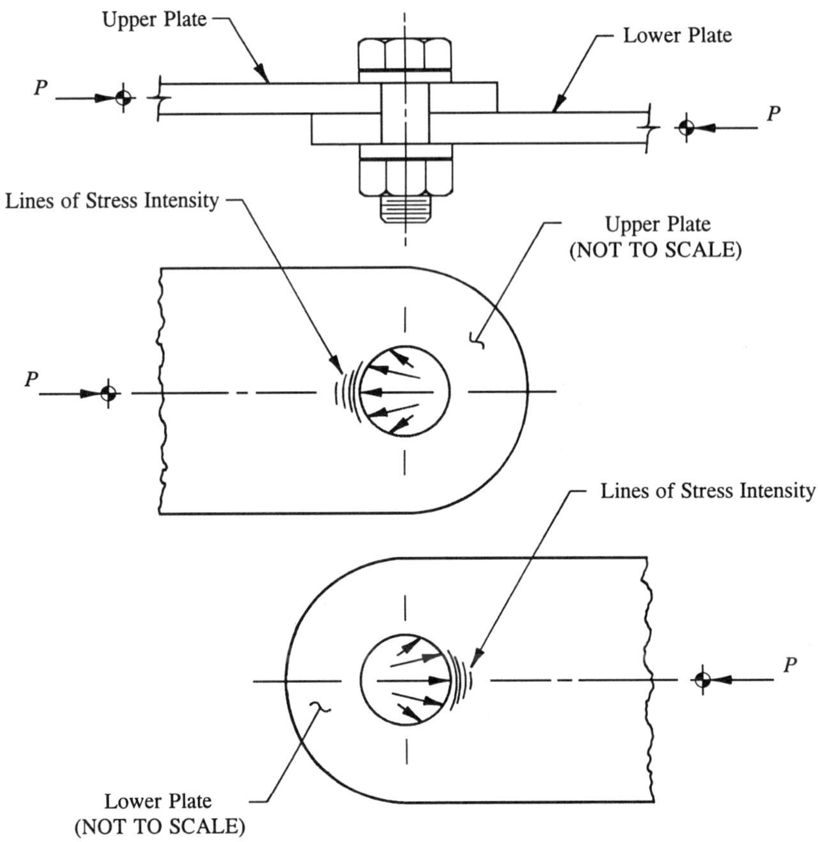

FIGURE 3-5 Diagram shows cylindrical bearing stress distribution.

bearing stress allowable F_{bru} than that of the connection plates), bearing failure will occur to the fastener before the plates. If this is the case here, bearing failure of the weaker strength fastener material will govern the bearing strength requirements (or failure) of the joint design, not that of the higher strength plate materials. The basis of this evaluation is made by simply comparing the bearing stress allowables of the fastener and plate materials.

Bearing stress allowables are established from structural test data, and their published values are documented in MIL-HDBK-5 for many different materials. For easy reference, the engineer is referred to the mechanical-property tables provided in Appendix E. The ultimate and yield bearing allowables found in these tables are based on a uniform distribution of stress acting on the projected area of the fastener onto the plate bearing area (or simply, $A_{br} = Dt$, where D is the diameter of the fastener and t is the thickness of the plate). Although bearing stresses are theoretically more complicated to describe than this, this mathematical

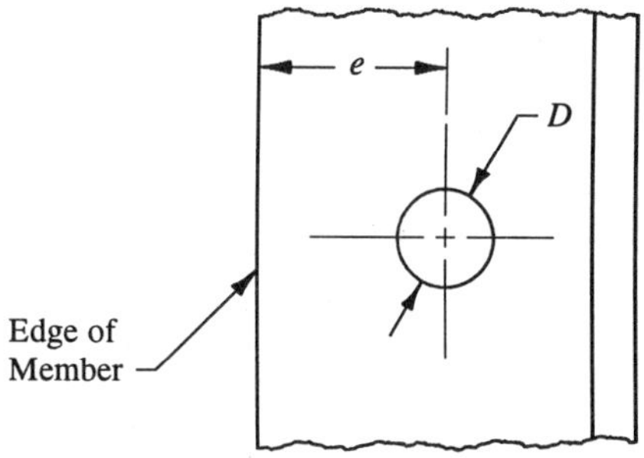

FIGURE 3-6 Edge distance measured from the center of the hole to the nearest free edge of the member.

interpretation is nonetheless correct: for its simplification is expressed and correlated with actual tested data to insure its accuracy and general load agreement.

The ultimate and yield allowable bearing stresses in MIL-HDBK-5 are given for fastener edge distances of $e/D = 1.5$ and $e/D = 2.0$, where e is the distance from the center of the hole to the nearest free edge of the member, Fig. 3-6, and D is the nominal hole diameter for a hole-filling fastener (rivet) and the nominal shank diameter for a nonhole-filling fastener (bolt or screw). Linear interpolation of allowable bearing stresses is permissible here for fastener edge distances ranging between these values; however, extrapolated values below 1.5 are not advised for actual design use, unless, of course, their values have been substantiated empirically. In general, when deciding upon a fastener for production use, the edge distance of the fastener chosen should allow for the next size fastener to be used. This allows for manufacturing errors, and for this reason, some aircraft companies recommend using a minimum edge distance of $2D + .030$ for structural detailing.[1] Thus, the ultimate allowable bearing strength of a plate or fastener, expressed in lb, is written:

$$P_{bru} = F_{bru}\, t\, D \tag{3-2}$$

where: F_{bru} = ultimate allowable bearing stress of the plate or fastener material
t = plate thickness
D = use the nominal hole diameter for a hole-filling fastener (rivet) and the nominal shank diameter for a nonhole-filling fastener (bolt or screw).

Bearing failure is then predicted by the following expression:

$$\text{Margin of Safety} = \text{M.S.} = \frac{P_{bru}}{p_s k} - 1$$

[1] The engineer should, however, follow specific company guidelines established for standard minimum edge distance requirements.

where: p_s = ultimate shear force of a fastener due to the applied force P and k = fitting factor for joint design (use 1.15 for commercial and military aircraft joint designs[1]).

In order to develop a format that is consistent with the static allowable joint strengths given in the tables throughout Sec. 8 of MIL-HDBK-5, the lowest value of either the ultimate allowable bearing stress F_{bru} or 1.5 times the yield allowable bearing stress F_{bry} is used for ultimate bearing strength computations.[2] If either of the above arguments are followed, no difficulty should then be encountered with permanent deformations of the structure at limit or operating design loads. Or mathematically, from their description, the following inequalities are thus formulated:

(1) If $F_{bru} < 1.5F_{bry}$, then use Eq. 3.2.

(2) If $1.5F_{bry} < F_{bru}$, then replace F_{bru} in Eq. 3-2 with $1.5F_{bry}$.

Direct substitution of 1.5 F_{bry} into Eq. 3-2 gives:

$$P_{bru} = 1.5F_{bry}tD \tag{3-3}$$

where P_{bru} is the ultimate allowable bearing strength of a plate or fastener (also see Eq. 3-2 for definition of terms).

Now, consider the single-shear lap joint and the double-shear lap joint structural arrangement of members shown in Fig. 3-7. The transfer of loads through these members can best be arrived at by depicting a joint made up of simple plate members. For the single-shear lap joint configuration, bearing failure of the web and tension clip is based on the full load that each member carries or $p_s = P$. However, if these members are made of similar materials, bearing failure need only be examined for the member having the thinner gage; since, the other member being thicker is therefore less critical (this is directly observed from the linearity of the function t in Eq. 3-2). For the double-shear lap joint configuration a slightly different situation occurs: here, the tension clips are investigated for bearing failure using $p_s = ½P$, while the web is analyzed for the full load that it carries or $p_s = P$. Example 3-1 will help to illustrate the application of Eqs. 3-2 and 3-3 to bearing failure of riveted connections (see ahead to page 165).

---

[1] A fitting factor may not be required for commercial and military aircraft when static testing is used to substantiate the basic structure.

[2] The design load factor (or ratio of ultimate to limit) for most military and commercial aircraft structures is 1.5. However, for outer space flight vehicles, design load factors can be different. Use only those design load factors that have been approved and specified by the appropriate federal or military procuring agencies for flight vehicle structures.

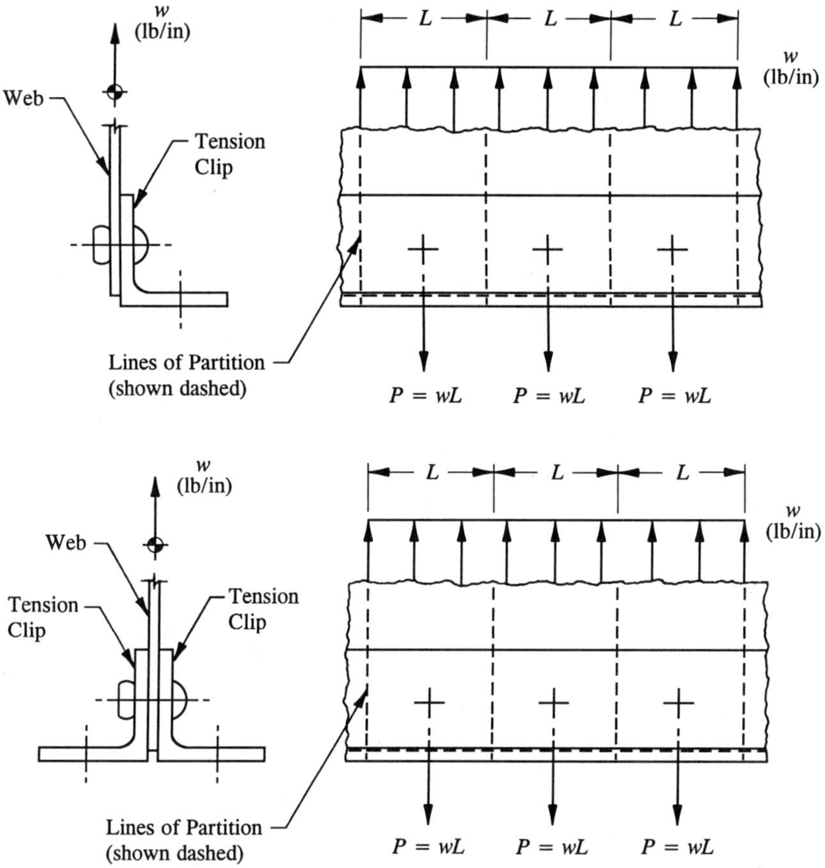

FIGURE 3-7 Bearing failure in various joint designs: (a) in a single-shear lap joint and (b) in a double-shear lap joint.

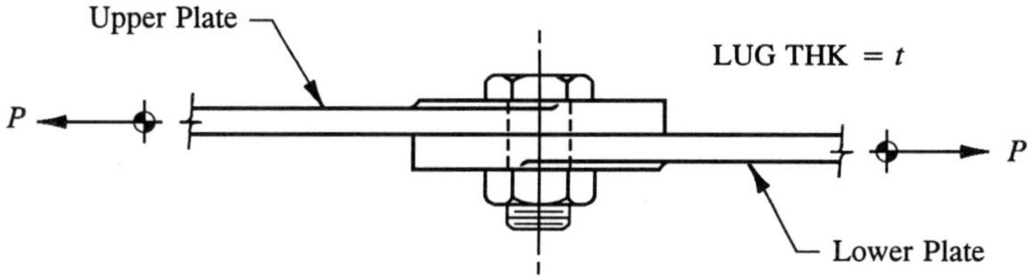

FIGURE 3-8 Mechanically fastened lap joint.

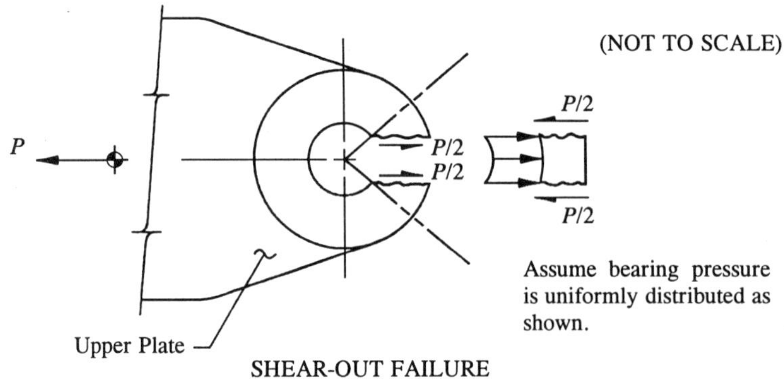

FIGURE 3-9 Shear failure of the lug material.

Shear-Out Failure of a Lug:

A mechanically fastened joint, such as the one shown in Fig. 3-8, may fail in shear by the physical bearing pressures created by the fastener onto the lug. This type of failure is viewed in Fig. 3-9, where a segment of lug is shown removed from the joint area in front of the hole. The wavy lines represent the lines of shear failure characterized by a sudden and abrupt failure of the lug material. The true cylindrical bearing pressure caused by the fastener bearing up against the lug is assumed to be uniformly distributed along the bearing surface of the fastener and lug. This assumption is valid in accordance with correlated tested data available in MIL-HDBK-5 for prescribed allowable bearing stresses of different materials. These data are established by dividing the actual test load of a fastener by its projected bearing area ($A_{br} = Dt$, where D = nominal hole diameter for a hole-filling fastener (rivet) and the nominal shank diameter for a nonhole-filling fastener (such as a bolt or screw) and t = lug thickness).

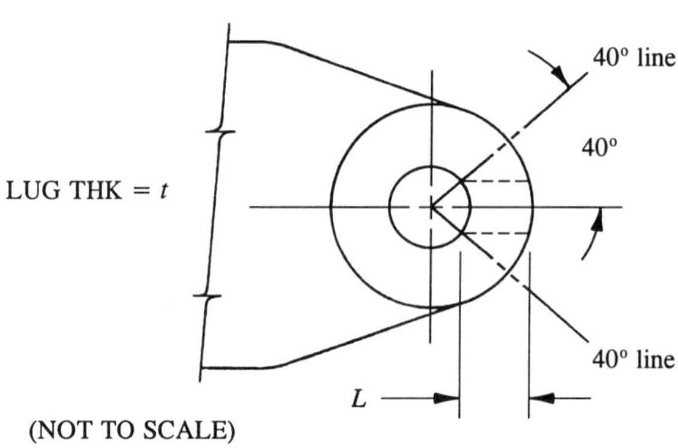

FIGURE 3-10 Sheared length of lug (shown by dashed lines).

The applied force P is resisted by the sheared areas of the lug which are bound by the 40° lines radiating from the center of the fastener. This can be seen in Fig. 3-10, where the actual sheared areas (shown by dashed lines) are measured horizontally from where these lines intersect the edge of the hole.

Assuming an average distribution of shearing stress across the sheared areas of the lug, the following equation is formulated from Eq. 4-9 of Chapter 4:

$$f_s = \frac{V}{A_{shr}} = \frac{P/2}{Lt} = \frac{P}{2Lt} \tag{3-4}$$

where: V = internal shear force

$A_{shr} = Lt$

L = sheared length of lug material (see Fig. 3-10)

t = lug thickness.

Shear-out failure is then predicted by making the following stress comparison:

$$\text{Margin of Safety} = \text{M.S.} = \frac{F_{su}}{f_s} - 1$$

where: F_{su} = ultimate allowable shear stress of the lug material (see the mechanical-property tables in MIL-HDBK-5 for specific listed values)

f_s = average shear stress (from Eq. 3-4).

Ultimate Allowable Tensile Strength $(P_t)_{\text{net}}$ of a Plate:

A mechanically fastened connection may fail in tension suddenly and abruptly across the net cross-sectional area of its connection plates caused by the discontinuity through which the fastener holes exist. For example, the single-shear lap

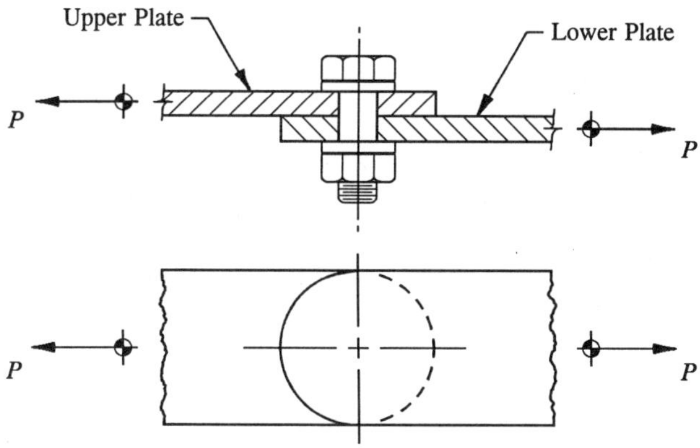

FIGURE 3-11 Single-shear lap joint in a tension-loaded joint.

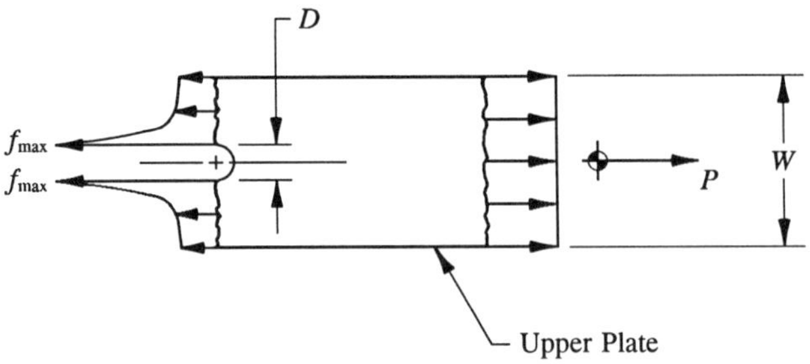

FIGURE 3-12 Tension failure of a plate across its net cross-sectional area through a hole.

joint of Fig. 3-11, tension failure will occur across the net (or least) section area of either the lower or upper plate (if necessary, see Sec. 2.2 for a brief review of net tension stresses). In retrospect, it was shown in that section that a flat plate will exhibit failure at the most critical combination of maximum load and minimum area. This usually occurs across the net area of the plate through the hole (for the analysis of tension-loaded members, $f_t = +P/A_{net}$). An actual tension failure or tear of the upper plate across its net cross-sectional area through the hole is viewed in Fig. 3-12.

Now, consider the adverse weakening effect of the fastener hole in such a connection at operating or limit stress levels. At these presumed levels, the true distribution of stress is more realistically described by stress-concentration factors[1] (predominant at the edges of the hole) than by the stresses represented by the solution of Eq. 2-3 (see page 61). For this reason, wherever possible, the aerospace design engineer should strive to streamline his designs by avoiding or at least minimizing joint irregularities, sharp breaks, and other joint discontinuities when they occur. While such conditions are not immediately detrimental to the structural airworthiness of most aircraft designs, their future implications could however be quite important. The magnitude of these peak stresses are based on the following general expression for localized stress concentrations at operating stress levels that are below the yield tension stress of the material F_{ty}:

$$f_{max} = K \frac{P}{A_{net}} \tag{3-5}$$

where: $A_{net} = (W - D)t$
K = stress-concentration factor (see footnote this page)

[1] Stress-concentration factors are very important in that branch of engineering concerned with "Fatigue and Fracture Mechanics." A considerable amount of graphs and charts have been accumulated and documented by Peterson, in his book *Stress-Concentration Factors*, for design use in a variety of practical design applications. Their empirical values are based on experimental verification using the "Photoelastic Method" of two-dimensional stress analysis problems.

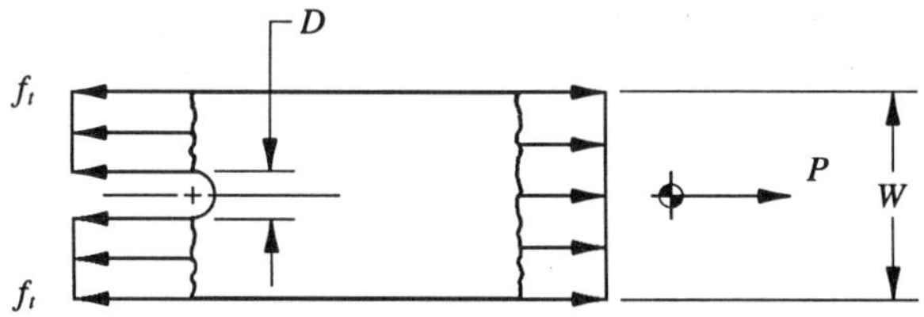

FIGURE 3-13 Uniform stress distribution across the hole is reached at the yield stress of the material (use $f_t = + P/A_{net}$ to calculate net stresses).

W = width of plate or sheet
D = actual hole diameter
t = thickness of plate or sheet.

Operating stress levels are established from actual flight loading conditions, and are used as a basis to determine the expected fatigue-life of a structure. However, the advanced nature of fatigue design is such that it is beyond the main intent or scope of this book to present a complete study of this subject here. Instead, it is hoped that an early and brief introduction to this subject will nevertheless help to enlighten and lead the engineer to a much better understanding and knowledge of net tension stresses in general. The engineer is again referred to Fig. 3-12, where the true elastic stress distribution across the net section area of the plate is illustrated.

In general, it can be said that stress concentrations predominantly occur at points of high stress intensity; of course, this presumes that peak stresses f_{max} have not exceeded the yield tension stress of the material F_{ty}. Since, if they do go above the proportional limit of the material, a more uniform stress distribution is likely to occur across the net section area of the plate, as shown in Fig. 3-13. The basis of this declaration is described as follows: Whenever initial operating tension loads are increased, the maximum peak stress (as diagrammed in Fig. 3-12 at the edges of the hole) will also increase until the yield tension stress of the material is reached. As the load is again increased, the yield stress of the material will hold constant at this point while the material of the plate at points of lower stress intensity continue to deform and strain to their initial yield values. A nearly uniform distribution of tension stress is reached when all points along the plate have yielded. Loading is resumed in this manner until failure is reached at the ultimate allowable tension stress of the material F_{tu}.

Written in terms of allowable values, Eq. 2-3 is redefined as follows for the ultimate strength of a plate in tension:

$$(P_t)_{net} = F_{tu} A_{net} \qquad \textbf{(3-6)}$$

where: $A_{net} = (W - D)t$

F_{tu} = ultimate allowable tension stress of the plate material
W = width of the plate
D = actual hole diameter
t = plate thickness.

To predict tension failure at ultimate load, the following load comparison is made for the plate:

$$\text{Margin of Safety} = \text{M.S.} = \frac{(P_t)_{\text{net}}}{p_t} - 1$$

where p_t is the applied ultimate tension load.

In addition to the above prediction, permanent set requirements must be satisfied at limit load. To accomplish this, the ultimate tension stress of the material F_{tu} must not exceed 1.5 times the yield tension stress of the material F_{ty}.[1] Hence, the following inequalities are formulated from this criterion:

(1) If $F_{tu} < 1.5 F_{ty}$, then use Eq. 3-6.

(2) If $1.5 F_{ty} < F_{tu}$, then replace F_{tu} in Eq. 3-6 with $1.5 F_{ty}$.

If we substitute 1.5 F_{ty} into Eq. 3-6, we obtain:

$$(P_t)_{\text{net}} = 1.5 F_{ty} A_{\text{net}} \tag{3-7}$$

where $(P_t)_{\text{net}}$ is the net ultimate allowable strength of a plate in tension (also see Eq. 3-6 for definition of terms). The obvious manifestations of using either Eq. 3-6 or 3-7 for limit load design are clear: permanent deformation requirements are satisfied at limit load which thereby renders and prevents fasteners from physically binding or jamming in their holes at operating design loads.

Yield Allowable Compressive Strength P_{cy} of a Plate:

A mechanically fastened connection may fail in compression across the gross cross-sectional area of the connection plates through which even fastener holes can exist. (See Sec. 2.2 for specific details and assumptions regarding the analysis of compression-loaded members, $f_c = -P/A_{\text{gross}}$.) It was previously demonstrated in that section (as it specifically relates to the analysis and design of connections here) that although fastener holes cause discontinuities in an actual connection, the gross (or full) cross-sectional areas of individual plate members can be used to perform compression stress calculations. In essence, the fasteners when installed in a

[1] See footnote (2) on page 152.

compression joint are considered to "fill the holes." This conclusion is mathematically consistent with the general theory that, at or below the proportional limit of the material, the gross yield allowable strength of a plate in compression is

$$P_{cy} = F_{cy} A_{\text{gross}} \quad (3\text{-}8)$$

[1]

where: $A_{\text{gross}} = Wt$
F_{cy} = yield allowable compression stress of the plate material
W = width of the plate
t = plate thickness.

Compression failure of the plate is predicted by making the following load comparison:

$$\text{Margin of Safety} = M.S. = \frac{P_{cy}}{p_c} - 1$$

where p_c is the applied ultimate compression load.

3.3 Concentrically Loaded Connections. A structural connection may be classified as one of the following types: (1) a concentrically loaded connection or (2) an eccentrically loaded connection. Both of these types are viewed in Fig. 3-14. If a joint is concentrically loaded, the applied force P passes through the center of gravity (CG)[2] of the fastener group and thereby physically prevents the joint from twisting. If, however, the applied load P does not lie in line with the centroid of area of the fastener group, the joint will twist. This twisting effect is characteristic of an eccentrically loaded connection (see Sec. 3.4 for the structural analysis methods used to analyze such joints). The center of gravity of the fastener group, which is also synonymous with the centroid of the fastener areas of the joint, is sometimes referred to as the center of resistance of the joint. The center of resistance is however only a theoretical abstraction; since, clearly, it is the shear areas of the joint fasteners that must provide the resisting forces to overcome the externally applied load.

To achieve an efficiently designed connection, one must strive to eliminate or at least attempt to minimize the eccentricities that occur in such designs. To do this, the arrangement of fasteners of a connection must be chosen so that the line of action of the externally applied load lines up with the centroid of area of the fastener group. The best designed connection is therefore one in which the path of the

---

[1] The application of this expression should, of course, preclude the affects of buckling and instability as a general consideration to the design of compression members. These topics are better treated when our study of the behavior of columns is presented in Chapter 7 (see Sec. 7.5, "Johnson-Euler Columns").

[2] For the actual computations of this quantity, the engineer is referred to Sec. 3.4, "Eccentrically Loaded Connections." (Specifically, see application of Eqs. 3-12 and 3-13 in that section.)

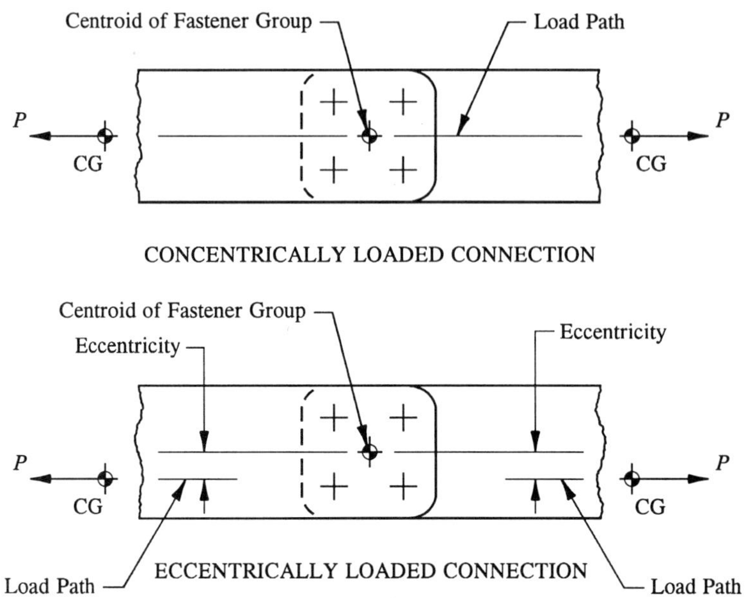

FIGURE 3-14 Mechanically fastened connections: (a) with a concentrically applied load and (b) with an eccentrically applied load.

applied load is most direct (that is, where the line of action of the load passes through the center of gravity of the fastener group). This eliminates the eccentricity of the joint and thereby prevents rotation or twisting of the joint altogether. On the other hand, the consequences of eccentricities are such as to invariably increase the structural weight of the overall connection design; this will affect the connection itself as well as influence the overall design aspects of the attaching structures. Each affected structure is increased in size in order to account for the applied load plus the additional moment that is produced by the eccentric effect of the applied load.

In analyzing a mechanically fastened connection, it is a generally accepted practice by industry professionals to assume that the frictional resistance between the joint fasteners and the plates of the connection are minimal at ultimate load. Generally speaking, if the frictional effects between the plates and fasteners of a joint have been overcome, the joint may be analyzed for its "ultimate strength capacity." Whether a connection is fastened together by rivets or bolts, the same structural definitions apply. Using Fig. 3-15, the theory of ultimate strength as it applies to a multiple riveted or bolted connection is presented. It assumes that the applied force P is equally distributed between joint fasteners of the same size and type (see Eq. 3-9), or proportionally distributed by a ratio of their allowable shear strengths if the joint fasteners are of different sizes and types (Eq. 3-10). The basis of this assumption is valid for joints stressed above the proportional limit of the

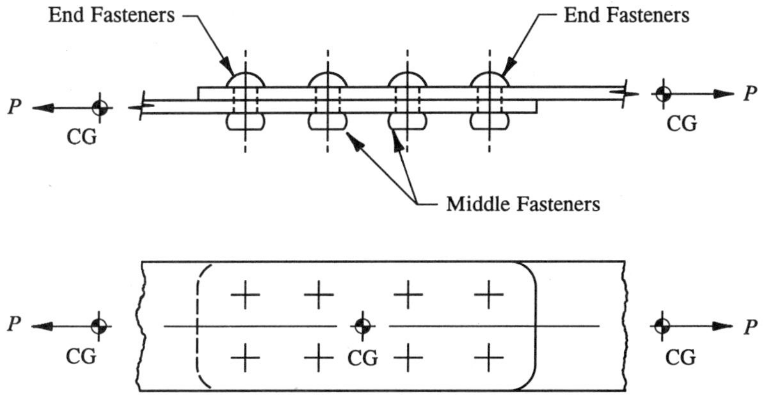

FIGURE 3-15 A multi-riveted connection.

material (this occurs in the inelastic range of stresses for a material).

Consider the fasteners of Fig. 3-15 to be of the same size and type. Theoretically, as the force P is initially applied to the plates, the end fasteners will begin to resist a much larger percentage of the applied force P than the middle fasteners. This of course assumes that all joint frictional effects have been overcome. As the force P is increased, the end fasteners will accept the increasing force until they reach their initial yield values. Then, they will hold this load as they yield while the increasing force is then carried by the middle fasteners to their initial yield values. The equal distribution of the force P to the six fasteners is then completed when all fasteners have yielded. Loading is again resumed until the ultimate strength or capacity of the joint is reached. Fundamentally, this provides the general theory that the applied force P (intrinsically, at higher loads) is equally distributed to joint fasteners of the same size and type. And thus, we can describe, mathematically, from this theory, the following structural tendency of these fasteners:

$$p_s = \frac{P}{n} \tag{3-9}$$

where: p_s = fastener shearing force
P = applied force (axial tension or compression)
n = number of joint fasteners.

If we now generalize our description of these fasteners for different sizes and types, a more general expression can be derived for the distribution of applied force P. Here, the distribution of load is based on a ratio of shear strengths of the joint fasteners:

$$p_s = \frac{P P_{su}}{\Sigma P_{su}} \tag{3-10}$$

where: p_s = fastener shearing force

$\Sigma P_{su} = (P_{su})_1 + (P_{su})_2 + (P_{su})_3 + \ldots + (P_{su})_n$

P_{su} = ultimate allowable shear strength of a fastener.

The actual computations using Eq. 3-10 are sometimes more conveniently done in tabular form, as shown in Table 3-3.

TABLE 3-3 FASTENER LOAD DISTRIBUTION FOR FASTENERS OF DIFFERENT SIZES AND TYPES

Fastener No.	D	P_{su}	p_s
1			
2			
3			
n			
	Total	ΣP_{su}	Σp_s*

* See table footnote next page.

The table is filled out with the given quantities listed (D and P_{su}) for each fastener type and the appropriate columns totaled (ΣP_{su} and Σp_s). If joint fasteners are not of the same size but are of the same type, Eq. 3-10 reduces to the following:

$$p_s = \frac{P A_{shr}}{\Sigma A_{shr}}$$

where: $A_{shr} = \frac{\pi}{4} D^2$

D = nominal pin or shank diameter for bolts and screws and the nominal hole diameter for rivets.

Since $\pi/4$ is common to both numerator and denominator of this equation, a further reduction of this expression is possible. Hence

$$p_s = \frac{P D^2}{\Sigma D^2}. \tag{3-11}$$

For this equation, fastener load distributions are also conveniently done in tabular form (here, the basic column format descriptions provided in Table 3-4 are used).

TABLE 3-4 FASTENER LOAD DISTRIBUTION FOR FASTENERS OF DIFFERENT SIZES BUT OF THE SAME TYPE

Fastener No.	D	D^2	p_s
1			
2			
3			
n			
	Total	ΣD^2	Σp_s*

* If the applied force P has been correctly distributed to each joint fastener, the sum of the individual fastener forces (Σp_s) should add up to this force P, or

$$\Sigma p_s = P.$$

This simple check will provide the engineer with a means of verifying the accuracy of his calculations, specifically, fastener load distributions.

To avoid the overlapping treatment and discussions of some parts of this section with those of Sec. 3.4, "Eccentrically Loaded Connections," the application of Eqs. 3-10 and 3-11 will be deferred for presentation until then. Although the assumptions of mechanically fastened connections are not precisely correct, their usage in the design of actual engineering hardware are nevertheless acceptable by aerospace industry standards. Experimental evaluation and experience of known connection types have shown that these assumptions correlate quite well with calculated values. The following assumptions as they were previously described in this section are summarized below:

(1) All frictional resistance between the plates and fasteners of a structural joint are neglected.

(2) All stress concentrations at the edges of the fastener holes are neglected at stresses above the proportional limit of the material.

(3) The applied force is equally distributed between joint fasteners of the same size and type, or proportionally distributed by a ratio of their allowable shear strengths if the joint fasteners are of different sizes and types. And, proportionally distributed by their shear areas if the joint fasteners are of different sizes but of the

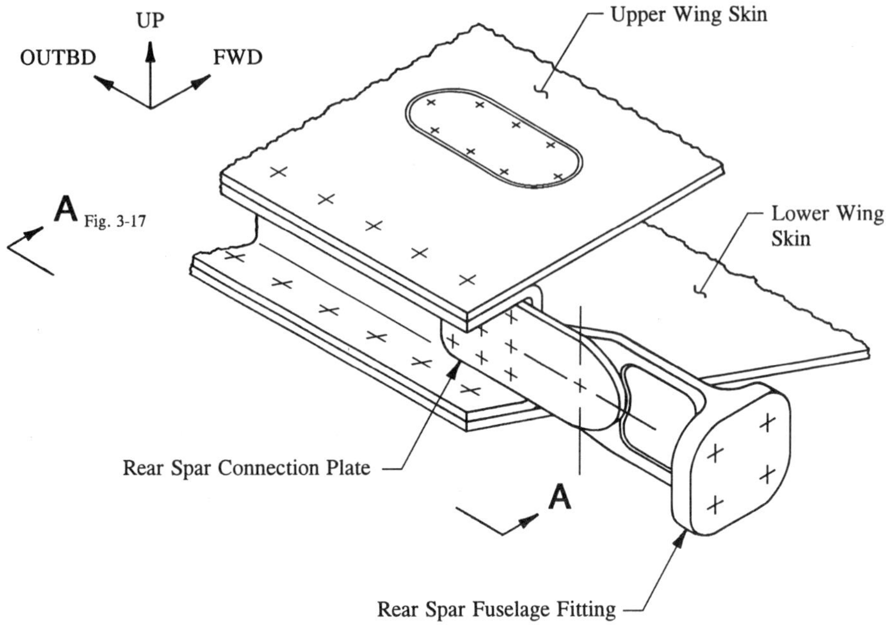

FIGURE 3-16 Wing rear spar to fuselage attachment.

same type.

(4) The bearing pressure between a fastener and a plate is assumed to be uniformly distributed over the plate bearing area.

(5) A tension joint is assumed to produce stresses which are uniformly distributed over the net area. For a compression-loaded member, the stresses are likewise uniformly distributed, but in this case, over the gross cross-sectional area of the plate.

(6) Shearing stresses are assumed to be uniformly distributed across the cross-sectional area of a fastener.

(7) The local bending effects of joint fasteners are neglected for relatively thin plate-like members.

The following example problem will help to illustrate the concepts and ideas of this section as it specifically relates to new, existing, and related structural joint designs. In particular, this example is chosen to exemplify the solution of concentrically loaded connections using Eq. 3-9. Its simplified loading format is presented now in an attempt to avoid the more difficult complexities associated with the solution of eccentrically loaded connections later. Too early of an exposure to these complexities now could jeopardize the engineer's later development and basic understanding of more complicated solutions. After the concepts and theory of concentrically loaded connections have been fully understood, the structural

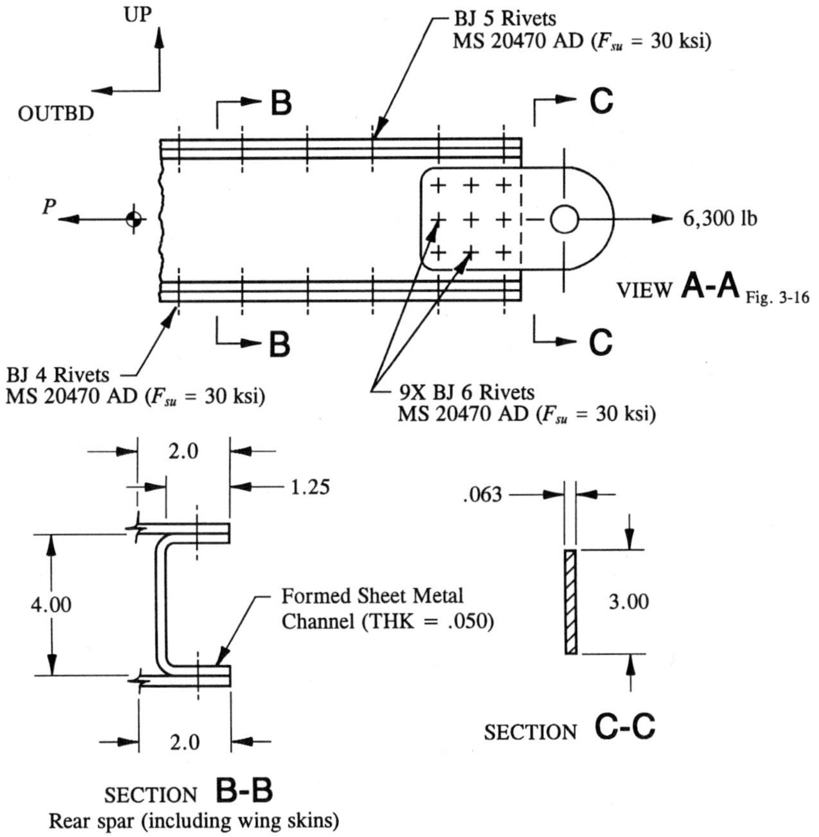

FIGURE 3-17 Concentrically loaded rear spar connection plate.

methods of analysis pertaining to the treatment of eccentrically loaded connections will be presented. It is much better to grasp certain basic concepts and fundamentals now than to lose sight of broader generalities of higher order complex solutions later.

Example 3-1 The aft wing-to-fuselage structure in Fig. 3-16 is considered critical for maximum wing forward-bending.[1] If the rear spar transmits a 6,300 lb force (ultimate) concentrically with its connection plate, as shown in View A-A of Fig. 3-17, what are the margins of safety for the different possible modes of failure that may occur for this structural design? Assume an effective width of skin of 2.0 in

[1] To simplify the loading condition of this example problem, wing torsion normally occurring simultaneously with wing forward-bending is neglected here. Its exclusion is intended to purposely simplify this problem solution by demonstrating an increasing progression to other solutions of more complicated connection types later. In Sec. 3.4, "Eccentrically Loaded Connections," this additional influence on the structural behavior of an eccentrically loaded connection will however be considered.

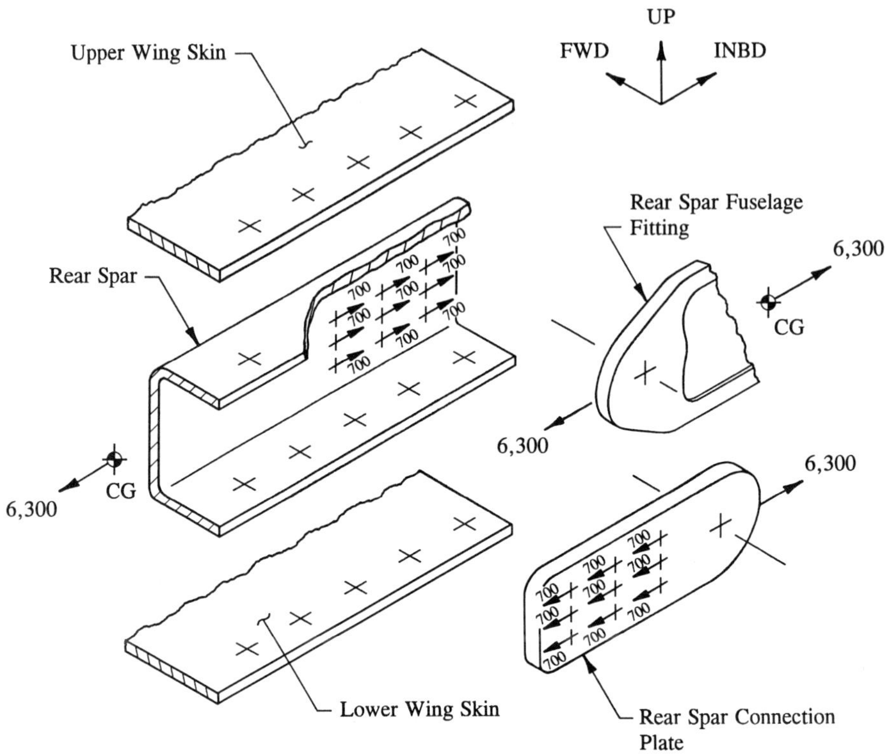

FIGURE 3-18 Diagram shows the internal distribution of fastener forces.

for the upper and lower wing skins. Also consider a fitting factor of 1.15 for joint design and a factor of safety of 1.5 for ultimate design (that is, a ratio of ultimate to limit = 1.5). All joint fasteners are of the same size and type and are assumed to have ample edge distance to prevent premature shear-out failure of the connection. In addition to satisfying the ultimate strength criteria of this connection design, be sure to verify permanent deformation requirements at limit load. Material: formed sheet metal channel, aluminum 2024-T42 (QQ-A-250/4); rear spar connection plate and upper and lower wing skins, aluminum 2024-T3 clad (QQ-A-250/5).

SOLUTION: The methods of analysis to the solution of this example are indicated by recognizing the various topics described in this section and how the pertinent relationships, assumptions, and idealizations were used to develop these formulations. On the basis of one of these earlier assumptions, that of distributing a concentric force equally between fasteners of the same size and type, the joint fasteners of this connection will each resist one-ninth (1/9) of the total applied load of 6,300 lb. Mathematically, this is determined from Eq. 3-9. Where

$$p_s = \frac{P}{n} = \frac{6,300}{9} = 700 \text{ lb.}$$

In Fig. 3-18, the actual fastener forces are drawn on an exploded view of the wing-to-fuselage structure.

The detailed solutions follow by applying the appropriate equations as they have appeared in different topics of this section. This means applying Eq. 3-1, $P_{su} = F_{su} A_{shr} C_r$, first and solving for the ultimate allowable shear strength of the connection rivets.

Ultimate Shear Failure of the Connection Rivets:

From the tabulated shear values of Table 3-1, we obtain $F_{su} A_{shr} = 862$ lb for the single-shear allowable strength of a BJ 6 rivet (MS 20470 AD, $F_{su} = 30$ ksi). As prescribed by MIL-HDBK-5, this value must also be corrected for high bearing stresses on the fastener. This correction factor is based on the thinner sheet thickness in a single-shear lap joint (for this example, this occurs in the .050 formed sheet metal channel). From Table 3-2, we obtain a single-shear strength correction factor of $C_r = .970$ for this particular rivet. The corrected allowable shear strength for this fastener is then computed using Eq. 3-1. Substituting the appropriate values into this expression gives:

$$P_{su} = F_{su} A_{shr} C_r = 862(.970) = 836 \text{ lb.}$$

The ultimate shear failure of all of the rivets of this fastener group is predicted from the following expression:

$$\text{Margin of Safety} = \text{M.S.} = \frac{P_{su}}{p_s k} - 1 = \frac{836}{700(1.15)} - 1 = +.04.$$

Now, the ultimate bearing failure of the rear spar and connection plate is determined.

Ultimate Bearing Failure of the Rear Spar:

Substituting the values given below into the bearing inequality of page 152, it can be shown that $1.5 F_{bry} < F_{bru}$. Hence, Eq. 3-3 is correctly chosen for the computation of ultimate bearing strength. Additionally, this will satisfy permanent deformation requirements of the rear spar at operating design loads. Thus, we obtain:

$$P_{bru} = 1.5 F_{bry}\, tD = 1.5(61,000)(.050)(.191) = 874 \text{ lb}$$

where: $F_{bru} = 118,000$ psi (QQ-A-250/4, $e/D = 2.0$)

$$F_{bry} = 61{,}000 \text{ psi (QQ-A-250/4, } e/D = 2.0)$$
$$t = .050 \text{ in}$$
$$D = .191 \text{ in (nominal hole diameter).}$$

$$\text{Margin of Safety} = \text{M.S.} = \frac{P_{bru}}{p_s k} - 1 = \frac{874}{(700)1.15} - 1 = +.09.$$

Ultimate Bearing Failure of the Rear Spar Connection Plate:

For this computation, it can be shown that $F_{bru} < 1.5\, F_{bry}$ (see values given below), and therefore to meet the ultimate and limit design requirements of this structural member, Eq. 3-2 is employed (see page 151).

$$P_{bru} = F_{bru}\, tD = 125{,}000(.063)(.191) = 1{,}504 \text{ lb}$$

where: $F_{bru} = 125{,}000$ psi (QQ-A-250/5, $e/D = 2.0$)
$F_{bry} = 84{,}000$ psi (QQ-A-250/5, $e/D = 2.0$)
$t = .063$ in
$D = .191$ in (nominal hole diameter).

$$\text{Margin of Safety} = \text{M.S.} = \frac{P_{bru}}{p_s k} - 1 = \frac{1{,}504}{(700)1.15} - 1 = +.87.$$

To gain a better perspective of the internal axial tension forces acting along the wing rear spar, axial load diagrams of individual members making up the rear spar are constructed, as shown in Fig. 3-19. These loading diagrams are easily verified at any section along the members by simply using the method of sections approach to internal loads analysis of Sec. 1.5 (use the free-body diagrams of isolated members for the actual computations). Observe the proper sequence of load transfers that occur for each member: that is, from connection plate to rivets, and then from rivets to rear spar. Also, note how the axial tension forces of one member increase while the axial forces of the other member decrease. In order to simplify the construction of these diagrams, the complex bearing pressures that normally exist between fasteners and plates of a connection have been assumed concentrated at fastener centerlines. For a more realistic description of theoretical bearing pressures that can occur at fastener holes, the reader is referred back to Sec. 2.2, Fig. 2-4.

With the possibility of tension failure occurring across the net section area of the connection, the ultimate strength of critical members in tension will require investigation. A comparison of axial diagrams for the rear spar and connection plate reveals that failure is likely to occur at locations of maximum axial tension. Assuming a uniform internal stress distribution across these members, the following computations are performed:

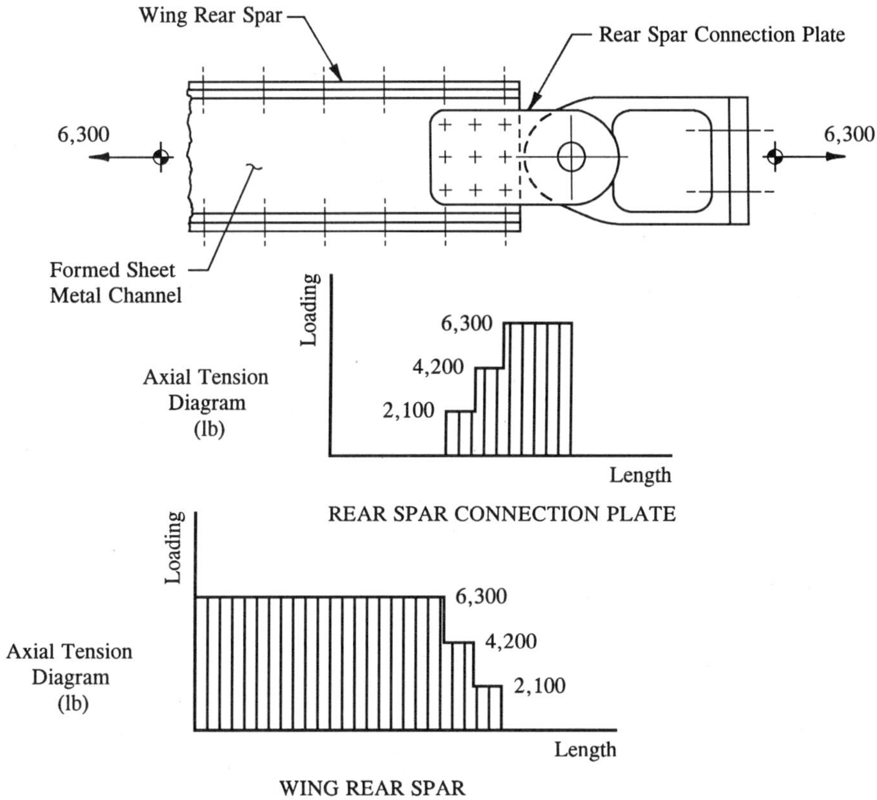

FIGURE 3-19 Axial tension diagrams: (a) rear spar connection plate and (b) wing rear spar.

Ultimate Tension Failure of the Rear Spar Connection Plate:

Since $F_{tu} < 1.5F_{ty}$, Eq. 3-6 is used to determine the ultimate strength of the rear spar connection plate in tension. This value is computed as follows:

$$(P_t)_{\text{net}} = F_{tu}A_{\text{net}} = 62,000(.153) = 9,486 \text{ lb}$$

where: $A_{\text{net}} = [3.00 - 3(.191)](.063) = .153 \text{ in}^2$ (see Fig. 3-20 for the actual dimensions used to compute this value)

$F_{tu} = 62,000$ psi (L), QQ-A-250/5

$F_{ty} = 45,000$ psi (L), QQ-A-250/5.

Using the axial diagram of the connection plate, a maximum tension load of 6,300 lb is found for this member. Substituting this value into the margin of safety expression for tension, we obtain:

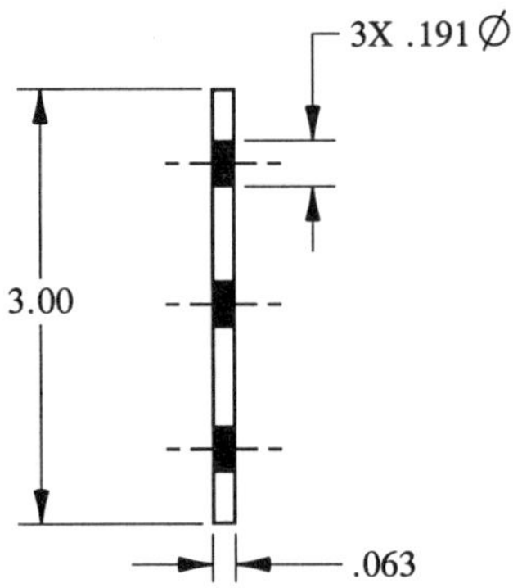

FIGURE 3-20 Net area of the rear spar connection plate.

$$\text{Margin of Safety} = \text{M.S.} = \frac{(P_t)_{\text{net}}}{p_t} - 1 = \frac{9,486}{6,300} - 1 = +.51.$$

Ultimate Tension Failure of the Rear Spar:

Here, the ultimate strength of the rear spar in tension will correspond to the sum of the material strengths of the individual members that make up the total section area (see Fig. 3-21 and to the mechanical-property values given for each member). Equations 3-6 and 3-7 are used to formulate a general expression for the actual computation of this quantity.

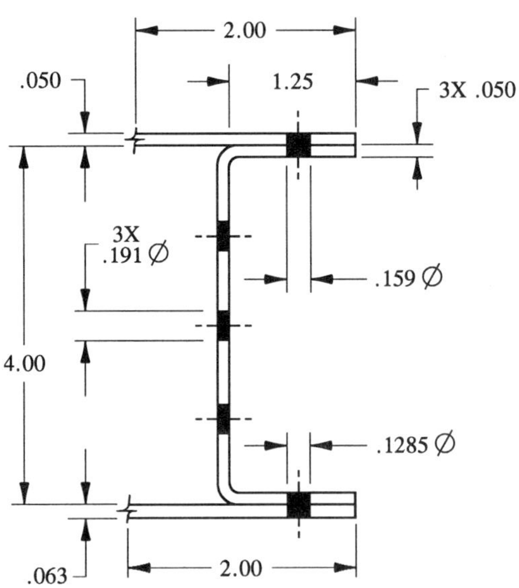

Mechanical Properties	
Upper Skin	F_{tu} = 60,000 psi (L)
	F_{ty} = 44,000 psi (L)
Lower Skin	F_{tu} = 62,000 psi (L)
	F_{ty} = 45,000 psi (L)
Rear Spar	F_{tu} = 62,000 psi (L)
	F_{ty} = 38,000 psi (L)

FIGURE 3-21 Net area of the wing rear spar.

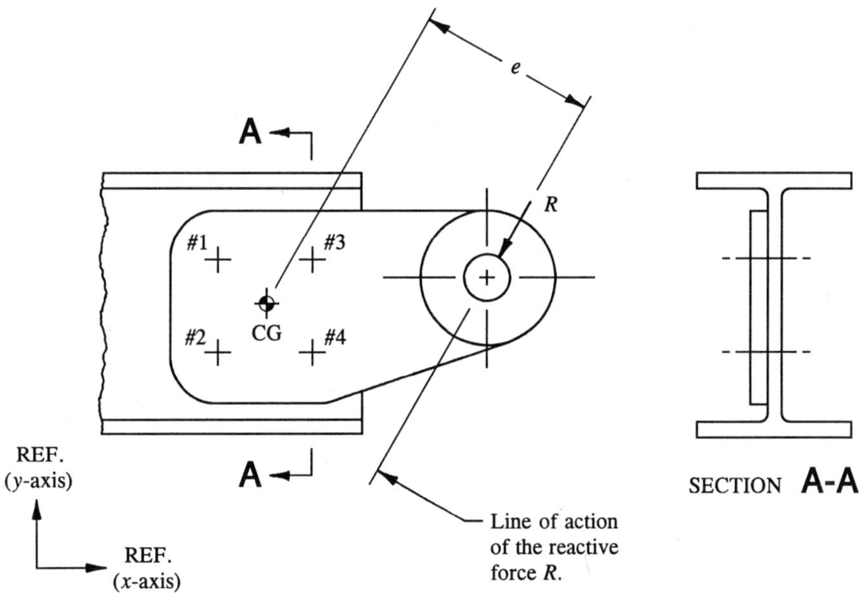

FIGURE 3-22 Eccentrically loaded connection. The line of action of the reactive force R does not pass through the center of gravity of the fastener group.

$$\begin{aligned}(P_t)_{net} &= (1.5F_{ty}A)_{channel} + (F_{tu}A)_{upper\ skin} + (F_{tu}A)_{lower\ skin} \\ &= 1.5(38,000)(.282) + 60,000(.092) + 62,000(.118) \\ (P_t)_{net} &= 28,910 \text{ lb}\end{aligned}$$

where: $A_{channel} = 4.00(.050) + 1.25(.050) + 1.25(.050) - .043 = .282 \text{ in}^2$
$A_{upper\ skin} = 2.00(.050) - .159(.050) = .092 \text{ in}^2$
$A_{lower\ skin} = 2.00(.063) - .1285(.063) = .118 \text{ in}^2.$

Substituting a maximum tension load of 6,300 lb for the rear spar into the margin of safety expression for tension, we obtain:

$$\text{Margin of Safety} = \text{M.S.} = \frac{(P_t)_{net}}{p_t} - 1 = \frac{28,910}{6,300} - 1 = +3.59.$$

Note that tension failure of the rear spar is not as critical as it is for the connection plate (compare results with the previous page).

3.4 Eccentrically Loaded Connections. In Sec. 3.3, mechanically fastened connections were restricted to the special case in which the line of action of the applied force had to pass through the centroid of the fastener group. This limitation prevented the connection from physically twisting and thus provided a simple way

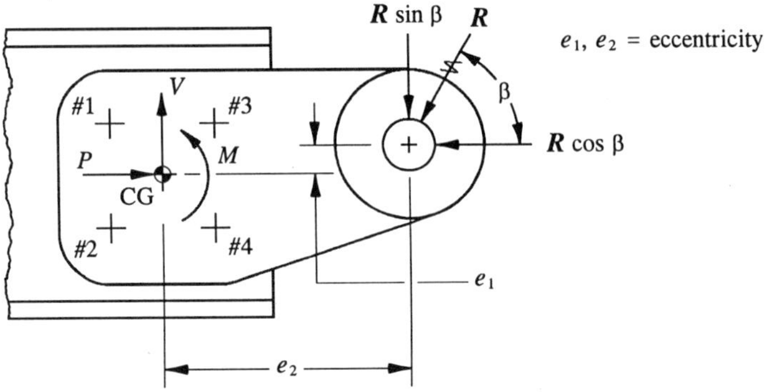

FIGURE 3-23 Eccentric load resolved into equivalent component forces.

of distributing the applied force in some prescribed manner to the fasteners of the connection. In this section, however, our discussions will emphasize the more general case where the applied force acting in the plane of the connection does not have to pass through the center of gravity of the fastener group (see Fig. 3-22 for this illustration). Such a connection, if it occurs, is referred to as being "eccentrically loaded." The resulting eccentricity of load will produce a twist or rotation of the entire joint around the centroid of the fastener group. Such a twist is what develops the torsional bending moment of the joint.[1]

The solution of such a connection is obtained by first resolving the reactive force R into equivalent horizontal and vertical components of force. This is done as shown in Fig. 3-23. Next, the internal loads V, P, and M necessary to establish equilibrium of the connection are computed at the center of gravity of the fastener group. To determine the magnitude of these internal forces, the equations of static equilibrium are applied. This corresponds to $\Sigma F_x = 0$, $\Sigma F_y = 0$, and $\Sigma M_{cg} = 0$ in separate solutions for the unknown quantities V, P, and M, respectively. Hence

$$\Sigma F_x = 0, \qquad P - R\cos\beta = 0, \quad P = R\cos\beta$$

$$\Sigma F_y = 0, \qquad V - R\sin\beta = 0, \quad V = R\sin\beta$$

$$\Sigma M_{cg} = 0, \qquad (+\!\circlearrowleft) \quad -M + (R\sin\beta)(e_2) - (R\cos\beta)(e_1) = 0$$

$$M = Re_2\sin\beta - Re_1\cos\beta.$$

The physical interpretation of these unknown forces is made by recognizing that it is the shear areas of the joint fasteners that resist the externally applied forces—not the internal loads V, P, and M idealized and represented at the

[1] Through structural testing, it can be shown that joints made by fastening their supported ends only through shear clips are considered simply-supported, while those additionally employing structural supports are considered rigid joints. Rigid joints are those which have the structural capability of preventing joint rotation. The amount of resistance they provide is conveniently measured by the magnitude of the torsional moment.

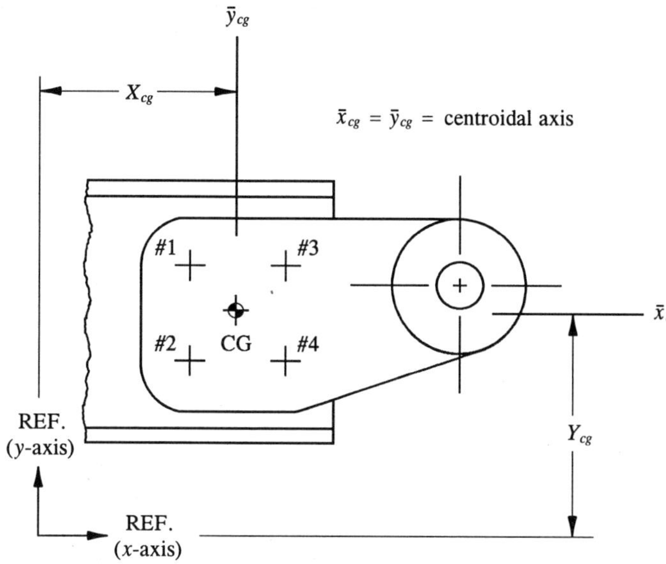

FIGURE 3-24 Centroid location of the fastener group.

(theoretical) centroid of the fastener group. Nevertheless, these internal forces do provide an expeditious and reliable way in which the solution of eccentrically loaded connections are described. Correlated from tests, the internal loads are described at the centroid of the fastener group where they will physically produce the desired shearing forces on the joint fasteners.

The remaining emphasis of this section is then to distribute these internal loads *V*, *P*, and *M* separately as shearing forces resisted by the fasteners of the connection. In this way, the connection, consisting of fasteners and plate-like members, can be fully investigated and analyzed by the strength criteria established for ultimate failure of joint designs (see Sec. 3.2). These failures are again listed here as they appeared in that section: (1) shearing failure of the fasteners, (2) bearing failure of the plates, (3) shear-out failure of the plates, (4) tension failure on the net cross-sectional area of the plates, and (5) yield compression failure on the gross cross-sectional area of the plates.

In order to establish the internal loads of an eccentrically loaded connection, the first step in the structural analysis solution is to firmly establish the centroid of area of the fastener group. By definition, the centroid (or center of gravity), from which the centroidal axes $\bar{x}_{cg}$ and $\bar{y}_{cg}$ must pass, is located from an arbitrarily chosen set of reference axes x and y (see Fig. 3-24). Using Table 3-5, the solution is set up in tabular form in which any pattern of different size fasteners can be used. After the table is completely filled out for each specific case, to locate the centroidal axes the following equations are applied:

$$X_{cg} = \frac{\Sigma\,(D^2x)}{\Sigma\,D^2} \tag{3-12}$$

$$Y_{cg} = \frac{\Sigma\,(D^2y)}{\Sigma\,D^2} \tag{3-13}$$

where: $\Sigma D^2 = D_1^2 + D_2^2 + D_3^2 + \ldots + D_n^2$

$\Sigma D^2x = D_1^2x_1 + D_2^2x_2 + D_3^2x_3 + \ldots + D_n^2x_n$

$\Sigma D^2y = D_1^2y_1 + D_2^2y_2 + D_3^2y_3 + \ldots + D_n^2y_n$

D = nominal hole diameter for rivets and the nominal shank diameter for bolts and screws

x = coordinate of a fastener measured along the reference x-axis

y = coordinate of a fastener measured along the reference y-axis.

The equations above are based on the shear areas of the fasteners ($A_{shr} = \pi D^2/4$). The reason that only the D^2 term appears in them is that the $\pi/4$ term happens to be common to both numerator and denominator, and therefore, this term cancels in each expression.

TABLE 3-5 CENTROID LOCATION FOR ANY PATTERN OF DIFFERENT SIZE FASTENERS

Fastener No.	D	x	y	D^2	D^2x	D^2y
1						
2						
3						
n						
		Total		ΣD^2	ΣD^2x	ΣD^2y

The values of X_{cg} and Y_{cg} represent the distances measured along the reference axes x and y, respectively, to locations corresponding to the centroidal axes $\bar{x}_{cg}$ and $\bar{y}_{cg}$ of the fastener group. The distances x and y are the coordinates of a fastener measured along the reference axes x and y, respectively, and, of course, in the shear plane of the connection. The reference axes are chosen completely arbitrarily; however, for convenience, they are purposely and conveniently chosen so that all of the fasteners in the fastener group considered will lie either along one of the axes or be contained somewhere within the first quadrant of the established coordinate system. In this way, the coordinates x and y of all fasteners in the fastener group will have positive values when listed in Table 3-5.

Further simplification of Eqs. 3-12 and 3-13 is possible if all joint fasteners are of the same size and type. In tabular form, these equations correspond to Table 3-6, as shown below:

TABLE 3-6 CENTROID LOCATION FOR ANY PATTERN OF THE SAME SIZE AND TYPE OF FASTENERS

Fastener No.	D	x	y
1			
2			
3			
n			
	Total	Σx	Σy

$$X_{cg} = \frac{\Sigma x}{n} \tag{3-14}$$

$$Y_{cg} = \frac{\Sigma y}{n} \tag{3-15}$$

where: n = number of joint fasteners
$\Sigma x = x_1 + x_2 + x_3 + \ldots + x_n$
$\Sigma y = y_1 + y_2 + y_3 + \ldots + y_n$.

In most design applications, it is customary to design a connection entirely composed of the same size and type of fasteners. Generally, selected mixed groups of rivets and bolts should be avoided, if possible. However, if they occur, their treatment should be handled conservatively using the methods and techniques of this chapter. Regardless of the actual arrangement of fasteners of a connection, the centroid can always be located by applying either set of Eqs. 3-12 and 3-13 or Eqs. 3-14 and 3-15. However, if the location of the centroid can be found by merely inspecting the fastener pattern of the connection, in such a case, there would be no need for actual centroid computations.

The basic approach to establish the structural integrity (or strength) of an eccentrically fastened connection is described as follows: a connection is divided into three separate problems in which three separate solutions are obtained. That is, the internal loads *V*, *P*, and *M* are each separately distributed as shearing forces to all of the fasteners of the fastener group. The resultant shearing forces are then obtained by simple superposition of the three separate solutions. Specifically, each solution is vectorially combined at each fastener. The resultant shearing forces are presumed acting in the plane of the connection; no out-of-plane tension forces are considered acting on a fastener. However, if they do occur, see Chapter 5, Eqs. 5-8, 5-9, and 5-10, for the interaction equations used to combine the simultaneous effects of shear and tension forces on a fastener.

TABLE 3-7 DISTRIBUTION OF DIRECT LOAD *V*

Fastener No.	D	P_{su}	$(p_s)_v$
1			
2			
3			
n			
	Total	ΣP_{su}	$\Sigma(p_s)_v$

TABLE 3-8 DISTRIBUTION OF DIRECT LOAD *P*

Fastener No.	D	P_{su}	$(p_s)_p$
1			
2			
3			
n			
	Total	ΣP_{su}	$\Sigma(p_s)_p$

TABLE 3-9 DISTRIBUTION OF TORSIONAL MOMENT *M*

Fastener No.	D	$\bar{x}$	$\bar{y}$	r	$P_{su}r$	$P_{su}r^2$	$(p_s)_m$
1							
2							
3							
n							
			Total		$\Sigma P_{su}r$	$\Sigma P_{su}r^2$	$\Sigma(p_s)_m$

To accomplish the distribution of internal loads *V*, *P*, and *M* to the fasteners of a joint made up of different sizes and types, Tables 3-7, 3-8, and 3-9 are each correspondingly filled out and the indicated column totals of these tables used as input data for actual numerical computations. The computations are performed by applying the following equations:

Distribution of Direct Shearing Force *V* (see Table 3-7):

$$(p_s)_v = \frac{V P_{su}}{\Sigma\, P_{su}}. \tag{3-16}$$

Distribution of Direct Axial Force *P* (see Table 3-8):

$$(p_s)_p = \frac{P P_{su}}{\Sigma\, P_{su}}. \tag{3-17}$$

Distribution of Torsional Moment *M* (see Table 3-9):

$$(p_s)_m = \frac{M P_{su}\, r}{\Sigma\, (P_{su} r^2)} \tag{3-18}$$

where: $\Sigma\, P_{su} = (P_{su})_1 + (P_{su})_2 + (P_{su})_3 + \ldots + (P_{su})_n$

$\Sigma(P_{su} r^2) = (P_{su} r^2)_1 + (P_{su} r^2)_2 + (P_{su} r^2)_3 + \ldots + (P_{su} r^2)_n$

P_{su} = ultimate allowable shearing strength of a fastener (use Eq. 3-1 for solid, protruding-head rivets; for all others, use prescribed published fastener specifications)

$r = \left[\bar{x}^2 + \bar{y}^2\right]^{1/2}$, from the Pythagorean theorem this distance represents the radial length from the fastener to the centroid of the fastener group

$\bar{x}$ = coordinate of a fastener measured from the centroid of the fastener group along the centroidal axis $\bar{x}_{cg}$

$\bar{y}$ = coordinate of a fastener measured from the centroid of the fastener group along the centroidal axis $\bar{y}_{cg}$.

If joint fasteners are of different sizes but are of the same type, Eqs. 3-16, 3-17, and 3-18 reduce to the following:

Distribution of Direct Shearing Force *V:*

$$(p_s)_v = \frac{V D^2}{\Sigma\, D^2}. \tag{3-19}$$

Distribution of Direct Axial Force *P:*

$$(p_s)_p = \frac{PD^2}{\Sigma D^2}. \tag{3-20}$$

Distribution of Torsional Moment *M:*

$$(p_s)_m = \frac{MD^2 r}{\Sigma (D^2 r^2)} \tag{3-21}$$

where: $\Sigma D^2 = D_1^2 + D_2^2 + D_3^2 + \ldots + D_n^2$

$\Sigma(D^2 r^2) = D_1^2 r_1^2 + D_2^2 r_2^2 + D_3^2 r_3^2 + \ldots + D_n^2 r_n^2$

D = nominal shank diameter for bolts and screws and the nominal hole diameter for rivets.

Tables 3-7, 3-8, and 3-9 are again used here, however, the term P_{su} is replaced by D^2 in each table. If joint fasteners are all of the same size and type, Equations 3-19, 3-20, and 3-21 are further reduced to the following:

Distribution of Direct Shearing Force *V:*

$$(p_s)_v = \frac{V}{n}. \tag{3-22}$$

Distribution of Direct Axial Force *P:*

$$(p_s)_p = \frac{P}{n}. \tag{3-23}$$

Distribution of Torsional Moment *M* (see Table 3-10):

$$(p_s)_m = \frac{Mr}{\Sigma r^2} \tag{3-24}$$

where: n = number of joint fasteners

$\Sigma r^2 = r_1^2 + r_2^2 + r_3^2 + \ldots + r_n^2.$

By comparing each term of Eq. 3-24 with each term in the torsional formula for beam structures (Tc/J), it can be seen that the basic theories of a connection in torsion can be analogized to those of a beam in pure torsion. Table 3-10 is used to arrange the tabular distribution of torsional moment M to all joint fasteners of a connection corresponding to this equation.

TABLE 3-10 DISTRIBUTION OF TORSIONAL MOMENT M

Fastener No.	r	r^2	$(p_s)_m$
1			
2			
3			
n			
	Total	Σr^2	

Let us now review the first equation of each set of equations presented thus far. These are, respectively: Eqs. 3-16, 3-19, and 3-22, and are each specifically used to distribute the direct shearing force V to all of the fasteners of the connection. The shearing force distributions are viewed in Fig. 3-25, where the direct shearing force V is shown resisted by the shearing forces of the joint fasteners. The second equation of each set of equations, Eqs. 3-17, 3-20, and 3-23, are used to distribute the direct axial force P to all of the fasteners of the connection. The actual distribution of this force is shown resisted by the shearing forces of the fasteners in Fig. 3-26.

The last equation of each set of equations, Eqs. 3-18, 3-21, and 3-24, are used to distribute the torsional moment M to all of the fasteners of the connection. The actual distributions are diagrammed as shown in Fig. 3-27. Here, the fasteners are shown resisting shearing forces which act perpendicularly to the lines drawn

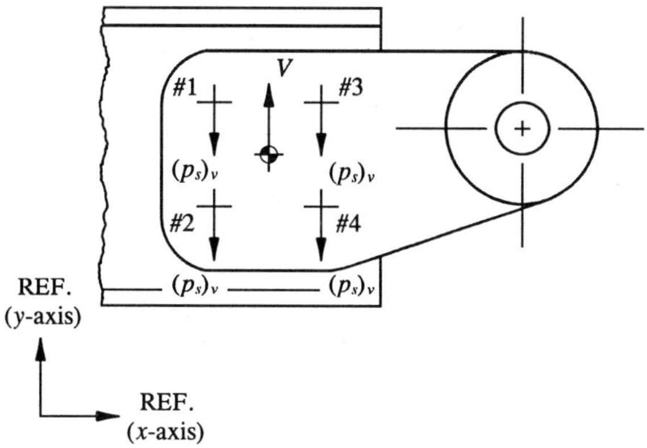

FIGURE 3-25 Distribution of direct shear force V resisted by the shearing forces of the joint fasteners.

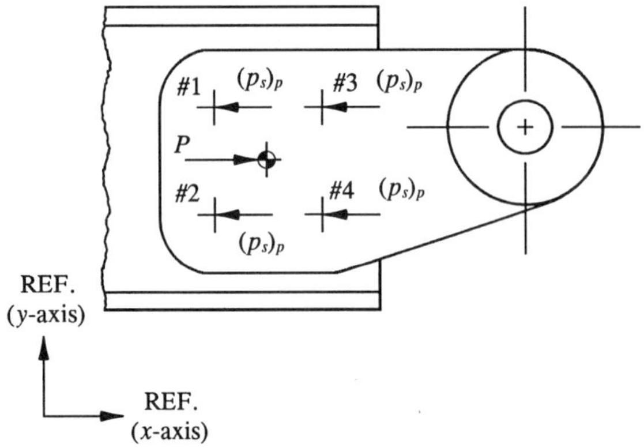

FIGURE 3-26 Distribution of direct axial force P resisted by the shearing forces of the joint fasteners.

connecting the centroid of the fastener group with each of the fastener centers. Also, note in particular how the resisting shearing forces are positioned in directions which directly oppose the moment M. Here, the rotation of M is depicted in a counterclockwise direction, therefore, to be consistent with the previous directions chosen for the shearing force distributions of V and P, the shearing forces of M must also be chosen as opposing forces. The magnitude of the shearing forces are directly proportional to their respective distances r from the centroid of the fastener group. Which means that fasteners situated farthest from the centroid of area will, by Eq. 3-18, 3-21, or 3-24, receive a larger distribution of the torsional

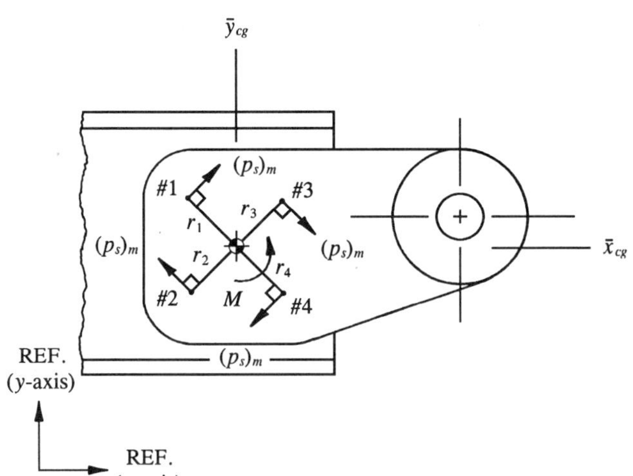

FIGURE 3-27 Distribution of torsional moment M resisted by the shearing forces of the joint fasteners.

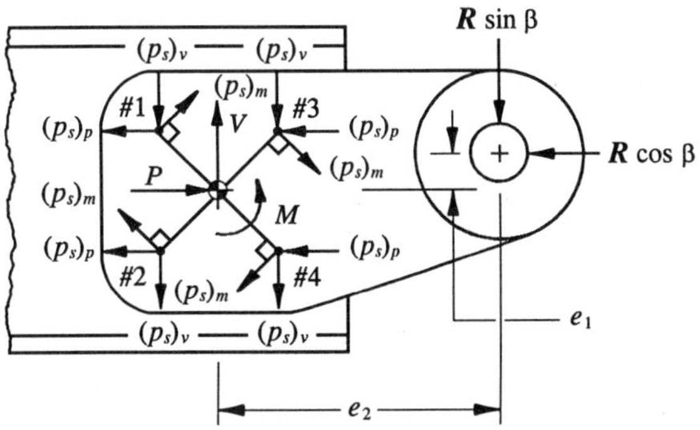

FIGURE 3-28 Superposition of rivet shearing forces due to the internal forces *V, P,* and *M.*

moment *M* than fasteners located nearest to the centroid (consider the distances defined by r_1, r_2, r_3, and r_4 as moment arms and the centroid as the pivot axis). Theoretically, then, if a fastener is located coincident with the centroid of area, by Eq. 3-18, 3-21, or 3-24, with $r = 0$, $(p_s)_m$ would also be zero. In actual fact, however, after the outer or most remote fasteners have received their proportionately larger shearing force distributions and have begun to yield, the inner fasteners, conceivably, could support the increasing load. Here lies the conservatism of this method. Nevertheless, however conservative this method may at first appear, it still remains the standard and accepted method of analysis of the aerospace industry in the design of mechanically fastened eccentrically loaded connections.

As long as the internal forces *V, P,* and *M* have been correctly described at the centroid of the fastener group, the method of superposition is applicable. The distributed shearing forces of their separate solutions are superimposed at each fastener location, as diagrammed in Fig. 3-28. It makes absolutely no difference whether all of the shearing forces are considered opposing, or for that matter, if all of them are not. What really does matter is that all of the shearing forces are consistently diagrammed in one prescribed direction or the other. In other words, in one case the fastener shearing forces are considered applied onto the fastener; in the other, the shearing forces are applied onto the plate. In either case, the shearing forces are of the same magnitude. And, since maximum strength is what a structure is normally designed for, the magnitude of the shearing forces are the desired quantities used to adequately represent and evaluate the structure for ultimate failure.

Superposition of Direct Forces *V, P,* and Torsional Moment *M:*

The final step in the analysis of an eccentrically loaded connection is to vectorially superimpose the shearing forces of the three separate solutions of *V, P,* and

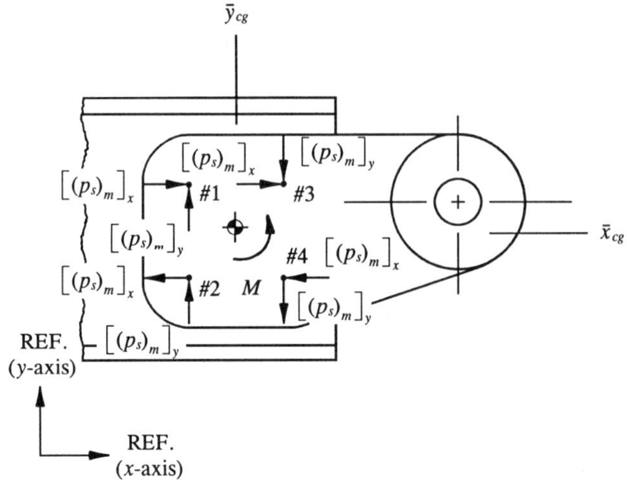

FIGURE 3-29 Pictorial representation of the component forces of the torsional moment *M*.

M into one resultant shearing force system acting at each fastener (for a review of these principles, the engineer is referred to Appendix A, "Resolution of Forces"). To simplify the vectorial superposition of these forces it is often more convenient to describe the shearing forces $(p_s)_m$ due to the torsional moment *M* by alternative expressions which can directly represent these forces into equivalent horizontal and vertical components. The pictorial diagram representing these components are viewed in Fig. 3-29. To determine their numerical values, Eqs. 3-18, 3-21, and 3-24 are each simplified into two alternative expressions based on an arbitrarily selected rectangular coordinate system. Hence, for a joint made up of different sizes and types of fasteners, the following general expressions are formulated to determine the components of shearing force due to the torsional moment *M:*

$$\left[(p_s)_m\right]_x = \frac{M P_{su} \bar{y}}{\Sigma\,(P_{su}\, r^2)} \tag{3-25}$$

$$\left[(p_s)_m\right]_y = \frac{M P_{su} \bar{x}}{\Sigma\,(P_{su}\, r^2)}. \tag{3-26}$$

Whereas, if the fasteners of the connection are of different sizes but are of the same type, these equations will reduce further to the following forms:

$$\left[(p_s)_m\right]_x = \frac{M D^2 \bar{y}}{\Sigma\,(D^2\, r^2)} \tag{3-27}$$

$$\left[(p_s)_m\right]_y = \frac{MD^2\bar{x}}{\Sigma\,(D^2 r^2)}. \tag{3-28}$$

And, if the fasteners are all of the same size and type, these equations will again simplify to:

$$\left[(p_s)_m\right]_x = \frac{M\bar{y}}{\Sigma\, r^2} \tag{3-29}$$

$$\left[(p_s)_m\right]_y = \frac{M\bar{x}}{\Sigma\, r^2}. \tag{3-30}$$

In general, Eqs. 3-25 through 3-30 are the preferred expressions used to express the torsional moment M into equivalent components of shearing force. In this form, resolution of shearing forces is not required at a fastener using trigonometric functions of any kind. Instead, the components of force are obtained directly, and are conveniently represented in a rectangular coordinate system which are then combined vectorially with the direct loads $(p_s)_v$ and $(p_s)_p$. Mathematically, this gives:

$$\Sigma\, p_x = (p_s)_p + \left[(p_s)_m\right]_x \tag{3-31}$$

$$\Sigma\, p_y = (p_s)_v + \left[(p_s)_m\right]_y. \tag{3-32}$$

From the Pythagorean theorem[1], an analogous expression for the resultant shearing force on a fastener is obtained. Thus

$$p_s = \left[(\Sigma\, p_x)^2 + (\Sigma\, p_y)^2\right]^{1/2}. \tag{3-33}$$

The distribution of torsional moment is an approximate method of analysis to a most complicated solution. However conservative it may seem, it should still serve the engineer well in the solution of most eccentrically loaded connection designs. To summarize the structural analysis method of this section, the following step-by-step procedure is presented here for the detailed solution of an eccentrically loaded connection:

(1) Resolve all of the applied forces acting on the connection into equivalent horizontal and vertical components.

(2) Locate the centroid (center of gravity) of the fastener group using one of the following set of equations depending on whether the fasteners are of different sizes (set a), or of the same size (set b):

---

[1] The Pythagorean theorem states that "the sum of the squares of the legs of a right triangle are equal to the square of the hypotenuse."

$$\text{(a)}\quad X_{cg} = \frac{\Sigma\,(D^2x)}{\Sigma\,D^2} \qquad \text{(b)}\quad X_{cg} = \frac{\Sigma\,x}{n}$$

$$Y_{cg} = \frac{\Sigma\,(D^2y)}{\Sigma\,D^2} \qquad Y_{cg} = \frac{\Sigma\,y}{n}.$$

(3) Indicate the equivalent forces V, P, and M at the centroid of the fastener group and then determine their values by applying the equations of static equilibrium:

(a) $\Sigma\,F_x = 0$ is used to solve for the direct axial force P.

(b) $\Sigma\,F_y = 0$ is used to solve for the direct shearing force V.

(c) $\Sigma\,M_{cg} = 0$ is used to solve for the torsional moment M.

(4) Calculate the shearing forces due to the forces V and P and then pictorially diagram these forces resisted by all of the fasteners of the connection using one of the following set of equations depending on whether fasteners are of different sizes and types (set a), of different sizes but of the same type (set b), or of the same size and type (set c):

$$\text{(a)}\quad (p_s)_v = \frac{V P_{su}}{\Sigma\,P_{su}} \qquad \text{(b)}\quad (p_s)_v = \frac{VD^2}{\Sigma\,D^2} \qquad \text{(c)}\quad (p_s)_v = \frac{V}{n}$$

$$(p_s)_p = \frac{P P_{su}}{\Sigma\,P_{su}} \qquad (p_s)_p = \frac{PD^2}{\Sigma\,D^2} \qquad (p_s)_p = \frac{P}{n}.$$

(5) Pictorially diagram the torsional moment M as shearing forces resisted by the fasteners of the connection. Then replace these forces by their corresponding horizontal and vertical components.

(6) Calculate the horizontal and vertical components of shearing forces (from step 5) resisted by all of the fasteners of the connection using one of the following set of equations depending on whether fasteners are of different sizes and types (set a), of different sizes but of the same type (set b), or of the same size and type (set c):

$$\text{(a)}\quad \left[(p_s)_m\right]_x = \frac{M P_{su}\,\bar{y}}{\Sigma\,(P_{su} r^2)} \qquad \text{(b)}\quad \left[(p_s)_m\right]_x = \frac{M D^2\,\bar{y}}{\Sigma\,(D^2 r^2)} \qquad \text{(c)}\quad \left[(p_s)_m\right]_x = \frac{M\bar{y}}{\Sigma\,r^2}$$

$$\left[(p_s)_m\right]_y = \frac{M P_{su}\,\bar{x}}{\Sigma\,(P_{su} r^2)} \qquad \left[(p_s)_m\right]_y = \frac{M D^2\,\bar{x}}{\Sigma\,(D^2 r^2)} \qquad \left[(p_s)_m\right]_y = \frac{M\bar{x}}{\Sigma\,r^2}.$$

(7) Vectorially superimpose the fastener shearing forces due to V, P, and M in their proper x and y rectangular coordinate directions using the following set of equations:

$$\Sigma p_x = (p_s)_p + \left[(p_s)_m\right]_x$$

$$\Sigma p_y = (p_s)_v + \left[(p_s)_m\right]_y .$$

(8) Calculate the magnitude of the resultant shearing force acting at each fastener using the following equation:

$$p_s = \left[(\Sigma p_x)^2 + (\Sigma p_y)^2\right]^{1/2}.$$

3.5 Important Remarks When Analyzing and Designing an Eccentrically Loaded Connection. Let us suppose that the highest loaded (or stressed) fastener of a connection can be found by simple inspection of the distributed quantities *V*, *P*, and *M*. This would of course make the computations of the remaining fasteners of the connection unnecessary. Generally, when comparing individual fastener load distributions of a connection, the maximum loaded fastener can usually be systematically figured out. Using Fig. 3-28 again to help illustrate and describe this technique, it can be seen that the distributed quantities indicated at each fastener there are critical at fastener #4. Hence, this fastener should correspond to the highest resultant shearing force of any fastener of the connection because the vectorial superposition of direct and torsional forces will combine more algebraically. After this and several more illustrative example problems of this nature have been thoroughly studied, the engineer will begin to acquire the mental judgment necessary to accurately evaluate those obvious critical combinations of shearing forces acting on a fastener. If the engineer can pinpoint the most critically stressed fastener of a particular fastener group, he can then avoid the many individual superfluous computations of lesser known loaded fasteners.

The reason that most groups of fasteners are not stressed to their maximum strengths simultaneously is principally due to the inherent way in which the torsional moment is distributed to joint fasteners as a whole. Remember, the ultimate capacity of a joint in torsion is based on the ultimate strength of those fasteners usually located farthest away from the centroid of the fastener group. And, for that reason, some residual strength is always available for fasteners located nearer to the centroid of the fastener group. This additional available capacity of a connection is entirely consistent however, even though the basic structural method of analysis of this chapter might clearly predict otherwise. Moreover, it should also be pointed out that, the absolute capacity of a connection can never be precisely determined from calculation. Only through careful and accurate monitoring of a connection during structural testing can precise fastener load distributions be accurately appraised. No proven method of analysis can demonstrate maximum load capacity better than through structural testing, or from independent comprehensive test data of similar or related designed structures. Sometimes even this simple technique can be used to conveniently avoid a rather costly redesign effort of joint designs unsubstantiated by empirical data or by analysis. In any case, their usage should be seriously contemplated as an alternative way in which an aircraft structure may be substantiated.

The engineer must consider all aspects and approaches to his structural designs: for it may be more prudent and less costly in the long run to initiate a structural test program for unsubstantiated regions of a structure than to spend additional engineering man-hours redesigning and reanalyzing unsubstantiated areas of that structure. An entire aircraft, conceivably, could be certified in this most direct way—using only preliminary, approximate, and comparative analysis techniques to verify and substantiate an aircraft for certification. The concept is quite simple: If a structure should fail prematurely during static testing, the failed structure would be beefed up (that is, eye-balled) and retested. If the reinforced structure should again prove to be understrength and fail unexpectedly, additional beef up would again be required. This process would continue until the structure would eventually meet all of the principal design requirements established for certification. This technique is not the most scientific, but, nevertheless, it can be a most reliable and formidable way to substantiate component parts of an aircraft, certainly worthy of engineering consideration.[1]

The following example will help to illustrate the specific structural analysis techniques outlined in this section as they specifically apply to the solution of an eccentrically loaded connection.

Example 3-2 A pulley bracket is fastened to an auxiliary beam structure of the same material by means of four solid, protruding-head rivets, as shown in Fig. 3-30. During installation of this bracket, rivets #1 and #3 were drilled out to the next larger size. Find the shearing force reacted by each rivet for a maximum cable tension load of 400 lb. Also discuss the different possible modes of failure that may occur for this installation.

SOLUTION: Before attempting the actual computations to the solution of this problem, the engineer should mentally prepare in his own mind the sequence of steps required to successfully substantiate the final design. For all intents and purposes, use past engineering experience to better understand and perceive all of the familiar and unfamiliar aspects of this problem. Then, use the summary on pages 183-185 to help project these perceived observations to its detailed solution.

Let us begin this solution by first resolving the cable tension load into horizontal and vertical components of force R_x and R_y acting at the center of the pulley. See Fig. 3-31 for the free-body diagram of the isolated pulley and the equilibrium forces necessary to balance this structural member. These forces are determined from the equations of statics as follows:

$$\Sigma F_x = 0, \qquad -R_x + 400 + 400\cos 35^\circ = 0, \quad R_x = 728 \text{ lb}$$

$$\Sigma F_y = 0, \qquad R_y - 400\sin 35^\circ = 0, \quad R_y = 229 \text{ lb}.$$

[1] This may well be the proper procedure for some problems of structural design, but a strong criticism of its overuse is noted when more efficient methods of structural analysis are available to the engineer.

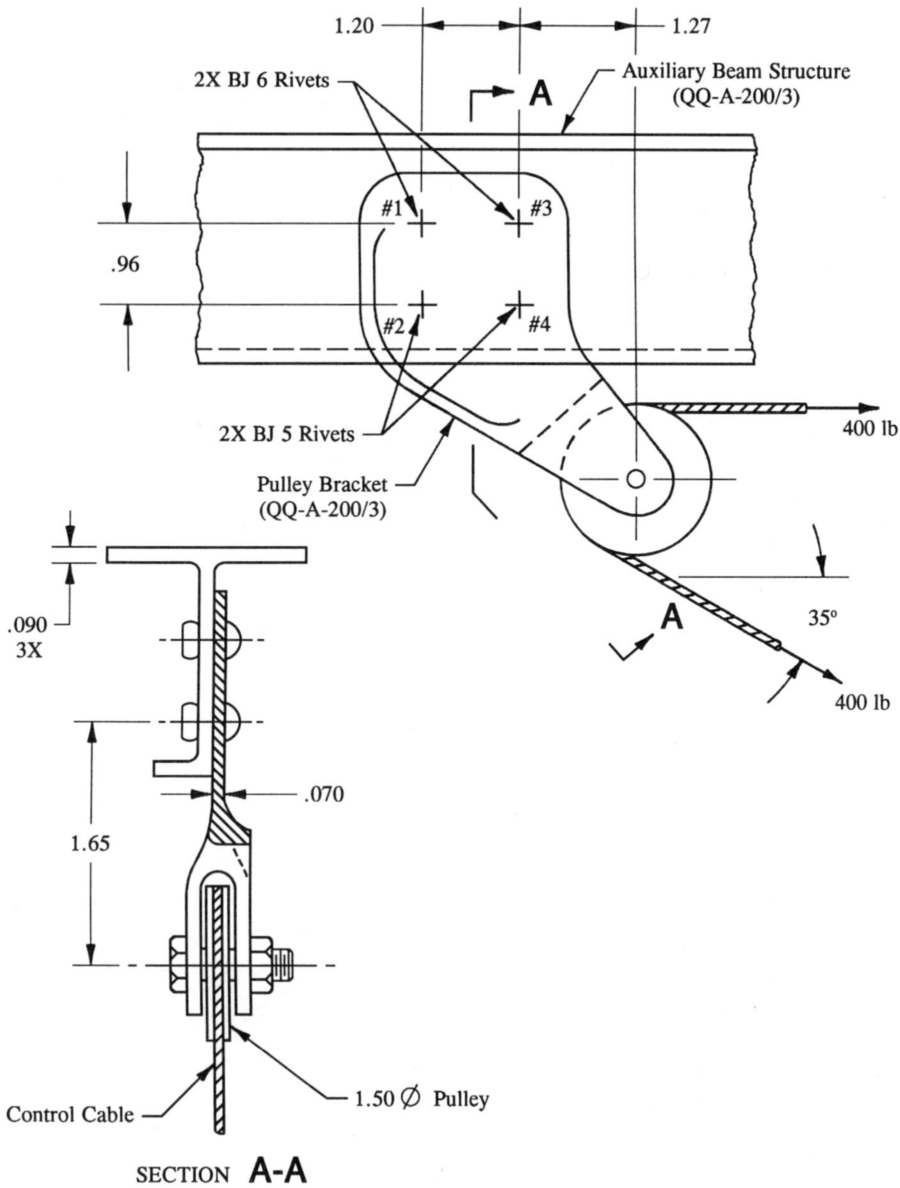

FIGURE 3-30 Pulley bracket installation for an auxiliary beam.

Note, in particular, how these forces then become applied loads on the bracket plate, as shown in Fig. 3-32. Next, the centroid of the rivet areas is located using the tabular format described in Table 3-5 (refer back to page 174).

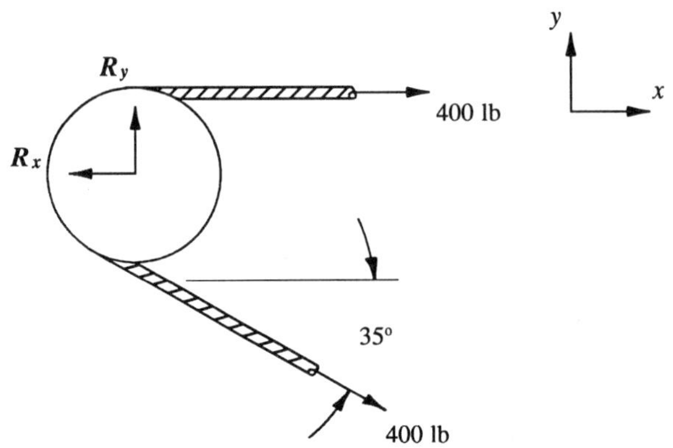

FIGURE 3-31 Free-body diagram of the isolated pulley and the equilibrium forces required to balance this member.

TABLE 3-11 CENTROID LOCATION OF RIVET AREAS

Fastener No.	D	x	y	D^2	D^2x	D^2y
1	0.191	0.000	0.960	0.0365	0.0000	0.035
2	0.159	0.000	0.000	0.0253	0.0000	0.000
3	0.191	1.200	0.960	0.0365	0.0438	0.035
4	0.159	1.200	0.000	0.0253	0.0303	0.000
			Total	0.1236	0.0741	0.070

For this connection, the rectangular coordinate axes x and y are chosen so that they conveniently intersect with the location of rivet #2. The location of the centroidal axes $\bar{x}_{cg}$ and $\bar{y}_{cg}$ are found by substituting the appropriate column totals of Table 3-11 into Eqs. 3-12 and 3-13. Hence

$$X_{cg} = \frac{\Sigma(D^2x)}{\Sigma D^2} = \frac{.0741}{.1236} = .600 \text{ in}$$

$$Y_{cg} = \frac{\Sigma(D^2y)}{\Sigma D^2} = \frac{.070}{.1236} = .566 \text{ in.}$$

Does this result seem reasonable with anticipated values estimated by just guessing at the location of the centroid? If they do, chances are pretty good that the computed values are probably correct—a little common sense logic now can go a long

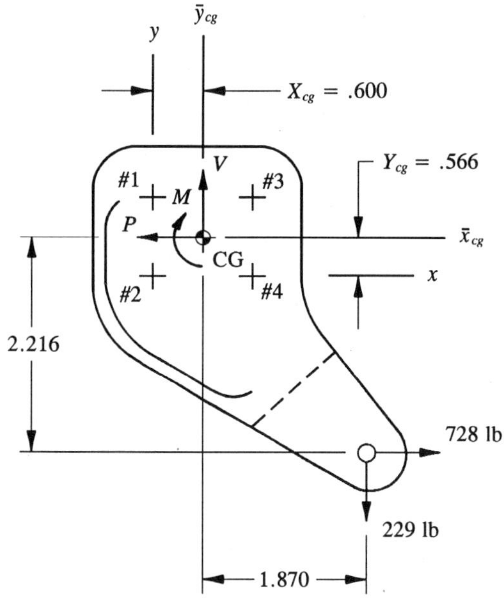

FIGURE 3-32 Free-body diagram of the pulley bracket and the internal forces *V, P,* and *M* at the centroid of the rivet group.

way in avoiding time-consuming repeat calculations later.

Now, with the centroid of the rivet group firmly established, the equilibrium forces *V, P,* and *M* at the centroid of the rivet group can be determined. These forces are indicated in Fig. 3-32, and their values are computed as follows using the equations of static equilibrium:

$$\Sigma F_x = 0, \qquad -P + 728 = 0, \quad P = 728 \text{ lb}$$

$$\Sigma F_y = 0, \qquad V - 229 = 0, \quad V = 229 \text{ lb}$$

$$\Sigma M_{cg} = 0, \qquad (+ \quad M + 229(1.87) - 728(2.216) = 0$$

$$M = 1,185 \text{ in-lb}.$$

Since these quantities are all positive values, the assumed directions of these forces have been correctly indicated in this figure. Only in the special case of a cantilevered beam structure, and the pulley bracket is considered just such a member here, are applied loads directly transferable to the centroid of a fastener group. In all other design cases, a beam would have to be free-bodied and the proper reaction forces described on the structure before the equilibrium forces *V, P,* and *M* at the centroid of a fastener group could actually be computed. The above argument will become clearer later in our study when these particular concepts have been reviewed and focused upon in more detail.

Rivet load distributions are achieved by distributing the forces *V*, *P*, and *M*, one at a time, as shearing forces resisted by all the rivets of the connection. For rivets of different sizes but of the same general type or category, distribution of rivet shearing forces is conveniently set up in tabular form (see Tables 3-12, 3-13, and 3-14 which follow).

TABLE 3-12 DISTRIBUTION OF DIRECT AXIAL FORCE *P*

Fastener No.	D	D^2	$(p_s)_P$
1	0.191	0.0365	215
2	0.159	0.0253	149*
3	0.191	0.0365	215
4	0.159	0.0253	149
	Total	0.1236	728

* Sample calculation for rivet #2:

$$(p_s)_P = \frac{PD^2}{\Sigma D^2} = \frac{728(.0253)}{.1236} = 149 \text{ lb.}$$

The shearing force distributions for the axial force *P* are pictorially diagrammed in Fig. 3-33.

TABLE 3-13 DISTRIBUTION OF DIRECT SHEARING FORCE *V*

Fastener No.	D	D^2	$(p_s)_V$
1	0.191	0.0365	68
2	0.159	0.0253	47*
3	0.191	0.0365	68
4	0.159	0.0253	47
	Total	0.1236	230

* Sample calculation for rivet #2:

$$(p_s)_V = \frac{VD^2}{\Sigma D^2} = \frac{229(.0253)}{.1236} = 47 \text{ lb.}$$

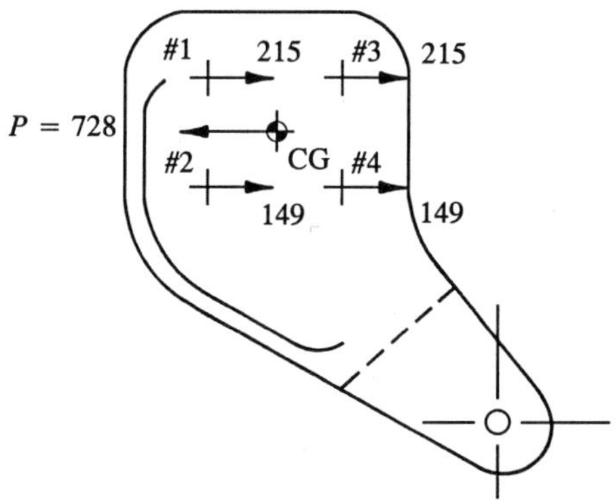

FIGURE 3-33 Distribution of the direct axial force *P*.

The shearing force distributions are drawn in Fig. 3-34. Note how each rivet is depicted here resisting the shearing force *V*. To maintain the same consistency of load distributions as those presumed for *V* and *P*, the torsional moment must also be shown in this same direction resisted by all of the rivets of the connection. The engineer is referred to Fig. 3-35, where the torsional shearing forces $(p_s)_m$ are shown individually diagrammed opposing the clockwise rotation of the torsional moment *M*. Since, in general, the solution of the torsional moment is more conveniently done in a rectangular coordinate axes system, these forces are not actually calculated. Instead, the horizontal and vertical components of these forces are computed (see Table 3-14).

TABLE 3-14 DISTRIBUTION OF TORSIONAL MOMENT *M*

Fast. No.	D	$\bar{x}$	$\bar{y}$	r	$D^2\bar{x}$	$D^2\bar{y}$	D^2r^2	$[(p_s)_m]_x$	$[(p_s)_m]_y$
1	0.191	0.600	0.394	0.718	0.0219	0.0144	0.0188	237	360
2	0.159	0.600	0.566	0.825	0.0152	0.0143	0.0172	235*	250*
3	0.191	0.600	0.394	0.718	0.0219	0.0144	0.0188	237	360
4	0.159	0.600	0.566	0.825	0.0152	0.0143	0.0172	235	250
						Total	0.0720		

* Sample calculations for rivet #2:

$$[(p_s)_m]_x = \frac{MD^2\bar{y}}{\Sigma(D^2r^2)} = \frac{1,185(.0143)}{.0720} = 235 \text{ lb}$$

$$[(p_s)_m]_y = \frac{MD^2\bar{x}}{\Sigma(D^2r^2)} = \frac{1,185(.0152)}{.0720} = 250 \text{ lb}.$$

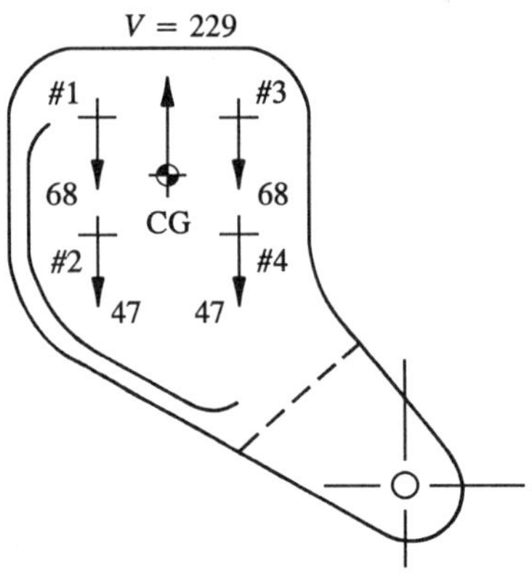

FIGURE 3-34 Distribution of the direct shearing force *V*.

The next step in the solution of this problem is to vectorially superimpose the three separate solutions for *V*, *P*, and *M* (see Fig. 3-36) into one resultant shearing force system. The actual computations are done in Table 3-15, and the results of that tabulation are shown in Fig. 3-37.

TABLE 3-15 SUPERPOSITION OF DIRECT AND TORSIONAL COMPONENT LOADS

Fastener No.	$(p_s)_v$	$(p_s)_p$	$[(p_s)_m]_x$	$[(p_s)_m]_y$	Σp_x	Σp_y	p_s
1	68	215	237	360	22	428	429
2	47	149	235	250	384	297	485*
3	68	215	237	360	22	292	293
4	47	149	235	250	384	203	434

* Rivet #2 is the maximum loaded rivet of the fastener group, and since it also has the smallest diameter, this critical combination, if substantiated by analysis, will also substantiate all of the other rivets of the pulley bracket installation not as critically loaded. Sample calculations for rivet #2:

$$\Sigma p_x = (p_s)_p + [(p_s)_m]_x = 149 + 235 = 384 \text{ lb}$$

$$\Sigma p_y = (p_s)_v + [(p_s)_m]_y = 47 + 250 = 297 \text{ lb}.$$

From the Pythagorean theorem,

$$p_s = [(\Sigma p_x)^2 + (\Sigma p_y)^2]^{1/2} = [(384)^2 + (297)^2]^{1/2} = 485 \text{ lb}.$$

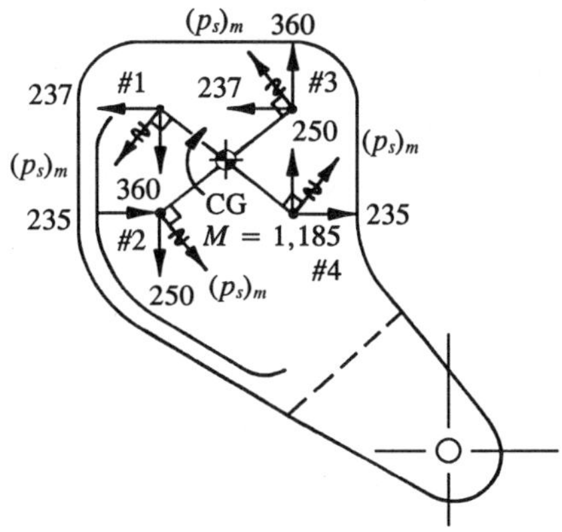

FIGURE 3-35 Distribution of the torsional moment M.

Possible Modes of Failure of the Pulley Bracket Installation:

(1) Check for shearing failure of rivet #2 (use Eq. 3-1 for this calculation).

(2) Substantiate the pulley bracket plate (see Fig. 3-30) for bearing failure at rivet #2 (bearing failure of the auxiliary beam web is not critical). This can be directly observed by comparing the linearity of the thickness dimensions of each member as described by Eqs. 3-2 and 3-3.

(3) To prevent shear-out failure of the pulley bracket plate, all rivets must have ample edge distance (check this condition by applying Eq. 3-4).

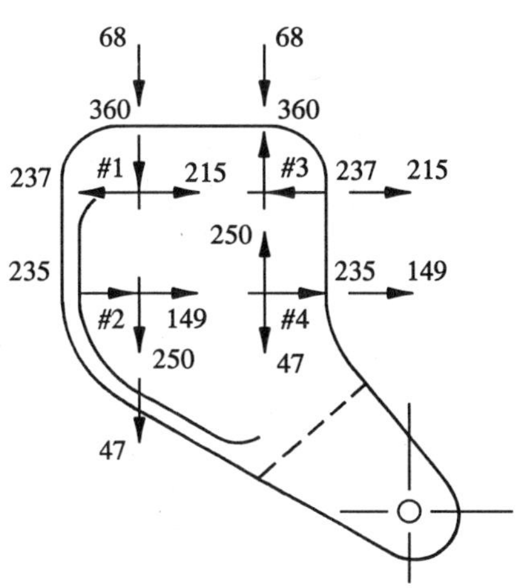

FIGURE 3-36 Rivet shearing forces (from Figs. 3-33, 3-34, and 3-35).

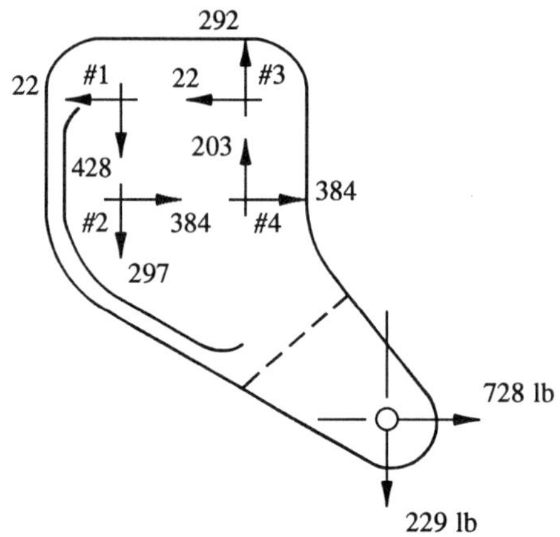

FIGURE 3-37 Superposition of direct and component shearing forces (from Table 3-15).

(4) Calculate the combined axial and bending stresses at critical points along the pulley bracket. Here, the equations of static equilibrium are applied at Sections A-A, B-B, and C-C, as shown in Fig. 3-38. Then, the internal loads found there are substituted into Eq. 2-9 and the maximum extreme fiber stresses are computed.

(5) Calculate the maximum shearing stress at Sections A-A, B-B, and C-C of the pulley bracket plate (see Chapter 4 for the method of analysis used to perform these evaluations).

(6) Perform a lug and pin analysis of the pulley bracket at point O (see a company structures manual for the step-by-step procedure used to substantiate these lug members).

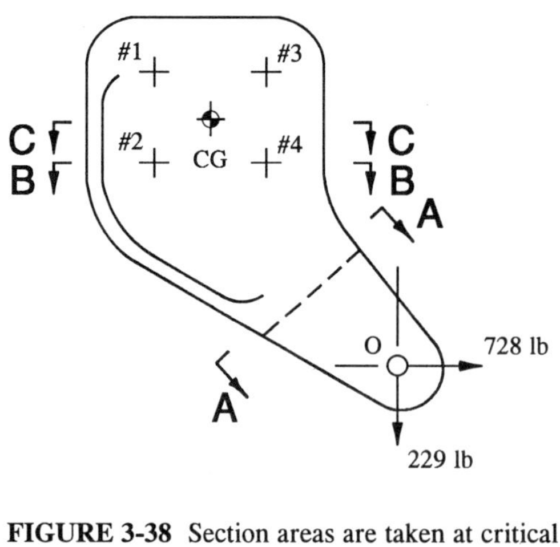

FIGURE 3-38 Section areas are taken at critical points along the pulley bracket.

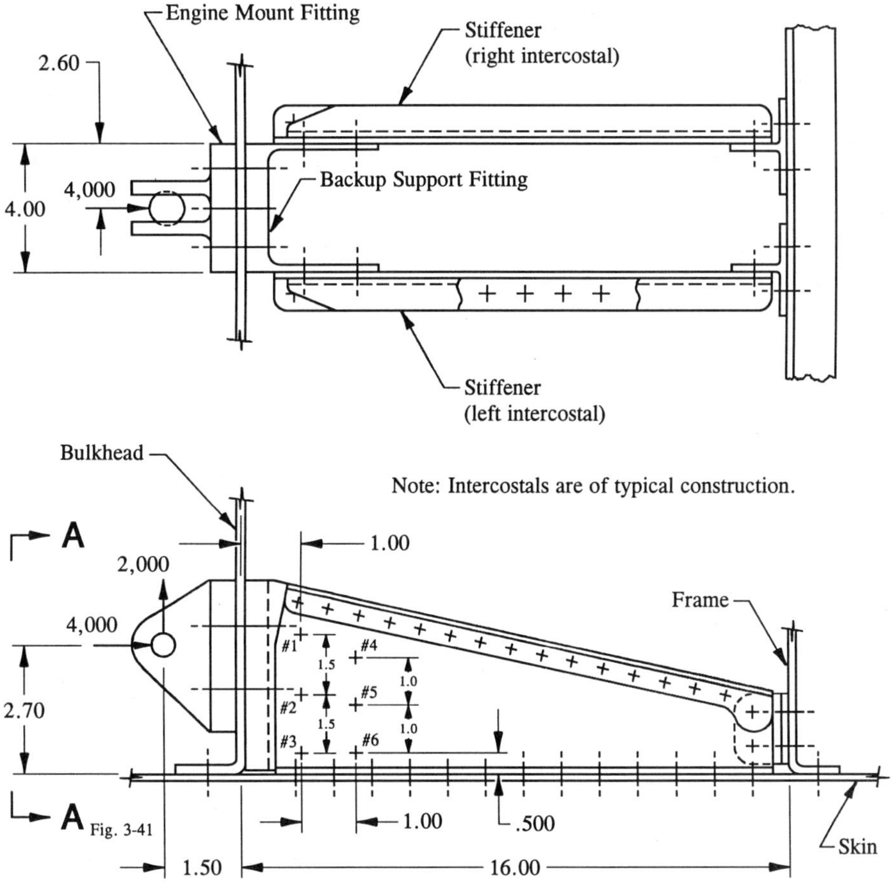

FIGURE 3-39 Structural arrangement of intercostals used to distribute concentrated loads more efficiently into the structure.

Example 3-3 The engine mount fitting of a production model aircraft is securely attached to its bulkhead structure as shown in Fig. 3-39. To prevent the bulkhead web from physically collapsing under the applied loads given, a backup structure consisting of a backup fitting and two identical intercostals is proposed for support of this member. For this structural arrangement, determine the shearing forces transmitted by the fasteners of the backup fitting structure (*Hint:* Isolate and compare intercostals first for maximum load combinations. Then, with the loads acting separately on the critical intercostal, determine the load distribution to joint fasteners.)

SOLUTION: Before each intercostal can be isolated and free-bodied for analysis, the applied loads must be properly distributed to each member. To do this, the

FROM FIGURE 3-39, INTERCOSTAL ASSEMBLY REMOVED FOR CLARITY.

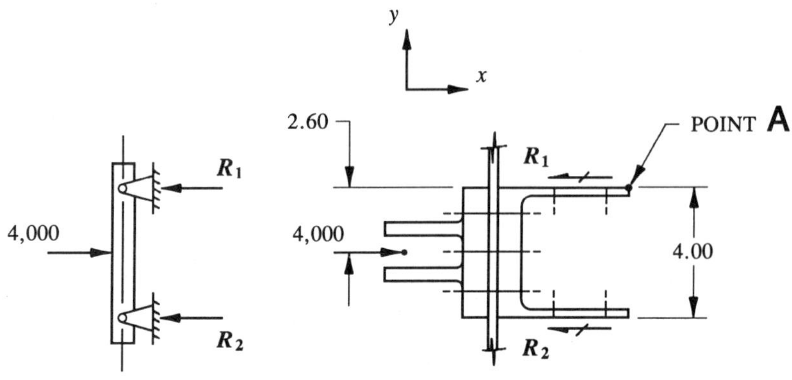

FIGURE 3-40 Distribution of horizontal applied load.

horizontal and vertical applied loads (4,000 lb and 2,000 lb, respectively) are each proportionately distributed to each intercostal in accordance with simple beam theory—so much of each load is reacted by the right intercostal and so much by the left. In other words, distribution is achieved by idealizing each intercostal as a support structure, and then distributing the applied loads to each respective member. To simplify our analysis further, let us assume that the intercostals are simply-supported. From this assumption, the distributed quantities (or shear forces) are easily found, as indicated by the unknown reaction forces R_1 and R_2, R_3 and R_4 in Figs. 3-40 and 3-41, respectively. To obtain the solution to these unknown quantities, the equations of equilibrium are applied. From statics, then, the following expressions are formulated:

$$\Sigma F_x = 0, \qquad 4,000 - R_1 - R_2 = 0$$

$$\Sigma M_A = 0, \qquad \circlearrowleft + \quad -4,000(2.6) + 4.0R_2 = 0, \quad R_2 = 2,600 \text{ lb}.$$

Substituting the value of R_2 into the first equation above, we obtain:

$$4,000 - R_1 - 2,600 = 0, \quad R_1 = 1,400 \text{ lb}.$$

For the vertically applied load (Fig. 3-41):

$$\Sigma F_z = 0, \qquad 2,000 - R_3 - R_4 = 0$$

$$\Sigma M_B = 0, \qquad \circlearrowleft + \quad -2,000(2.6) + 4.0R_4 = 0, \quad R_4 = 1,300 \text{ lb}.$$

And, substituting this value back into the first expression gives:

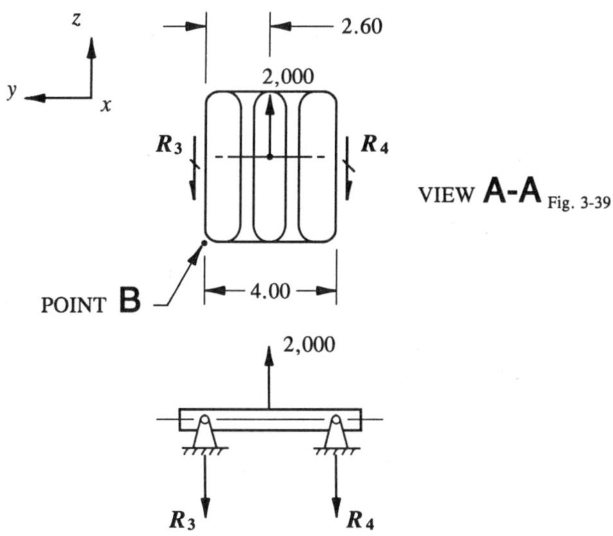

FIGURE 3-41 Distribution of vertical applied load.

$$2,000 - R_3 - 1,300 = 0, \quad R_3 = 700 \text{ lb}.$$

Now, comparing intercostal loads, it is rather clear that the left intercostal, with $R_2 = 2,600$ lb and $R_4 = 1,300$ lb, will have the maximum combination of distributed loads to its structure; consequently, the right intercostal, with the lower loads $R_1 = 1,400$ lb and $R_3 = 700$ lb, is not as critically loaded. Keeping this point in mind, and noting the fact that both intercostals are identical structures, this means that the left intercostal (with its higher loads) must be structurally more critical. And therefore, this member is chosen to represent the structural analysis solution of both members. In effect, what this says is that, with the critical combination of applied loads known for the left intercostal, the analytical substantiation of this member is sufficient to presume the structural integrity and substantiation of the other intercostal. A complete free-body diagram of the left intercostal with the proper orientation of reaction forces indicated is shown in Fig. 3-42.

However, before solving for these unknown reactions, let us review and evaluate the structural capabilities of the shear clip, bulkhead, and skin members representing these unknown quantities. For instance, it is common knowledge that a shear clip will provide very little axial restraint capability, tension or compression, compared to its primary function governed by its ability to support vertical shear loads (thus, the reaction R_2 is denoted for the structural capability of this member). Also, too flexible to afford much horizontal restraint is the bulkhead web itself—since its primary capability is to carry shear loads in-plane (thus, the

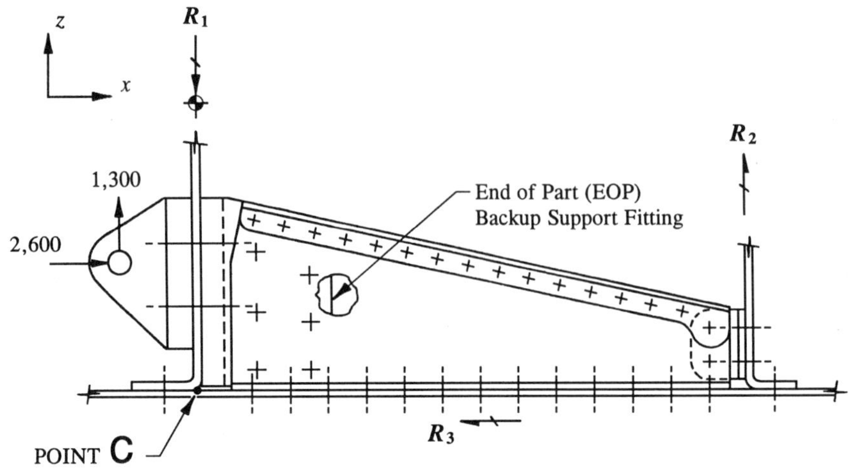

FIGURE 3-42 Free-body diagram of the left intercostal with the proper orientation of reaction forces. (Dimensions pertinent to the analysis are shown in Fig. 3-39.)

reaction symbol R_1 is denoted for this member). Now consider what structural member will provide the horizontal restraint capability required to stabilize the engine mount from side movement? Answer: The skin does by physically shearing the axial load through its skin fasteners (here, the symbol R_3 is used to denote and thus represent the physical restraint capability of this member).

Now, with all of the reactions having been defined in terms of the support capabilities of the structure, the equations of equilibrium can be directly applied to the left intercostal.

$$\Sigma F_x = 0, \quad 2,600 - R_3 = 0, \quad R_3 = 2,600 \text{ lb}$$

$$\Sigma F_z = 0, \quad -R_1 + R_2 + 1,300 = 0$$

$$\Sigma M_C = 0, \quad \circlearrowleft\!+ \quad 2,600(2.7) + 1,300(1.5) - 16.0R_2 = 0, \quad R_2 = 561 \text{ lb.}$$

And substituting R_2 back into the second equation of equilibrium gives:

$$-R_1 + 561 + 1,300 = 0, \quad R_1 = 1,861 \text{ lb.}$$

The completely balanced structure is shown in Fig. 3-43. Note, in particular, that the reaction R_3 could have been expressed in terms of individual skin rivet loads. This is accomplished by assuming an equal distribution of shear to each rivet. From Eq. 3-9, the following rivet shear loads would then be obtained:

$$p_s = \frac{P}{n} = \frac{2,600}{13} = 200 \text{ lb.}$$

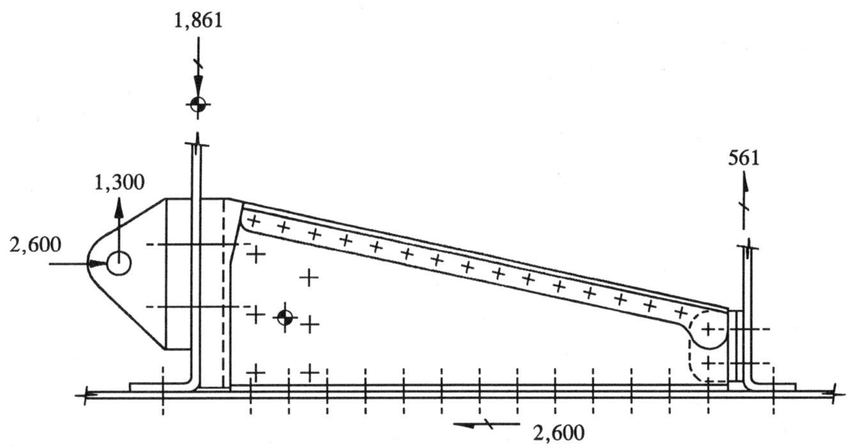

FIGURE 3-43 Left intercostal is shown with reaction forces determined.

Shearing failure is then predicted for these rivets by using Eq. 3-1 and the appropriate (substitution of values) into the margin of safety expression.

Next, with all reaction forces determined, the internal loads *V, P,* and *M* at the centroid of the rivet group are determined. But first, before this can be done, from the structural arrangement of fasteners indicated in Fig. 3-39, the exact location of the rivet group centroid must be found. This is done by simple inspection of the rivet coordinates at the fastener group. (However, should this technique completely elude the engineer, Eqs. 3-14 and 3-15 can help with a review of these principles: that is, to formulate certain aspects or distinct features of these equations which can then help us determine the way in which the centroid location is arrived at or problems like this are more expeditiously solved.) To evaluate these loads, a vertical section cut (or slice) is taken through the centroid of the rivet group, Fig. 3-44, and the equations of equilibrium applied in the usual way as follows:

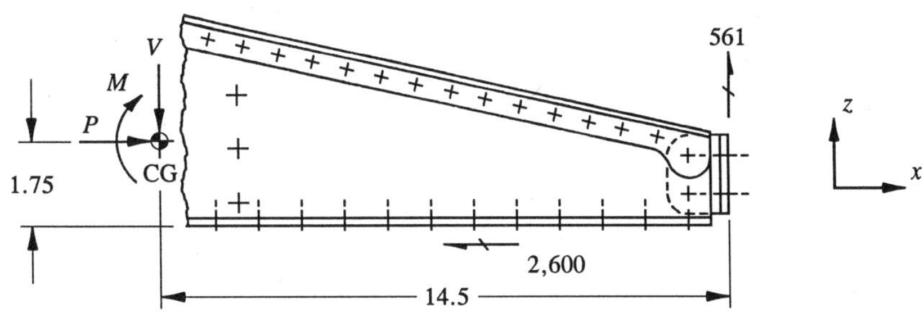

FIGURE 3-44 Internal forces *V, P,* and *M* across the intercostal through the centroid of the rivet group.

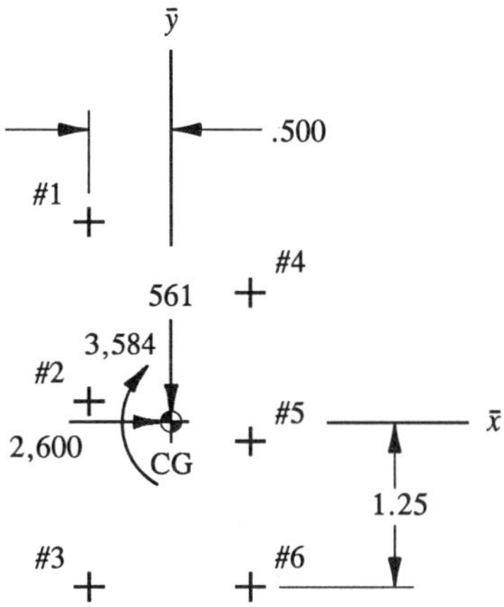

FIGURE 3-45 Internal forces *V, P,* and *M* at the centroid of the rivet group.

$$\Sigma F_z = 0, \qquad 561 - V = 0, \quad V = 561 \text{ lb}$$
$$\Sigma F_x = 0, \qquad -2,600 + P = 0, \quad P = 2,600 \text{ lb}$$
$$\Sigma M_{cg} = 0, \qquad 2,600(1.75) - 561(14.5) + M = 0$$
$$M = 3,584 \text{ in-lb.}$$

These quantities are correctly diagrammed in Fig. 3-45.

Since all rivets are of the same size and type, rivet load distributions are greatly simplified. Hence, the following equations are employed for these computations:

Distribution of Direct Shearing Force *V* (see Eq. 3-22):

$$(p_s)_v = \frac{V}{n} = \frac{561}{6} = 93 \text{ lb.}$$

Distribution of Direct Axial Force *P* (see Eq. 3-23):

$$(p_s)_p = \frac{P}{n} = \frac{2,600}{6} = 433 \text{ lb.}$$

These distributions are pictorially diagrammed in Fig. 3-46(a) as rivet shearing forces.

Distribution of Torsional Moment *M* (see Eqs. 3-29 and 3-30):

$$\left[(p_s)_m\right]_x = \frac{M\bar{y}}{\Sigma r^2}$$

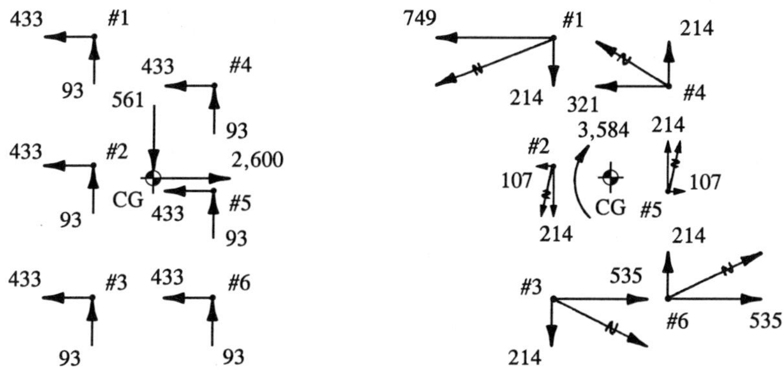

(a) Distribution of Direct Loads *V* and *P*.

(b) Distribution of Torsional Moment *M*.

FIGURE 3-46 Rivet shearing forces: (a) for the direct loads *V* and *P* and (b) for the torsional moment *M*.

$$\left[(p_s)_m\right]_y = \frac{M\bar{x}}{\sum r^2}.$$

The actual computations are done in tabular form (refer to Table 3-14 for some of the appropriate column headings to use for this tabulation).

TABLE 3-16 DISTRIBUTION OF TORSIONAL MOMENT *M*

Fastener No.	$\bar{x}$	$\bar{y}$	r	r^2	$[(p_s)_m]_x$	$[(p_s)_m]_y$
1	0.500	1.75	1.820	3.312	749*	214*
2	0.500	0.25	0.559	0.312	107	214
3	0.500	1.25	1.346	1.812	535	214
4	0.500	0.75	0.901	0.812	321	214
5	0.500	0.25	0.559	0.312	107	214
6	0.500	1.25	1.346	1.812	535	214
			Total	8.372		

* Sample calculations for rivet #1:

$$\left[(p_s)_m\right]_x = \frac{M\bar{y}}{\sum r^2} = \frac{3,584(1.75)}{8.372} = 749 \text{ lb}$$

$$\left[(p_s)_m\right]_y = \frac{M\bar{x}}{\sum r^2} = \frac{3,584(.500)}{8.372} = 214 \text{ lb}.$$

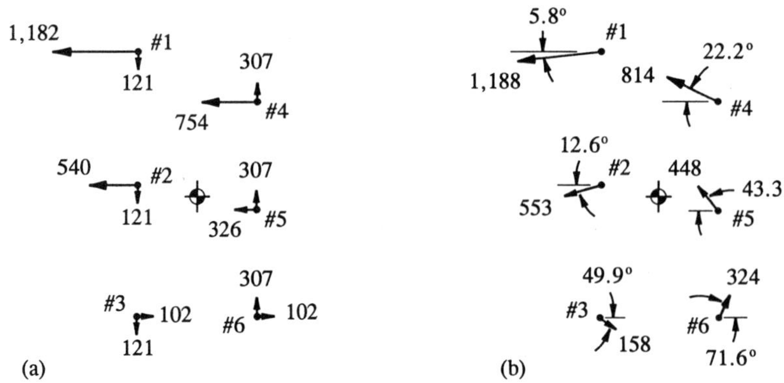

FIGURE 3-47 (a) Summation of direct and component shearing forces (from Table 3-17). (b) Resultant fastener shearing forces (see last column of Table 3-17).

The component torsional shearing forces are shown diagrammed in Fig. 3-46(b). Next, the three separate solutions of *V*, *P*, and *M* are vectorially superimposed into a horizontal and vertical component shearing force system. This is conveniently done in tabular form in Table 3-17, and the results of that tabulation are diagrammed in Fig. 3-47(a).

TABLE 3-17 SUPERPOSITION OF DIRECT AND TORSIONAL COMPONENT LOADS

Fastener No.	$(p_s)_v$	$(p_s)_p$	$[(p_s)_m]_x$	$[(p_s)_m]_y$	Σp_x	Σp_y	p_s
1	93	433	749	214	1,182*	121*	1,188
2	93	433	107	214	540	121	553
3	93	433	535	214	102	121	158
4	93	433	321	214	754	307	814
5	93	433	107	214	326	307	448
6	93	433	535	214	102	307	324

* Sample calculations for rivet #1:

(a) Summation of forces in the *x*-direction:

$$\Sigma p_x = (p_s)_p + [(p_s)_m]_x = 433 + 749 = 1,182 \text{ lb.}$$

(b) Summation of forces in the *y*-direction:

$$\Sigma p_y = (p_s)_v + [(p_s)_m]_y = -93 + 214 = 121 \text{ lb.}$$

And then from these values, based on the critically stressed rivet, the resultant shearing force of rivet #1 is computed:

$$p_s = \left[(\Sigma\, p_x)^2 + (\Sigma\, p_y)^2\right]^{1/2} = \left[(1,182)^2 + (121)^2\right]^{1/2} = 1,188 \text{ lb.}$$

Reapplying these same equations again, but this time, to the rest of the rivets of the fastener group, the resultant shearing forces of the remaining rivets are calculated. Their values are tabulated in the last column of Table 3-17. This then completes the required solution to this problem: that of calculating the rivet shearing forces of the backup fitting support structure, Fig. 3-47(b).

Although the particular requirement of this example problem has been met, and the engineer fully understands the details of its solution, the structural integrity of the final design must of course also include the static strength requirements for mechanically fastened connections as established in Sec. 3.2. As a review of these criteria, a connection should always include the basic structural evaluations of (1) shearing failure of the connection rivets and (2) bearing failure of the connection plates. In most cases, unless specifically calculated for by the engineer, all other analytical checks possible for the structure are presumed to be unnecessary (that is, not a serious consideration or necessary requirement for structural substantiation). This occurrence, conceivably, might result from either a condition of the internal loads being too low or the structure being too heavy (overstrength). In either case, it remains the engineer's prerogative to determine whether these superfluous computations actually warrant his personal stress evaluation of the structure.

Now consider what other possible structural failures could conceivably occur in this design? Answer: To completely substantiate the structural integrity of this entire design, the engineer must also include in his analytical investigations the preliminary stress checks of the following structures: (1) shear clips, (2) engine mount fitting, (3) intercostals, (4) bulkhead, (5) frame, (6) skin, and (7) backup support fitting. The engineer is encouraged to mentally prepare or review in his mind those detailed, step-by-step stress evaluations that he may deem necessary and appropriate for general substantiation of these structural members. Or, alternatively, simply list each equation used (from Chapters 1, 2, and 3) with its corresponding margin of safety expression. After subsequent chapters of this text have been fully treated, this mental preparation should again be attempted, but this time, expanded to include the material of these newer chapters.

3.6 Analysis of a Fuselage Frame Splice Using Computer-Generated Output Loads. Many different types of mechanically fastened connections are possible in aircraft design. Among these, the most common types that are most frequently encountered by the aircraft design engineer will be discussed in this section. It is hoped that from these specific example problems, the engineer will gain a better understanding to the solution of complex structures, and, from this knowledge, demonstrate the ability to act effectively in similar or related design situations. The first of these examples will illustrate the basic principles of frame splice design

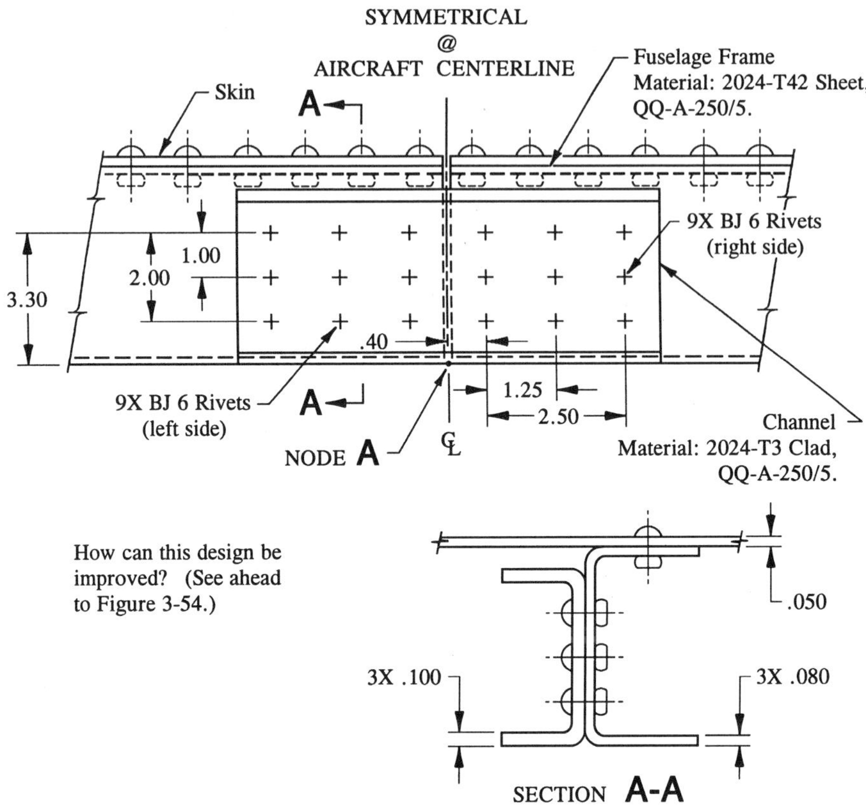

FIGURE 3-48 Fuselage centerline frame splice.

using output loads given from a computer model analysis of a fuselage frame.

Example 3-4 A channel section is used to splice a fuselage frame across its centerline, as shown in Fig. 3-48. The internal loads given from a computer model solution of this structure for fuselage down-bending are shown on isolated segments of the frame structure in Fig. 3-49. These loads are defined at node point A as follows: $P = 1,500$ lb, $V = -1,200$ lb, and $M = -650$ in-lb. The sign convention adopted below was used to correctly represent these loads on exposed sections of the fuselage frame (the engineer is encouraged to verify these loads on the structure).

(1) P is a tension load if its value is positive.
(2) V acts inward towards the center of the fuselage on the left-hand side of an exposed section if its value is positive.
(3) M produces compression on the skin side if its value is positive.

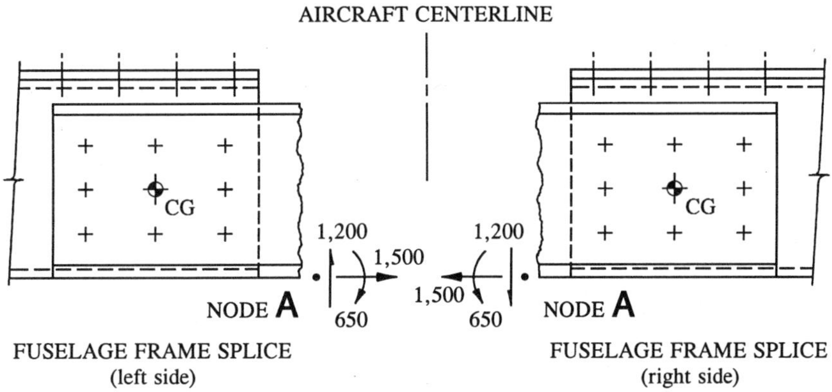

FIGURE 3-49 Internal loads at Node A for isolated segments of the frame structure.

Consider the frame splice symmetrical about the centerline of the aircraft and determine the appropriate bearing and shearing margins of safety for the most critical rivet group. (*Hint:* pinpoint the critical rivet group by comparing internal frame loads *V*, *P*, and *M* at the centroid of each rivet group.)

Discussion: In many computer-generated solutions, internal loads are not normally indicated at the centroid of a fastener group. In such cases, the engineer must transfer these loads there, to structurally duplicate the true behavior of the connection design. For the most part, these loads are very similar to hand-calculated loads, in that, they (program loads) are also uniquely derived from load manipulations—that is, through the application of the equations of equilibrium, these loads may conveniently be represented at arbitrary points acting anywhere on or off the structure (e.g., the leading edge of a wing is sometimes used to describe the location of wing loads, although they do not however realistically occur there). Consequently, for this reason, such loads are normally transferred to certain specified points on the structure that will more realistically represent the true physical loading effect of the structure under load. As a matter of fact, no matter where these loads have been depicted, on or off the structure, they must always be transferred back to their proper location on the structure before proceeding ahead with structural computations using their values. For the analysis of mechanically fastened connections this location, commonly referred to as "the centroid of the rivet group," is of particular importance to the eventual correct solution of the connection.

SOLUTION: Using the sign convention given for each loading, and from basic definitions used to describe internal loads existing at a section of beam, the following loads are indicated for the left- and right-hand sides of the frame structure. The engineer should have no difficulty describing these loads there using the sign convention given for each particular loading. These loads are indicated on each section of frame structure in Fig. 3-49. However, before using their values to determine rivet shearing forces, each loading system must be correctly defined at the centroid of their respective rivet groups. Only then can the true stress behavior of the fuselage splice joint be accurately duplicated by the structural analysis methods discussed in this chapter.

The pertinent formulas necessary to make these simple transformations are found throughout this book. The engineer is referred in particular to specific details and background information in Chapter 1, Sec. 1.5. Basically, though, it should be recalled from this chapter that internal loads can generally be described at any point on or off a structure. And, since only one particular location can correctly describe the true structural behavior of a connection design under load. In accordance with the procedure outlined in this chapter, to determine rivet shearing forces, this location must correspond to the centroid of the rivet group. This is most easily accomplished by performing simple transformations of load using the equations of static equilibrium.

Now, to gain additional insight into the structural behavior of the fuselage centerline frame splice, let us briefly describe the proper sequence of load transfers that should occur across the centerline of this splice arrangement: Quite simply, the internal loads from one side of the frame structure (this includes both the skin and basic frame section) are transferred by nine (9) BJ 6 rivets to the channel section across the centerline splice to the other side of the frame structure by the other nine (9) BJ 6 rivets. Then, according to the discussions outlined above, to describe these load transfers correctly, the loads given for each side diagrammed in Fig. 3-49 must be transferred to the centroid of each rivet group. (By inspection, the centroids are located at the centers of the rivet groups.) From statics, the numerical computations of these transformations for the left- and right-hand sides of each rivet group are shown below (see also Figs. 3-50 and 3-51, respectively).

$$\Sigma F_x = 0, \qquad -P + 1,500 = 0, \quad P = 1,500 \text{ lb}$$

$$\Sigma F_y = 0, \qquad -V + 1,200 = 0, \quad V = 1,200 \text{ lb}$$

$$\Sigma M_{cg} = 0, \qquad \circlearrowleft + \quad 650 + M - 1,200(1.65) - 1,500(2.30) = 0$$

$$M = 4,780 \text{ in-lb.}$$

$$\Sigma F_x = 0, \qquad P - 1,500 = 0, \quad P = 1,500 \text{ lb}$$

$$\Sigma F_y = 0, \qquad V - 1,200 = 0, \quad V = 1,200 \text{ lb}$$

$$\Sigma M_{cg} = 0, \qquad \circlearrowleft + \quad -650 - M - 1,200(1.65) + 1,500(2.30) = 0$$

$$M = 820 \text{ in-lb.}$$

The equivalent forces *V*, *P*, and *M* at each centroid are then compared, and the critical set producing the maximum combination of rivet shearing forces is chosen for the actual connection analysis. The other, which is analytically more favorable, is less critical, and therefore structurally obvious—and thus, enveloped by simple logic and reasoning. For this example, this will occur for the left-hand side since for this particular rivet group the moment is slightly higher (4,780 in-lb for the left-

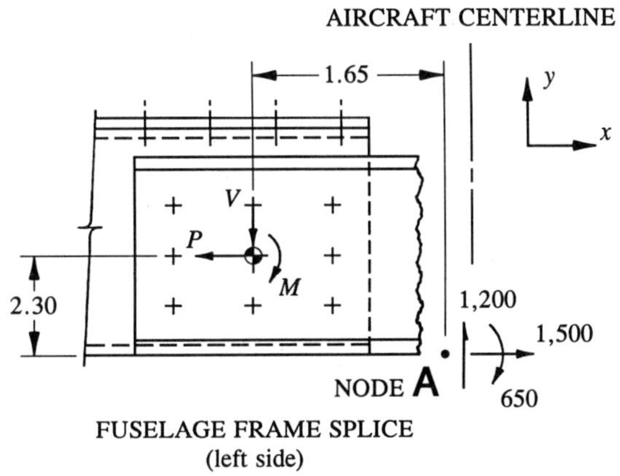

FIGURE 3-50 Internal forces at the centroid of the fuselage frame splice (left side).

hand side versus 820 in-lb for the right-hand side).

Distribution of rivet shearing forces for the equivalent forces *V*, *P*, and *M* are viewed in Fig. 3-52 for each rivet of the left-hand side; where, pictorially, these forces have been diagrammed at all of the rivet locations. For rivets of the same size and type, the shearing forces are evaluated by applying Eqs. 3-22, 3-23, and 3-24 (the engineer is also referred to Eqs. 3-29 and 3-30). The results of these computations are tabulated in Tables 3-18, 3-19, and 3-20, respectively. Since the direct shearing forces of *V* and *P* will divide equally between all fasteners of the rivet group, the most critical fastener becomes the one for which the distribution of torsional component forces combine algebraically in the same direction as those indicated for the direct shearing forces. Both components of torsion are observed to do just that for rivet #9 (see Fig. 3-52).

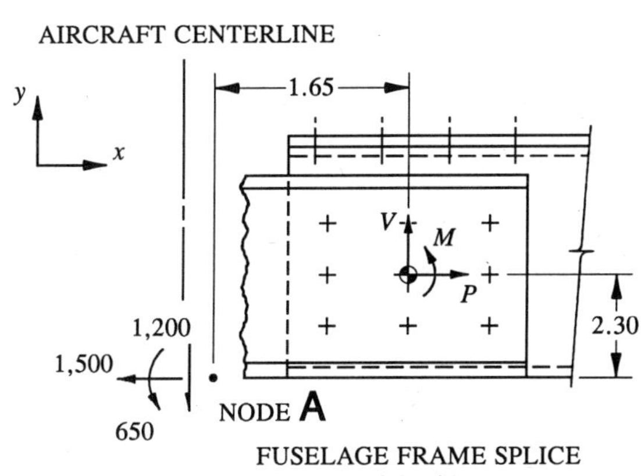

FIGURE 3-51 Internal forces at the centroid of the fuselage frame splice (right side).

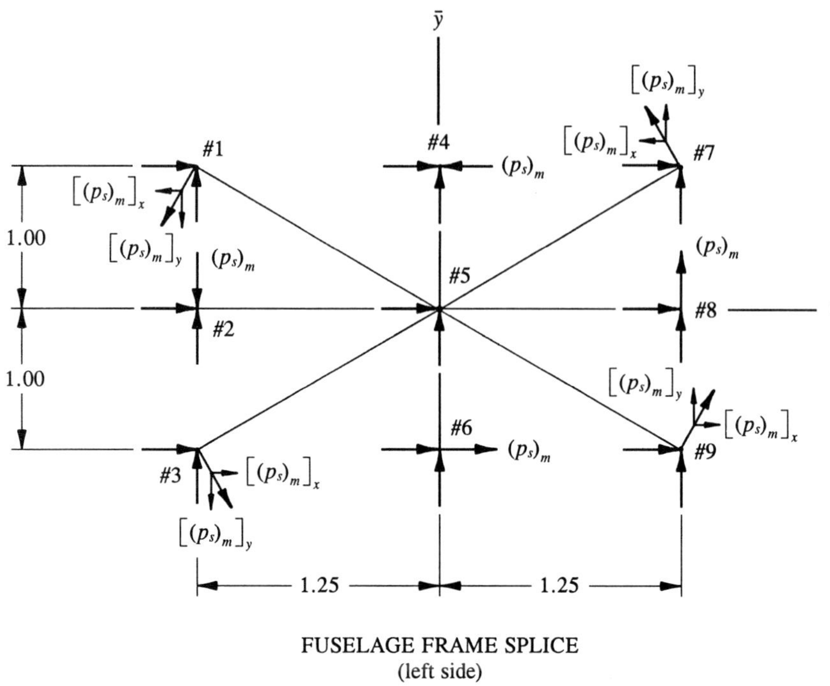

FIGURE 3-52 Distribution of rivet shearing forces for the internal forces *V*, *P*, and *M*. (Component shearing forces of the torsional moment shown labeled.)

TABLE 3-18 DISTRIBUTION OF DIRECT SHEARING FORCE *V*

Fastener No.	D	D^2	$(p_s)_v$
1	0.191	0.036	133
2	0.191	0.036	133
3	0.191	0.036	133
4	0.191	0.036	133
5	0.191	0.036	133
6	0.191	0.036	133
7	0.191	0.036	133
8	0.191	0.036	133
9	0.191	0.036	133*
		Total	1,197

* Sample calculation for rivet #9: $(p_s)_v = \dfrac{V}{n} = \dfrac{1,200}{9} = 133$ lb.

TABLE 3-19 DISTRIBUTION OF DIRECT AXIAL FORCE P

Fastener No.	D	D^2	$(p_s)_p$
1	0.191	0.036	167
2	0.191	0.036	167
3	0.191	0.036	167
4	0.191	0.036	167
5	0.191	0.036	167
6	0.191	0.036	167
7	0.191	0.036	167
8	0.191	0.036	167
9	0.191	0.036	167*
		Total	1,503

* Sample calculation for rivet #9:

$$(p_s)_p = \frac{P}{n} = \frac{1,500}{9} = 167 \text{ lb}.$$

TABLE 3-20 DISTRIBUTION OF TORSIONAL MOMENT M

Fastener No.	D	$\bar{x}$	$\bar{y}$	r	r^2	$[(p_s)_m]_x$	$[(p_s)_m]_y$
1	0.191	1.25	1.0	1.60	2.56	311	389
2	0.191	1.25	0.0	1.25	1.56	0	389
3	0.191	1.25	1.0	1.60	2.56	311	389
4	0.191	0.00	1.0	1.00	1.00	311	0
5	0.191	0.00	0.0	0.00	0.00	0	0
6	0.191	0.00	1.0	1.00	1.00	311	0
7	0.191	1.25	1.0	1.60	2.56	311	389
8	0.191	1.25	0.0	1.25	1.56	0	389
9	0.191	1.25	1.0	1.60	2.56	311*	389*
			Total		15.36		

* Sample calculations for rivet #9:

$$\left[(p_s)_m\right]_x = \frac{M\bar{y}}{\Sigma r^2} = \frac{4,780(1.0)}{15.36} = 311 \text{ lb} \quad \text{(from Eq. 3-29)}$$

$$\left[(p_s)_m\right]_y = \frac{M\bar{x}}{\Sigma r^2} = \frac{4,780(1.25)}{15.36} = 389 \text{ lb} \quad \text{(from Eq. 3-30)}.$$

Having found the most critical fastener, it then remains to compute the resultant shearing force of this rivet. The vectorial superposition of direct and torsional shearing forces into one resultant shearing force system for each rivet of the connection is tabulated as shown in the last column of Table 3-21.

TABLE 3-21 SUPERPOSITION OF DIRECT AND TORSIONAL COMPONENT LOADS (see Fig. 3-53)

Fastener No.	$(p_s)_v$	$(p_s)_p$	$[(p_s)_m]_x$	$[(p_s)_m]_y$	Σp_x	Σp_y	p_s
1	133	167	311	389	144	256	294
2	133	167	0	389	167	256	306
3	133	167	311	389	478	256	542
4	133	167	311	0	144	133	196
5	133	167	0	0	167	133	213
6	133	167	311	0	478	133	496
7	133	167	311	389	144	522	541
8	133	167	0	389	167	522	548
9	133	167	311	389	478	522	708*

* Sample calculations are performed for rivet #9 as follows:

$$\Sigma p_x = (p_s)_p + [(p_s)_m]_x = 167 + 311 = 478 \text{ lb}$$

$$\Sigma p_y = (p_s)_v + [(p_s)_m]_y = 133 + 389 = 522 \text{ lb}.$$

And then, the resultant shearing force is obtained from the solution of the Pythagorean theorem:

$$p_s = [(\Sigma p_x)^2 + (\Sigma p_y)^2]^{1/2} = [(478)^2 + (522)^2]^{1/2} = 708 \text{ lb}.$$

The last step in this solution is to determine the bearing and shearing margins of safety for the connection. Again using the location of rivet #9, the following checks are made:

Ultimate Allowable Shearing Strength of Rivet #9:

$$P_{su} = F_{su} A_{shr} C_r = 862(1.0) = 862 \text{ lb}$$

where: $F_{su} A_{shr} = 862$ lb (from Table 3-1)

$C_r = 1.0$ (from Table 3-2 in .080 in sheet thickness).

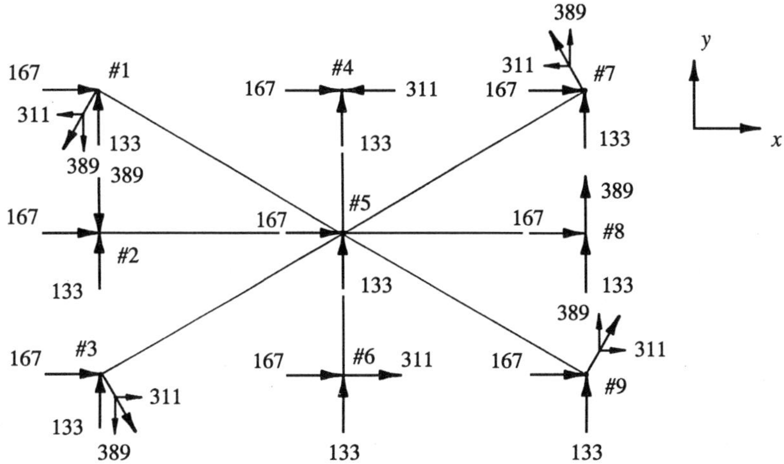

FUSELAGE FRAME SPLICE
(left side)

FIGURE 3-53 Summary of rivet shearing forces (from Table 3-21).

Shearing failure is then predicted by:

$$\text{Margin of Safety} = \text{M.S.} = \frac{P_{su}}{p_s k} - 1 = \frac{862}{(708)1.15} - 1 = +.06.$$

Ultimate Allowable Bearing Strength of the Channel Web:

Since $F_{bru} < 1.5 F_{bry}$, Eq. 3-2 is applied for the computation of ultimate allowable bearing strength of the channel web (see Table A-4, page 649, in Appendix E for this material).

$$P_{bru} = F_{bru} t D = 125,000(.100)(.191) = 2,387 \text{ lb}$$

where: $F_{bru} = 125,000$ psi (QQ-A-250/5, $e/D = 2.0$)
$F_{bry} = 84,000$ psi (QQ-A-250/5, $e/D = 2.0$)
$t = .100$
$D = .191.$

Bearing failure is then predicted by:

$$\text{Margin of Safety} = \text{M.S.} = \frac{P_{bru}}{p_s k} - 1 = \frac{2,387}{(708)1.15} - 1 = +1.93.$$

Ultimate Allowable Bearing Strength of the Fuselage Frame Web:

This time, $F_{bru} > 1.5F_{bry}$. Hence, Eq. 3-3 is used for the computation of ultimate allowable bearing strength of the fuselage frame web (see mechanical-property table for this material in MIL-HDBK-5F).

$$P_{bru} = 1.5F_{bry}tD = 1.5(58,000)(.080)(.191) = 1,329 \text{ lb}$$

where: $F_{bru} = 114,000$ psi (QQ-A-250/5, $e/D = 2.0$)
$F_{bry} = 58,000$ psi (QQ-A-250/5, $e/D = 2.0$)
$t = .080$
$D = .191.$

Bearing failure is predicted by:

$$\text{Margin of Safety} = \text{M.S.} = \frac{P_{bru}}{p_s k} - 1 = \frac{1,329}{(708)1.15} - 1 = +.63.$$

The ultimate shearing and bearing allowables computed above are listed in Table 3-22. The margins of safety are listed in Table 3-23.

TABLE 3-22 ULTIMATE SHEARING AND BEARING ALLOWABLES

Fastener No.	p_s	P_{su}	$(P_{bru})_{\text{channel}}$	$(P_{bru})_{\text{frame}}$
1	294	862	2,387	1,329
2	306	862	2,387	1,329
3	542	862	2,387	1,329
4	196	862	2,387	1,329
5	213	862	2,387	1,329
6	496	862	2,387	1,329
7	541	862	2,387	1,329
8	548	862	2,387	1,329
9	708	862	2,387	1,329

In addition to the shearing and bearing requirements of the connection, basic strength checks along the frame splice at critical sections must also be investigated. Their importance to a successful solution of the overall structure is, without exception, immediate and relevant to the problem-at-hand. Their solutions should be arrived at by careful deliberation. The engineer is encouraged to list only those possible structural failures discussed in previous chapters of this text.

TABLE 3-23 ULTIMATE SHEARING AND BEARING MARGINS OF SAFETY

Fastener No.	Shearing Failure MS	Bearing Failure $(MS)_{channel}$	Bearing Failure $(MS)_{frame}$
1	+ 1.55	+ 6.06	+ 2.93
2	+ 1.45	+ 5.78	+ 2.78
3	+ 0.38	+ 2.83	+ 1.13
4	+ 2.82	+ 9.59	+ 4.90
5	+ 2.52	+ 8.74	+ 4.43
6	+ 0.51	+ 3.18	+ 1.33
7	+ 0.39	+ 2.84	+ 1.14
8	+ 0.37	+ 2.79	+ 1.11
9	+ 0.06	+ 1.93	+ 0.63

3.7 Analysis of Connections Having Mechanical Fasteners Installed in Two Different Planes. Thus far, in our discussions of mechanically fastened connections, we have identified those particular connection types having mechanical fasteners installed in just one plane. To simplify those discussions, this plane usually coincided with the plane of the web of a conventional beam structure. In this section, however, we will expand our discussions of this subject to include the analysis of connections having fasteners installed in two different planes. Such connections are common in aircraft design where additional fastener strength across a splice joint or connection is required.

To help us illustrate these connections in two different planes, we will again consider a fuselage centerline splice arrangement (see Fig. 3-48, page 204). But this time, to the basic fuselage frame structure, two rather simple alternative redesign choices will be incorporated. They are: (1) a splice channel designed to nest in the basic fuselage frame structure, Fig. 3-54, and (2) two reinforcement straps fastened along the inner and outer fuselage frame caps, Fig. 3-55. The choice of redesigns will depend upon the particular design criteria and requirements established by the U.S. Government military armed forces or by the appropriate federal agency in charge of aircraft certification. For example, in some cases, even during the preliminary stages of structural testing, it may be far more economical to use temporary reinforcement straps on the tested structure than to initiate a costly redesign effort of that structure for the conformity of the production aircraft structure. Essentially, the basis of this argument is formulated by comparing the corresponding critical stresses of each structure. Written as an inequality, this comparison corresponds to the following mathematical formulation:

$$f_{\text{test structure}} \geq f_{\text{production model structure}}\,.$$

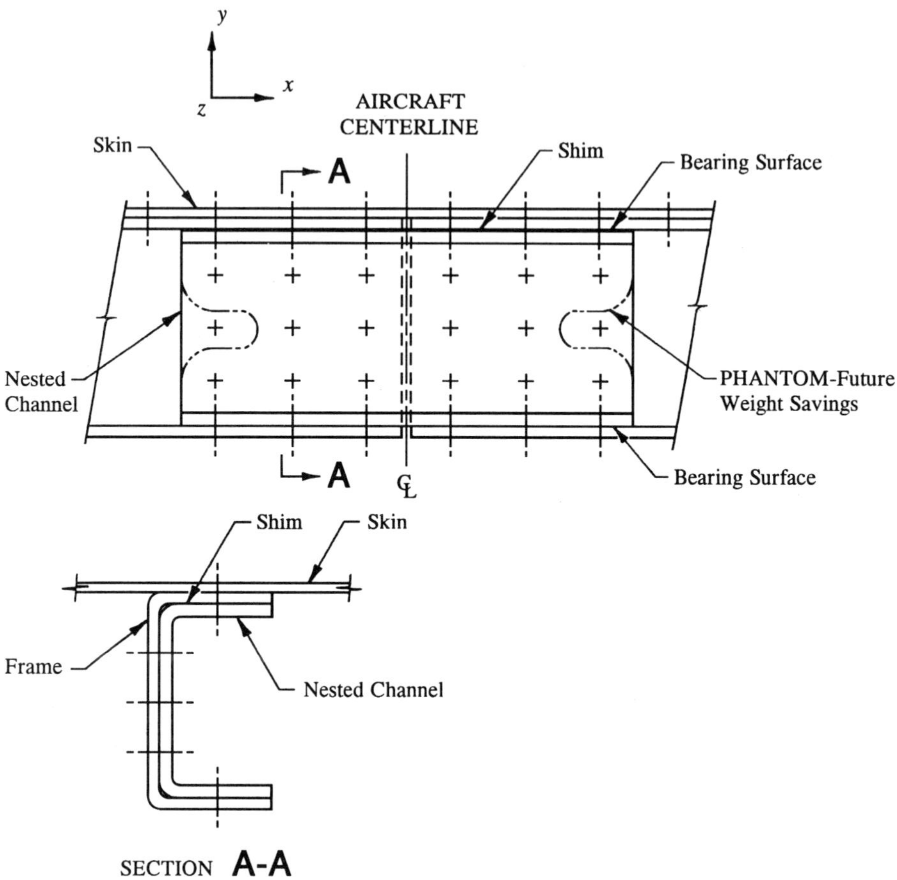

FIGURE 3-54 Fuselage centerline frame splice redesigned using a nested channel.

From this expression derives the following statement: If the basic frame structure with temporary reinforcement straps can be shown through structural testing to be of sufficient strength, then the preferred design of the nested splice channel could later be incorporated into the production model aircraft structure so long as that structure was shown analytically to be of equal or slightly greater strength than the actual tested structure. To gain a better perspective and understanding of this comparative method of analysis, the engineer is referred specifically to Chapter 6, Example 6-5. This rather simple, straightforward approach to stress analysis is highly recommended and worthy of special attention in situations where redesigning of the actual test structure would not be easily accomplished otherwise. In the final analysis, no matter which redesign choice is selected, in this illustration, temporary straps or a nested splice channel, the actual stress computations of the basic rivet design would not appreciably change. And, regardless of which design was

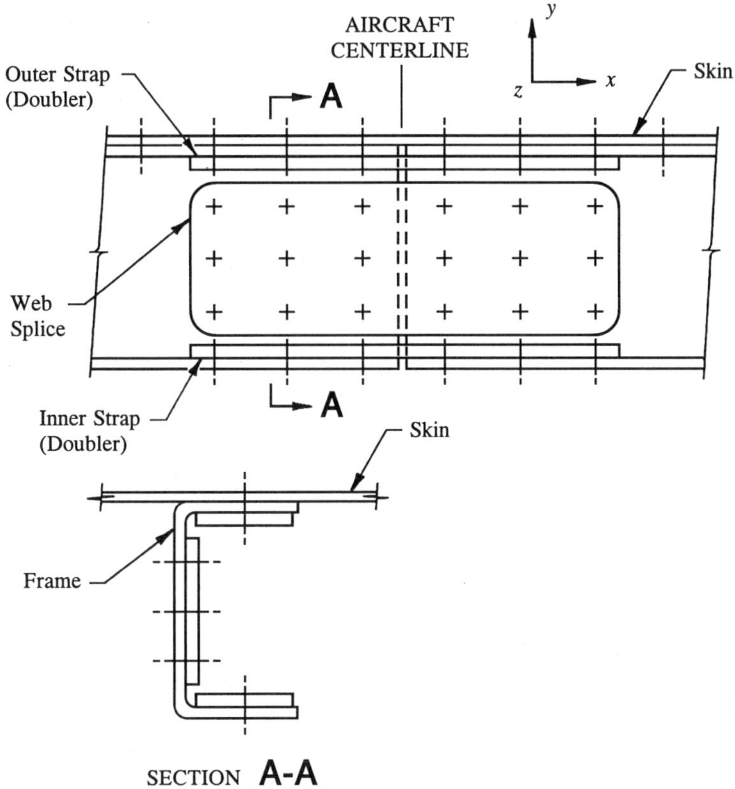

FIGURE 3-55 Fuselage centerline frame splice redesigned with reinforcement straps.

ultimately used for the final production design, the overall fastener strength of the centerline splice would be considerably improved.

Now, let us focus our attention back to the main subject of this section: that of analyzing connections having fasteners installed in two different planes. In accordance with the analysis procedure of connections, this is accomplished by distributing the internal frame loads V, P, and M described at the centroid of the fastener group to those fasteners capable of resisting shear loads. Considering this solution in two planes, then, this distribution will now also include the frame cap rivets (see nested splice channel, Fig. 3-54).

Before actually performing the numerical computations, however, the restraint capabilities of these rivets must be discussed. For example, the aircraft industry will recommend that rivets loaded in tension be avoided as primary load-carrying members. Hence, tension should not be directly applied to a rivet. Of course, secondary effects in aircraft design are quite common, i.e., buckling of the wing and fuselage skin panels which can in these cases induce secondary tension loads in the skin rivets; also, lap joints where the built-in effects of the joints themselves can

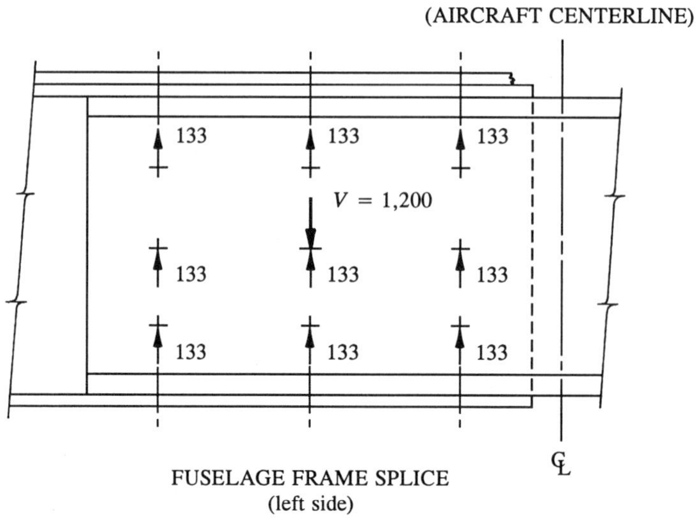

FIGURE 3-56 Distribution of rivet shearing forces due to the vertical shear force V (see internal loads calculated on page 206).

also induce secondary tension loads in the rivets. However, to account for their increased stress effect on the basic joint design, fitting factors are normally incorporated in the stress analysis. Additionally, when the frame structure is loaded, the nested splice channel will provide some frictional resistance by bearing up against the frame structure. Although this is possible, in general, the effects of this condition are considered quite small, and therefore, are usually neglected by the design engineer. Hence, no expected resistance is offered by the frame cap rivets in the vertical direction—that is, no bearing capability of the nested channel itself.

Essentially, we have now described the physical restraints of the splice joint from which the internal loads V, P, and M can be distributed: that is, the frame cap rivets will react shear loads in the plane of the frame cap (or x-z plane), while the web rivets will react shear loads in the plane of the frame web (or x-y plane). Let us now begin the distribution of these internal loads. Since the joint vertical shear force V also acts in the shear plane of the web rivets, this load is distributed as shear through the resistance offered by the 9 web rivets of this joint. This is diagrammed in Fig. 3-56 for these rivets. Mathematically, we obtain:

$$(p_s)_v = \frac{V}{n} = \frac{1,200}{9} = 133 \text{ lb}.$$

For the joint horizontal axial force P, both the web and cap rivets can provide the ability to resist horizontal shear loads. As such, the axial force P is distributed to all 15 rivets of this fastener group (i.e., 9 web and 6 frame cap rivets). This

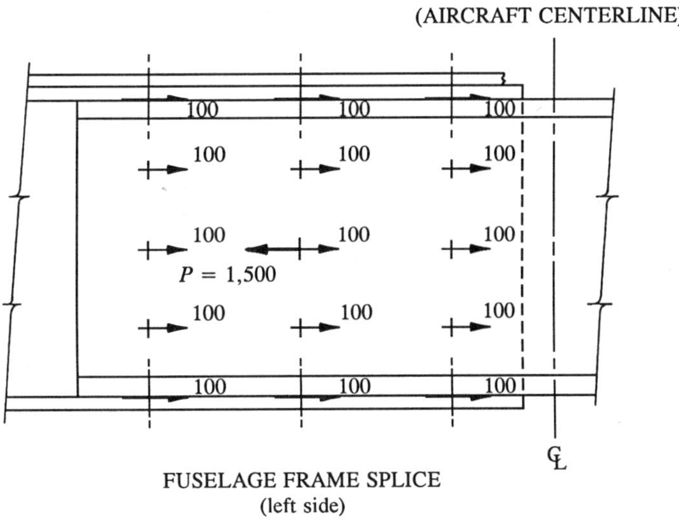

FIGURE 3-57 Distribution of rivet shearing forces due to the horizontal axial force P (see internal loads calculated on page 206).

distribution is viewed in Fig. 3-57. And, for each rivet, we obtain the following shearing forces:

$$(p_s)_p = \frac{P}{n} = \frac{1,500}{15} = 100 \text{ lb.}$$

Now, for the distribution of moment M, the following iteration method is proposed. Here, the moment is distributed as shear to the entire fastener group in the usual way—that is, by drawing radial lines to each rivet from the centroid of the rivet group and indicating the shearing forces of that distribution, see Fig. 3-58. Based on the arguments previously mentioned in this section, the frame cap rivets can not effectively resist the vertical components of $(p_s)_m$. Instead, their values must be redistributed back to the entire rivet group capable of sustaining such loads. Remember, the frame cap rivets are assumed to only react shear in the x-z plane (horizontally), not in the y-z plane (vertically).

To accomplish the actual redistribution of load to these rivets, the vertical components $\left[(p_s)_m\right]_y$ are evaluated in terms of a second moment M_1 (each component contributes a moment value to M_1 at the centroid of the rivet group, see Fig. 3-59). Here, from statics, this evaluation is performed as follows:

$$\Sigma M_{cg} = 0, \qquad (+ \quad M_1 - \Sigma\left[(p_s)_m\right]_y d = 0,$$

and therefore

$$M_1 = \Sigma\left[(p_s)_m\right]_y d$$

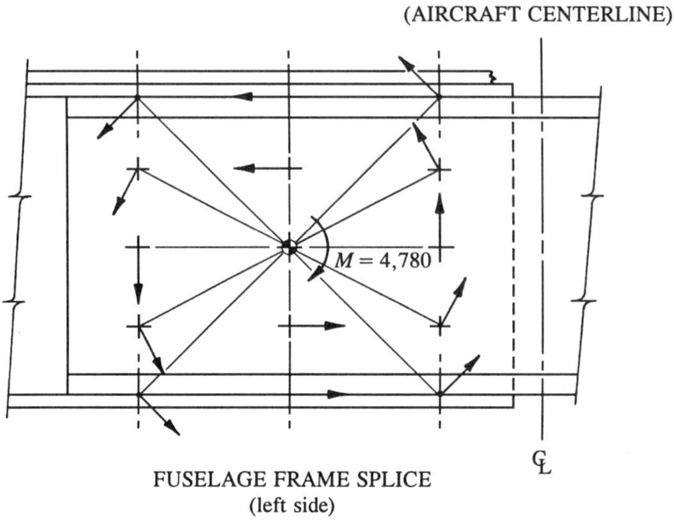

FIGURE 3-58 Distribution of rivet shearing forces due to the torsional moment M (see internal loads calculated on page 206).

where the value of M_1 represents the moment at the rivet group centroid due to the vertical components of the frame cap rivets. The moment M_1 is then distributed again to the entire group of rivets. As before, this distribution will again produce additional components of shearing force $\left[(p_s)_m\right]_x$ and $\left[(p_s)_m\right]_y$ at each fastener. And, based upon our previous reasoning for the redistribution of $\left[(p_s)_m\right]_y$, which basically stipulates that the vertical components of $(p_s)_m$ cannot be effectively resisted by the frame cap rivets, these components must again be evaluated by accumulating their contributions to a third moment M_2 at the centroid of the rivet group. The magnitude of this new moment is then distributed again to the entire rivet group. And so the procedure goes: for each successive iteration, a new moment is generated, and from this value, a new system of rivet shearing forces is produced.

Each iteration helps to contribute to the final system of rivet forces. In general, though, convergence is quickly achieved after the first iteration, as the vertical components of $(p_s)_m$ will generally produce a small enough moment at the centroid to be mathematically insignificant for further distribution of this load to the rivet group. The final solution is obtained when the rivet shearing forces for each separate loading system are algebraically superimposed in accordance with their proper orientations: horizontally and vertically. (From our discussions here, this should include the accumulative contributions from the following loads: $P + V + M + M_1 + M_2 + \ldots + M_n$.) The numerical computations are left as an exercise for the engineer to complete.

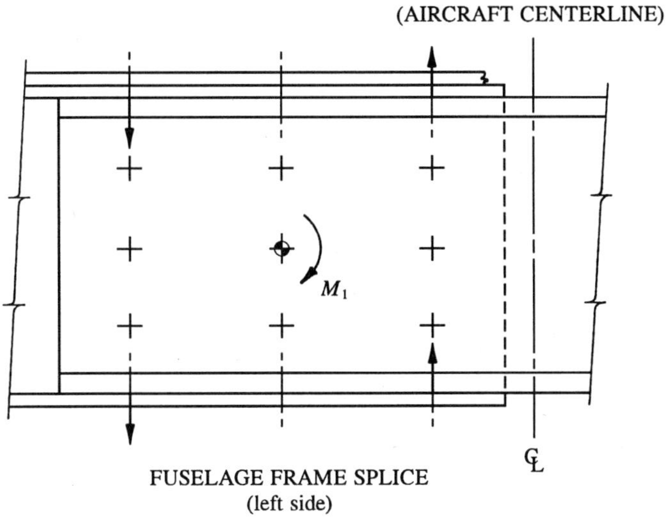

FIGURE 3-59 Moment at the centroid of the rivet group due to the vertical components of the frame cap rivets.

In general, as far as acceptable designs go, a connection should, if possible, be securely fastened to its main structure—this is done through the use of both web and frame cap rivets at the connection. Such a design is far superior to its preceding design-type (see structural arrangement of members in Example 3-4). Where, in that problem, the splice channel was not designed to nest in the basic fuselage frame structure.

3.8 Problem for Solution. For the latch track fitting shown in Fig. 3-60, determine the ultimate margin of safety for the most critically loaded fastener. The fasteners are ¼ in diameter titanium bolts. Assume a fastener edge distance $e/D = 2.0$ and a fitting factor of 1.15 for commercial aircraft design. From page 347, use the interaction equation $R_s^3 + R_t^2 = 1$ for the analysis of these bolts in combined shear and tension and Fig. 5-59 for the graphical solution. The ultimate strength allowables of this fastener are $P_{su} = 4,650$ lb in single-shear and $P_{tu} = 3,700$ lb in tension. Consider a fitting factor k to meet FAA requirements for commercial aircraft design. (*Note:* Before investigating for the critical fastener, the fitting must first be balanced in each plane. Then, the loads determined there, distributed as bearing forces on the fitting and as tension forces in the fasteners. Assume that the applied load is uniformly distributed as indicated in the views provided.)

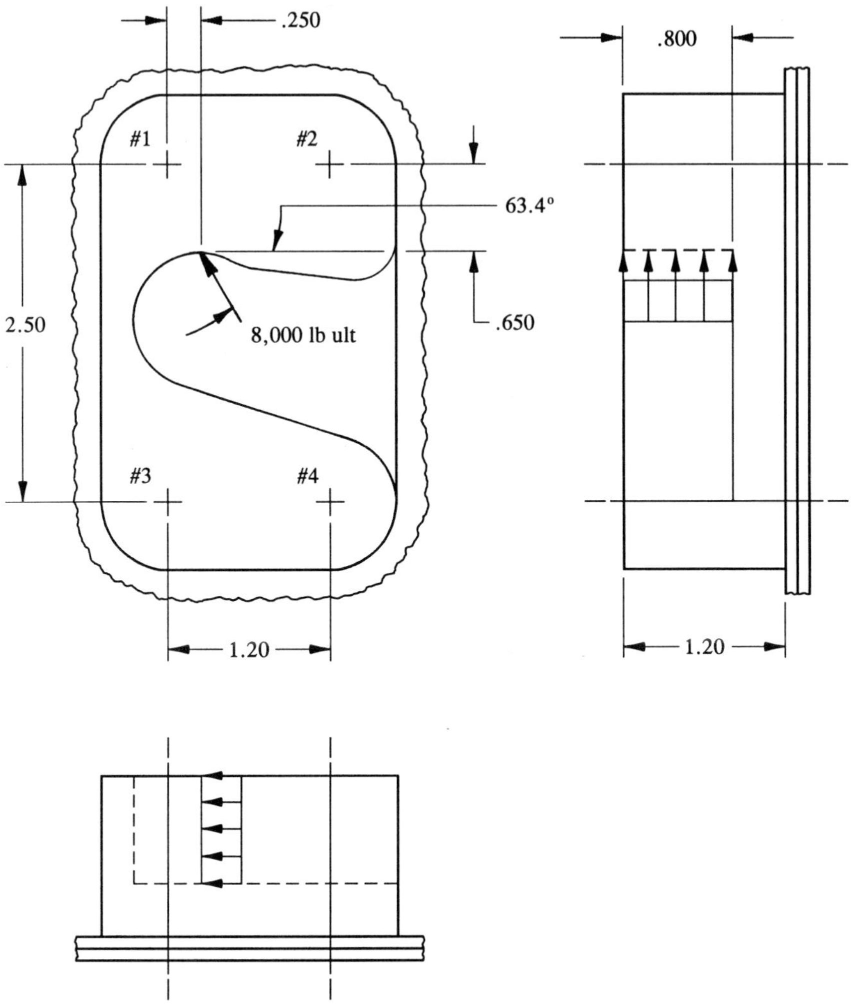

FIGURE 3-60 Latch track fitting for a passenger door installation.

CHAPTER 4

Shearing Stresses

4.1 Introduction. Except for Sec. 2-9 of Chapter 2, up to now in our discussions of aircraft stress analysis, we have primarily concerned ourselves with symmetrical beam sections[1] or with those sections they depicted were forced, by the stabilizing nature of their attached skins, to bend about either a horizontal or vertical axis of their cross-sectional areas. In Fig. 4-1, such an arrangement of members is shown where the skin is observed to do just that: stabilize the unsymmetrical zee section by forcing it to bend about the horizontal bending axis of their combined section areas. This axis, more appropriately referred to as the "failure axis," or "principal axis," must also pass through the neutral axis of the skin and zee section combination.

Now, consider the zee section in Fig. 4-2. Without the stabilizing effect of the skin, the beam will physically bend around the failure axes (principal axes x_p and y_p). For such a case, the internal shear V normally expected at an exposed section of beam is resolved into planes containing the principal bending axes x_p and y_p.[2] Thereby physically duplicating the true bending action of the loaded structure. Fortunately, most aircraft structural members are stabilized, and therefore, do not fall into this latter category. The stabilizing effect of the skin should save the analyst considerable engineering time, and thus economically prove by requiring

[1] Refer to Chapter 2, Sec. 2.3, Fig. 2-7, for their disposition and description.

[2] The engineer is referred to the complex bending theory of beams with unsymmetrical beam sections in Chapter 2, Sec. 2-9, or to an advanced college textbook on this particular subject for comparative study.

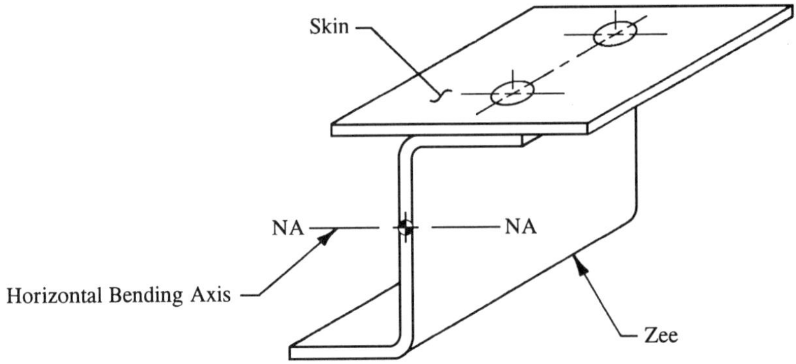

FIGURE 4-1 Beam (in composite) consisting of a zee section member and skin. Bending occurs about an axis parallel to the skin line.

fewer analytical computations, the structural adequacy and reliability of his designs.

When a beam bends, the material fibers on the concave side will shorten while the material fibers on the convex side will lengthen. This is diagrammed in Fig. 4-3 where $x =$ the original material fiber lengths on the upper and lower surfaces of the beam before flexural bending occurs. At any point between the neutral axis and the extreme fibers of the concave side, the beam undergoes compression (or contraction), and anywhere between the neutral axis and the extreme fibers of the convex side the beam undergoes tension (or elongation). These stresses were studied in depth in Chapter 2, where the elastic stress design of an initially straight homogeneous beam undergoing flexural bending was considered.

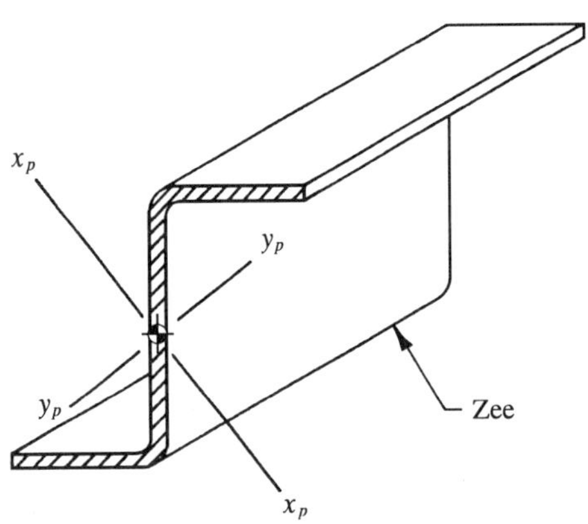

Beam Composed of a Zee Section Member
(no axis of symmetry)

FIGURE 4-2 Zee section physically bends around the principal axes x_p and y_p.

Concave Side (compression fibers contract)

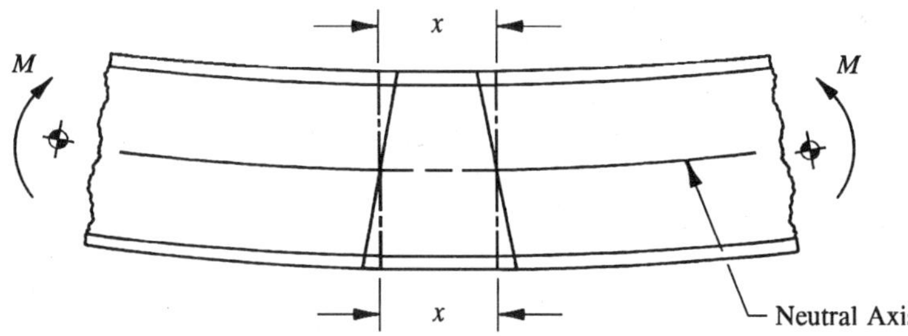

Convex Side (tension fibers elongate)

FIGURE 4-3 Beam undergoing flexural bending.

Also described in that same chapter was how to derive stress from a single applied axial force; such a force usually produces either tension or compression axial stresses. However, if the line of action of the applied force is found not to line up with the centroid of the cross-sectional area, the resulting eccentricity of load path created by such an effect (or offset) will produce a combined stress system of axial and bending stresses. The nature of axial, bending, and combined axial and bending stresses, as they were presented in that chapter, are again presumed and carefully considered here in our study of shearing stresses in this chapter. As a review of these limitations, the following assumptions are summarized below:

(1) The beam material is homogeneous.

(2) The beam is straight or at worst only slightly curved.

(3) The beam material has a similar stress-strain curve in tension and compression.

(4) The cross-sectional area of the beam is constant throughout its entire span.

(5) The beam has at least one axis of symmetry or is known to be stabilized in at least one plane.

(6) Stresses are assumed to be elastic whether or not they actually occur below the proportional limit of the material.[1]

Essentially, if these assumptions are followed closely in the solution of shearing stresses, the limitations which they impose on some structural designs should not for the most part diminish the accuracy and reliability of their final solutions.

In summary, then, up to this point in our study of elastic stress design, we have mainly considered the following stress types: (1) stresses due to an internal axial force P, (2) stresses due to an internal bending moment M, and (3) a com-

[1] The justification for this last assumption is based on the logical inference or presumption that inelastic bending design, assumed to be elastic, is conservative.

bination of stresses occurring simultaneously due to (1) and (2). As yet, we have not fully described those stresses which are produced by an internal shearing force V at an exposed section of beam, viz., shearing stresses. Such stresses, not yet considered in our study of stress design, will be conveniently expressed in equation form in Sec. 4.2 of this chapter. Their solutions are needed to properly design and select a structure at critical sections based on this particular failure mode. In Chapter 1 it was shown how to painstakingly apply the equations of static equilibrium at sections of a beam to find the internal shears acting there.[1] The design shear is then the maximum internal shear V found from the constructed shear diagram of the applied loading structure.[2]

The engineer is cautioned not to use the maximum applied forces acting on the structure as maximum internal shears. Instead, to describe the internal loads picture of the structure correctly, draw the shear loading diagram of the entire structure first and then verify the maximum internal shears from this completed diagram. A simple sketch will usually suffice in most cases to pinpoint the critical shears. This can usually be done by simple inspection of the critical sections along the structure. Then, from these values or critical combinations, the maximum shearing stresses $(f_s)_{\max}$ are computed by evaluating Eq. 4-2 (see page 227). The required beam section is selected by comparing this value to the ultimate allowable shear stress F_{su} of the material used. Expressed as an equation, the required selection is made as follows:

$$\text{Margin of Safety} = \text{M.S.} = \frac{F_{su}}{(f_s)_{\max}} - 1 .$$

Also described in this chapter is the concept of shear flow q. A term which is closely related to our previous discussions of shear stress f_s. Its value is however alternatively expressed by considering the change in bending moment that occurs at different sections along a beam. The change in bending moment is explained in the following way: If different bending moments occur at different, but yet neighboring, sections of a beam, then there must also exist between these sections couple-forces[3] of different magnitudes; it is this difference that must be counteracted by what is commonly referred to as "shear flow" between the sections. Conversely, if instead, identical bending moments were to occur at these same sections, no shear flow would result between the sections considered since

[1] The design engineer is referred to Sec. 1.5, "Method of Sections Approach to Internal Loads Analysis," for the basic approaches and fundamental concepts necessary to perform internal loads analysis on exposed segments of a beam. As it specifically relates to our study of shearing stresses in this section, how to determine the maximum internal shears V occurring at critical sections of a beam?

[2] The applied forces must interact locally into the structure first before a clear representation of the internal loads of the structure can be accurately appraised.

[3] See Appendix B, "Couple-Force Relationship of Moments," where from Eq. A-7 or $P_{\text{couple}} = M/H$ a moment can be represented at an exposed section of beam by an equivalent couple-force located at the centroid of its upper and lower cap areas.

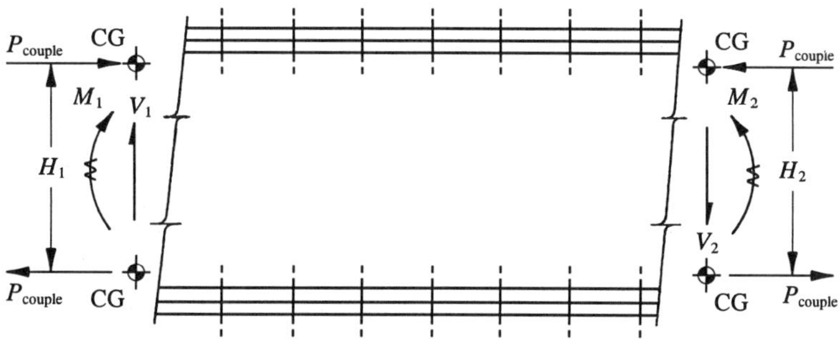

FIGURE 4-4 Isolated segment of beam in equilibrium. Internal loads shown at exposed sections of beam.

identical bending moments would also produce identical couple-forces. To illustrate this graphically, section cuts are taken perpendicular to the axis of the beam shown in Fig. 4-4. The internal bending moments occurring there are replaced by equivalent couple-forces, and their values proportionally distributed to members according to their respective cross-sectional areas, Fig. 4-5. (Or, see Sec. 2.6, "Member Forces," for specific details of how to establish internal member forces from an internal bending stress distribution across an exposed section of beam.)

For clarity, the upper and lower structural members with their corresponding internal member forces P_1 and P_2, P_3 and P_4, respectively, are shown separated from the beam structure in this sketch. This can be seen in the figure where the individually attached members have been completely isolated and free-bodied from the main structure. Such forces are required to maintain static equilibrium of these members. Their difference $P_2 - P_1$ and $P_4 - P_3$ is what constitutes the resistance (in terms of shearing forces) by the fasteners attaching these members together. Hence, using the equations of equilibrium, the following expressions for shear flow q are written for each member:

FOR THE UPPER MEMBER

$$\Sigma F_x = 0, \qquad P_1 + q_{\text{upper}} L - P_2 = 0$$

$$q_{\text{upper}} = \frac{P_2 - P_1}{L}.$$

FOR THE LOWER MEMBER

$$\Sigma F_x = 0, \qquad -P_3 - q_{\text{lower}} L + P_4 = 0$$

$$q_{\text{lower}} = \frac{P_4 - P_3}{L}.$$

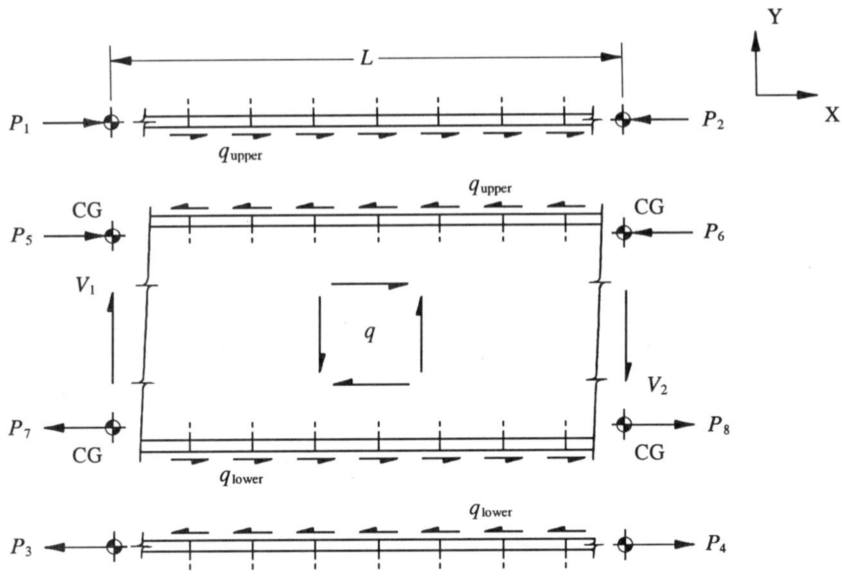

FIGURE 4-5 Diagram shows the interconnection shearing forces (or shear flow) between attached members of the beam.

The equations above can then be written as a general expression for shear flow q as follows:

$$q = \frac{\Delta P}{L} \tag{4-1}$$

where: ΔP = difference between the internal forces of a member at adjacent sections along a beam

L = distance measured between the section areas considered along the beam (see Fig. 4-5)

q = design shear flow.

The shear flow q is then used to properly size and space the fasteners of each attached member (see page 254). This is normally done by trial and error assuming different values of fastener spacing s in Eq. 4-10 to arrive at a solution. For easy reference, this equation is written below:

$$p_s = qs$$

where: p_s = fastener shearing force

q = design shear flow

s = fastener spacing.

For example, with the value of q known, and the value of s assumed, the fastener shearing force p_s as determined by this expression is found. Then, with the value of p_s computed, and the shearing properties of the fasteners P_{su} and bearing properties of the material P_{bru} known, the shearing and bearing failures of the connection are predicted (see specific equations used in the solution of Example 3-1 in Chapter 3). Prescribed allowable values are conveniently found in MIL-HDBK-5, company manuals, or from the appropriate governing agency in charge of issuing such documents or disclosures.

The equations described in this brief introduction are fully treated in the following sections of this chapter. Also, specific example problems are provided to fully illustrate their applications. In Sec. 4.2, a more convenient approach to computing shear flow q for beam design will be presented: specifically, that is, by solving Eq. 4-3 instead of Eq. 4-1. Note, in particular, how similar Eq. 4-3 is expressed to the shearing stress formula, Eq. 4-2. Also, note in particular, the fact that both formulas are independently derived of bending moment M. More about this as we continue our study of shearing stresses in the next section.

4.2 Shearing Stresses (shear flow). Although beams may be attached together by means of different methods, e.g., mechanical fasteners, adhesive-bonds, or by welding, the basic theories and fundamental concepts which they portend do not change. Essentially, only the "allowables" are different for each particular method of attachment. This is also basically true for the general methods of analysis for beam design that are used in this section to solve for (1) shearing stresses f_s and (2) shear flow q.

A detailed development of shear stress and shear flow will not be formally introduced in this section. Instead, formulas used in the solution of these quantities are presented without derivation or proof. Thus in keeping with the main intent and purpose of this book: that is, to avoid unwieldy, complex, and rigorous type of mathematical derivations. Hence, the following expressions are written for shear stress f_s and shear flow q:

$$f_s = \frac{VQ}{I_{na}\, t} \tag{4-2}$$

and

$$q = \frac{VQ}{I_{na}} \tag{4-3}$$

where V = internal shearing force, Q = static moment of area (see ahead to Eq. 4-8 for the mathematical description and evaluation of this property), I_{na} = moment of inertia of the total cross-sectional area around the neutral axis of a beam section, and t = beam web thickness.

A detailed treatment of Eq. 4-3 will be postponed until Sec. 4.4, where the design theory of shear flow will be applied to prismatic beams, i.e., beams of a constant cross-sectional area. The main intent of this section is therefore to establish the design procedures which are used to determine the required internal shearing stresses permissible in a beam undergoing internal shear deflection[1]. Such procedures form the basis for the strength design of members in flexural shear; that is, where a beam is chosen strong enough to resist the internal maximum shearing stresses $(f_s)_{max}$ occurring during flexural bending. The required section is then selected based on the ultimate allowable shear stress F_{su} of the material. The design theory of shearing stresses, as given by Eq. 4-2, was derived from the same fundamental concepts and principles developed in our formulation of the flexure formula (Eq. 2-5) in Sec. 2.3. Therefore, all conditions and limitations imposed on its application in that section are again presumed and imposed fully on the solution of shearing stresses (or shear flow) here in this section. The following predicted failure in shear is then written:

$$\text{Margin of Safety} = \text{M.S.} = \frac{F_{su}}{(f_s)_{max}} - 1 \qquad \textbf{(4-4)}$$

where: F_{su} = ultimate allowable shearing stress of the material (see MIL-HDBK-5 for commonly used materials)

$(f_s)_{max}$ = maximum applied ultimate shearing stress.

Note particularly how Eqs. 4-2 and 4-3 are expressed: each one is described independently of the internal bending moment M from which these expressions were originally derived. Here, the internal shear force V which can also occur at different sections during flexural bending is used exclusively. These equations were derived from the well-known flexure formula Mc/I_{na} (refer to Sec. 2.3), and, as such, are directly linked to the internal bending moment M. That is, the shear is treated independent of bending moment in these equations although the physical action of a beam is directly influenced by the change in bending moment that actually occurs at different sections along that structure. This of course is consistent with theoretical interpretations and the general understanding of beam behavior, and thereby allows the engineer a more direct and flexible approach to the design solution of such members.

Equations 4-2 and 4-3 are restricted, however, to the special case of shearing stresses that are calculated in the elastic range of a stress-strain curve of a material. Fortunately, such a restriction is usually considered conservative anyway. Inelastic (or plastic) beam design will not be considered in our study of shearing stresses. Since, a more advanced study of this subject now would only lead to additional confusion and complication in what is considered here only a rudimentary

[1] Internal shear deflection is a technical term that is used to describe the resulting effect attributed to the shearing forces which occur within a beam subjected to bending.

introductory discussion of this subject for design engineers. It then follows from the limitation imposed that if calculated shearing stresses are elastic, the neutral axis must therefore be coincident with the centroidal axis of the cross-sectional area. This notion is, of course, consistent with elastic beam design theory. And, thus, the following conclusions can be drawn: that

$$Y_{na} = Y_{cg}$$

and, from this, it also follows that

$$I_{na} = I_{cg}\,.$$

Furthermore, it can be reasoned out that if internal bending moments between adjoining sections of a beam are constant, the beam physically resists no internal shears between the sections considered. This can be easily verified for the beam loaded as shown in Fig. 4-6 between points *B* to *C*. However, if internal bending moments are not constant between adjoining sections, such is the case seen between points *A* to *B* and *C* to *D*, then a constant internal shear will also develop between the adjoining sections. Consequently, if such a beam does resist both shear and bending, its design and analysis becomes slightly more involved, requiring two separate stress computations instead of one.

These rather simple relationships can always be verified by comparing other shear and moment diagrams of actual loading structure. The engineer is referred to those additional cases provided in Appendix D. Use this appendix as a guide to the different interrelationships that are possible between shears and bending moments along a beam.

To summarize our findings, we can describe our observations of shears and bending moments in the following simple and descriptive way:

(a) If a linear change in bending moment (i.e., first order variable bending moment) occurs between two adjoining sections of a beam, then a constant shear will develop between these adjoining sections.[1] That is,

$$\Delta M = \text{constant } V.$$

(b) If a constant bending moment occurs between two adjoining sections of a beam, then zero shear will develop between these adjoining sections, or

$$\text{constant } M = \text{zero } V.$$

[1] If a higher order change in bending moment (n) occurs between two adjoining sections of a beam, then a lower order shear (n - 1) will develop between these adjoining sections. For example, a second order variable bending moment will have a first order variable shear (this relationship that exists between shears and bending moments can be seen in Fig. 1-35).

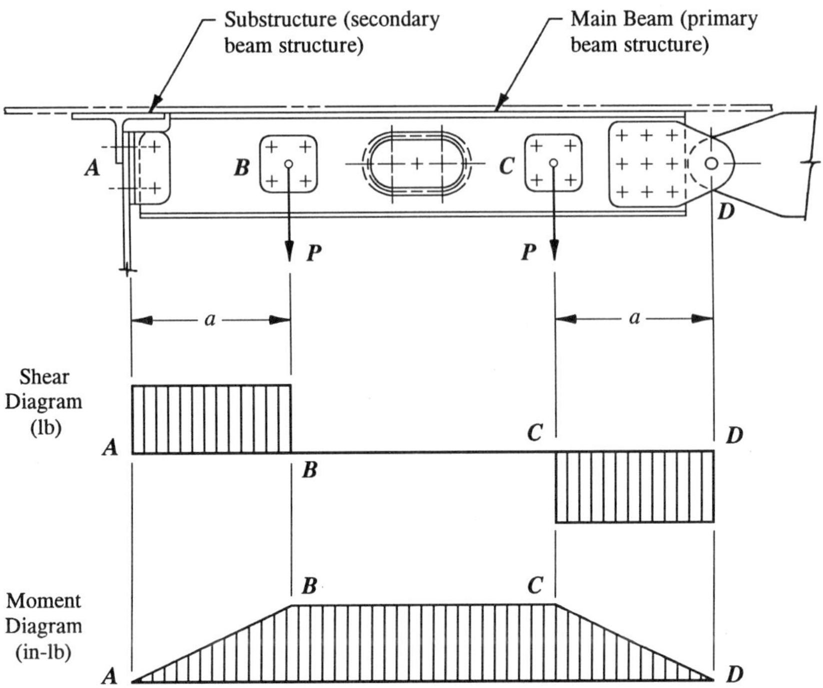

FIGURE 4-6 Relationship between shears and bending moments in a loaded beam.

This then establishes the simple interrelationship between bending moments M and shearing forces V along a beam. These principles can be used as a guide to a better understanding of more complex loaded structures.

Now, an alternative expression, very useful in subsequent sections of this book, is formulated below. By dividing Eq. 4-2 by Eq. 4-3 and rearranging terms, we obtain:

$$f_s = \frac{q}{t} \tag{4-5}$$

where: f_s = design shearing stress
q = design shear flow
t = beam web or panel thickness.

Computer model program solutions of actual designed structures are quite common; generally, load output shears from these solutions are generated and described in terms of either shear flows, shearing stresses, or both. As such, Eq. 4-5 becomes a very powerful expression—the engineer can transform reliable output data given in terms of shear flow q into shearing stresses f_s, or vice versa, without laborious and detailed computations required from the more complicated, involved solutions of Eqs. 4-2 and 4-3. On the other hand, computer-derived program shearing stresses, if they are to be correctly applied to the actual conformity of the structure, must first be converted to design shear flows using (compatible) program input thicknesses. Mathematically, the above argument is expressed like this:

$$(f_s)_{\text{program}} = \frac{q}{t_{\text{program}}} \quad \text{(developed from Eq. 4-5)}$$

where: $(f_s)_{\text{program}}$ = program output shearing stress
t_{program} = program input web or panel thickness
q = design shear flow.

Solving for q, we obtain:

$$q = (f_s)_{\text{program}}\, t_{\text{program}}\,. \tag{4-6}$$

Thus, when converting program shearing stresses to design shear flows be sure to use corresponding program input thicknesses—not actual drawing thicknesses. However, once design shear flows have been converted, drawing changes, if made, can then be utilized in new revised solutions: simply by reevaluating Eq. 4-5 for each proposed new drawing change. This is done by substituting the value of q from Eq. 4-6 into Eq. 4-5 which then gives the design shearing stress applicable to the actual conformity of the structure. Using this method of reasoning, the following expression is written:

$$f_s = \frac{(f_s)_{\text{program}}\, t_{\text{program}}}{t} \tag{4-7}$$

where: f_s = design shearing stress
t = design web or panel thickness.

Also note, for instance, if $t_{\text{program}} = t$, then Eq. 4-7 reduces to

$$f_s = (f_s)_{\text{program}}\,,$$

and therefore no conversion in program shearing stress is necessary. Lastly, shearing stress failure is predicted as follows:

$$\text{Margin of Safety} = \text{M.S.} = \frac{F_{su}}{f_s} - 1$$

where: F_{su} = ultimate allowable shearing stress of the material
f_s = design ultimate shearing stress (from Eq. 4-7 above).

Structural designs are constantly being modified and changed by the engineer, and if program shearing stresses are used instead of design shear flows, final design solutions can be erroneously figured. The localized effects of redesign, for instance, on the magnitude of computer output design shear flows is minuscule at most because of the redistribution effects at higher design loads that usually accompany inelastic stress behavior[1]. For this reason, shear flows normally require no conversion of their values even though drawing changes have been made subsequent to current computer runs. Of course, redistribution is also a function of the magnitude of these design changes. However, changes in web and panel thicknesses of 10% to 30% are quite common in preliminary design stages, and should pose no real problem on final design solutions.

In Chapter 8, Eq. 4-7 will again become very useful to us in the solution of shearing stresses occurring in aircraft panels[2] subjected to shear loads. Until then, however, our main emphasis will be concentrated on the following general topics: (1) design and analysis of beam webs and (2) design and analysis of fasteners used in the construction of metallic, built-up beams (i.e., the interconnection forces occurring between individually attached members making up a built-up beam section).

Before an example problem is introduced in this section illustrating the principles and practical applications of shearing stress design, the nature or properties associated with the computation of Q, as given by Eqs. 4-2 and 4-3, will first be demonstrated. Essentially Q is a term based upon theoretical interpretations and general observations closely linked to our study of elastic bending stresses. Its value is usually computed around one side or the other of the neutral axis of a partial cross-sectional area of a beam (refer ahead to Fig. 4-8), where, for the majority of practical design cases, this should prove to be the desired location for optimum shearing stress design. To arrive at a numerical value for Q, the following expression is formulated below:

$$Q = \Sigma A\bar{y} = A_1\bar{y}_1 + A_2\bar{y}_2 + A_3\bar{y}_3 + \ldots + A_n\bar{y}_n \tag{4-8}$$

where: Q = static moment of area
A = element areas
$\bar{y}$ = distance measured from the neutral axis of the total cross-sectional area to the centroidal axis of individual element areas.

To design a member for shear, the maximum shear stress $(f_s)_{max}$ of that member must be determined. Fortunately, for most members encountered in actual

[1] Plasticity or inelastic stress behavior refers to the property of materials known as yielding (or permanent set or deformation). This condition can occur without actually incurring failure of the plastic member.

[2] Aircraft panels are designed to carry shear, axial, and bending loads, while nonstructural panels carry only pressurized loads (see Chapter 9, Sec. 9.5, "Design and Analysis of Doors in Pressurized Aircraft").

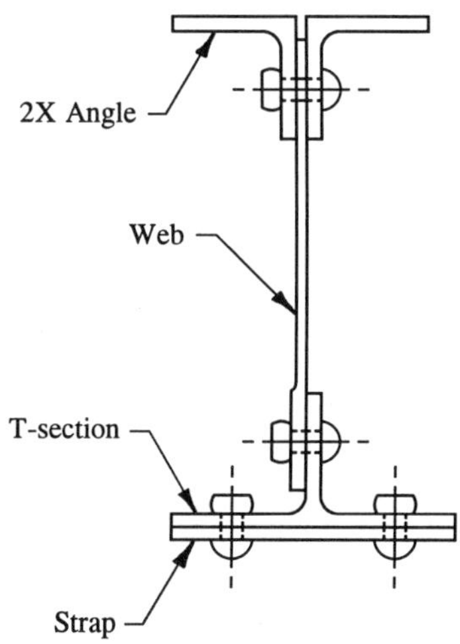

FIGURE 4-7 Built-up beam section fastened together with rivets.

production design, shearing stresses are maximum at the centroidal axis of the cross-sectional area of the member.[1] This observation can then greatly simplify the computation of Q by making this quantity more definite to determine—thus avoiding the time-consuming computations by trial and error. In general, regardless of how a beam is constructed, e.g., one could use individually attached members, such as angles, straps, and doublers to construct a built-up beam section, the basic theoretical computations of Q for such a composite section would not change.

Now let us consider an I-beam made up of several members all of which are fastened together by rivets or bolts. Such a beam section is shown in Fig. 4-7, where the members making up the composite beam section are each clearly identified. The maximum shearing stress for this beam section will occur at the neutral axis. To obtain this value, one must either consider the partial area above or below this axis, as shown in Fig. 4-8. Personal preference will dictate which partial area to use when performing the actual computations. In most cases, the choice is obvious: the partial area made up of fewer element areas is chosen. Look ahead now to Fig. 4-9, where our beam section (I-beam) is shown partitioned into rectangular element areas. Note that fewer element areas are required to define the lower part of this beam. If this section (lower partial area) is then used in subsequent computations of shear stress, the resulting analysis should prove less complicated since fewer actual computations to determine the total static moment of area Q would be required. The shearing stresses developed in such a beam are now considered and

[1] Not expressly covered by the material of this book, the maximum shearing stress of a curved beam (elastic or plastic design) occurs at the neutral axis of the cross-sectional area of the member, and not at the centroidal axis of the section area. The reason for this is quite clear: the neutral axis is determined from the loading characteristics across an exposed section area of a beam, while the centroidal axis is solely a function of the geometric shape of the beam section area.

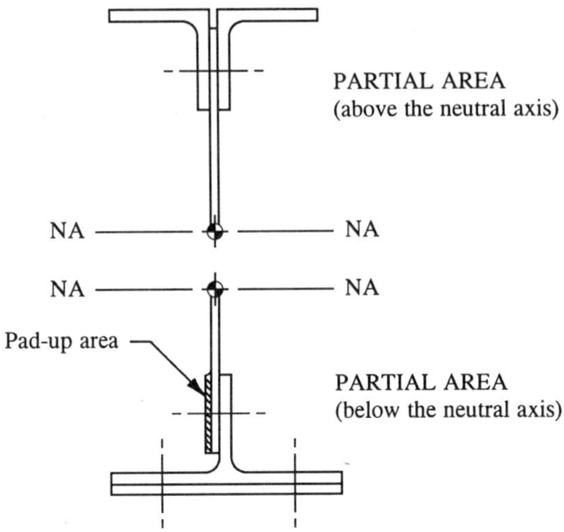

FIGURE 4-8 Section area above and below the neutral axis. Pad-up area (shown cross-hatched) ignored for clarity.

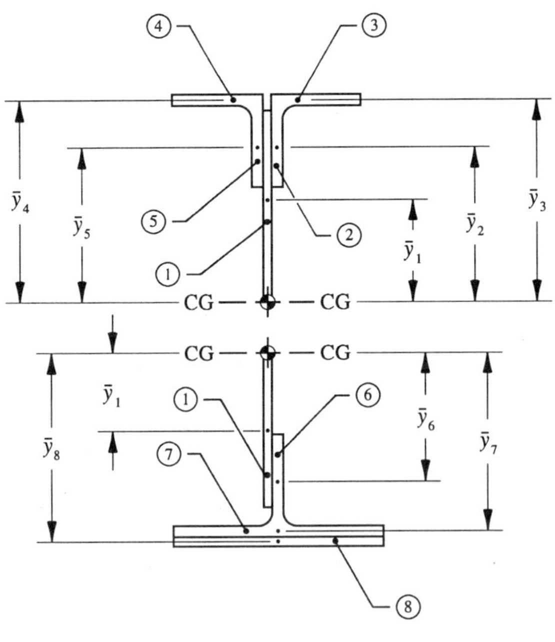

FIGURE 4-9 Beam section is partitioned into rectangular element areas.

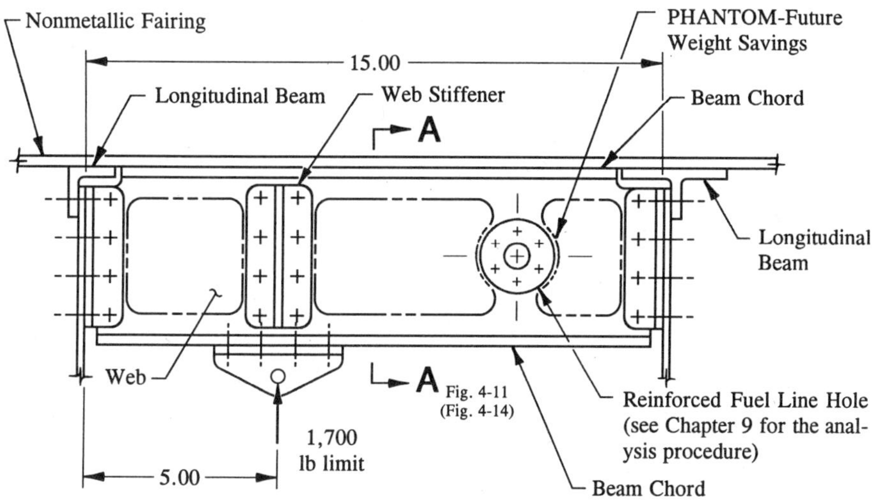

FIGURE 4-10 Beam structure for Example 4-1.

fully described in the example problem which follows. This example will best illustrate the general concepts and theoretical background ascribed to in our study of shearing stresses thus far in this section. Follow along if you will for the specific details of its solution.

Example 4-1 For the beam structure loaded as shown in Fig. 4-10, determine the maximum shearing stress for the section area indicated in Fig. 4-11 for this structure (use Eq. 4-2 for this computation). Then with this maximum value, predict the shear failure of the section at ultimate load.[1] That is, compare the ultimate allowable shearing stress F_{su} of the material to the maximum ultimate shearing stress $(f_s)_{max}$ calculated for the critical section of the beam. Make your prediction using Eq. 4-4.

SOLUTION: First, the reactions necessary to establish equilibrium of this beam are found, Fig. 4-12:

$$\Sigma F_y = 0, \qquad -R_1 - R_2 + 1,700 = 0$$

$$\Sigma M_A = 0, \qquad \circlearrowleft^{+} \quad -1,700(5) + R_2(15) = 0, \quad R_2 = 567\,\text{lb}.$$

Then substituting $R_2 = 567$ lb into the first equation gives:

[1] Today, all commercial aircraft vehicles are regulated by the FAA (Federal Aviation Administration) to oversee the substantiation and verification to codes of an aircraft structure at ultimate load. Ultimate load is usually 1.5 times limit load. Sometimes, however, even this factor can be slightly deviated from . . . as military requirements are sometimes less than 1.5 for some aircraft flight vehicle structures.

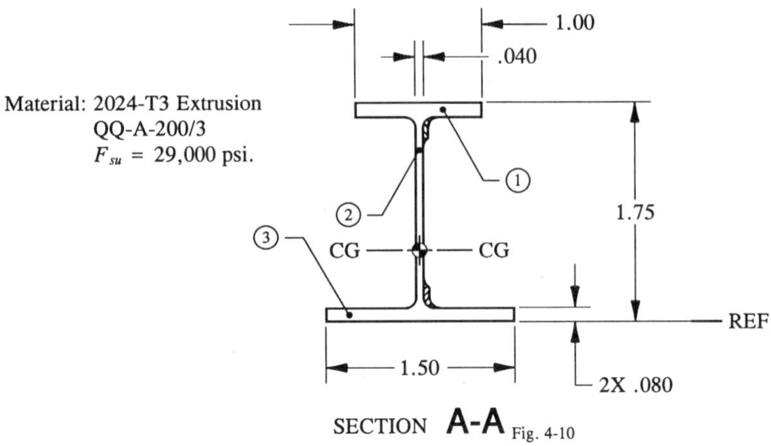

FIGURE 4-11 Cross-sectional area of beam. Pad-up areas (shown cross-hatched) ignored for clarity.

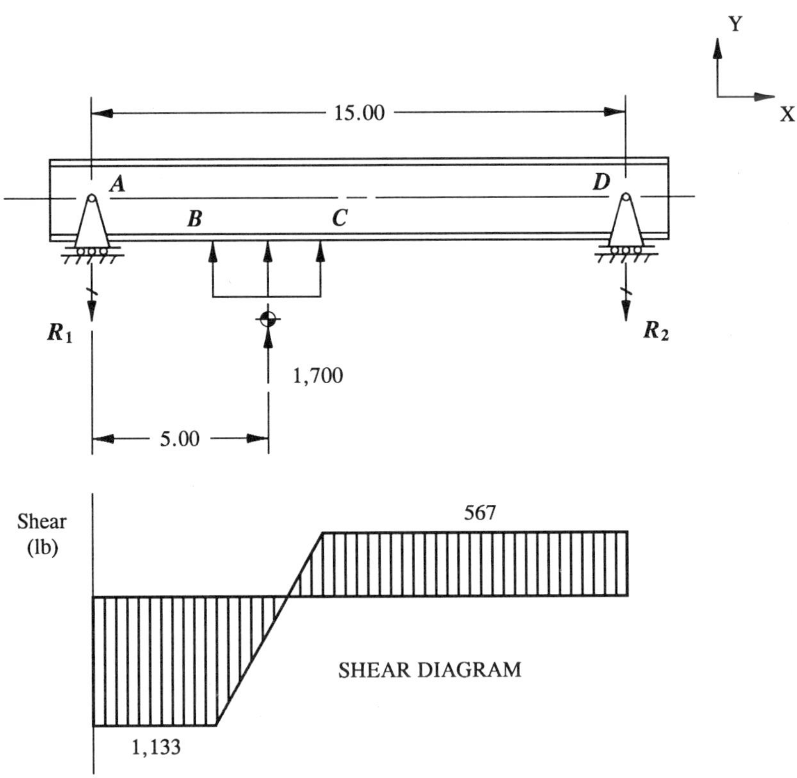

FIGURE 4-12 Free-body diagram of the beam and accompanying shear diagram constructed.

$$-R_1 - 567 + 1,700 = 0, \quad R_1 = 1,133 \text{ lb.}$$

Before the maximum shearing stress for the beam can be determined, the maximum internal shear acting along the beam must be found. This is most easily done by establishing a shear diagram of the beam for the given loading. Then, from this diagram, constructed here as shown in Fig. 4-12, the maximum internal shear can easily be pinpointed. The detailed construction of this diagram, however, has been left as an exercise for the engineer to complete. A review of the basic principles of its construction, if necessary, are found and discussed in Chapter 1, in particular, the engineer is referred to Sec. 1.6. Since the construction of this beam is essentially homogeneous (identical in form, composition, etc.) throughout the entire length of the beam, design of this member is straightforward: the beam is analyzed for that portion of its structure which carries the maximum shear. This occurs for the left-hand portion of the structure, as shown from A to B in this figure, where the value of shear is 1,133 lb. All lesser known shear values are, of course, not critical and therefore require no analytical substantiation.

Now, with the maximum internal shear known for this beam, the shear stress formula, Eq. 4-2 ($f_s = VQ/I_{na}t$) may be solved for the maximum shearing stress $(f_s)_{\max}$. Of course, the values of Q, I_{na}, and t must also be known before the actual computations can be performed. Here, the moment of inertia I_{na} is set up in the usual way: in tabular form as shown in Table 4-1. Refer back to Fig. 4-11 for the partitioning used to segment the I-beam section into designated rectangular element areas.

TABLE 4-1 MOMENT OF INERTIA I_{na}*

Element	b	h	y	A	Ay	Ay^2	I_o
1	1.000	0.080	1.710	0.080	0.137	0.234	0.000
2	0.040	1.590	0.875	0.064	0.056	0.049	0.013
3	1.500	0.080	0.040	0.120	0.005	0.000	0.000
			Total	0.264	0.198	0.283	0.013

* The engineer is referred back to Fig. 4-11, Section A-A, for pertinent dimensions.

$$Y_{cg} = \frac{\Sigma\, Ay}{\Sigma\, A} = \frac{.198}{.264} = .750 \text{ in.}$$

If we assume that $Y_{na} = Y_{cg}$ for elastic design, it directly follows from this that $I_{na} = I_{cg}$. Solving for these quantities gives:

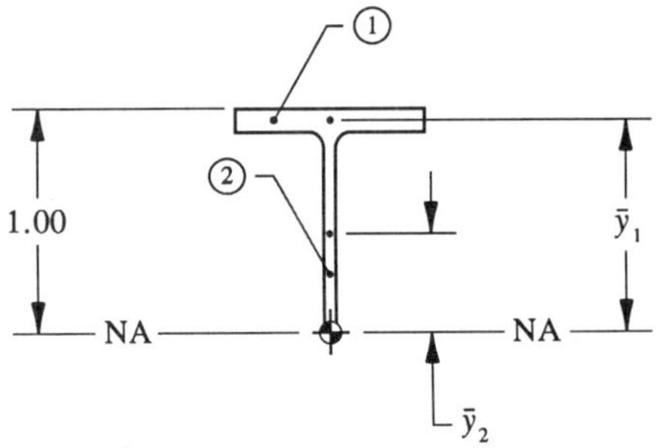

FIGURE 4-13 Partial area above the neutral axis of Section A-A.

$$I_{na} = I_{cg} = \Sigma I_o + \Sigma Ay^2 - Y_{cg}(\Sigma Ay) = .013 + .283 - .750(.198)$$
$$I_{na} = .147 \text{ in}^4.$$

Next, the value of Q is determined. Here, to obtain the "maximum" shearing stress, the partial area above the neutral axis of Section A-A is chosen (see Fig. 4-13). Of course, the lower partial area could also have been chosen for this computation.[1] All numerical computations of this quantity are performed in tabular form (see Table 4-2 below).

TABLE 4-2 STATIC MOMENT OF AREA Q

Element	A	$\bar{y}$	$A\bar{y}$
1	0.080	0.960	0.077
2	0.037	0.460	0.017
		$Q = \Sigma A\bar{y} =$	0.094

Then, substituting all quantities into the general expression for shear stress gives:

$$(f_s)_{\max} = \frac{VQ}{I_{na}t} = \frac{1,133(.094)}{.147(.040)} = 18,113 \text{ psi limit.}$$

At ultimate (or 1.5 times limit), we obtain the following predicted shear failure of

[1] Logically and rationally one can deduce that since only one value of shearing stress can occur at any one point on a structure (here, this refers to the beam web), and, if V, I_{na} and t do not change in Eq. 4-2 for the computation of Q, then it must also follow that $Q_{\text{upper}} = Q_{\text{lower}}$.

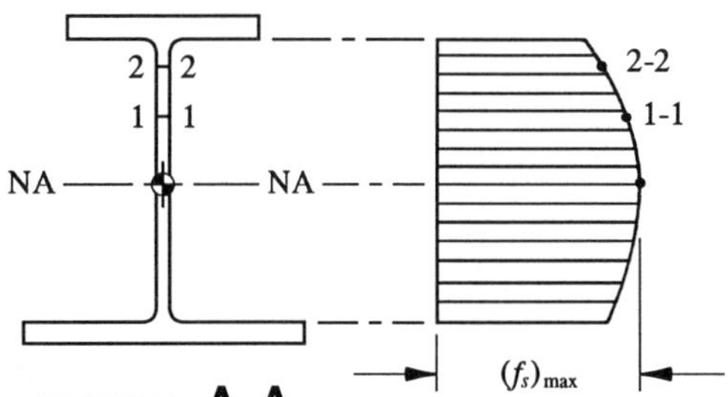

FIGURE 4-14 Shearing stress distribution is shown mainly carried by the web.

the web:

$$\text{Margin of Safety} = \text{M.S.} = \frac{F_{su}}{(f_s)_{max}} - 1 = \frac{29,000}{18,113(1.5)} - 1 = +.07.$$

As an alternative solution to this problem, it is now left as an exercise for the engineer to prove that the same predicted maximum shearing stress will result if the partial area below the neutral axis of the I-beam section were instead used to predict shearing failure of the web structure.

Before going any further in this chapter, let us expand our ideas related to our study of shearing stresses by making certain broad interpretations and general observations of shearing stresses across a section of beam area. For instance, in our example problem, if imaginary cuts were taken at different levels from the neutral axis of our I-beam section, what shearing stresses at these levels would develop? Using the same principles and logic employed thus far in our computations of "maximum" shearing stress, the shearing stresses at intermediate levels can also be found—consider the partial areas either above or below these imaginary levels. Then, to establish a general trend (or curve), each value determined is appropriately plotted on graph paper. Such a plot is viewed in Fig. 4-14. As expected, the variation of shearing stresses across the I-beam section is observed to reach a maximum value at the neutral axis. This occurrence is convenient and should help the engineer in the selection of viable alternative design candidates. Simply by focusing the attention on beams of "adequate" web shear strength; that is, selection of web designs based on the ultimate shearing stress F_{su} of the material, convergence of beam selections are quickly achieved. Simply put, convergence is possible by a simple increase in web thickness of the basic beam structure until adequate strength of the underlining web design has been fully achieved. Mathematically speaking, until a positive shear margin of safety for the web structure itself has been adequately designed for. For the most part, beams are constructed of thin webs, and their designs are easily negotiated by merely solving the shearing stress formula, Eq. 4-2, for $(f_s)_{max}$. Other typical cross-sectional areas frequently encountered in shearing stress design of aircraft structures are depicted in Table 4-3 (more about this table in the next section).

4.3 Maximum Shearing Stress of Common Aircraft Sections. From the variation of shearing stresses established across the I-beam section of the previous example problem (review distribution of shearing stresses given in Fig. 4-14), it can be seen that the total vertical shear V is mainly carried by the web of the basic beam section. No vertical shear is actually carried by the beam chords themselves. For this reason, it follows that the maximum shearing stress of an I-beam, normally calculated by the shear stress formula, Eq. 4-2, can be conveniently approximated by dividing this total by the web cross-sectional area between beam flanges ($A_{web} = ht$). This very useful and unique relationship for shear stress is expressed in equation form as follows:

$$(f_s)_{max} = \frac{V}{A_{web}} = \frac{V}{ht} \quad \text{(approximate solution)} \tag{4-9}$$

where: V = total vertical shear
A_{web} = web cross-sectional area between beam flanges
h = height measured between beam flanges (see Table 4-3, Case d, page 241)
t = web thickness.

Now, if we take the web cross-sectional area of our previous example problem, and the maximum internal vertical shear of 1,133 lb, the maximum shearing stress for the I-beam section used in the solution of that problem can be approximated. Substituting the appropriate values into the equation above, we obtain:

$$(f_s)_{max} = \frac{1,133}{.064} = 17,703 \text{ psi limit} \quad \text{(approximate solution)}$$

where: $A_{web} = (1.75 - .080 - .080)(.040) = .064 \text{ in}^2$ (see Section A-A, Fig. 4-11).

The accuracy of our solution will depend upon how well the beam flanges of our I-beam are geometrically defined with respect to the total section area of the beam. For example, if the beam flanges are well-defined members, beefy, the approximate method of analysis becomes quite accurate. For most preliminary and investigative stages of design work this accuracy is sufficient and should prove highly reliable. However, one must keep in mind that approximate solutions may not always yield conservative results. For instance, as can be seen from our comparison solution here, the approximate method (maximum shearing stress of 17,703 psi limit) is slightly less than the true maximum shearing stress originally obtained by the exact method of analysis (i.e., the shearing stress formula). That

TABLE 4-3 MAXIMUM SHEARING STRESS FOR COMMON AIRCRAFT SECTIONS

a. Rectangular Section

$$(f_s)_{max} = \frac{VQ}{I_{na}t} = \frac{3V}{2A}$$

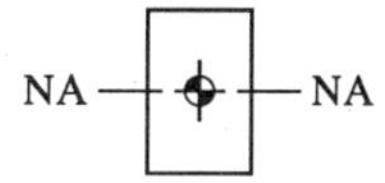

b. Solid, Circular Section

$$(f_s)_{max} = \frac{VQ}{I_{na}t} = \frac{4V}{3A}$$

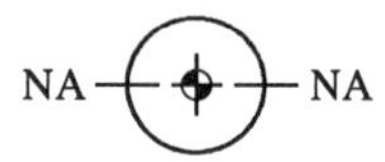

c. Tubular Section

$$(f_s)_{max} = \frac{VQ}{I_{na}t} = \frac{4V}{3A}\left[1 + \frac{Dd}{D^2 + d^2}\right]$$

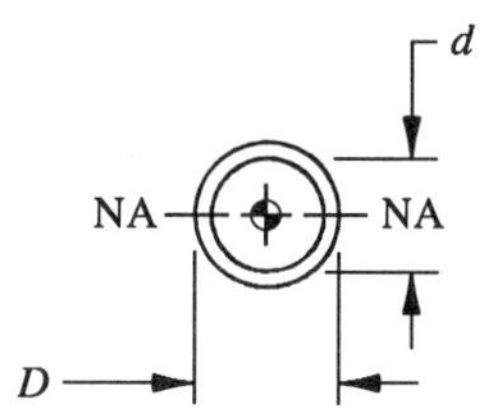

d. I-beam or C-beam Section

$$(f_s)_{max} = \frac{VQ}{I_{na}t} \quad \text{(exact solution)}$$

$$(f_s)_{max} = \frac{V}{A_{web}} = \frac{V}{ht} \quad \text{(approximate solution)}$$

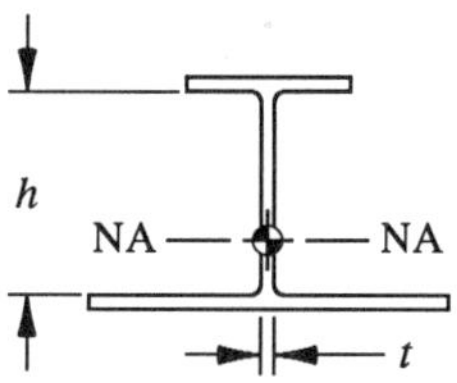

solution gave a shearing stress of 18,113 psi limit. Nonetheless, such accuracy is usually sufficient to accurately check, even predict, those computations made by more rigorous or detailed methods of analysis. For our comparison solution, the approximate method of analysis differs by about 2% from those values computed earlier. This comparison is made as follows:

$$\%\ \text{Error} = \frac{18,113 - 17,703}{18,113}(100) = 2\% \quad \text{(slightly unconservative).}$$

The engineer should not be lulled into complacency by using the approximate method of analysis arbitrarily, as this comparison clearly shows that true maximum shearing stresses can sometimes be slightly higher. In fact, in some cases, where the beam flanges of a structure are not well-defined members, perhaps that approaching a rectangular beam cross-sectional area, the maximum shearing stress calculated by the approximate method can be as much as 50% off (this is 50% less than the true maximum shearing stress obtained from the shearing stress formula solution). See Table 4-3 for the maximum shearing stress of a rectangular beam section. There, $(f_s)_{max} = 3V/2A$.

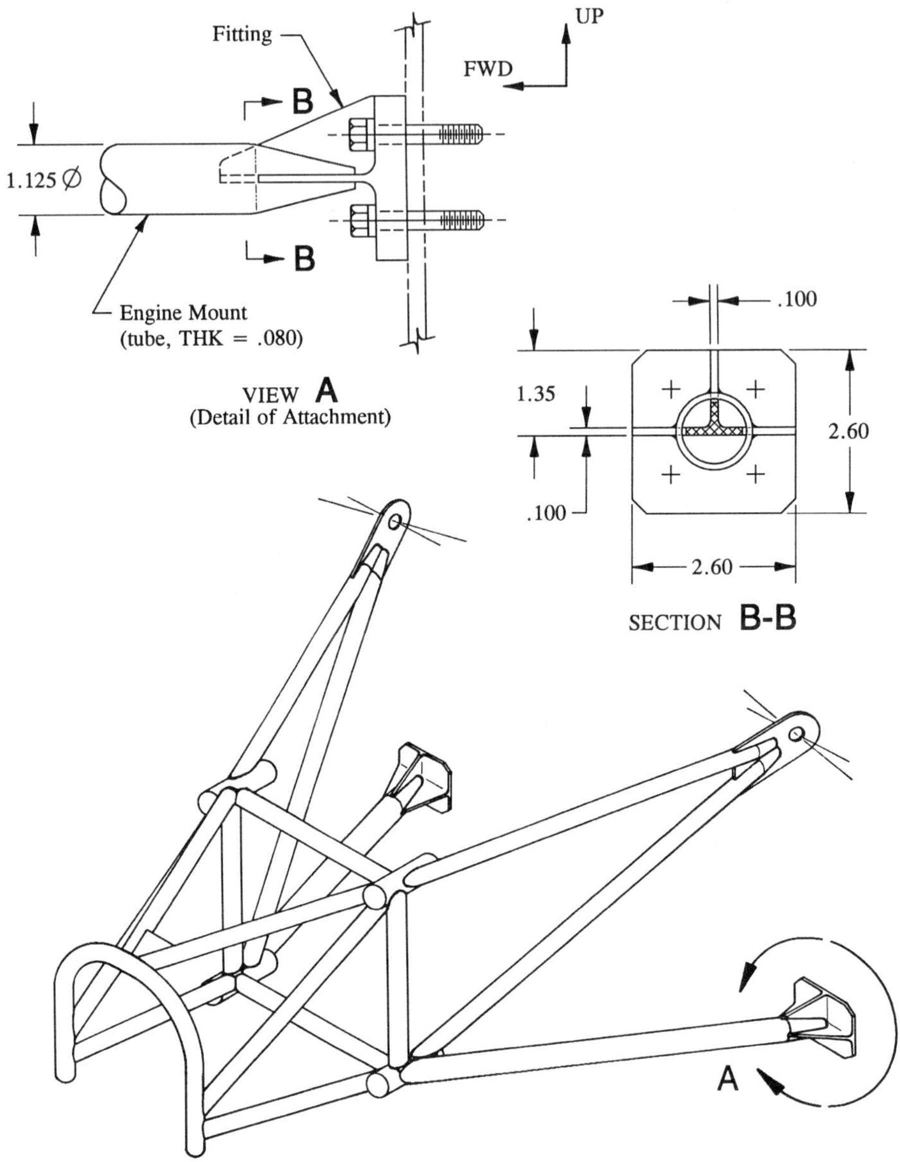

FIGURE 4-15 Engine support structure.

Example 4-2 The engine support structure is constructed of 4130 steel tubes welded to 4130 steel fittings, as shown in Fig. 4-15. Find the maximum shearing stresses for the tube and fitting members? Make your stress predictions (margin of safety evaluations) at ultimate load using a maximum internal shear of 3,500 lb ultimate acting in the vertical direction. Note: The entire assembly is heat treated to 125 ksi subsequent to welding.[1]

SOLUTION: Suffice it to say that when a member is heat treated subsequent to welding, it should fully develop its entire spectrum of material allowable strengths: F_{tu}, F_{ty}, F_{cy}, F_{su}, F_{bru}, F_{bry}, etc. A slight reduction in allowables, however, is sometimes recommended by industry because a welded structure generally is more brittle and therefore less resistant to shock, impact, vibration, and fatigue loads. These unknown perimeters of a welded structure are exactly why experienced engineers recommend a purely subjective reduction of 20% in material allowable strengths in those design cases where a structure is heat affected[2]. The actual degree of conservatism used for a welded structure should however be verified by the appropriate analysis department or by the particular governing military or commercial agencies in charge of overseeing production design criteria. The actual weld material used to structurally bond the engine mount assembly structure together must also be analyzed. The engineer is referred to MIL-HDBK-5, Sec. 8.2, for a discussion of "Metallurgical Joints."

To find the ultimate allowable shearing stress F_{su} of 4130 steel needed to solve the particular details of this problem, refer specifically to the mechanical-property table given in MIL-HDBK-5F for this material. In this table, the ultimate allowable shearing stress of 4130 steel is found by referring to the ultimate allowable shearing stress corresponding to an ultimate allowable tension stress of 125 ksi. This gives $F_{su} = 75$ ksi.

The formulas in Table 4-3 can be used to determine the maximum shearing stresses for the tube and fitting members of the engine support structure. These expressions have been verified countless times and therefore require no further substantiation or proof; they are presumed to be correct. Follow along now for the analytical evaluations of these members for ultimate shear failure. For the tubes (see View A):

$$(f_s)_{\max} = \frac{4V}{3A}\left[1 + \frac{Dd}{D^2 + d^2}\right] \quad \text{(see Table 4-3, Case c)}$$

where: $V = 3,500$ lb

$D = 1.125$ in

$d = 1.125 - (2)(.080) = .965$ in

$$A = \pi\left[\frac{D}{2}\right]^2 - \pi\left[\frac{d}{2}\right]^2 = .263 \text{ in}^2.$$

These values are then substituted into the general expression above, and the maximum shearing stress for the tubes is found.

[1] Such a note on an engineering drawing generally indicates the ultimate allowable tension strength of the material.

[2] The heat-affected zone refers to both the "parent" and "weld" materials of the welded structure.

$$(f_s)_{\max} = \frac{4(3,500)}{3(.263)}\left[1 + \frac{1.125(.965)}{(1.125)^2 + (.965)^2}\right]$$

$$(f_s)_{\max} = 26,513 \text{ psi ultimate.}$$

Predicted ultimate shear failure of the tubes:

$$\text{Margin of Safety} = \text{M.S.} = \frac{.80\,F_{su}}{(f_s)_{\max}} - 1 = \frac{60,000}{26,513} - 1 = +1.26$$

where: F_{su} = 75,000 psi (refer to MIL-HDBK-5F)
$.80\,F_{su}$ = 60,000 psi (reduction factor of 20% in material strength due to welding).

For the fittings (see also View A):

$$(f_s)_{\max} = \frac{VQ}{I_{na}\,t} \quad \text{(see Eq. 4-2 for definition of terms).}$$

The maximum shearing stress of the steel fitting (T-beam section) is found by applying the same basic principles that were used to solve the shearing stress formula in the previous example problem for an I-beam section (for specific details of these computations, refer back to Example 4-1). It was graphically shown in that problem how the maximum (or peak) shearing stress for an I-beam section is concentrated along the neutral axis of its section area. Thus, the solution of Eq. 4-2 need only be performed once: that is, at the neutral axis. Generally speaking, other intermediate shearing stresses may occur within the beam structure itself, but their values, usually less critical, need not be investigated: A beam subjected to shear is normally designed by its maximum shearing stress only. For the present, no rapid method of analysis, approximate or otherwise, has been devised to determine the maximum shearing stress of a T-beam section. Consequently, our solution here must involve the more detailed treatment or evaluation of these stresses using Eq. 4-2. In Table 4-4, the moment of inertia I_{na}, stiffness property of a beam, is tabulated for the T-beam section. Proper sectioning of its cross-sectional area is viewed in Fig. 4-16.

TABLE 4-4 MOMENT OF INERTIA I_{na}

Element	b	h	y	A	Ay	Ay^2	I_o
1	2.600	0.100	0.050	0.260	0.013	0.001	0.000
2	0.100	1.250	0.725	0.125	0.091	0.066	0.016
			Total	0.385	0.104	0.067	0.016

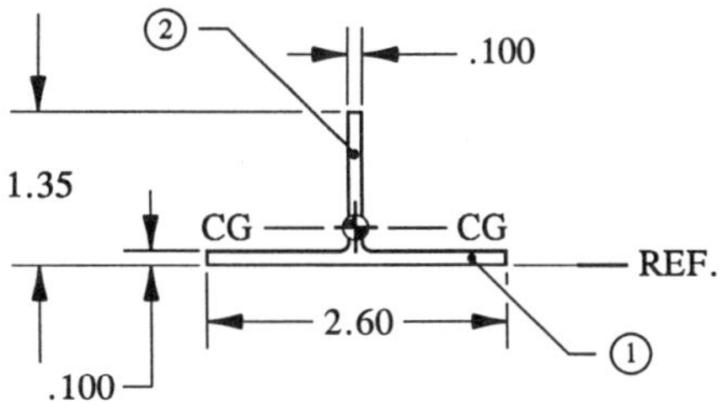

FIGURE 4-16 Engine mount fitting is partitioned into rectangular element areas.

$$Y_{cg} = \frac{\Sigma Ay}{\Sigma A} = \frac{.104}{.385} = .270 \text{ in}$$

$$I_{cg} = \Sigma I_o + \Sigma Ay^2 - Y_{cg}(\Sigma Ay) = .016 + .067 - .270(.104) = .055 \text{ in}^4.$$

For elastic stress design, $Y_{na} = Y_{cg}$, and the following property of the section also holds true, that

$$I_{na} = I_{cg} = .055 \text{ in}^4.$$

Now, the static moment of area is determined. To simplify our computations of this quantity, the partial area above the neutral axis of the beam section area is prepared, as shown in Fig. 4-17. The result of this evaluation is formulated as follows:

$$Q = \Sigma A\bar{y} = A_2\bar{y}_2 = (1.08)(.100)\left[\frac{1.08}{2}\right]$$

$$Q = .058 \text{ in}^3 \quad \text{(upper partial area of the T-section).}$$

This value can also be verified by using the partial area of the lower section, as shown in Fig. 4-18. The following expression is formulated for this partial area:

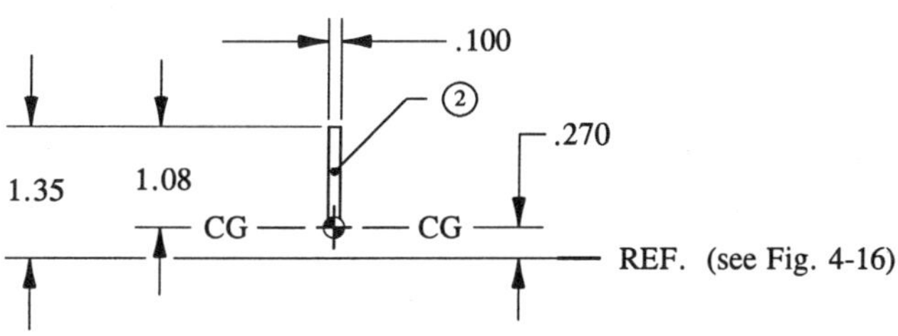

FIGURE 4-17 Partial area above the neutral axis.

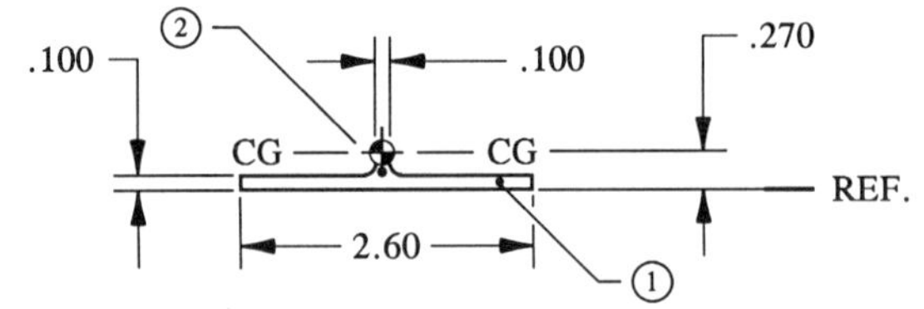

FIGURE 4-18 Partial area below the neutral axis.

$$Q = \Sigma A\bar{y} = A_1\bar{y}_1 + A_2\bar{y}_2 = (2.60)(.100)(.220) + (.100)(.170)\left[\frac{.170}{2}\right]$$
$$Q = .058 \text{ in}^3 \quad \text{(lower partial area of the T-section).}$$

This again demonstrates the consistency of this method: the static moments of area Q are the same for the partial areas considered on either side of the neutral axis of the total section area.

Then substituting all known values into the shearing stress formula, the desired maximum is found. Here, this gives:

$$(f_s)_{\max} = \frac{VQ}{I_{na}\,t} = \frac{(3,500)(.058)}{(.055)(.100)} = 36,909 \text{ psi.}$$

Predicted ultimate shear failure of the steel fittings:

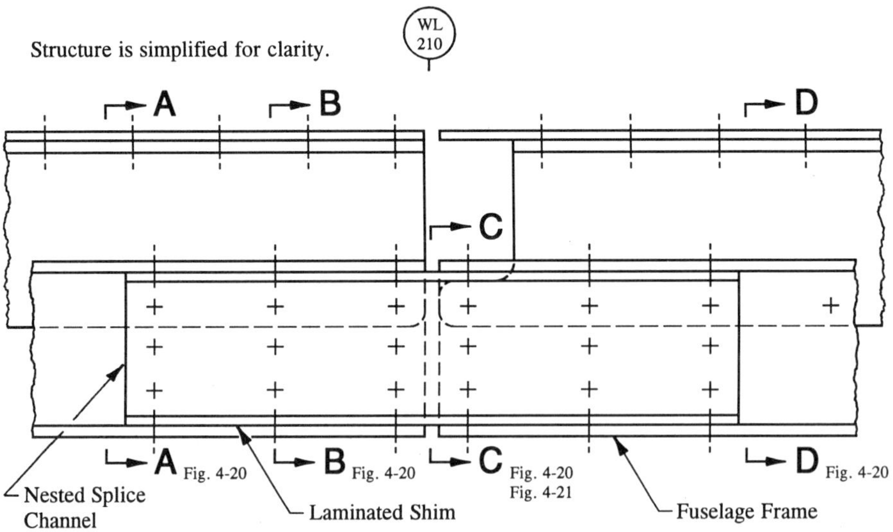

FIGURE 4-19 Fuselage frame splice at WL 210.

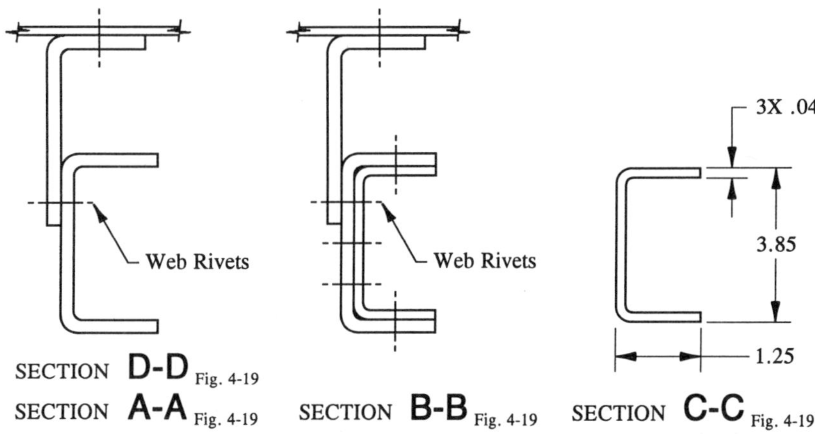

FIGURE 4-20 Fuselage frame splice beam sections.

$$\text{Margin of Safety} = \text{M.S.} = \frac{.80\,F_{su}}{(f_s)_{max}} - 1 = \frac{60,000}{36,909} - 1 = +.63$$

where: $F_{su} = 75,000$ psi (see MIL-HDBK-5F or refer to discussion on p. 243)
$.80\,F_{su} = 60,000$ psi (reduction factor of 20% in material strength due to welding).

Example 4-3 The fuselage frame structure in Fig. 4-19 is spliced at WL 210 using an arrangement of members as shown. If the basic frame structure carries a maximum constant shear of 1,200 lb ultimate, find the maximum shearing stress developed by the web of the most critical frame section (include Sections A-A through D-D along the frame structure in your preliminary determination of critical sections). Isolated cross-sectional areas along the frame are drawn in Fig. 4-20. Discuss other failures that might occur and their solutions. In other words, substantiate the basic frame structure in general. Also include the splice channel in your preliminary investigations. Use a value of $F_{su} = 47,000$ psi for the frame structure (refer to the mechanical-property table for 7075-T6 aluminum in MIL-HDBK-5F, QQ-A-250/12, THK = .040 in).

SOLUTION: The approximation of maximum shearing stresses using Eq. 4-9 is again considered here in our frame solution. If our findings are, say, within 30% of the allowable shearing stress of the material, then a more detailed approach to the analysis would be advised. However, if shearing stresses are shown to be below those in the acceptable range, no further analysis, detailed or otherwise, would be required.

It is the engineer's prerogative to avoid needless and superfluous computations if he so chooses when logic and rationale for their exclusion are justified.

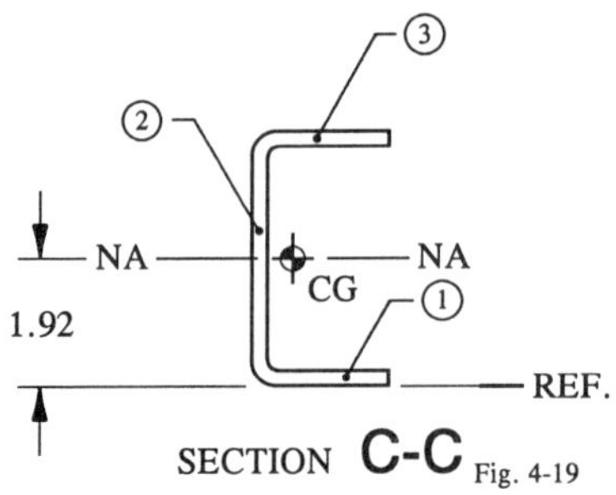

FIGURE 4-21 Section area is partitioned into rectangular element areas.

Sometimes, just a simple written statement or stipulation of obvious conclusions is all that is necessary for substantiation of an otherwise complicated alternate. This technique often eliminates the more lengthy evaluations made of obvious and intuitive design candidates. The time saved can then be better spent on more productive and important considerations.

From Table 4-3, Case d, the simplified expression for a C-section is used to approximate the maximum shearing stress for the critical frame section (at Section C-C). By inspection, Section C-C is deemed critical because the smaller shear area at this section must also carry the full design shear. Such a critical design combination should produce a maximum shearing stress that ultimately governs the basic design criterion of the frame structure in shear.[1] Hence, the following computation is made:

$$(f_s)_{\max} = \frac{V}{A_{\text{web}}} = \frac{1,200}{(3.85 - .040 - .040)(.040)}$$

$$(f_s)_{\max} = 7,958 \text{ psi} \quad \text{(approximate solution)}.$$

Compare this value with the much higher ultimate allowable shear strength of the basic frame material or $F_{su} = 47,000$ psi. For the sake of completeness of our general study of shearing stresses, the following suggestion is made: state your conclusions of structural integrity as a mathematical expression predicting shear failure. For the analyzed frame structure, let this comparison be expressed like this:

$$\text{Margin of Safety} = \text{M.S.} = \frac{F_{su}}{(f_s)_{\max}} - 1 = \frac{47,000}{7,958} - 1$$

$$\text{M.S.} = +\,4.91 \quad \text{(approximate solution)}.$$

[1] Of course, our approximate method of analysis can also be applied to substantiate the beefier (less critical) cross-sectional areas at A-A, B-B, and D-D. But, as a general rule, these rather superfluous computations, of seemingly lower stress intensities, are simply disregarded.

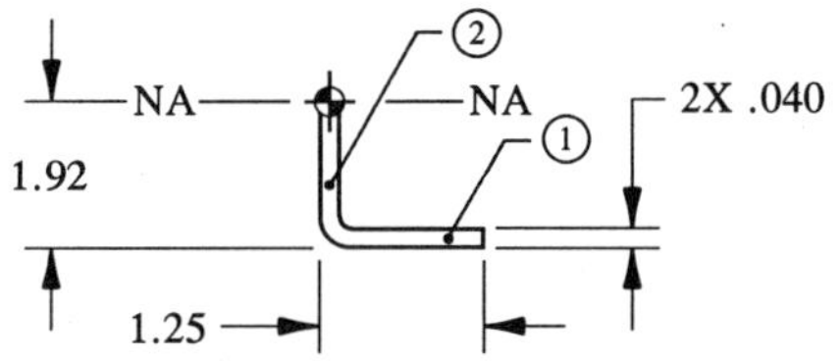

FIGURE 4-22 Partial area below the neutral axis.

Let us now see just how accurate our findings have been up to this point in our investigation of maximum shearing stresses by considering the more exact solution (see application of the shearing stress formula, Eq. 4-2). Refer to Fig. 4-21 for the proper sectioning of element areas used to calculate the moment of inertia of Section C-C and also to Table 4-5 for the actual computations employed. The static moment of area is computed for the lower partial area of Section C-C as follows:

$$Q = \Sigma A\bar{y} = A_1\bar{y}_1 + A_2\bar{y}_2 = (1.25)(.040)(1.90) + (1.88)(.040)(.94)$$
$$Q = .166 \text{ in}^3.$$

Refer to Fig. 4-22 for the dimensions pertinent to the analysis.

TABLE 4-5 MOMENT OF INERTIA I_{na}

Element	b	h	y	A	Ay	Ay^2	I_o
1	1.250	0.040	0.020	0.050	0.001	0.000	0.000
2	0.040	3.770	1.925	0.151	0.290	0.559	0.179
3	1.250	0.040	3.830	0.050	0.191	0.733	0.000
			Total	0.251	0.482	1.292	0.179

$$Y_{cg} = \frac{\Sigma\, Ay}{\Sigma\, A} = \frac{.482}{.251} = 1.920 \text{ in}$$

$$I_{na} = \Sigma\, I_o + \Sigma\, Ay^2 - Y_{cg}(\Sigma\, Ay)$$
$$I_{na} = .179 + 1.292 - 1.920(.482) = .546 \text{ in}^4.$$

Since $Y_{na} = Y_{cg}$ for elastic design,

$$I_{na} = I_{cg} = .546 \text{ in}^4.$$

To proceed now with the solution of maximum shearing stresses, we obtain from Eq. 4-2:

$$(f_s)_{max} = \frac{VQ}{I_{na}\,t} = \frac{(1,200)(.166)}{(.546)(.040)} = 9,121 \text{ psi}.$$

From this, we can now accurately predict, essentially verifying our approximate solution, that shearing stresses are not critical for any section along the fuselage frame structure. Although most aircraft designs are analyzed by exact (detailed) methods of analysis,[1] an approximate solution nonetheless provides a wealth of reliable information from its application.

GENERAL DISCUSSION: All possible failure modes of a structure must be considered by the design engineer. The following suggestions are made below to help the engineer accomplish a complete and thorough examination of the basic frame structure and splice:

(1) The internal frame loads (*P* and *M*), normally expected along a fuselage frame structure, are transferred across the frame splice by the nested channel shown in Fig. 4-19. The combined loading effects of these loads on the splice channel at Section C-C must be considered by investigating the bending and axial compression or tension stresses which they produce at this location. Equation 2-9 is applied for this evaluation (see page 77). This will also substantiate the beefier sections at A-A, B-B, and D-D. Strength allowables are based on F_{tu} and F_{cy}. However, if crippling failure (Chapter 6) is deemed a more critical design consideration for these sections, the crippling allowable strength F_{cc} of their composite areas would then govern their solutions.

(2) The splice connection is analyzed for the combined transfer of internal frame loads (*V*, *P*, and *M*) across the splice at WL 210. This means analyzing for joint failures which are governed by shearing failure of the connection rivets and bearing failure of the nested channel and fuselage frame. The allowable strength, either P_{su} or P_{bru}, will govern the solution to their designs. The solution is performed by the analysis methods of Chapter 3 (see also Example 3-4 for the solution of a related example problem).

(3) The spacing and sizing of rivets along the web rivet line for Sections A-A, B-B, and D-D are determined by the solution of (a) Eq. 4-3 or $q = VQ/I_{na}$ and (b) Eq. 4-10 or $p = qs$. The static moment of area Q in the first of these expressions, part (a), is defined as described in Table 4-7 (see ahead to page 260), Case n, where $Q = \Sigma A\bar{y} = Q_1 + Q_2 + Q_3 = A_1\bar{y}_1 + A_2\bar{y}_2 + A_3\bar{y}_3$ for the channel section. Consider that the channel, in effect, shears completely off (at the web rivet line) from the rest of the cross-sectional area. The same situation occurs at Section

[1] This is true because of the nature of aircraft designs. For the most part, an aircraft undergoes many different flight conditions and, as such, at least one of these conditions will usually produce shearing stresses critical enough to warrant such a detailed investigation.

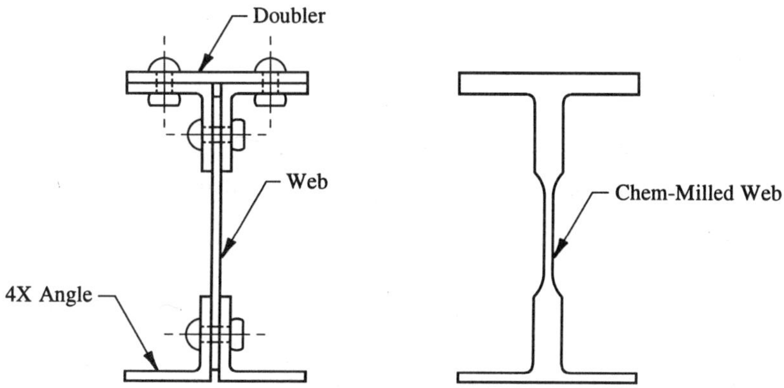

FIGURE 4-23 (a) Built-up beam section. (b) Simulated integral beam section.

B-B, however, the combination of back-to-back channels here, somewhat beefier cross-sectional area, makes this section structurally less critical. And therefore, the analysis of this section, as far as rivet shear and plate bearing evaluations go, would not be required. These computations (and observations) will become more apparent as our study of interconnection shearing forces and their applications to built-up beam structures is formally introduced in the next section.

4.4 Interconnection Shearing Forces of Built-up Beams. The general concepts and principles used in the solution of shearing stresses in Sec. 4-2 are again utilized in part here in this section in our study of interconnection shearing forces (or shear flow) of built-up beams. In general, an aircraft structure is constructed of many different types of members, such as angles, straps, doublers, and reinforcing plates, all of which are held together to the main structure by means of structural fasteners. This is viewed in Fig. 4-23(a) where several individual members have been joined together to form a built-up beam section. Conditionally, the fasteners of this beam must also provide the additional function of making each member act in concert (together) with all of the other attached members of the built-up structure. Thus, theoretically simulating an integral beam section, as shown in Fig. 4-23(b). Hypothetically, if fasteners of such a built-up beam are not provided in sufficient numbers or sizes along the full span of beam, sliding between the surfaces of individual members will occur. This sliding action will prevent the built-up structure from physically acting in composite with its attached members, thereby making the proposed arrangement of members less desirable as far as efficient and acceptable designs go. In effect, the bending stiffness[1] of the beam is reduced from the maximum value that would normally be expected from a section having no such limitation imposed like this. A well-designed, built-up beam will

[1] Bending stiffness is a property of a beam that is conveniently measured by the moment of inertia of the beam.

therefore have all of its fasteners properly sized and spaced according to the shear flow acting between the individually attached members. Only then can the full bending stiffness I_{na} of such a beam, as demonstrated by the methods of Appendix F of this book, be accurately appraised and used for designing (sizing) purposes.

The interconnection shearing forces necessary to make such members act together effectively with the main structure will be the main focus of attention in this section. The procedure for calculating such forces is of course related to our previous study of shearing stresses and, therefore, all the information available to us from that section will again be used here to help us understand more clearly the foregoing discussions and concepts used in this section.

Let us now review the development of our original shear flow equation, Eq. 4-1 ($q = \Delta P/L$), in Sec. 4.1. Essentially, a change in bending moment occurring at different sections along a beam was used to derive this simple expression. In particular, it was found that if different magnitudes of bending moments were developed at different sections of a beam, their difference in terms of equivalent couple-forces[1] or ΔP would be totally resisted by the interconnection shearing forces of the fasteners occurring between the sections considered.

Hypothetically then, if the couple-forces were of the same magnitude, no apparent interconnection forces would actually develop between the sections. The fasteners would then perform a nominal function of keeping the members together. Theoretically, the fasteners would not resist or develop any horizontal shearing forces. They would, in effect, be unloaded. However, if the couple-forces were not of the same magnitudes at neighboring sections, then more push would develop at one section than the other. This difference would be resisted by the fasteners between the sections considered. Thus, equilibrium would be maintained, and the individual members would be considered fully effective.

The above line of reasoning is exactly how our shear flow equation was developed earlier in this chapter (see Sec. 4-1). For easy reference, this equation is again written here below:

$$q = \frac{\Delta P}{L} \quad \text{(from Eq. 4-1)}$$

where: ΔP = difference between the internal forces of a member at adjacent sections along a beam

L = distance measured between the section areas considered along the beam (see Fig. 4-5)

q = design shear flow.

In this form, Eq. 4-1 is not particularly obvious to use nor is it very practical to apply. Instead, the shear flow equation in alternative form, that which was presented in Sec. 4.2 for composite beams will be utilized in this section. This

[1] Refer back to Fig. 4-4 where couple-forces were diagrammed as concentrated forces acting at the cap area centroids of a beam section.

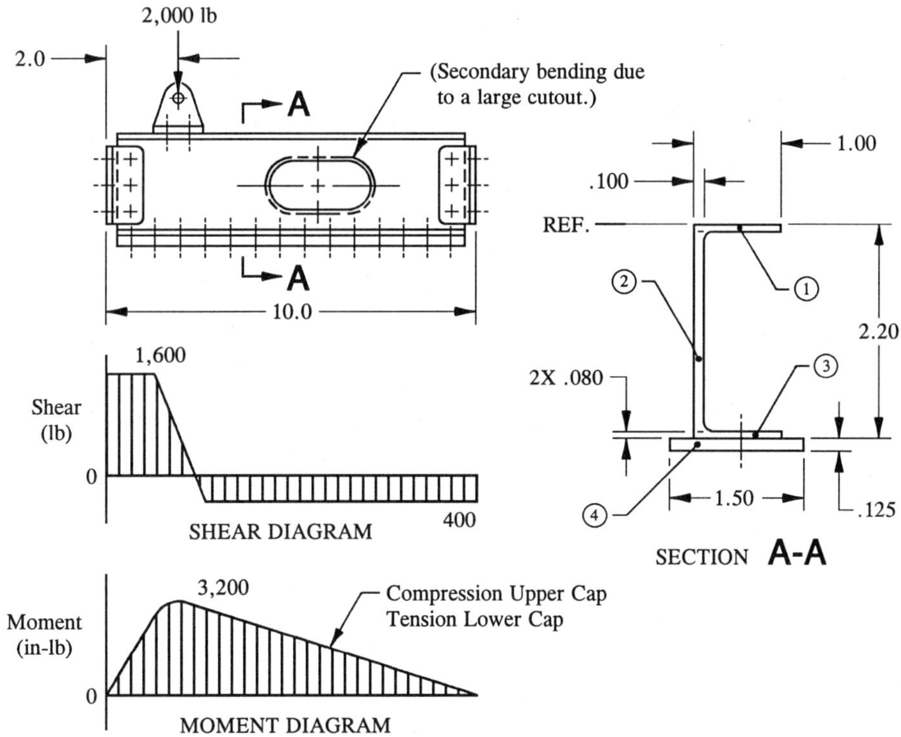

FIGURE 4-24 Aluminum beam structure is subjected to a maximum ultimate force of 2,000 lb at the location indicated.

equation is again written as follows:

$$q = \frac{VQ}{I_{na}}$$

where: V = internal shearing force

Q = static moment of area (as defined by Eq. 4-8 for the attached members of a composite beam)

I_{na} = moment of inertia of the total cross-sectional area around the neutral axis of a beam section.

The importance of this equation is further emphasized in Appendix H, where the moment of inertia of a built-up beam section was found to be structurally more effective in bending resistance than the sum of the bending resistances offered by the individual members of the section acting separately. Although a beam may be attached together by means of adhesive-bonds, screws, welding, or bolts and rivets, the basic procedure for calculating "loads" or "shear flows" for these attachment types remains essentially the same. Intrinsically, however, different attachment types will develop different allowable shear strengths.

The strength of a joint is either based on its resistance to shear of its fasteners or its resistance to bearing of its attached members of the joint. The required spacing of fasteners in a built-up beam is therefore directly determined from the shear flow equation ($q = VQ/I_{na}$). All members that make up the built-up beam must then be securely attached by fasteners that can fully develop the design shear flow q between them. This criterion is essential to make the beam act structurally together (as a unit). To find the magnitude of the interconnection shearing forces acting between such members, the following expression as a function of shear flow and fastener spacing is employed:

$$p_s = qs \tag{4-10}$$

where: q = design shear flow (for beams, use $q = VQ/I_{na}$)
s = fastener spacing along the span of beam.

The application of this equation will now be illustrated by several example problems.

Example 4-4 An aluminum beam structure of a constant cross-sectional area is subjected to a maximum ultimate force of 2,000 lb, as shown in Fig. 4-24. If the beam is simply-supported at its ends by shear clips, what required spacing of BJ 6 aluminum rivets (F_{su} = 30,000 psi) would be recommended for the attached reinforcement strap? See Table 3-1, page 146, where the allowable single-shear strength of this particular rivet is tabulated (P_{su} = 862 lb ult). Also calculate the maximum shearing stress for this beam. The moment of inertia I_{na} is defined on the basis of the total cross-sectional area (see Table 4-6). This tabulation includes the reinforcement strap and channel section acting together as a unit, which, as such, presumes the proper size and spacing of fasteners for the attached reinforcement (and applied loads given).

SOLUTION: Before actually performing the numerical computations to solve this problem, let us formulate in our minds the necessary sequence of steps involved to accomplish its design solution. Like an experienced cabinet maker who must bring his hammer, nails, and saws to work with him, the engineer must have at his fingertips the proper dimensions, allowables, and general-approved aerospace methods and techniques of analysis required to accomplish a favorable design objective. The accomplished, well-seasoned engineer will therefore take the necessary additional time to prepare his preliminary investigations, sometimes simply as thoughts, general ideas, notions, etc., in advance of detailed formulations and derivations. The time spent early in the preliminary design effort will usually save him additional man-hours later. It is good design practice well worth the initial investment now than to spend valuable man-hours later making tedious and nebulous design changes of a structural nature. In the next few paragraphs, the general solution description and equations of this section pertinent to rivet and web design of this example problem are formulated.

TABLE 4-6 MOMENT OF INERTIA I_{na}

Element	b	h	y	A	Ay	Ay^2	I_o
1	1.000	0.080	0.040	0.080	0.003	0.000	0.000
2	0.100	2.040	1.100	0.204	0.224	0.247	0.071
3	1.000	0.080	2.160	0.080	0.173	0.373	0.000
4	1.500	0.125	2.262	0.187	0.424	0.959	0.000
			Total	0.551	0.824	1.579	0.071

$$Y_{cg} = \frac{\Sigma\, Ay}{\Sigma\, A} = \frac{.824}{.551} = 1.495 \text{ in}$$

$$I_{cg} = \Sigma\, I_o + \Sigma\, Ay^2 - Y_{cg}\,(\Sigma\, Ay)$$
$$I_{cg} = .071 + 1.579 - 1.495(.824) = .418 \text{ in}^4.$$

From elastic beam theory,

$$Y_{na} = Y_{cg} = 1.495 \text{ in}$$

and

$$I_{na} = I_{cg} = .418 \text{ in}^4.$$

For rivet design, Eq. 4-3 ($q = VQ/I_{na}$) and Eq. 4-10 ($p_s = qs$) are applied in a simultaneous solution to determine the interconnection forces p_s acting between the reinforcement strap and the channel section. The shear diagram in Fig. 4-24 will help locate the appropriate maximum internal design shear V to use in the first of these required evaluations. The maximum shear is 1,600 lb and this same value can also be used to design the basic web structure for static shear strength. By the methods of Sec. 4.2, specifically, the solution of Eq. 4-2 or $(f_s)_{\max} = VQ/I_{na}t$, this evaluation is accomplished.

Web Design:

Let us now perform the computation of maximum shearing stress, but in two different ways: (1) using the approximation for an I-beam section as given in Table

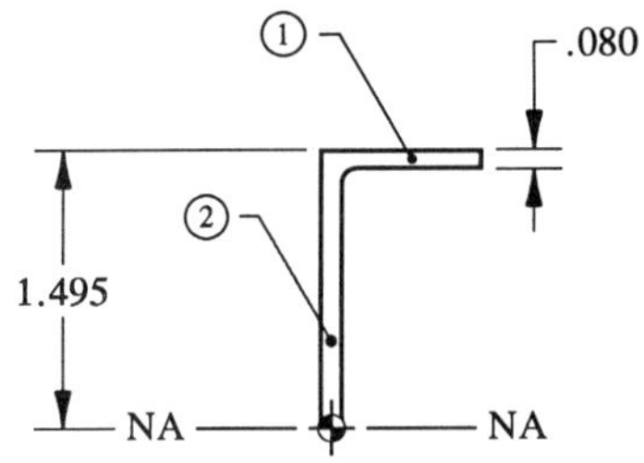

FIGURE 4-25 Partial area above the neutral axis of Section A-A. Refer back to Fig. 4-24 for pertinent dimensions.

4-3, Case d, and (2) using the conventional shearing stress formula. From Table 4-3, the solution proceeds as follows:

$$(f_s)_{\max} = \frac{V}{A_{\text{web}}} = \frac{1,600}{(2.20 - .080 - .080)(.100)}$$

$$(f_s)_{\max} = 7,843 \text{ psi ultimate} \quad \text{(approximate solution)}.$$

This analysis is crude but nevertheless provides a quick and reliable reference tool for analyzing more geometrically difficult design cases such as our particular beam section here. Since most aluminum materials exhibit an allowable shearing stress of around 36,000 psi, the web (THK = .100 in) is not critical. In fact, unless other design parameters actually control the design of this web, one could conceivably initiate some future weight reduction and cost-savings[1] for this area of the structure. For instance, the web could be pocketed, say from .100 to .080 in thick, or possibly a better choice might be a lighter weight channel section altogether.

Further, it can also be argued that if bending stresses[2] are maintained considerably below allowable compression and tension strength levels of the material, the reinforcement itself could be entirely eliminated. This would prove highly desirable, since by eliminating the reinforcement altogether, no rivets would be needed, and therefore, no fastener analysis would be required. Such cases are common where the loads from a critical loading condition have been significantly reduced from higher design levels. No matter what the reasons are, changes in criteria,

[1] The engineer should make a special effort to list for his own personal reference those potential areas of weight reduction and cost-savings of a structure worth initiating a future redesign effort on. Potential weight reduction and cost-savings in a down economy, and this is usually the case at or near industry market bottoms, could mean postponement of an engineer's eventual lay-off (or termination) long enough until more favorable economic forces begin to reshape these markets around again. Since all forces of nature, as governed by supply-and-demand economics, are presumed cyclical, an economic turnaround is most likely just around the corner. Job security begins when the engineer can effectively prepare himself for future industry market bottoms long before they actually occur.

[2] Bending stresses are verified by the method of analysis of Sec. 2.3. For their approximations, see also Sec. 2.4.

overdesign, testing or changes in basic design philosophies, or what, the engineer must have the flexibility to quickly adapt to these constantly changing design situations. At this point in our preliminary investigations of the web structure, no further elaboration is necessary; the web capacity is more than structurally adequate for the design loads given. It is also interesting to note that the exact solution, as demonstrated below, will have nearly the same shearing stresses as that computed for our approximate solution (see previous page), once again verifying the reliability and simplicity of our approximate method of analysis. Hence

$$(f_s)_{\max} = \frac{VQ}{I_{na}\,t} = \frac{(1,600)(.216)}{(.418)(.100)} = 8,268 \text{ psi} \quad \text{(exact solution)}$$

where: $V = 1,600$ lb ultimate

$I_{na} = .418 \text{ in}^4$

$t = .100$ in

$Q = \Sigma A\bar{y} = A_1\bar{y}_1 + A_2\bar{y}_2$ (see Fig. 4-25)

$= (1.00)(.080)(1.495 - .040) + (1.495 - .080)(.100)\left[\frac{1.495 - .080}{2}\right]$

$Q = .216 \text{ in}^3.$

Rivet Design of the Reinforcement Strap:

For most practical design cases, the same spacing of rivets is normally expected along the entire span of a structure. This is true even though the shear might be much less in other regions of that same structure.[1] For this problem, rivet design is achieved by first substituting the known values of V, Q, and I_{na} into the shear flow equation. Here, this gives:

$$q = \frac{VQ}{I_{na}} = \frac{1,600(.144)}{.418} = 551 \text{ lb/in ultimate}$$

where the static moment of area Q is defined as the area of the reinforcement strap (element #4) around the neutral axis of the total beam section, see Fig. 4-26. Or, just simply consider that the strap actually shears off from the total cross-sectional area. Mathematically, the following expression is formulated and the value of Q is solved for:

$$Q = \Sigma A\bar{y} = A_4\bar{y}_4 = .187\left[2.2 + \frac{.125}{2} - 1.495\right] = .144 \text{ in}^3.$$

[1] Of course, the engineer has the freedom of designing rivet spacing as he wishes. For example, a greater refinement in spacing could be achieved for the region of lower shear, say, where $V = 400$ lb (refer to the shear diagram on page 253). In most realistic problem situations encountered in the industry however, this kind of refinement in spacing is not recommended, and, in most cases, is ill-advised and should be avoided (for the ease of fabrication).

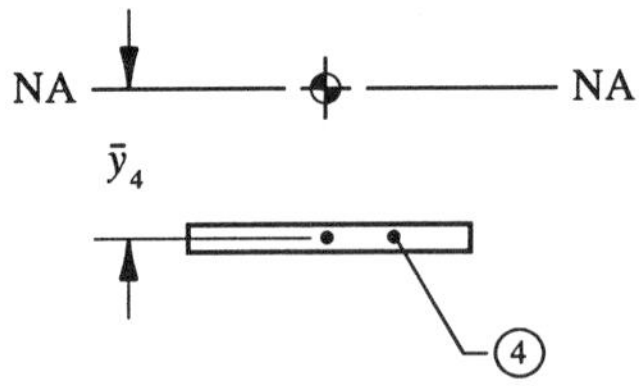

FIGURE 4-26 Static moment of area defined for the reinforcement strap. Refer back to Fig. 4-24 for pertinent dimensions.

Lastly, the required rivet spacing is computed from Eq. 4-10. Using the allowable single-shear strength of a BJ 6 rivet in .080 in thick sheet material, we obtain the required rivet spacing for the reinforcement strap:

$$p_s = qs \quad \text{(see Eq. 4-10 for term definitions).}$$

Solving for the required spacing of rivets, this equation takes the following special form.[1]

$$s_{\text{required}} = \frac{P_{su}}{qk} = \frac{862}{551(1.15)} = 1.36 \text{ in}$$

where: $P_{su} = F_{su} A_{shr} C_r = 862$ lb (from Eq. 3-1)

$F_{su} A_{shr} = 862$ lb (single-shear strength of a BJ 6 rivet, see Table 3-1)

$C_r = 1.0$ (single-shear strength correction factor for a solid, protruding-head rivet in .080 in thick sheet material, see Table 3-2)

$k = 1.15$ (fitting factor for joint or connection design).

For actual production design, use fasteners spaced 1.25 in center-to-center. This also meets the acceptable design range established for aircraft production fasteners, i.e., spacing of fasteners between $4D$ and $8D$. For our solution, therefore, if $s = 1.25$ and $D = 6/32$ (use a nominal hole diameter of .191 from Table 3-1), this gives a spacing-to-diameter ratio of 6.5 diameters or $6.5D$, which is within acceptable design limits.

The bearing resistance of the reinforcement and channel has not been specifically treated in this solution; nor may such an investigation prove or govern the ultimate design behavior of these members in bearing. Nevertheless, the engineer should for the sake of completeness of his analysis still make the appropriate

---

[1] If the engineer has some difficulty in understanding how this expression was formulated, try, instead, a trial-and-error approach to arrive at the same solution by assuming different values of s in Eq. 4-10 and then with the value of p_s zero in on a margin of safety using M.S. $= (P_{su}/p_s k) - 1$. A margin of safety of "zero" should pinpoint the same fastener spacing of 1.36 in. This solution, of course, assumes that the effects of bearing stresses are not critical.

TABLE 4-7 STATIC MOMENT OF AREA Q FOR COMMON BUILT-UP SECTIONS

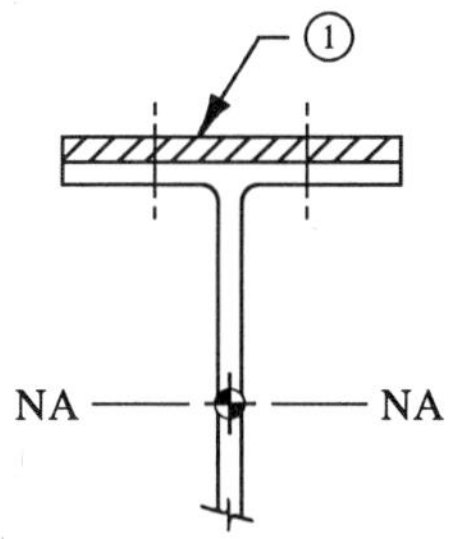

(a) $Q = Q_1$

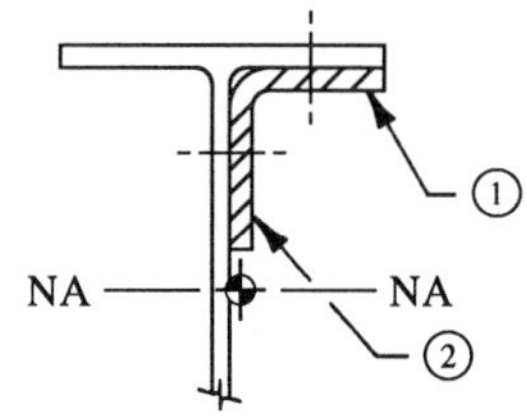

(b) $Q = Q_1 + Q_2$

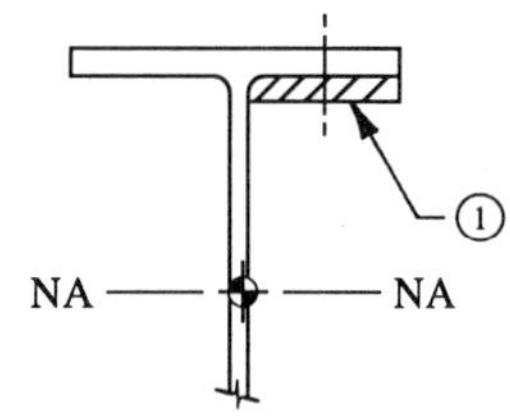

(c) $Q = Q_1$

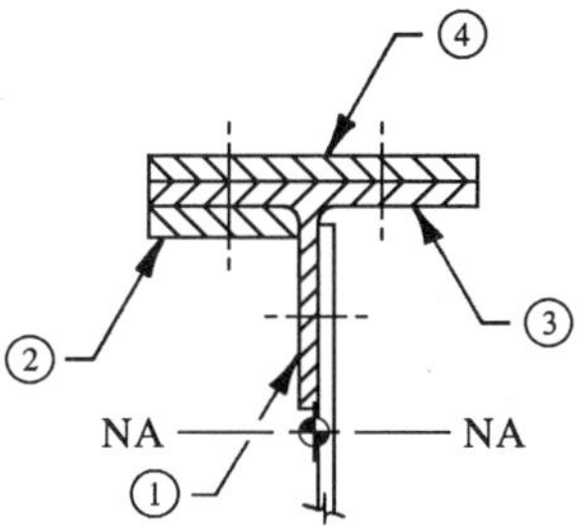

(d) $Q = Q_1 + Q_2 + Q_3 + Q_4$

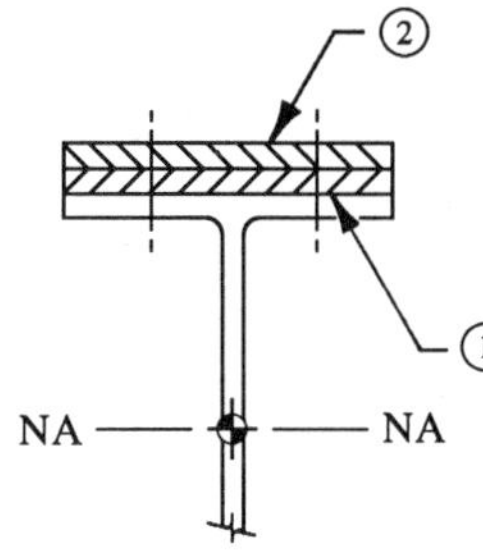

(e) $Q = Q_1 + Q_2$

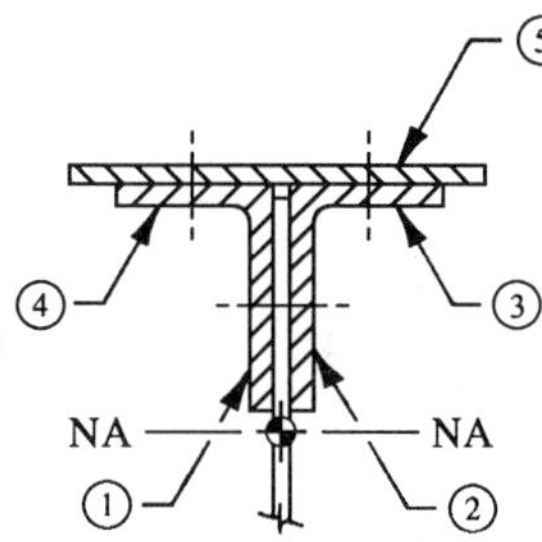

(f) $Q = Q_1 + Q_2 + Q_3 + Q_4 + Q_5$

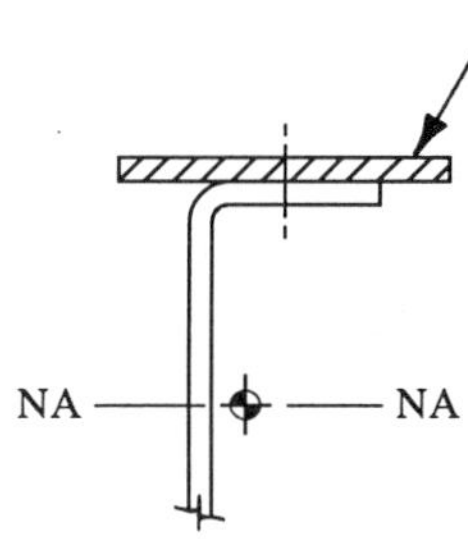

(g) $Q = Q_1$

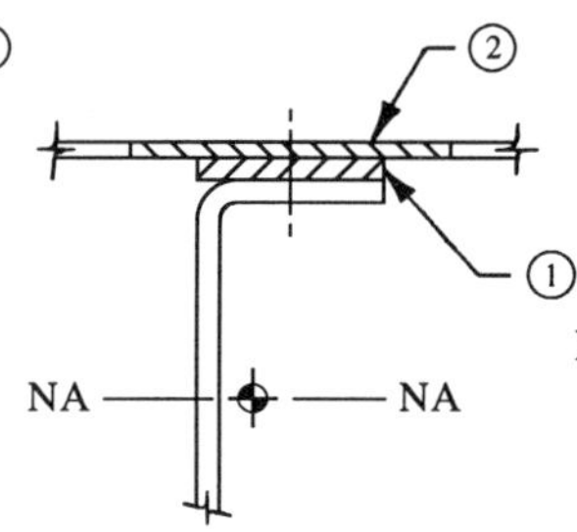

(h) $Q = Q_1 + Q_2$

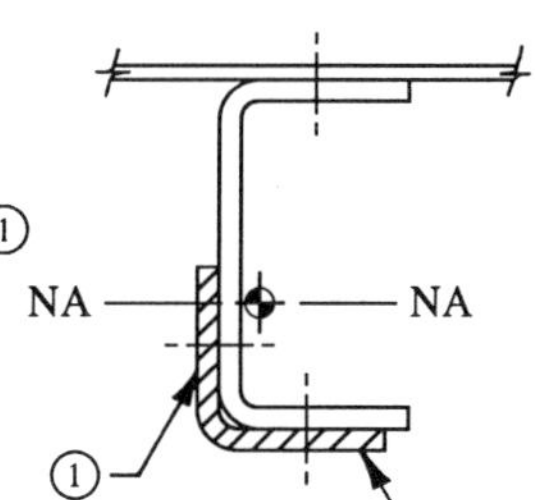

(i) $Q = Q_1 + Q_2$ ②

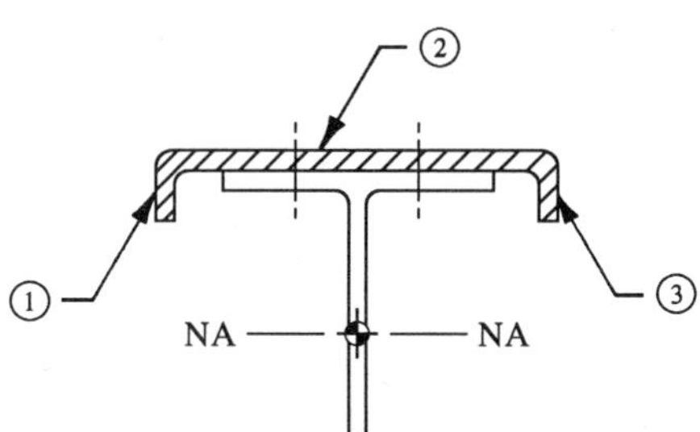

(j) $Q = Q_1 + Q_2 + Q_3$

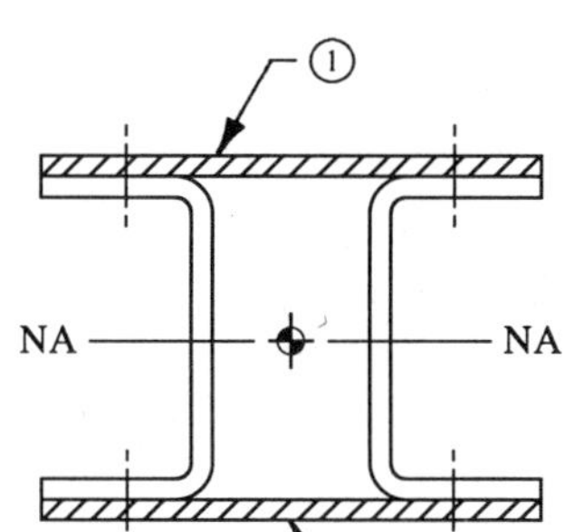

(k) $Q = Q_1$
$Q = Q_2$ ②

TABLE 4-7 STATIC MOMENT OF AREA Q FOR COMMON BUILT-UP SECTIONS (continued)

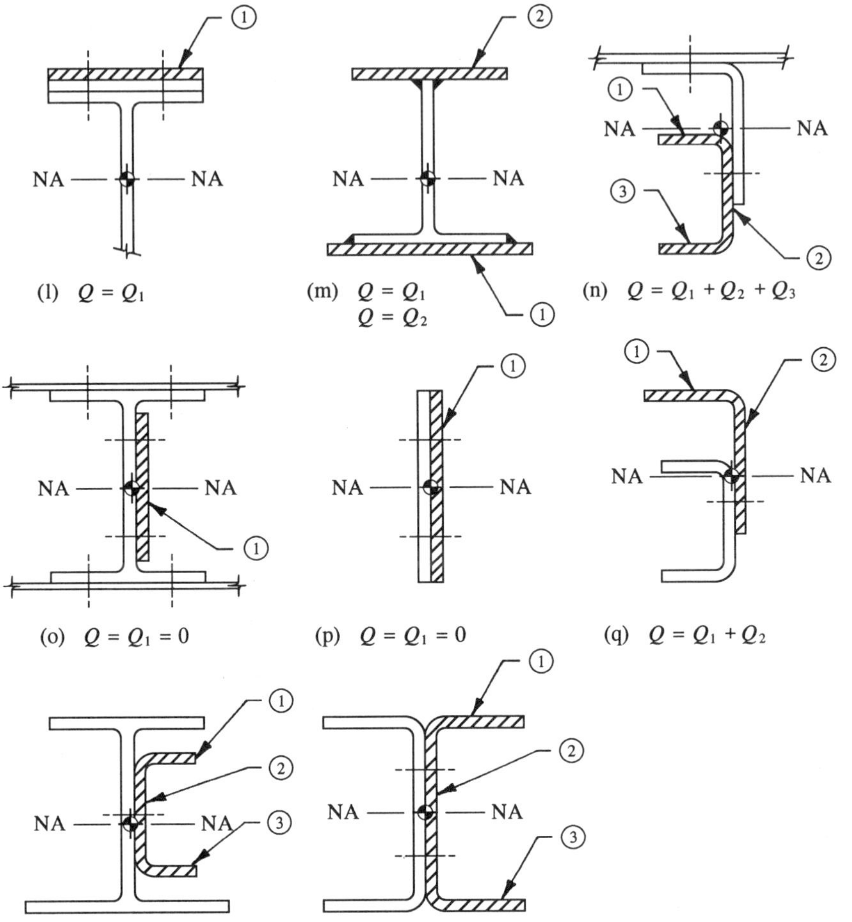

(l) $Q = Q_1$

(m) $Q = Q_1$
$Q = Q_2$

(n) $Q = Q_1 + Q_2 + Q_3$

(o) $Q = Q_1 = 0$

(p) $Q = Q_1 = 0$

(q) $Q = Q_1 + Q_2$

(r) $Q = Q_1 + Q_2 + Q_3$

(s) $Q = Q_1 + Q_2 + Q_3 = 0$

bearing evaluations of each structural member.[1]

Let us now look at a hypothetical case. Suppose Section A-A of our example problem was composed of "two reinforcement straps" instead of one, probably as a result of, let us say, high bending stresses, how would the previous computations of spacing of rivets differ? Here, the physical action of "both reinforcements" acting together will govern the basic rivet design for our hypothetical solution.[2] This

[1] Review pertinent equations fundamental to bearing strength computations in Sec. 3.2.

[2] The outer reinforcement is not usually critical by itself for the installed fasteners of multiple attached reinforcements.

means that, as a unit, the members act in concert with each other and therefore also shear together as a unit from the total cross-sectional area. Such an arrangement of members is diagrammed in Table 4-7, Case e. The proper choice of members to use when calculating Q has been predetermined in this table for different types of built-up beam sections. Consider in all cases the cross-hatched members physically shearing off from the total cross-sectional area by the fasteners holding these members to the main structure. For our hypothetical case, the rivet interconnection forces are indicated at the interface or mating surfaces of the beam flange and both reinforcements. This is also valid for any multiple system of reinforcements. The same line of reasoning follows for their solutions.

In Cases a, b, e, i, j, k, and l the design shear flow ($q = VQ/I_{na}$) divides equally between multiple rows of fasteners of equal size and strength. If, however, the rows of fasteners are of either different sizes or different types, a ratio of their allowable shear strengths P_{su} is instead used to proportionately distribute the design shear flow between their rows. Mathematically, this ratio is described as follows:

$$q_{\text{row}\,\#1} = \frac{q(P_{su})_{\text{row}\,\#1}}{(P_{su})_{\text{row}\,\#1} + (P_{su})_{\text{row}\,\#2}} \tag{4-11}$$

where: q = design shear flow (for beams, use $q = VQ/I_{na}$)
$q_{\text{row}\#1}$ = design shear flow for the fasteners in the first row
$q_{\text{row}\#2}$ = design shear flow for the fasteners in the second row (see Eq. 4-12)
$(P_{su})_{\text{row}\,\#1}$ = allowable shear strength for the fasteners in the first row
$(P_{su})_{\text{row}\#2}$ = allowable shear strength for the fasteners in the second row.

Since $q = q_{\text{row}\,\#1} + q_{\text{row}\,\#2}$, we obtain:

$$q_{\text{row}\,\#2} = q - q_{\text{row}\,\#1}. \tag{4-12}$$

In all of the other cases described in this table, the members shear along one row of fasteners. Of these cases, only in Case f are the fasteners in double-shear. Double-shear allowable values are given in Table 3-1, page 146, for some commonly used rivets. Other sources, such as MIL-HDBK-5 or company-approved fastener manuals, may also provide current available information on approved fasteners for design.

Example 4-5 A beam constructed of several attached members, each securely fastened to its composite structure to form a built-up I-beam section, is shown in Fig. 4-27. Indicate for the extruded angle members how many rows of BJ 5 rivets (F_{su} = 30,000 psi), spaced 6.3 rivet diameters between centers, should be used to structurally fasten these members to the composite structure. Use an ultimate design shear of 3,950 lb for this evaluation. For the sake of completeness of your

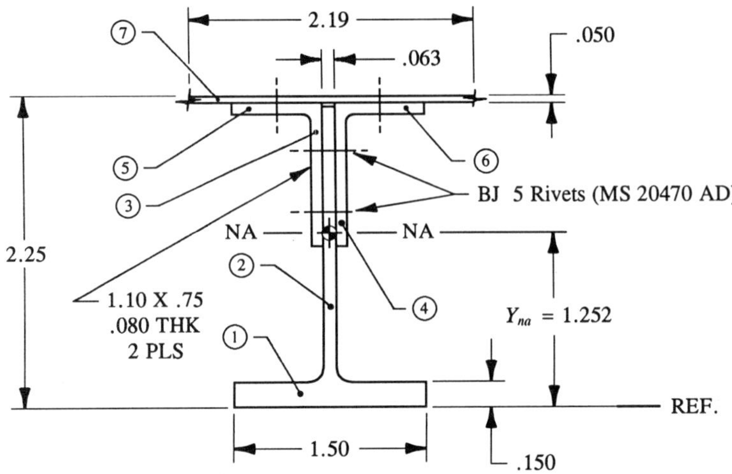

FIGURE 4-27 Built-up beam section.

analysis solution, also investigate other possible failure modes that may occur for this built-up section, such as the critical shearing stress of the web, the critical shear strength of the web rivets, and the bearing strength of the web and extruded angle members. Consider the extruded members made of 2024-T3510 aluminum alloy material. From the mechanical-property tables in MIL-HDBK-5F, we find: $F_{su} = 29,000$ psi, $F_{bru} = 108,000$ psi, and $F_{bry} = 71,000$ psi (see also Appendix E, Table A-2, page 647).

SOLUTION:

Web Design:

The first step in our solution of this problem is to compute the maximum web shearing stress of the I-beam section. Before actually attempting a complete and detailed investigation of this quantity however, let us first determine our solution by approximation. This should hopefully provide us with some relative measure of just how well (or maybe just how critical) the web structure is designed. For our beam section, shear failure of the web structure is approximated by solving the following equation below (see Table 4-3, page 241, Case d):

$$(f_s)_{\max} = \frac{V}{A_{\text{web}}} = \frac{3,950}{.124} = 31,855 \text{ psi ultimate}$$

where: $V = 3,950$ lb

$$A_{\text{web}} = (2.25 - .050 - .080 - .150)(.063) = .124 \text{ in}^2.$$

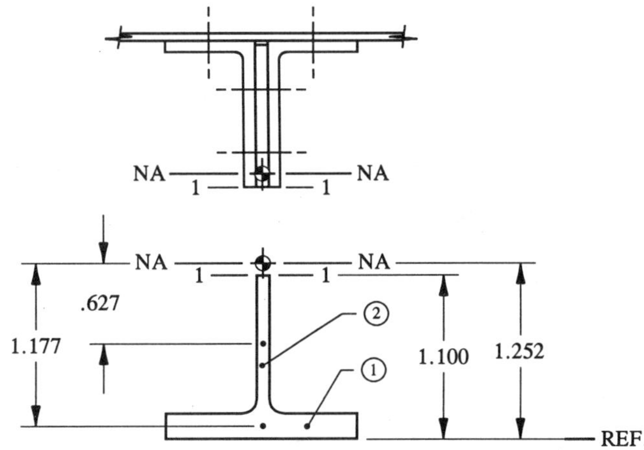

FIGURE 4-28 Lower partial area partitioned into rectangular element areas.

A high shearing stress, indeed. Although this value does exceed the allowable shearing stress of the material (compare this value with $F_{su} = 29,000$ psi), remember that our solution here is approximate and could conceivably be on the conservative side. It therefore behooves us further to reexamine our solution, but this time, using a more accurate method of analysis at our disposal. Never just start beefing up a structure based on the results of an approximation unless that structure is known with greater certainty to be understrength. For our particular case study, the approximate solution (as shown above) is close enough to the allowable shearing stress of the material to warrant such a detailed investigation. In general, a well-designed I-beam section will tend to have well-defined, beefy cap members, and therefore will normally give better approximate results for maximum shearing stresses than for those sections that are not so beefed up. Remember, our solution above is only "an approximate indication," and only that, and therefore should only be considered in that light. A greater refinement of the analysis is thus found by applying the shearing stress formula, Eq. 4-2, for $(f_s)_{\max}$.

To do this, the moment of inertia I_{na} is computed for the whole cross-sectional area of the I-beam section, as shown in Table 4-8. Note that the centroidal axis (this also corresponds to the neutral axis Y_{na} for an elastic structure) is located a distance $Y_{cg} = 1.252$ in from the reference axis, which meets the cross-section at a location through the combined thickness of the materials at this level. Because of the combined thickness of the web and extruded angles, the required maximum shearing stress usually prevalent at the neutral axis will not occur at this level. But instead, the web thickness t by itself, which is indicated just below the neutral axis of the section at a distance 1.100 in from the reference axis (or level 1-1) will produce the desired maximum value. The engineer should recall that shearing stresses at different levels of a cross-sectional area are different because the values of Q and sometimes t at these levels are different.

The static moment of area Q is chosen for the partial area below level 1-1, as fewer element areas are needed there in the computations of this section property. Alternatively, the partial area above level 1-1 could also have been chosen for this computation. But no matter which partial area is used, in either case, the value of Q would be exactly the same (the engineer is encouraged to verify this simple assertion). In Fig. 4-28, the lower partial area describing these element areas are diagrammed. And so, we obtain:

$$Q = \Sigma A\bar{y} = A_1\bar{y}_1 + A_2\bar{y}_2 = (1.5)(.150)(1.177) + (.95)(.063)(.627)$$
$$Q = .302 \text{ in}^3.$$

TABLE 4-8 MOMENT OF INERTIA OF THE I-BEAM SECTION*

Element	b	h	y	A	Ay	Ay^2	I_o
1	1.500	0.150	0.075	0.225	0.017	0.001	0.000
2	0.063	2.050	1.175	0.129	0.152	0.178	0.045
3	0.080	1.020	1.610	0.082	0.131	0.212	0.007
4	0.080	1.020	1.610	0.082	0.131	0.212	0.007
5	0.750	0.080	2.160	0.060	0.130	0.280	0.000
6	0.750	0.080	2.160	0.060	0.130	0.280	0.000
7	2.190†	0.050	2.225	0.109	0.244	0.542	0.000
			Total	0.747	0.935	1.705	0.059

* Refer to Fig. 4-27.

† This value corresponds to the effective sheet width of the .050 in aluminum sheet (2024 series) in compression. The engineer is referred to specific guidelines and equations for effective sheet area computations in Chapter 6, Sec. 6.3.

$$Y_{cg} = \frac{\Sigma Ay}{\Sigma A} = \frac{.935}{.747} = 1.252 \text{ in.}$$

Since $Y_{na} = Y_{cg}$ for elastic stress design, it follows directly that

$$I_{cg} = I_{na} = \Sigma I_o + \Sigma Ay^2 - Y_{cg}(\Sigma Ay) = .059 + 1.705 - 1.252(.935)$$
$$I_{cg} = I_{na} = .593 \text{ in}^4.$$

All values are then substituted into Eq. 4-2, which gives the true working or operating stress level.

$$(f_s)_{\max} = \frac{VQ}{I_{na}\,t} = \frac{(3,950)(.302)}{(.593)(.063)} = 31,931 \text{ psi ultimate.}$$

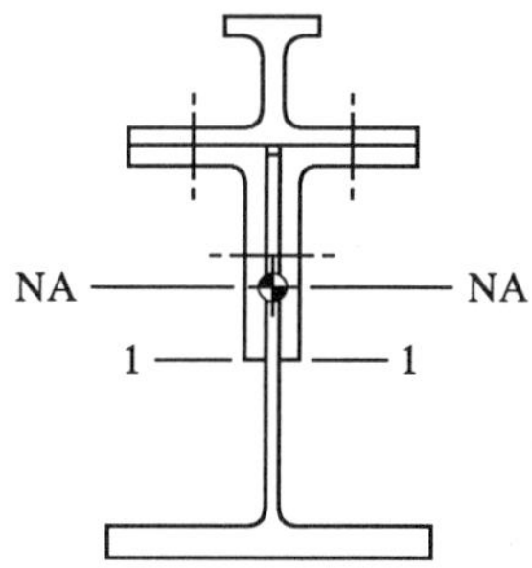

(a) Check level 1-1 (use the minimum web thickness).

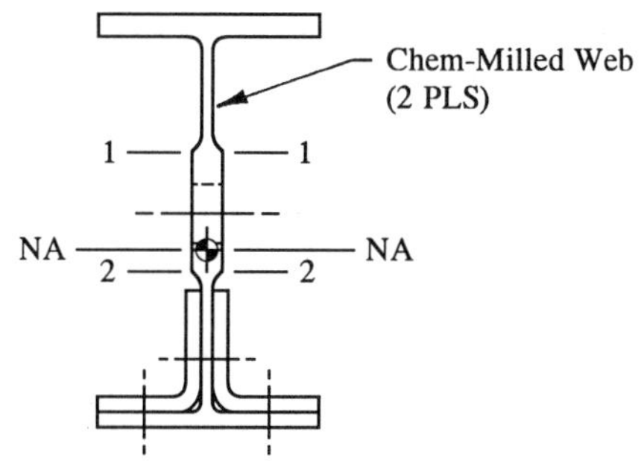

(b) Check levels 1-1 and 2-2 (use the minimum web thickness).

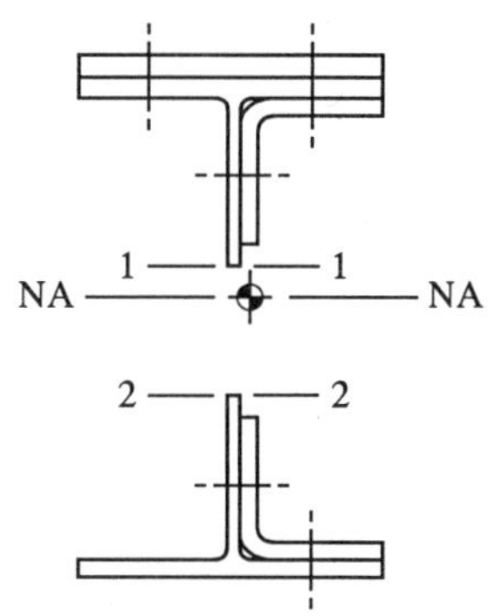

(c) Check levels 1-1 and 2-2.

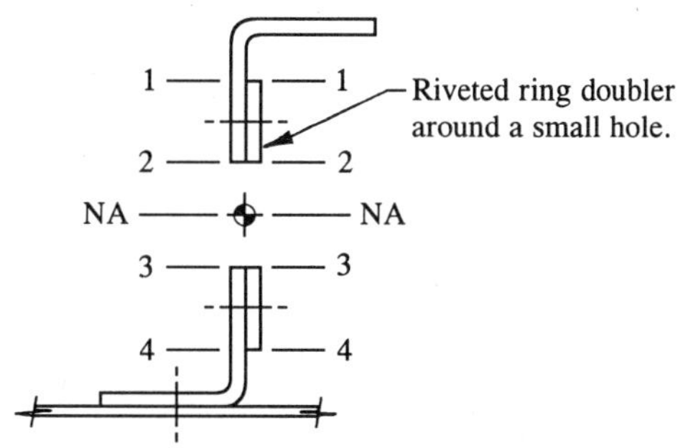

(d) Check levels 1-1, 2-2, 3-3, and 4-4.

FIGURE 4-29 Locations of possible maximum shearing stress not necessarily occurring at the neutral axis.

Failure at ultimate is then predicted by:

$$\text{Margin of Safety} = \text{M.S.} = \frac{F_{su}}{(f_s)_{\max}} - 1 = \frac{29,000}{31,931} - 1 = -.09.$$

And so it seems, at least as far as this prediction is concerned, our web structure is understrength as we had first calculated from our preceding results of approximate shearing stresses. Other cross-sectional areas where maximum shearing stresses may not necessarily occur at the neutral axis are depicted in Fig. 4-29.

Rivet Design:

The rest of our solution follows by finding the shear flow along the web rivet line(s) and then making the appropriate failure analysis predictions based on the joint capacity of the structure: (1) shearing of the web rivets and (2) bearing of the web structure and attached extruded angles. From the procedure outlined in this

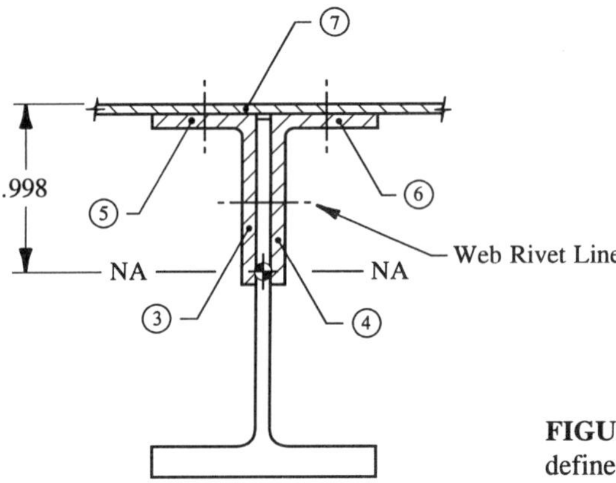

FIGURE 4-30 Static moment of area defined for the beam section (areas shown cross-hatched).

section, the rivet analysis begins by solving the shear flow equation, Eq. 4-3 or $q = VQ/I_{na}$. Here, the values of V and I_{na} are known from our previous computations of shearing stress. So, it then remains to determine Q. If the partial area shown cross-hatched in Fig. 4-30 is used for this purpose, the following expression for Q is formulated:

$$Q = \Sigma A\bar{y} = A_3\bar{y}_3 + A_4\bar{y}_4 + A_5\bar{y}_5 + A_6\bar{y}_6 + A_7\bar{y}_7.$$

The engineer should not be overly concerned with the location of the neutral axis, just consider that the extruded angles and skin (element areas #3 thru #7) acting together (in composite) theoretically shear from the remaining structure. See T-section in Fig. 4-30. Then make the appropriate computations as specified by the equation above for Q. This equation is conveniently set up in columns (see format used in Table 4-9). From definition, the distance $\bar{y}$ is measured from the centroid of each element area to the centroid of the total cross-sectional area.

TABLE 4-9 STATIC MOMENT OF AREA Q

Element	A	$\bar{y}$	$A\bar{y}$
3	0.082	0.358	0.029
4	0.082	0.358	0.029
5	0.060	0.908	0.054
6	0.060	0.908	0.054
7	0.109	0.973	0.106
		$Q = \Sigma A\bar{y} =$	0.272

Therefore,

$$q = \frac{VQ}{I_{na}} = \frac{3,950(.272)}{.593} = 1,812 \text{ lb/in ultimate.}$$

A very high shear flow, indeed, to consider for a structure having just one row of BJ 5 rivets. Through many years of engineering experience and practical study one can develop the foresight and intuitive skills to predict the various impacts certain loads (or loading conditions) may have on a structure. Using these skills here for our particular design case: an additional row of BJ 5 rivets is recommended along the web rivet line. Then, the computed shear flow (from above) will divide equally between the two rows of web rivets, i.e., $q = 1,812/2 = 906$ lb/in per row. The interconnection shearing forces of these rivets along the horizontal web plane are then computed from Eq. 4-10,

$$p_s = qs = 906(1.002) = 908 \text{ lb}$$

where: s = rivet spacing at $6.3D$ or $6.3(.159) = 1.002$ in
D = rivet nominal hole diameter = .159 in.

Ultimate Shear Strength of the Web Rivets:

Since both rows of 5/32 in diameter web rivets are in double-shear, the rivets are evaluated for their allowable double-shear strengths. This is done using Eq. 3-1 as follows:

$$P_{su} = F_{su} A_{shr} C_r = 30,000(.0397)(.872) = 1,039 \text{ lb}$$

where: $A_{shr} = 2A = 2\left[\frac{\pi}{4}D^2\right] = 2\left[\frac{\pi}{4}(.159)^2\right] = .0397 \text{ in}^2$
D = .159 in (nominal hole diameter for a 5/32 in diameter rivet, refer to Table 3-1)
C_r = .872 (double-shear strength correction factor for a 5/32 in diameter protruding-head rivet in .063 in gage material, see Table 3-2)
$F_{su} = 30,000$ psi.

Ultimate shear failure is then predicted by:

$$\text{Margin of Safety} = \text{M.S.} = \frac{P_{su}}{p_s k} - 1 = \frac{1,039}{908(1.15)} - 1 = +.00$$

where: $P_{su} = 1,039$ lb (from above)
p_s = 908 lb (interconnection shearing force)
k = 1.15 (fitting factor for joint or connection design).

Ultimate Bearing Strength of the Extruded Angles:

For the extruded angles, we have $1.5F_{bry} < F_{bru}$ (see values given below). Therefore, to meet both the ultimate and limit (permanent set) bearing strength criteria for these members, the following equation is employed (see Eq. 3-3):

$$P_{bru} = 1.5F_{bry}\,tD = 1.5(71,000)(.080)(.159) = 1,355 \text{ lb}$$

where: F_{bru} = 108,000 psi (QQ-A-200/3, $e/D = 2.0$)
F_{bry} = 71,000 psi (QQ-A-200/3, $e/D = 2.0$)
t = .080 in
D = .159 in (see Table 3-1).

Bearing failure is then predicted by:

$$\text{Margin of Safety} = \text{M.S.} = \frac{P_{bru}}{p_s k} - 1 = \frac{1,355}{454(1.15)} - 1 = +1.60$$

where: P_{bru} = 1,355 lb (from above)
p_s = 908/2 = 454 lb (interconnection shearing force; like a double-shear lap joint, the total shear load divides equally between the extruded angles)
k = 1.15 (fitting factor for joint or connection design).

Bearing Strength of the Web:

Here, the full shear load p_s = 908 lb is carried by the web. Clearly, a more critical loading condition by far. A simple check of bearing allowables for the material also indicates that $1.5F_{bry} < F_{bru}$. Hence

$$P_{bru} = 1.5F_{bry}\,tD = 1.5(71,000)(.063)(.159) = 1,067 \text{ lb}$$

where: F_{bru} = 108,000 psi (QQ-A-200/3, $e/D = 2.0$)
F_{bry} = 71,000 psi (QQ-A-200/3, $e/D = 2.0$)
t = .063 in
D = .159 in (nominal hole diameter for a 5/32 in diameter rivet, refer to Table 3-1).

Bearing failure is then predicted by:

$$\text{Margin of Safety} = \text{M.S.} = \frac{P_{bru}}{p_s k} - 1 = \frac{1,067}{908(1.15)} - 1 = +.02$$

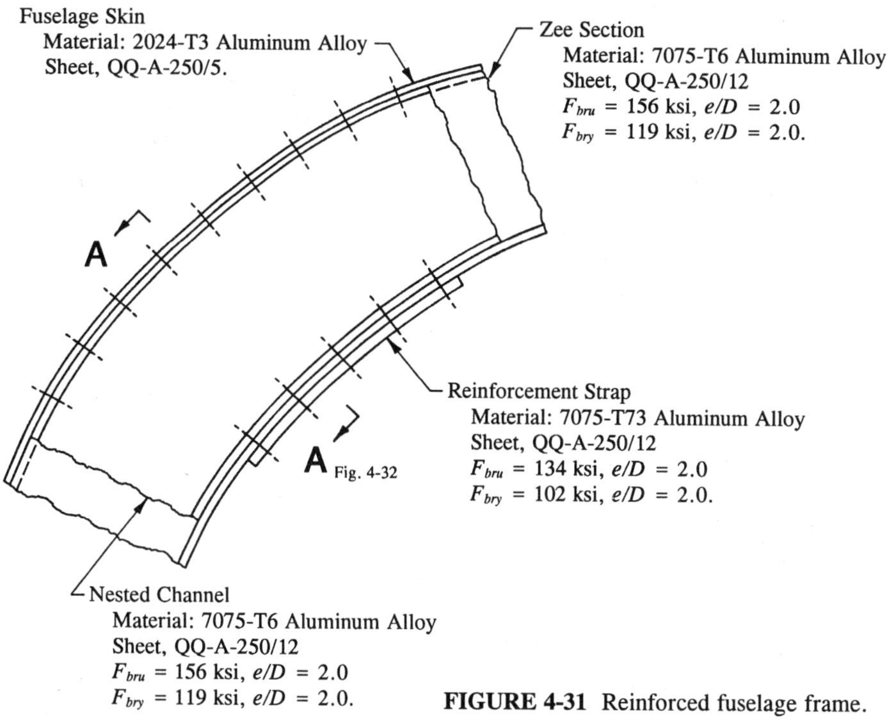

FIGURE 4-31 Reinforced fuselage frame.

where: $P_{bru} = 1,067$ lb (from the previous page)
$p_s = 908$ lb (interconnection shearing force)
$k = 1.15$ (fitting factor for joint or connection design).

Example 4-6 Using the principles and techniques outlined in earlier parts of this section, determine the proper spacing of BJ 5 (MS 20470 AD) rivets for the reinforcement strap shown in Fig. 4-31. The strap was added to the fuselage frame to increase the overall bending stiffness of the frame in this region of the structure. Assume that computations have already substantiated this structure (including the strap) for design bending stresses across the basic frame section to acceptable strength levels. (See Sec. 2.5 for the elastic design of combined axial and bending members, $f = \pm P/A \pm Mc/I_{na}$.) A computer maximum search routine of all flight and landing conditions in this region of the fuselage has determined a maximum internal shearing force of 3,160 lb ultimate acting in the plane of the frame web. Shearing stresses are not critical (verify this claim by approximation; use $(f_s)_{\max} = V/A_{\text{web}}$ as a simple check).

SOLUTION: To solve this problem for rivet spacing requires the solution of the shear flow equation ($q = VQ/I_{na}$). First, the unknowns I_{na} and Q are found. Then, commensurate with our study of this section, once their values have been determined, the actual shear flow occurring in the horizontal plane of the reinforcement strap along the span of beam may be computed. The moment of inertia is determined from the cross-sectional area shown in Fig. 4-32. Here, the total cross-sectional area, including the reinforcement strap, is used and broken down into simpler rectangular elements. All computations are done in tabular form (see Table 4-10). The static moment of area Q is computed for the reinforcement strap. This member theoretically shears along the lower frame cap rivet line and therefore (the rivets) must develop the shear flow at this level to effectively overcome part of the internal bending resistance capable of being developed by the total section area. Thus, any reduction in moment of inertia I_{na} of the total cross-sectional area is precluded. Such is the nature of efficient designs. Hence

$$Q = Q_1 \quad \text{(for the strap only; see also Case g, Table 4-7)}$$

$$Q = A_1\bar{y}_1 = .150\left[1.561 - \frac{.125}{2}\right] = .225 \text{ in}^3.$$

Substituting this and all known values (Q and I_{na}) into Eq. 4-3, the horizontal shear flow q along the strap rivet line is determined.

$$q = \frac{VQ}{I_{na}} = \frac{3,160(.225)}{1.407} = 505 \text{ lb/in}$$

where: $V = 3,160$ lb ultimate
$Q = .225 \text{ in}^3$ (from above)
$I_{na} = 1.407 \text{ in}^4$ (from Table 4-10).

TABLE 4-10 MOMENT OF INERTIA OF SECTION A-A

Element	b	h	y	A	Ay	Ay^2	I_o
1	1.200	0.125	0.062	0.150	0.009	0.001	0.000
2	1.200	0.050	0.150	0.060	0.009	0.001	0.000
3	1.150	0.050	0.200	0.057	0.011	0.002	0.000
4	0.050	3.100	1.775	0.155	0.275	0.488	0.124
5	0.050	3.150	1.750	0.157	0.276	0.482	0.130
6	1.150	0.050	3.350	0.057	0.193	0.645	0.000
7	1.200	0.050	3.350	0.060	0.201	0.673	0.000
8	1.920*	0.032	3.391	0.061	0.208	0.706	0.000
			Total	0.757	1.182	2.998	0.254

* This value is determined from the equation, $W_e = 30t$, which approximates the effective width of skin of aluminum alloy materials (series 2024). For a more accurate formula to compute this value, the engineer is referred to Chapter 6, Eq. 6-10, for the solution of effective sheet areas of built-up compression members.

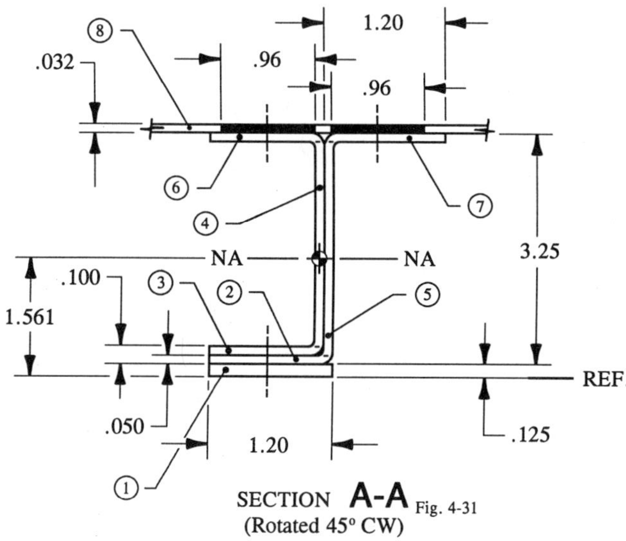

FIGURE 4-32 Fuselage frame cross-sectional area.

$$Y_{cg} = \frac{\Sigma Ay}{\Sigma A} = \frac{1.182}{.757} = 1.561 \text{ in}$$

$$I_{cg} = \Sigma I_o + \Sigma Ay^2 - Y_{cg}(\Sigma Ay)$$
$$I_{cg} = .254 + 2.998 - 1.561(1.182) = 1.407 \text{ in}^4.$$

For elastic beam design,

$$Y_{na} = Y_{cg},$$

and therefore

$$I_{na} = I_{cg} = 1.407 \text{ in}^4.$$

Next, the interconnection shearing forces for the reinforcement rivets are computed from Eq. 4-10 by trial and error. For instance, if we assume a 1.0 in spacing for our first trial solution, this gives:

$$p_s = qs = 505(1.0) = 505 \text{ lb}.$$

Shearing Strength of the Reinforcement Rivets:

$$P_{su} = F_{su} A_{shr} C_r = 596(1.0) = 596 \text{ lb}$$

where: $F_{su} A_{shr}$ = 596 lb (single-shear allowable for a 5/32 in diameter solid, protruding-head rivet, see Table 3-1)

C_r = 1.0 (single-shear strength correction factor for a 5/32 in diameter solid, protruding-head rivet in .100 in thick sheet material, i.e., the combined thickness of the .050 in channel and the .050 in zee is used for the sheet thickness of the thinnest gage material in a single-shear lap joint).

Shearing failure is predicted by:

$$\text{Margin of Safety} = \text{M.S.} = \frac{P_{su}}{p_s k} - 1 = \frac{596}{505(1.15)} - 1 = +.03.$$

Bearing Strength of the Reinforcement Strap:

$$P_{bru} = F_{bru}\, t D = 134,000(.125)(.159) = 2,663 \text{ lb}$$

where: F_{bru} = 134,000 psi, e/D = 2.0

F_{bry} = 102,000 psi, e/D = 2.0

t = .125 in (thickness of the reinforcement strap)

D = .159 in (nominal hole diameter for a 5/32 in diameter rivet from Table 3-1).

Bearing failure is predicted by:

$$\text{Margin of Safety} = \text{M.S.} = \frac{P_{bru}}{p_s k} - 1 = \frac{2,663}{505(1.15)} - 1 = +3.59.$$

Bearing Strength of the Lower Fuselage Frame Flanges:

$$P_{bru} = F_{bru}\, t D = 156,000(.100)(.159) = 2,480 \text{ lb}$$

where: F_{bru} = 156,000 psi, e/D = 2.0

F_{bry} = 119,000 psi, e/D = 2.0

t = .100 in (combined thickness of the lower flanges)

D = .159 in (nominal hole diameter for a 5/32 in diameter rivet from Table 3-1).

Bearing failure is predicted by:

$$\text{Margin of Safety} = \text{M.S.} = \frac{P_{bru}}{p_s k} - 1 = \frac{2,480}{505(1.15)} - 1 = +3.27.$$

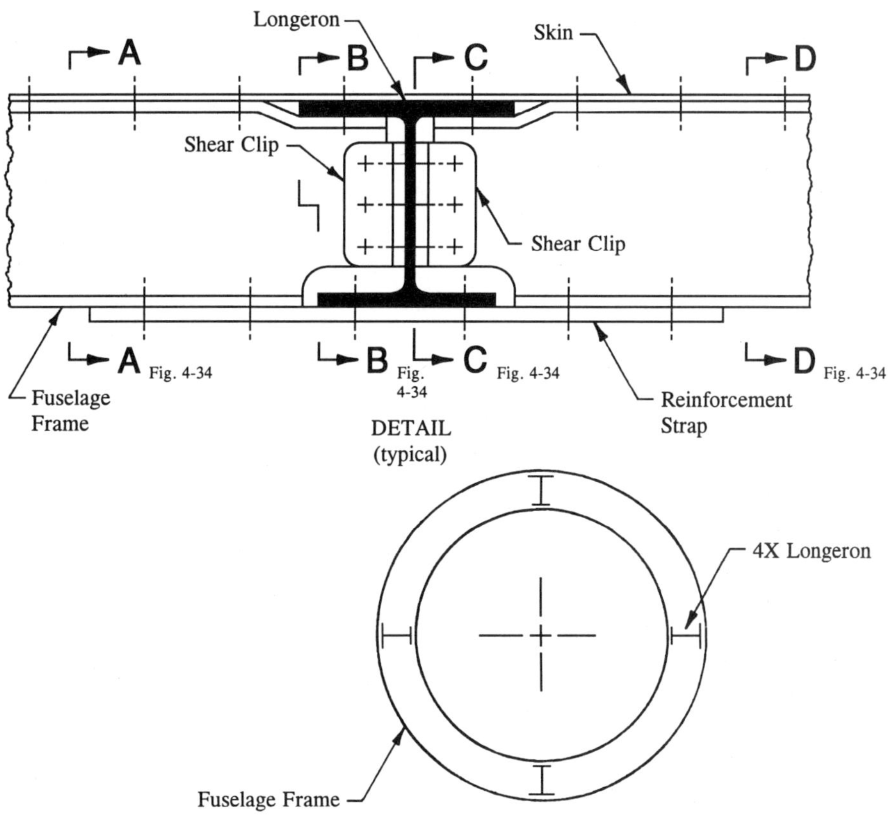

FIGURE 4-33 Fuselage frame and longeron intersection.

From our predicted failures above, the reinforcement rivets are clearly shear critical, inasmuch as a slightly positive shear margin of safety (M.S. = + .03) was arrived at for the 5/32 in diameter rivets. This means that the shearing failure of the rivets, as opposed to the bearing failure of the reinforcement strap and lower frame flange members, will govern the design of the reinforcement. Hence, no other trial solutions are deemed necessary. This then completes the solution to our example problem: to install BJ 5 rivets spaced 1.0 in center-to-center along the reinforcement strap. Generally speaking, this also meets the recommended design criterion of the aerospace industry as far as acceptable fastener designs go (i.e., rivets should be spaced between $4D$ and $8D$ center-to-center).[1]

Example 4-7 The fuselage frame in Fig. 4-33 consists of four main longeron members. Each longeron is allowed to pass through the cutouts in the frame as

[1] For our example, $s = 1.0$ and $D = 5/32$ (using a nominal hole diameter of .159 from Table 3-1), thus, this gives a spacing-to-diameter ratio of 6.3 diameters or $6.3D$.

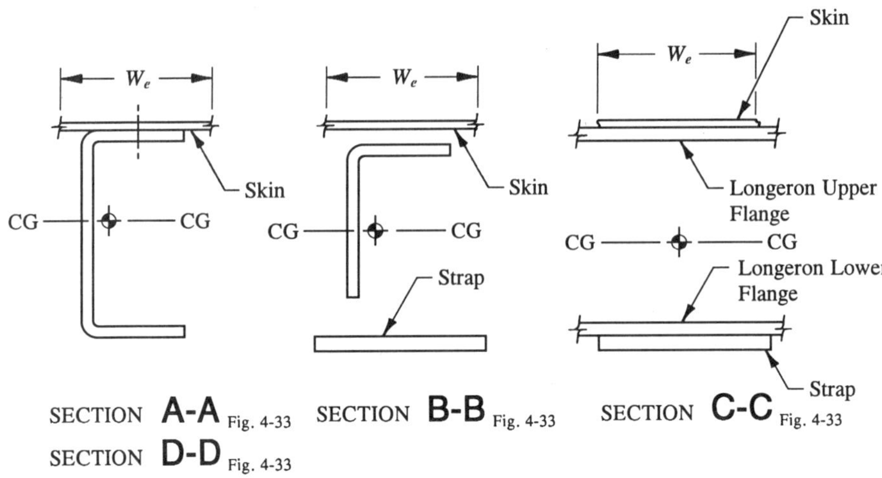

FIGURE 4-34 Beam sections for the fuselage frame of Example 4-7. The effective sheet width W_e is determined from Eq. 6-10, Sec. 6.3.

continuous members as shown. For this arrangement of members, describe the possible stress failures that may occur. Do not perform actual numerical computations however, just state the appropriate equations to use for substantiation.

SOLUTION: Problems similar to this commonly occur in actual fuselage frame design. Their solutions are based on a complete and careful study and evaluation of the behavior of a frame under ultimate loading conditions: specifically, the ultimate stresses produced by a system of internal loads *V*, *P*, and *M* acting at different sections along the structure. These stresses are then compared to the strength allowables of the material that are used to design the basic frame structure. Consider the internal loads physically applied at the centroidal axis of the frame sections investigated. This is consistent with internal loads analysis (computer-generated output) normally given from a computer model solution of actual fuselage frame structure. This is also compatible with the notion that operating or working stress levels of a fuselage frame are low enough to be considered elastic. If they are not, the stresses which they produce are inelastic and the structure is designed according to those principles of "inelastic or plastic stress design."

If, however, the inelastic stress design of a member should be ignored by the analyst, the consequences should not be that burdensome—the analysis is considered merely conservative. In all cases, elastic stresses (like those computed from the flexure formula $f_b = \pm Mc/I_{na}$) are nearly exact to slightly higher than those that would ordinarily be found by inelastic stress methods. Elastic design of a structure means that operating stresses are below the proportional limit of the material. For such cases, the centroidal axis is coincidental with the neutral axis of the cross-sectional area. If the above arguments have not been clearly understood, a brief review illustrating these points should again be reviewed in Chap. 2, Sec. 2.3.

To begin our investigation of the fuselage frame, let us determine the maximum shearing stresses occurring at Sections A-A, B-B, and D-D. These sections are viewed in Fig. 4-34. The computations are straightforward using Eq. 4-2, $(f_s)_{\max} = VQ/I_{na}t$. For a similar and related problem solution, the engineer should follow the detailed solution of Example 4-3 for its application.

Now let us look at a slightly different situation not yet considered up to this point in our investigation of joint shear failure. Consider the transfer of shear V across the joint at Section C-C. Physically, no web exists there. Therefore, how is the internal shear actually transferred across the joint of the fuselage frame? Answer: The fuselage frame web will transfer the shear across the joint (in the area of Section C-C) through the back-to-back shear clips provided at the longeron. The design and analysis of shear clips are covered in Chapter 5. Until then, let us assume that the shear clips designed here are of sufficient strength to provide a continuous load path to accomplish the transfer of shear load across the cutout region.

The reinforcement strap is held together along the inner frame flange by six rivets. However, only the two end rivets of the reinforcement strap on each side of the longeron are actually considered in the transfer of loads across the joint. See Chapter 2, Sec. 2.6, for the analysis method used to distribute the internal loads P and M across a joint to individual members of a built-up beam section. This was the analysis method of that chapter. In this chapter, the same results can be obtained, but instead, by shear flow calculations. Here, consider that the reinforcement strap theoretically shears from the fuselage frame structure at Section A-A or D-D (these section areas are chosen for the analysis because they are considered the most representative sections carrying internal loads along the basic frame structure). The largest shear flow, calculated from these sections, governs the rivet design (size and spacing requirements). Equation 4-3, $q = VQ/I_{na}$, is used to determine the shear flow q, while Eq. 4-10, $p_s = qs$, is used for the actual determination of rivet spacing (use Table 4-7, Case g, to establish the value of Q for the reinforcement strap member). The strap theoretically shears from the total cross-sectional area along the inner frame cap rivets. Margins of safety are then formulated for (1) shearing failure of the rivets, (2) bearing failure of the reinforcement strap, and (3) bearing failure of the inner frame flange.

If the longeron cutouts are typical at the four locations indicated in Fig. 4-33, the maximum internal loads V, P, and M at any one critical location will suffice for the substantiation of structure at the other three locations. However, if the basic structure or loading combinations are different at these locations, the engineer must perform duplicate analyses at each longeron. Hopefully, even in these cases, some intuitive reasoning can be made to eliminate those less critical (or trivial) combinations. If this cannot be done, the engineer must instead perform the analysis four separate times—with each of the corresponding force systems (V, P, and M) applied at the longeron locations.

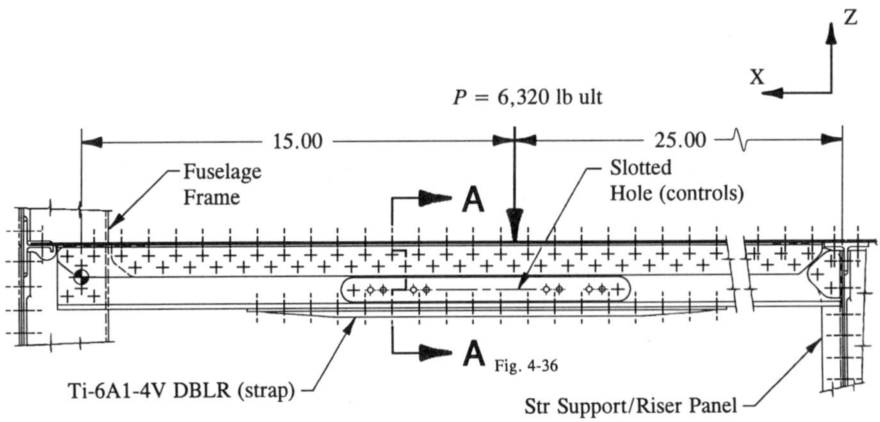

FIGURE 4-35 Cargo bay floor beam modification.

This then concludes the various stress checks made for this structure as they would pertain to the subject matter of this chapter. Other possible checks required should of course be done in accordance with those predicted failures established in other sections of this book. For instance: (1) the stringer outer flange rivets in shear and bearing (see stringer cutout in Sec. 2.6), (2) the shear clips and fasteners, and (3) the basic strength of the frame structure along various sections described along the frame, i.e., specifically, combined axial and bending stresses occurring across the frame structure at Sections A-A, B-B, C-C, and D-D (see Eq. 2-9, $f = \pm P/A \pm Mc/I_{na}$, in Sec. 2.5). Additionally, compression members must be evaluated for inter-rivet buckling, Sec. 6.2; effective sheet areas of built-up sections, Sec. 6.3; and crippling of built-up sections, Sec. 6.4.

4.5 Problem for Solution. A portion of web was removed from a floor beam, Fig. 4-35, to allow clearance for control routing. A titanium strap along the cutout region was proposed to increase the loss of bending stiffness due to the reduced cross-sectional area of the beam. Complete the following: (a) Assuming adequate bending stiffness for the modified section proposed (see Fig. 4-36), what is the required shear flow for the attached titanium strap? (b) Is the calculated shear flow, answer to question (a), a true or fictitious value? (*Hint:* verify by equating VQ/I_{na} to $\Delta P/L$.) (c) Formulate a general expression to determine the required fastener spacing for the strap installation (consider a fitting factor k to meet FAA requirements for commercial aircraft). Material: titanium strap, $E = 16.4 \times 10^6$ psi; aluminum I-beam, $E = 10.5 \times 10^6$ psi.

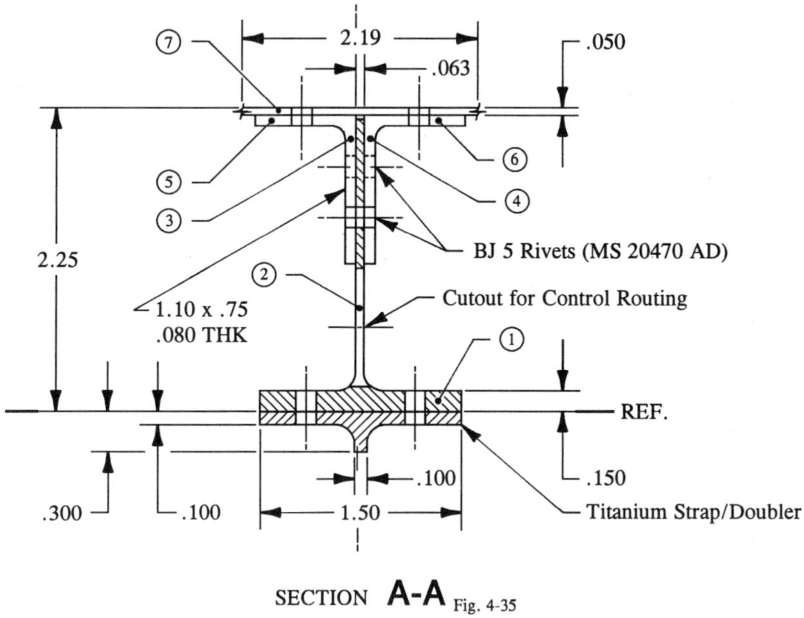

FIGURE 4-36 Cargo bay floor beam MOD sectional area detail.

CHAPTER

5

Shear and Tension Clip Supports

5.1 Introduction. Shear and tension clip supports will be the main emphasis of study of this chapter.[1] They are principally used as "support structure" for the purpose of joining together one structural member to another. The shear clip is the most utilized type of the two joining such members together. This particular support is identified by its ability to transfer (or react) shear from an externally applied system of forces on a structure. The shear clip resists shear only, while the tension clip, as its name also implies, principally transfers axial tension loads. Physically, however, their construction is the same. In Secs. 5.2 and 5.3, three main supports are considered for our discussion: (1) single angle clips, (2) back-to-back angle clips, and (3) tee clips. Their applications as support structures are illustrated in Figs. 5-1(a), (b), and (c), respectively.

Sometimes overlooked because of their simplicity, shear and tension clip supports can become critical design areas which can sometimes result in or be the cause of inadequate or faulty main structural designs. Many engineering structural failures can be eliminated if sufficient strength to the support structure of a beam is

[1] Compression clips do sometimes occur in certain aircraft design applications. For the time being, however, let us say that for the same magnitude of loading and construction, a compression clip is considerably less critical than a tension clip, and therefore is automatically substantiated. This will become more obvious to the engineer after a complete study of tension clip supports has been presented in Sec. 5.3.

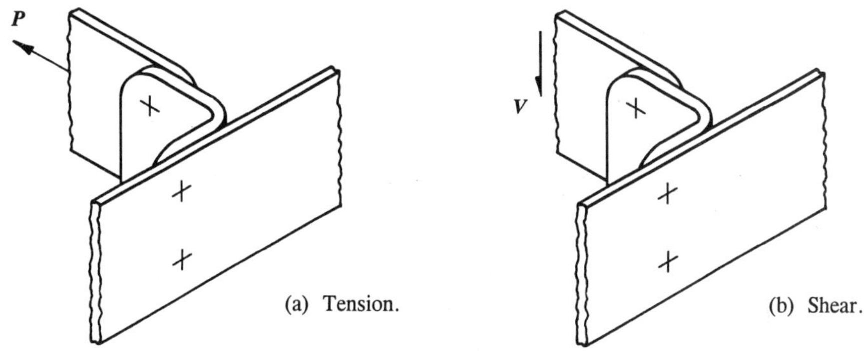

FIGURE 5-1(a) Single angle clips: (a) in tension and (b) in shear.

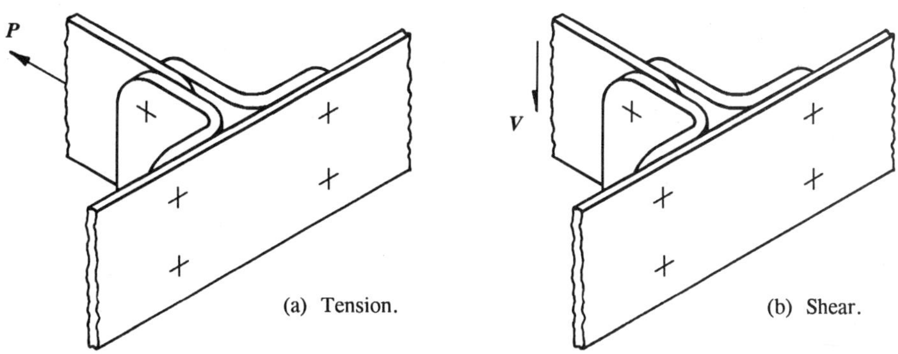

FIGURE 5-1(b) Back-to-back angle clips: (a) in tension and (b) in shear.

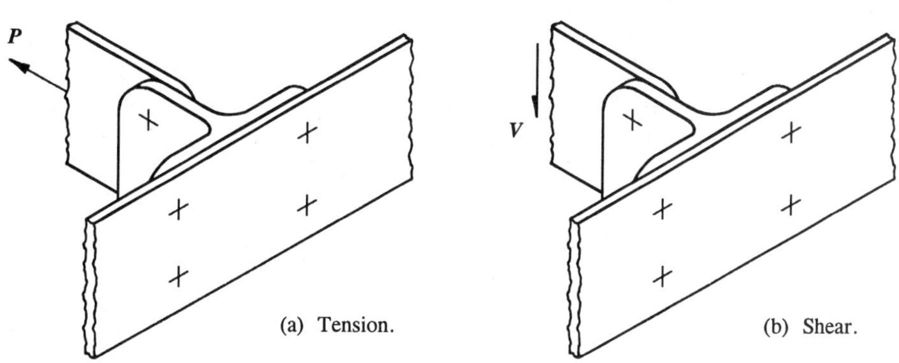

FIGURE 5-1(c) Tee clips: (a) in tension and (b) in shear.

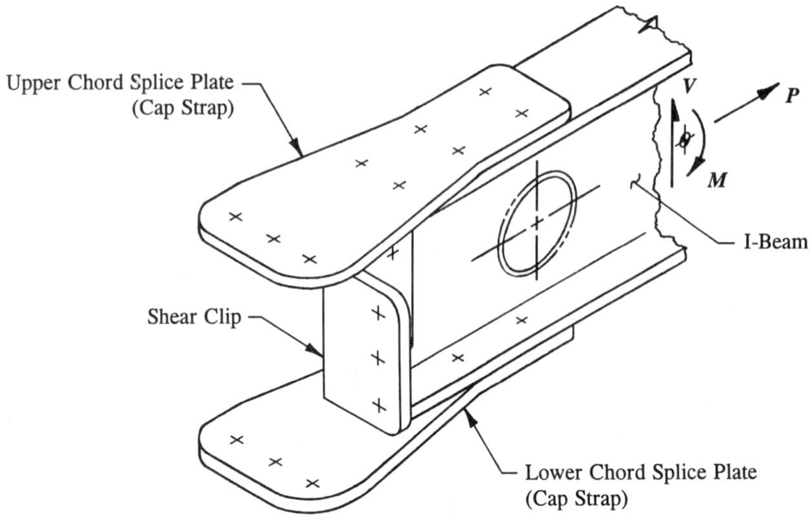

FIGURE 5-2 Fixed-support structure using upper and lower chord splice plates.

provided. In some applications, they (shear and tension clips) may be conveniently used as mounting brackets to support electrical wiring harnesses, electrical and mechanical equipment hardware, gauges, indicators, instruments, etc.

The purpose of this chapter is to relate the externally applied forces of a main member (longeron, gear beam, etc.) to the forces which are transmitted to the support structure of that beam. These forces may be classified into two distinct support groups. The first group provides the shear restraint of the main structure in the vertical direction or "shear clips," while the second group provides the axial tension restraint of the main structure in the horizontal direction or "tension clips." These are the main forces to which shear and tension clip supports will be considered subjected to in this chapter.[1]

A shear clip is designed to rotate under load an amount without inducing or causing failure. Therefore, a shear clip connection must be made flexible (in other words, "simply-supported"), otherwise, the connection (or simply-supported end) will build up an end moment causing the joint to become overstressed. If, however, a stiffer support structure is desired, upper and lower chord splice plates can be added. This alternative arrangement of members is commonly referred to as a "fixed support." Its structural arrangement is viewed in Fig. 5-2. For this new support configuration, the shear clip will still provide a continuous load path for the basic web structure to carry (or transfer) its full vertical internal shear loading, while the splice plates carry the bending and axial (tension or compression) loads

[1] In addition, a shear clip can also prevent the main structure from physically sliding or moving horizontally under relatively light loading, unlike its diagrammatical representation would have you believe (see idealized representation of a support shear clip in Sec. 1.2, Fig. 1-3, commonly referred to as a roller support).

across the joint.

In general, although a fixed-supported beam is a redundant structure, its overall design is still more efficient than a simply-supported (determinate) structure. The reason for this is explained in the following way: the internal shears and bending moments that are normally generated in a fixed beam structure are better distributed along the entire span of that beam. A better distribution of loading along the entire beam structure (including the support members) is why the overall weight of a fixed beam structure is usually less, and therefore more desirable for actual production model consideration. Unlike the fixed beam, a simply-supported beam will peak or concentrate its internal bending moments at or near its applied loading points. For this reason, and because most beams are designed by the peak bending moments that are developed along their spans, a simply-supported structure is not as efficient. This of course assumes that the properties of both beams are homogeneous (of a constant construction) throughout their entire lengths. To verify the above arguments, the engineer is encouraged to compare the different beam loading solutions provided in Appendix D. For example, given the same magnitude of loading, compare the internal loads (shear and bending moments) of a fixed beam structure with the internal loads of a simply-supported beam structure. What are your findings? Are they in agreement with those facts previously mentioned?

If no alternative means can be provided than to carry support loads in tension from one member to another, then only in these special situations should tension clips be actually contemplated for design use. In most cases, the experienced design engineer will purposely install a support member by orienting its position in a structure in shear applications only. Tension clips are to be avoided, if possible. If they can be avoided, the support and the main structure to which they are joined together can generally avoid a high weight penalty. Although a tension clip is far less efficient structurally than a shear clip, their practical applications are nevertheless very important since they are often utilized in actual production designs.

If there is any reason to doubt the restraining action (or capability) of a support structure, the analysis of that support should be performed on a logical and conservative basis. One way to do this is to assume overlapping design assumptions for the actual support structure in question. For example, one could design the main structure twice assuming two different support structures: (1) a simply-supported structure and (2) a fixed-supported structure. However, if such a proposal seems too drastic a measure or weight penalty to pay, an alternative procedure might be to assume just an average or maybe some partial degree of restraint for the unknown support structure. For additional review of beams with partial restraining support structures, the engineer is referred to Sec. 1.9, "Partial Degree of Restraint of Support Types." For the most part, though, these concerns are often exaggerated, even misguided, since most aircraft structures are structurally tested under simulated flight and landing conditions anyway. Essentially, by monitoring the structural behavior of these questionable areas of a support structure under actual test loading conditions, the engineer can always corroborate his original design assumptions of the actual support structure. The information derived from these structural tests can also be used to design other unknown support types.

The study of this chapter will also consider the concepts related to prying action and its effects at the interface of various structural members, and those limitations that must also be imposed on their solutions will also be elaborated upon. Our study will conclude by analyzing bolts, screws, and rivets for combined (or interaction) shear and tension effects. To help the engineer design shear and tension clip supports with more confidence and self-assurance of their reliability and strength, the following recommended design parameters (rules-of-thumb) have been formulated:

(1) No form of welding is to be used for tension clip designs.

(2) Provide sufficient edge distance for metallic structures: $e/D = 2D + .030$ (or 1/32 for tolerance) to allow the next larger size fastener to be installed, if necessary. Composites are treated more conservatively based on inserted attachment configuration of joint attachments, i.e., $e/D = 3D$.

(3) Design shear and tension clips made of extruded sections with nominal fillet radii and formed sections with minimum bend radii.

(4) Reduce or eliminate all eccentricities by installing fasteners as close as possible to the bend radii of formed sheet metal angles and to the fillets of extruded angles.

(5) Do not mix bolts and rivets in the same fastener pattern.

(6) Avoid discontinuities or joggles to prevent cracking where possible.

In general, a conservative approach to the stress analysis of shear and tension clips should be followed. The FAA requires a fitting factor of 1.15 to comply with shear and tension clip support designs, their fasteners, and bearing upon the joined members when no structural test data has been proved.

The importance of shear and tension clips to an aircraft structure cannot be overemphasized. The engineer should not underestimate their simple design details. Frequently a structural failure may start by so-called "unimportant" details of a structure. Before proceeding ahead any further with the material of this chapter, the engineer is encouraged to review those principles outlined in Sec. 1.2 of Chapter 1, "Conventional Support Types," where in that section we primarily concerned ourselves with specific types of restraints that were supplied by different support structures.

5.2 Design and Analysis of Shear Clip Supports. Localized regions of a primary structure, such as shear clip supports, require the same detailing and investigation (sizing) as do the main members of that same structure. Shear clips are often treated as secondary members and too often are not given the proper importance and close scrutiny that they merit. As a consequence, their weakening effect can cause the structural failure in other critical areas of the primary structure, even though the shear clip itself may not have actually failed. More about this in later

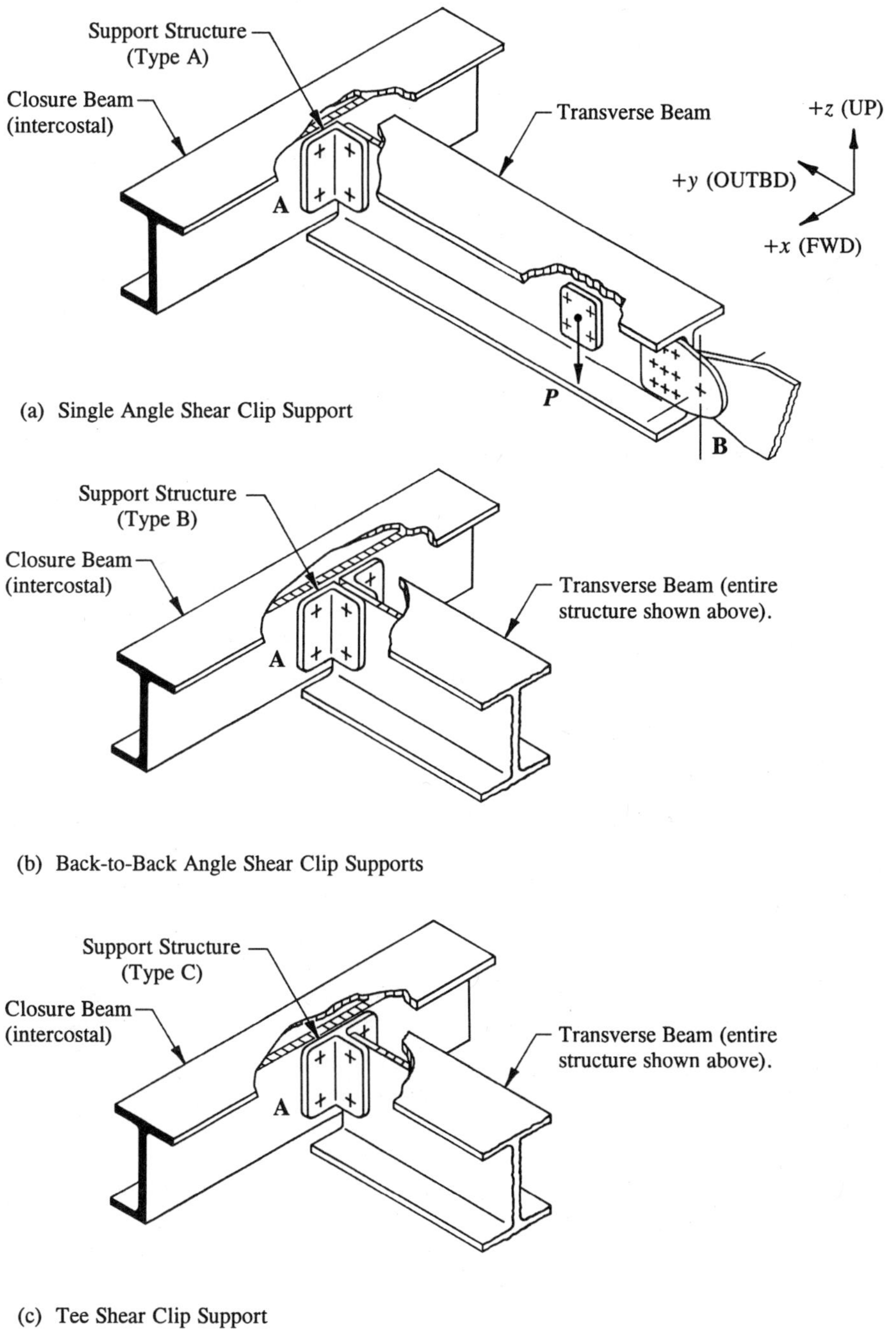

FIGURE 5-3 Various types of shear clip supports: (a) the single angle shear clip, (b) back-to-back angle shear clips, and (c) the tee clip.

parts of this section.

Shear clips are designed in various shapes and sizes. Among these, three main support types, Fig. 5-3, are investigated in this section: (1) a single angle clip, (2) back-to-back angle clips, and (3) a tee clip. From the structural arrangement of members depicted in Fig. 5-3(a), it can be seen that the vertical shear load that is carried by the transverse beam is transferred through the support structure to the closure beam. Of these structural supports, the tee clip is by far the most efficient. This will become apparent when our investigation reveals the structural performance and behavior of these particular supports under load. Their solutions are systematically arrived at by balancing their structures one plane at a time.

A shear clip is a support structure primarily used to transfer (or react) a shear load from one structural member to another; no axial, bending, or twisting is considered for such a support member. Supports of this kind are used in many structural applications of major aircraft designs and usually require the same special consideration by the engineer for their successful design. It can be said that a well-designed structure is no better than its support structure. Overdesign of the main structure is useless and unnecessary if the support structure to which the main structure is attached is inadequately designed for static strength, fatigue, etc. Therefore, to avoid premature failure of these members (shear clips), it would serve the engineer well to pay particular attention to their simple design details. Sometimes overlooked because of their simplicity, shear clips are frequently considered only secondary components of a main structure. Even so, they can still dramatically influence the structural behavior and performance of the overall structure. They can cause unnecessary structural deficiencies of the main structure if their designs are not adequately treated. In the final analysis, however, the capacity of a shear clip is governed either by bearing failure of its joined members[1] or by shearing failure of its fasteners. Both failure modes must be anticipated and predicted if the reliability and strength of the shear clip is to be assured.

A shear clip provides the ability to restrain the end of a beam from physically moving in the plane of the attached web (vertically, that is, as shown in Fig. 5-3). Any axial or bending across the support region itself is more effectively resisted by other structural support types or considerations. For instance, upper and lower splice plates could be used, as was shown in Fig. 5-2. Although shear clips may appear to provide some degree of resistance or restraint axially, or by rotating or twisting, none is normally considered by the engineer. Essentially, very little actual resistance can be offered, if any, and so none is presumed for such a support member. The question here may involve complex theoretical considerations and unknowns which, because they are truly subjective and cannot be quantitatively verified, are not capable of analysis. Since we cannot attain "perfect results," we need to consider our value judgments (basic assumptions) only to the extent that they may affect our final design solutions. However, our conservatism does not need to cause a severe weight penalty of the structure as a whole if we can operate on a well-tested and well-proved method in which we have good reason to have

[1] This includes the adjacent structure to which the shear clip is also attached.

confidence as to the final results.

Although our comments above seem to indicate a rather crude deviation from theoretical considerations, their solutions of shear clip supports are nevertheless very reliable and predictable. The reason is that many years of engineering experience, mostly through physical testing and general observation of a structure, have gone into corroborating our basic design assumptions. No better proof of the true strength and structural integrity of a member can be obtained than through its physical testing: no matter what results have been shown before by rigorous or sophisticated theoretical methods of stress analysis.

To summarize our findings up to this point, we can reasonably predict the structural behavior of a shear clip as follows: that, the primary load-carrying ability of this structural member in the vertical shear plane[1] direction of its attached legs significantly exceeds the loading capabilities of other forms of resistance that might be possible for such a support member. Therefore, none is usually considered in these other directions. Of course, if the shear clip is forced to bend, rotate, or to be pulled in other than its intended direction, then it must also be designed according to the procedures and strength requirements established for the design of these additional loads (be that axial, bending, or torsion).

When designing shear clip supports, it is important to understand how they work, and how they react to their intended applied shear loads. A better understanding of how externally applied loads of a structure are transferred through support shear clips from one structural member to another will be fully described in detail in the remaining paragraphs of this section. The following supports will be considered (refer again to Fig. 5-3): (1) a single angle shear clip (Type A), (2) back-to-back angle clips (Type B), and (3) a tee clip (Type C).

Let us begin our investigation of these supports by first considering the single angle shear clip support (Type A). After its detailed solution has been determined and all appropriate margins of safety are written for its anticipated structural failures, other structural considerations of its design will be discussed. From statics, a vertical shear reaction R_1 is denoted at the supported end (see Fig. 5-4). Thus, if the shear clip and the attached web can accomplish the transfer of shear load without structural failure, the magnitude of the reaction R_1, as would normally be determined from a statics solution of beam reactions at this support, would be correctly predicted. Otherwise, something more or less than a simply-supported condition for the support structure, as originally perceived by the analyst in his preliminary evaluation (or assumption) of the support structure, would occur. This condition would cause some redistribution of support loads to other critical areas of the structure. The over-loading effects of these areas (which would also include the support at B) could ultimately cause some premature failure of the structure, although the shear clip (or joined members at support A) was the real cause of failure in the first place, but did not fail.

[1] Although a shear clip may be installed vertically, inclined, or horizontally in actual structure, for the purposes of analysis and discussion, the shear clips described in this section will be physically and purposely oriented vertically.

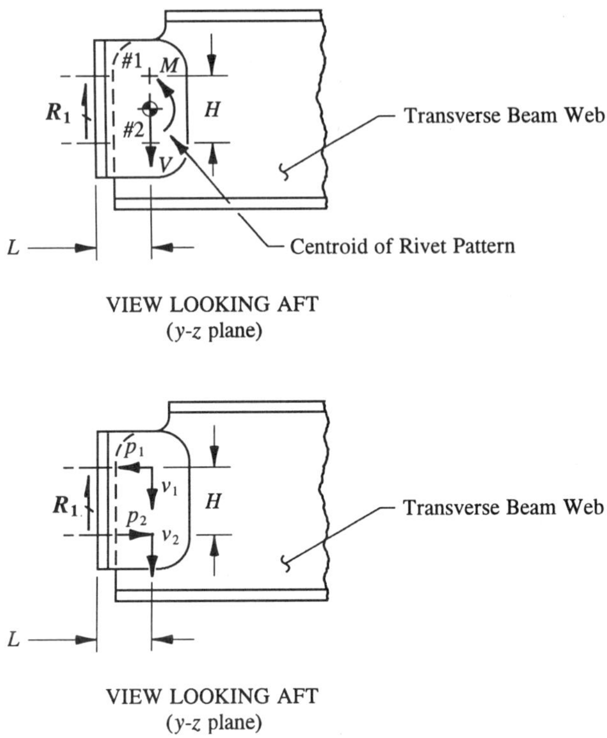

FIGURE 5-4 Equilibrium forces to balance the shear clip in the *y-z* plane.

Let us now determine the equilibrium forces to balance the shear clip in the *y-z* plane (this is shown in Fig. 5-4). The shear reaction R_1 is distributed to the two fasteners in the *y-z* plane according to the basic concepts of joint analysis used in Chapter 3 to distribute eccentric loads to connection designs.[1] First, the reaction R_1 is balanced at the centroid of the rivet pattern (this is done by inspection or by the procedure of Sec. 3.4, where the equations of statics are employed to balance the shear clip in static equilibrium). Then, the equilibrium forces V and M obtained at the centroid from this transfer of load are further distributed to the individual fasteners as equivalent shearing forces. Their values are determined from rapid techniques of connection analysis used to distribute equilibrium forces to connection rivets. The shear V and bending moment M divide equally between equal size and strength fasteners.[2]

---

[1] See "Couple-Force Relationship of Moments" in Appendix B. For shear clip supports having more than two fasteners in one plane, use Eqs. 3-22, 3-23, and 3-24 in Chapter 3.

[2] Distribution of shearing forces to fasteners of unequal size and strength was explained in Chapter 3, Sec. 3.4.

Hence

$$v_1 = v_2 = \frac{V}{2}$$

and

$$p_1 = p_2 = \frac{M}{H} \quad \text{(from Eq. A-7, Appendix B)}$$

where: $V = R_1$
$M = R_1 L$
H = distance measured between fastener centers
L = distance measured from the rivet line to the shear plane of the attached leg.

The final solution is obtained by combining shearing forces into a single force system or resultant at each fastener location. From the Pythagorean theorem, the general expression used to determine resultant forces, the following equations are written:

Resultant shearing force for fastener #1:

$$P_1 = (v_1^{\,2} + p_1^{\,2})^{1/2}.$$

Resultant shearing force for fastener #2:

$$P_2 = (v_2^{\,2} + p_2^{\,2})^{1/2}.$$

The final step in our solution is to predict the shearing and bearing failures of the shear clip and joined members (use Eqs. 3-1, 3-2, and 3-3 in Sec. 3.2 for this determination). These equations are summarized below:

Shearing failure:

$$\text{Margin of Safety} = \text{M.S.} = \frac{P_{su}}{p_s k} - 1$$

where: P_{su} = ultimate shear allowable of the fastener[1]
p_s = resultant shearing force of the fastener
k = 1.15 (fitting factor used in joint and connection designs).

---

[1] Compute allowable values from Eq. 3-1 for solid, protruding-head rivets. Otherwise, for all other type rivets, including bolts, screws, etc., use only published values.

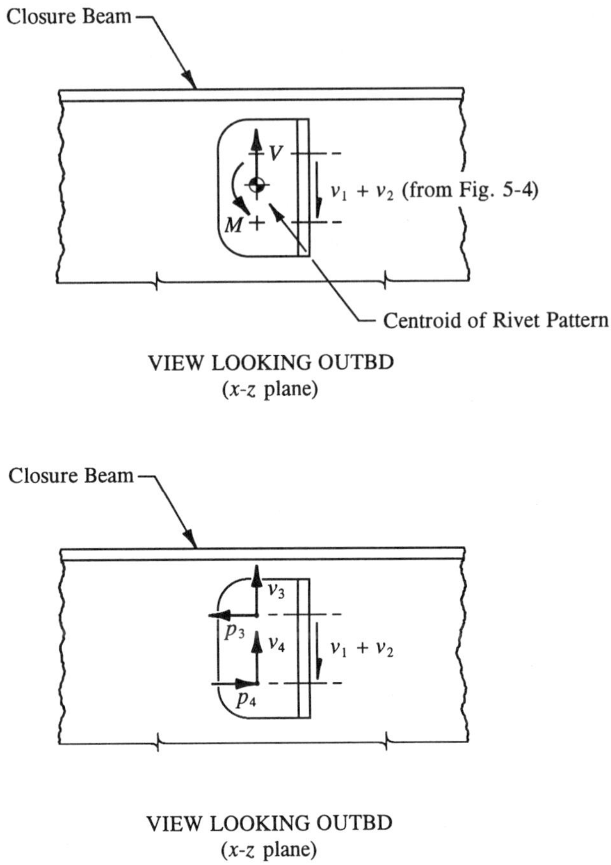

FIGURE 5-5 Equilibrium forces to balance the shear clip in the x-z plane.

Bearing failure:

$$\text{Margin of Safety} = \text{M.S.} = \frac{P_{bru}}{p_s k} - 1$$

where: P_{bru} = ultimate bearing allowable of the material (use either Eq. 3-2 or 3-3 for this computation)

p_s = resultant shearing force of the fastener

k = 1.15 (fitting factor used in joint and connection designs).

The fundamental factor on which this analysis was based on was formed by correctly idealizing the support structure of the beam; essentially, that is, the restraint capability that the support member (a shear clip) can offer to its main structure. If the underlying assumptions of a beam support have somehow been erroneously assumed or arrived at, its final design solution, which also includes all adjacent structures to which the supports are attached, will also be erroneously figured. The reason why this is so is that the equations of static equilibrium are based on a correct evaluation of the support capability of a beam. For a shear clip, a simply-supported restraint member, this resistance is measured by its ability to resist shear only.

Now, let us rotate the shear clip in Fig. 5-4 in the *x*-*z* plane, as shown in Fig. 5-5. If we do this, a similar arrangement of loads for the shear clip is indicated. Our solution in this plane begins by distributing the reaction shear $v_1 + v_2$ (which equals R_1 in Fig. 5-4) from the *y*-*z* plane to the centroid of the rivet pattern. The final resultant force system of fastener shearing forces is obtained as we did before in our previous solution for fastener shearing forces in the *y*-*z* plane. The shear V and bending moment M (expressed as a couple-force) again divide equally between equal size and strength fasteners. The results are summarized below:

$$v_3 = v_4 = \frac{V}{2}$$

$$p_3 = p_4 = \frac{M}{H}$$

where: $V = R_1$
$M = R_1 L$
H = distance between fastener centers
L = distance measured from the rivet line to the shear plane of the attached leg.

Resultant shearing force for fastener #3:

$$P_3 = (v_3^2 + p_3^2)^{1/2}.$$

Resultant shearing force for fastener #4:

$$P_4 = (v_4^2 + p_4^2)^{1/2}.$$

Predicted shearing and bearing failures then follow by using the appropriate equations described earlier in this section.

Before concluding our discussions here, let us look at the transverse beam web and the closure beam web to which the shear clip support is also attached. In Fig. 5-6, an exploded view of the support area is constructed to help us view the internal system of shearing forces occurring in equilibrium. The shearing forces are indicated in directions in agreement with established convention for their adoption.

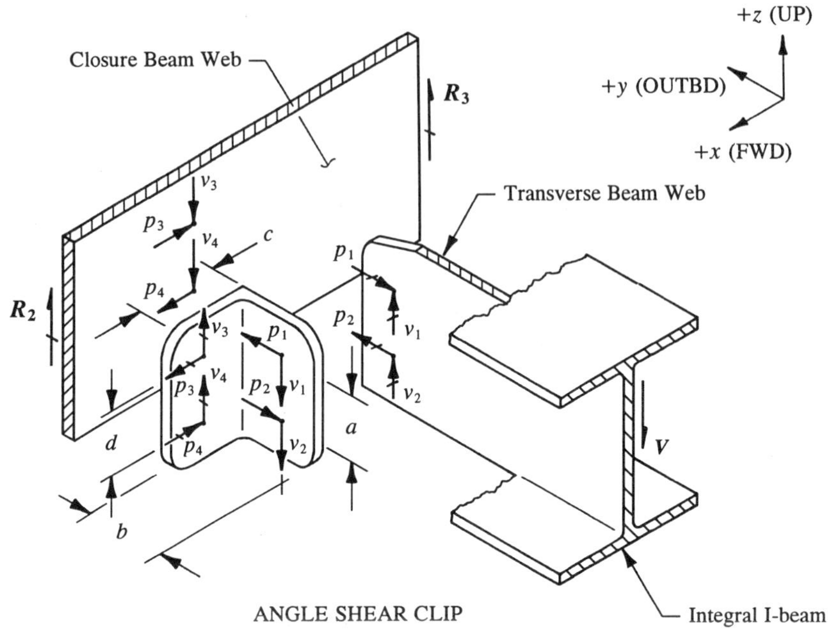

FIGURE 5-6 Transfer of load through an angle shear clip (Type A).

And thus, from their description on the isolated shear clip, the following equations are formulated:

(1) $v_1 = v_2 = v_3 = v_4 = V/2$

(2) $p_1 = p_2 = Vb/a$ (based on the couple-force relationship of moments M/H in Appendix B)

(3) $p_3 = p_4 = Vc/d$ (also based on the couple-force relationship of moments M/H in Appendix B).

Note that the web structure of each attached member will carry an equal and opposite shearing force from those values indicated for the shear clip. For this reason, these members must also be investigated for predicted bearing failure (see ahead to Example 5-1, page 303).

Shearing stresses and bending stresses occurring in the legs of the shear clip are usually neglected by the engineer if the shear clip has been previously substantiated by analysis for those particular structural failures associated with connection designs.[1] Or, we could also say that the internal stresses due to the

[1] Basically, this says that Mc/I_{na} and $VQ/I_{na}t$ are not applicable to beams of low span-to-depth ratios. Shear clip supports fall into this low range category of beam design (see Fig. 5-7). The analysis

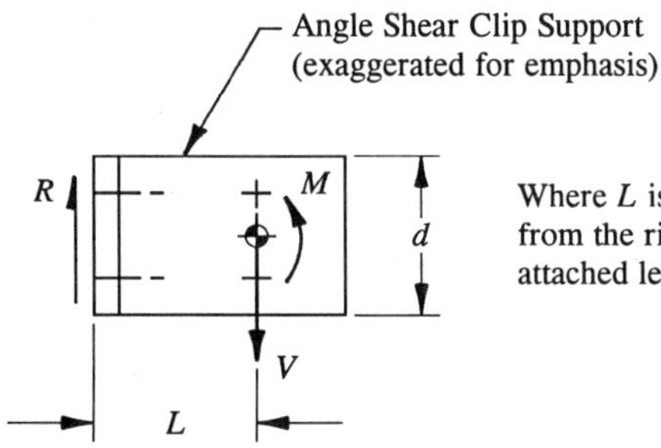

Where L is the distance (or span) measured from the rivet line to the shear plane of the attached leg and d is the beam depth.

FIGURE 5-7 Beam of low span-to-depth ratio.

shears and bending moments occurring in the legs (or rectangular sections) of the shear clip are essentially enveloped by other design criteria: namely, shearing failure of the fasteners and bearing failure of the joined members. In addition, each rivet used in a structural design is limited by a minimum sheet thickness requirement. For example, the minimum design thickness of a shear clip leg permissible if a 3/16 in diameter rivet is used is .036 in (see Table 3-2, "Shear Strength Correction Factors for Solid, Protruding-Head Rivets"). This limitation (minimum design sheet thickness for rivets) and the effect of eccentricity on shearing and bearing failures, in effect, control the basic design of the shear clip. That is, a shear clip, if used for shear applications only, is primarily designed by either shearing failure of its fasteners or bearing failure of its joined members, not by shearing and bending of its attached legs.

To summarize: the main design function of a shear clip is purposely limited to carrying and transferring loads in the shear plane of its attached legs; horizontally, however, it can only prevent the overall structure from physically moving or sliding in that direction under light loading. No appreciable build-up of end moment should occur for this support member if this limitation is directly imposed on its design. A shear clip support is therefore principally designed for its main intended purpose: that of transferring shear from one structural member to another; and, therefore, if this can be accomplished, the support structure can be used in actual production designs. So long as the engineer has provided the necessary load paths for a simply-supported structure, as given from a statics solution of reactions for the support structure, the main structure, attached structure, and support structure itself should provide a reliable and predictable indicator of their structural design solutions. Thereby avoiding a redistribution of loads to other critical regions of the structure in cases of nonconformal supports.

In general, a shear clip support is unnecessarily beefed up (overdesigned) if that support member is used for the express purpose of transferring axial tension

---

of beams (i.e., shear clip supports) having low span-to-depth ratios is beyond the scope of this book. Engineers that are interested are referred to *Formulas for Stress and Strain* by Raymond J. Roark, McGraw-Hill Book Company, 1965, Fourth Edition, Article 35, "Beams of Relatively Great Depth."

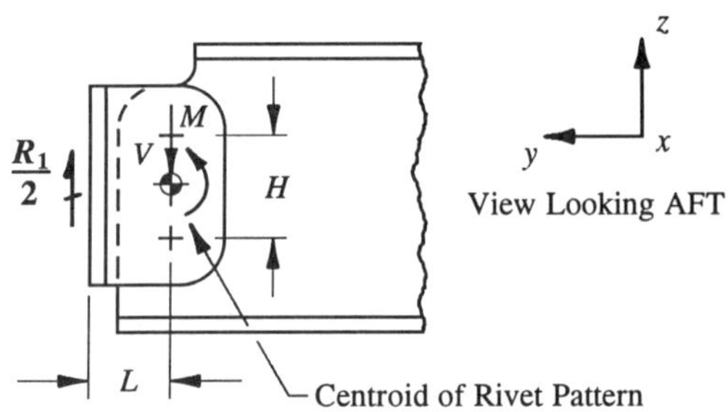

(a) FWD SHEAR CLIP

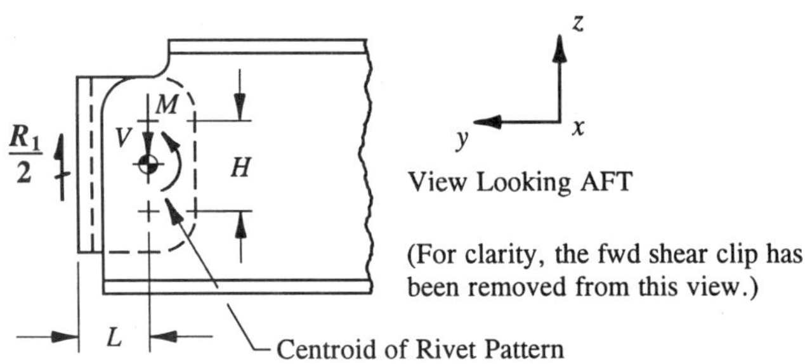

(b) AFT SHEAR CLIP

FIGURE 5-8 Equilibrium forces V and M indicated for (a) the fwd shear clip and (b) the aft shear clip.

loads (this, of course, includes a bending moment since compression and tension are simultaneously produced from its loading effect). A tension clip is, however, such a poor design alternative that the engineer should reconsider any other alternative choices for redesign. A better redesign alternative would be to, instead, consider continuous beam caps to stiffen the support area (see Fig. 5-2, where significant weight reduction and cost-savings may be realized by also making use of splice plates to carry the basic tension loads across the support area).

The second type of support structure considered in this section is called back-to-back angle shear clips (Type B). Using this support for the support structure in Fig. 5-3(b), the following unknown reaction R_1 is again denoted there.[1] As before, in our investigations of a single angle clip support structure, a back-to-back system of angle shear clips also assumes a simply-supported restraint condition. Therefore, the basic theories outlined in our previous solution of a single angle clip support are also applicable here to our present discussions of back-to-back angle shear clip supports, except that for the structural arrangement of support members

[1] Its real value is, of course, verifiable once the equations of equilibrium are applied to the main structure under simulated flight and landing conditions.

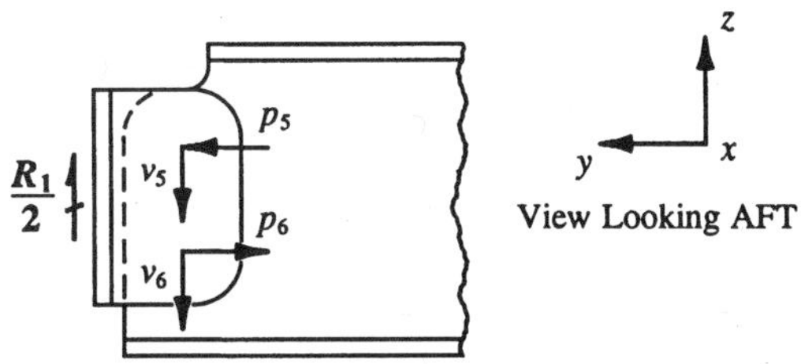

(a) FWD SHEAR CLIP

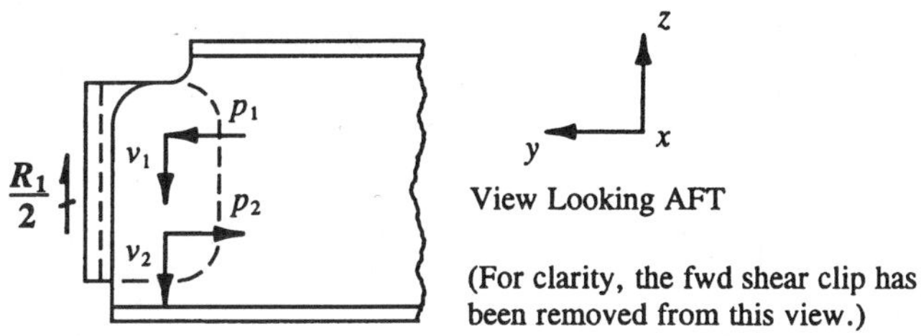

(b) AFT SHEAR CLIP

FIGURE 5-9 Vertical shears and bending moments (from Fig. 5-8) are distributed as shearing forces to the rivets of (a) the fwd shear clip and (b) the aft shear clip.

considered here, the reaction shear R_1, applied eccentric to each angle, will divide equally between the forward and aft shear clips. Assuming, of course, that the shear clips are of identical construction and material, which for most aircraft structures this should prove to be the case. Here, the web of our design beam carries the full design shear R_1, while the shear clips themselves carry only one-half of this design value or $\frac{1}{2}R_1$. Bearing failure is then more likely to occur in the web, since this member carries twice the design shear as do either of the individual shear clips. The detailed solution of a back-to-back system of unsymmetrically loaded angle shear clips is deferred until later when our minds can better grasp the additional complexities associated with their solutions.[1] For now, let us determine the equilibrium forces to balance the shear clips at support A, as shown in Fig. 5-8. The equilibrium shears and bending moments for each support structure in the plane of the transverse beam web are carefully represented at the centroid of their respective fastener patterns; and then, in accordance with prescribed methods of analysis for their distribution, distributed as horizontal and vertical shearing forces to individual fasteners of their respective rivet groups, as shown in Fig. 5-9. For each shear clip, the shear V and bending moment M (expressed as an equivalent couple-force) divide equally between equal size and strength fasteners:[2]

[1] Refer to Example 5-2 on page 309 for the solution of unsymmetrically loaded back-to-back angle shear clips.

[2] Refer again to footnote (2) on page 286.

For the fwd shear clip:

$$v_5 = v_6 = \frac{V}{2}$$

$$p_5 = p_6 = \frac{M}{H}$$

where: $V = \dfrac{R_1}{2}$ and $M = \left[\dfrac{R_1}{2}\right]L$

H = distance measured between fastener centers

L = distance measured from the rivet line to the shear plane of the attached leg.

For the aft shear clip:

$$v_1 = v_2 = \frac{V}{2}$$

$$p_1 = p_2 = \frac{M}{H}$$

where: V, M, H, and L are the same quantities as defined above for the forward shear clip.

All horizontal and vertical shearing forces in the plane of the transverse beam web are shown on an exploded view of the support structure in Fig. 5-10. From the Pythagorean theorem, these forces are combined mathematically into a single resultant force at each fastener location. This gives:

Resultant shearing force for fastener #1:

$$P_1 = \left[(p_1 + p_5)^2 + (v_1 + v_5)^2\right]^{1/2} \quad \text{(this fastener is in double-shear).}$$

Resultant shearing force for fastener #2:

$$P_2 = \left[(p_2 + p_6)^2 + (v_2 + v_6)^2\right]^{1/2} \quad \text{(this fastener is also in double-shear).}$$

Since the fasteners are of the same size and strength,[1] their resultants are of the same magnitude, that is,

$$P_1 = P_2.$$

[1] If rivets are not of the same size and strength, distribution of fastener shearing forces is instead achieved by the methods of Chapter 3, "Connection Analysis." However, in such cases, you need only base your findings on the most critical fastener.

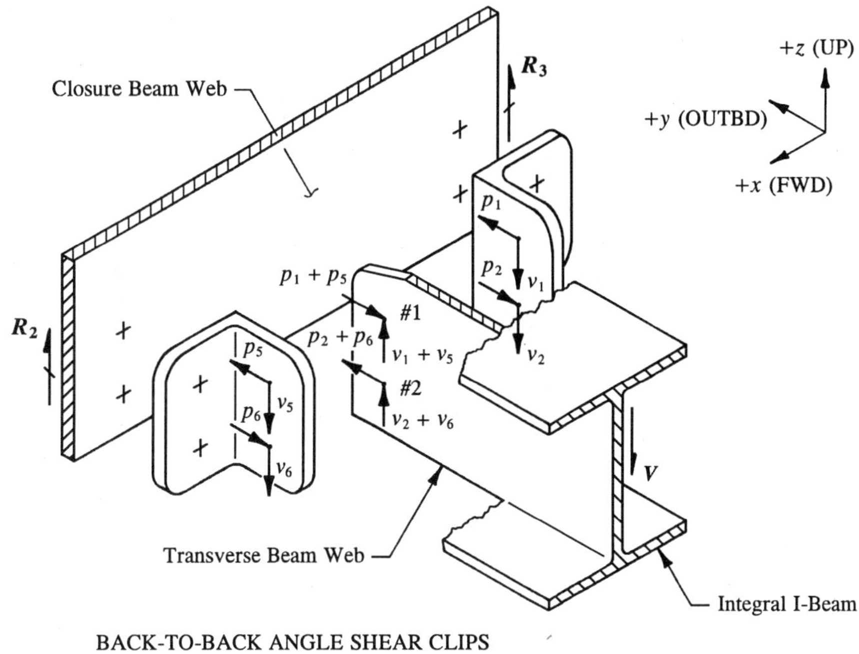

FIGURE 5-10 Transfer of load through back-to-back angle shear clips (Type B).

The fasteners in this plane are in double-shear and are analyzed by the methods of Sec. 3.2. Bearing and shearing failures are formulated as follows:

Shearing failure:

$$\text{Margin of Safety} = \text{M.S.} = \frac{P_{su}}{p_s k} - 1$$

where: P_{su} = ultimate double-shear allowable of the fastener[1]
$p_s = P_1 = P_2$
$k = 1.15$ (fitting factor used in joint and connection designs).

Bearing failure of the aft shear clip:

$$\text{Margin of Safety} = \text{M.S.} = \frac{P_{bru}}{p_s k} - 1$$

where: P_{bru} = ultimate bearing allowable of the material (Use either Eq. 3-2 or 3-3 for this computation.)

[1] See footnote on page 287.

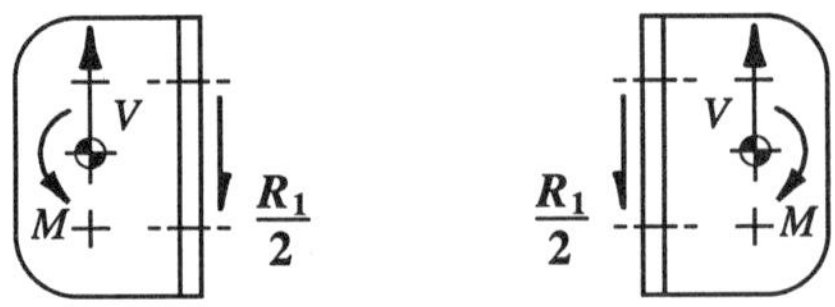

Fwd Shear Clip Aft Shear Clip

VIEW LOOKING OUTBD
(x-z plane)

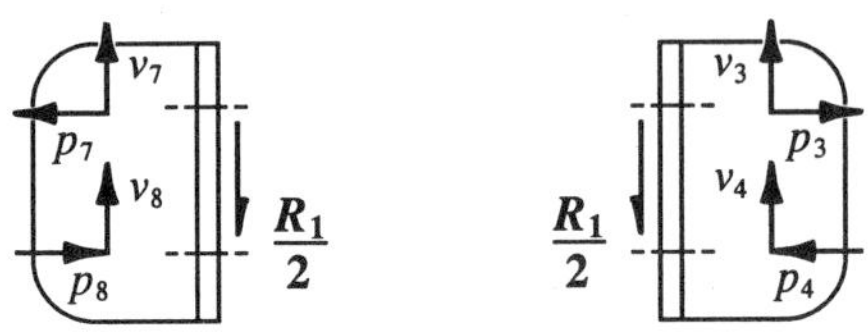

Fwd Shear Clip Aft Shear Clip

VIEW LOOKING OUTBD
(x-z plane)

FIGURE 5-11 Back-to-back shear clips are isolated from the transverse beam and free-bodied in the x-z plane.

$$p_s = \tfrac{1}{2} P_1 = (v_1^2 + p_1^2)^{1/2} = (v_2^2 + p_2^2)^{1/2}$$

k = 1.15 (fitting factor used in joint and connection designs).

Bearing failure of the fwd shear clip:

$$\text{Margin of Safety} = \text{M.S.} = \frac{P_{bru}}{p_s k} - 1$$

where: P_{bru} = ultimate bearing allowable of the material (Use either Eq. 3-2 or 3-3 for this computation.)

$$p_s = \tfrac{1}{2} P_2 = (v_5^2 + p_5^2)^{1/2} = (v_6^2 + p_6^2)^{1/2}$$

k = 1.15 (fitting factor used in joint and connection designs).

Bearing failure of the transverse beam web:

$$\text{Margin of Safety} = \text{M.S.} = \frac{P_{bru}}{p_s k} - 1$$

where: P_{bru} = ultimate bearing allowable of the web material (Use either Eq. 3-2 or 3-3 for this computation.)

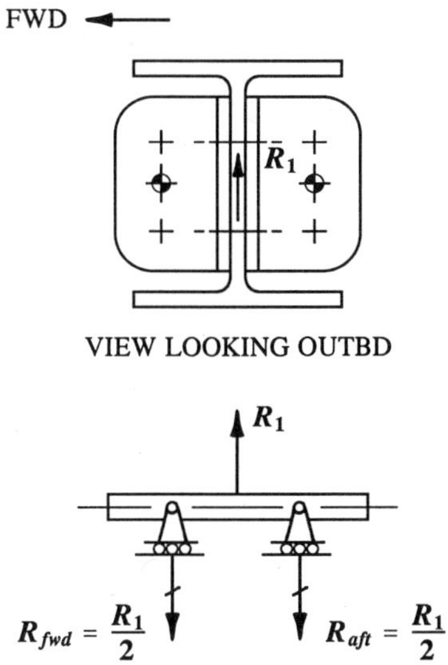

FIGURE 5-12 Idealized representation of back-to-back shear clips.

$p_s = P_1 = P_2$
$k = 1.15$ (fitting factor used in joint and connection designs).

Isolating each support clip once again, but this time in the plane of the closure beam web, we obtain the following system of shearing forces in equilibrium, as shown in Fig. 5-11. Since the shear clips, in effect, tend to separate under load, they function very much independently of each other, like two separate members, each one individually loaded carrying with it a proportionate share of the shear reaction R_1. Why does the shear reaction R_1 divide equally between each support clip? Answer: If the rivet centroids are considered points of support for each group of rivets, from statics, the solution is obvious: that is, since the distances from the web reaction shear R_1 to each centroid rivet group are the same, the shear divides equally between the shear supports or ½ R_1.[1] See Fig. 5-12 for this illustration. Distribution is then easily achieved by inspection: the shear V and bending moment M divide equally between equal size and strength fasteners. Then, the following expressions for the actual distribution of these quantities are used:

$$v_3 = v_4 = \frac{V}{2} \qquad v_7 = v_8 = \frac{V}{2}$$

$$p_3 = p_4 = \frac{M}{H} \qquad p_7 = p_8 = \frac{M}{H}$$

[1] The same line of reasoning is used to determine individual support loads for unsymmetrically loaded back-to-back shear clips.

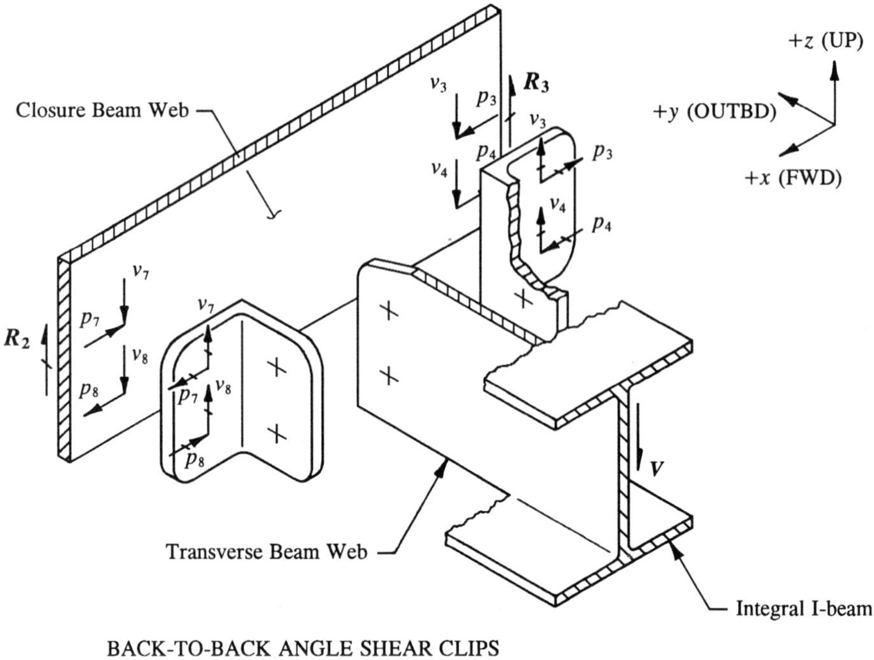

FIGURE 5-13 Transfer of load through back-to-back angle shear clips (Type B).

where: $V = \dfrac{R_1}{2}$ and $M = \left[\dfrac{R_1}{2}\right]L$

H = distance between fastener centers

L = distance measured from the rivet line to the shear plane of the attached leg.

The horizontal and vertical system of shearing forces in the plane of the closure beam web are summarized in Fig. 5-13. From these distributions, resultant shearing forces at each rivet location are determined and their values used to predict the following failures:

(1) shearing failure of the closure beam rivets,
(2) bearing failure of the closure beam web, and
(3) bearing failure of the shear clips.

Our third and final support member, a tee clip (Type C), is by far the most efficient of the three types of support members considered up to this point in our study of shear clip support members. Here is how a tee shear clip arrangement for the support structure in Fig. 5-3(c) would actually work. First, let us answer this basic question: How much of the reaction shear R_1 is reacted by each rivet group?

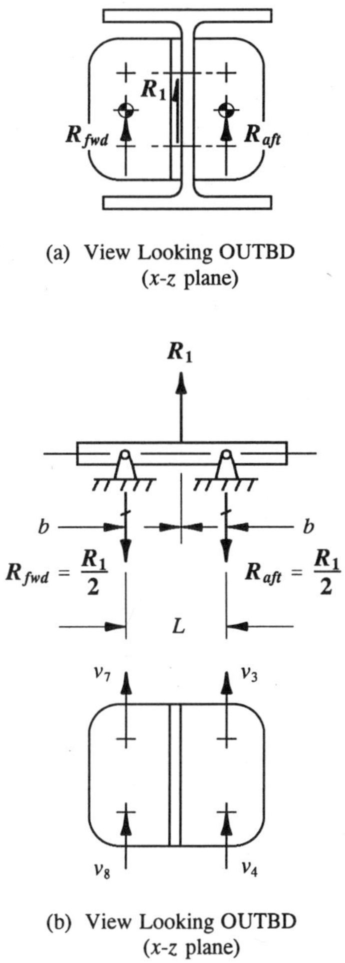

FIGURE 5-14 (a) Symmetrically loaded tee clip support. (b) Distribution of rivet shearing forces.

Answer: Since the support is symmetrically loaded, one-half (½) of the reaction shear R_1 is reacted by each rivet group (see Fig. 5-14). Unlike back-to-back angle shear clips, a tee shear clip is structurally a better design candidate because it develops no bending moments at the centroid of each rivet group. The support is statically in equilibrium. The shears R_{fwd} and R_{aft} from each centroid are then distributed to the rivets of each fastener group, Fig. 5-14(b) as follows:

$$v_3 = v_4 = \frac{R_{aft}}{2} = \frac{R_1/2}{2} = \frac{R_1}{4}$$

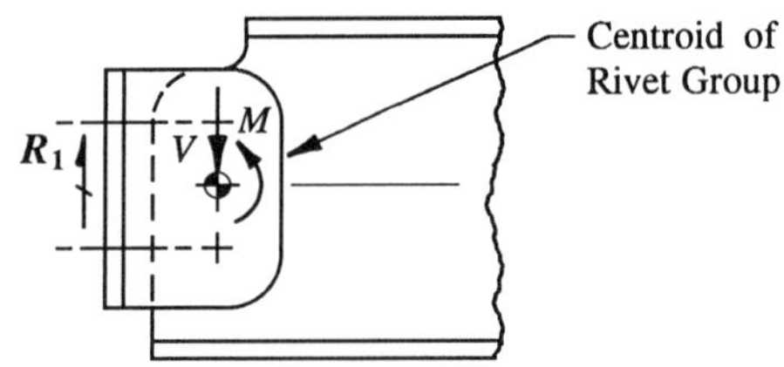

(a) View Looking AFT

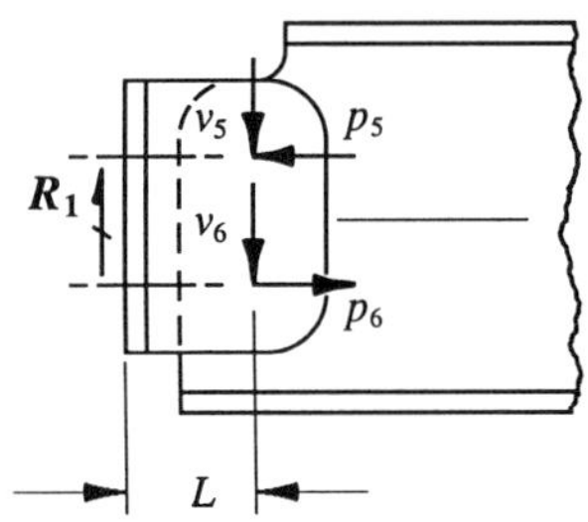

(b) View Looking AFT

FIGURE 5-15 (a) Equilibrium forces V and M in the x-z plane for the tee clip support. (b) Distribution of rivet shearing forces in the x-z plane.

$$v_7 = v_8 = \frac{R_{fwd}}{2} = \frac{R_1/2}{2} = \frac{R_1}{4}.$$

The appropriate failure checks are determined from these values:

(1) shearing failure of the closure beam rivets,
(2) bearing failure of the tee clip, and
(3) bearing failure of the closure beam web.

Now, in the other plane, that is, looking aft in Fig. 5-3, we obtain the equilibrium forces V and M, and from their values determine the corresponding rivet shearing forces, as shown in Figs. 5-15(a) and (b). Rivet shearing forces are determined from earlier techniques of this section that were used to distribute equilibrium forces to connection rivets. Here, this gives:

$$v_5 = v_6 = \frac{V}{2}$$

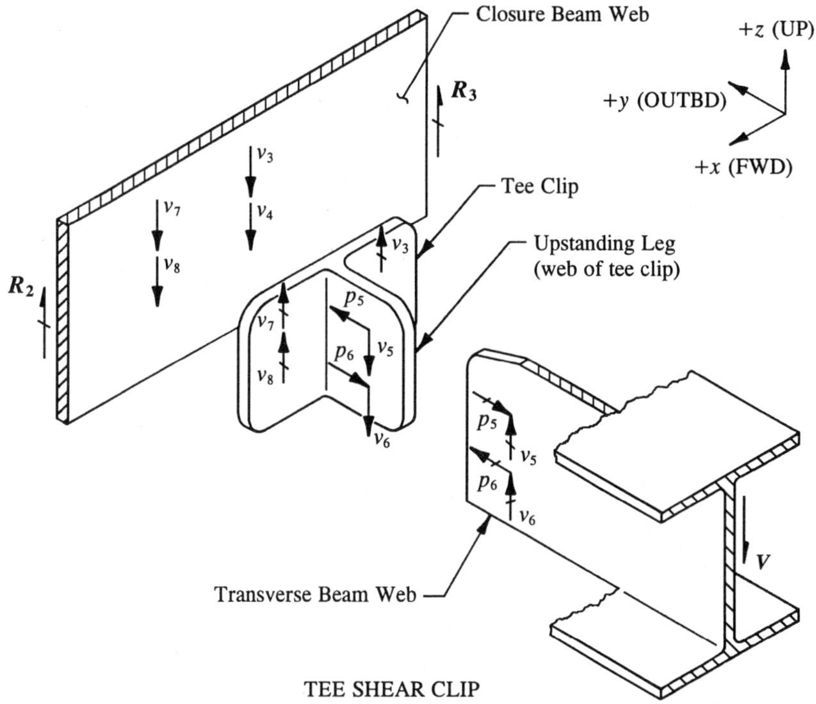

FIGURE 5-16 Transfer of load through a tee shear clip (Type C).

$$p_5 = p_6 = \frac{M}{H}$$

where: $V = R_1$
$M = R_1 L$
H = distance measured between fastener centers
L = distance measured from the rivet line to the shear plane of the attached leg.

All rivet shearing forces are drawn on a companion diagram (see Fig. 5-16 for the final system of shearing forces). From these, resultant shearing forces are computed as follows:

$$p_5 = (v_5^2 + p_5^2)^{1/2}$$

$$p_6 = (v_6^2 + p_6^2)^{1/2}.$$

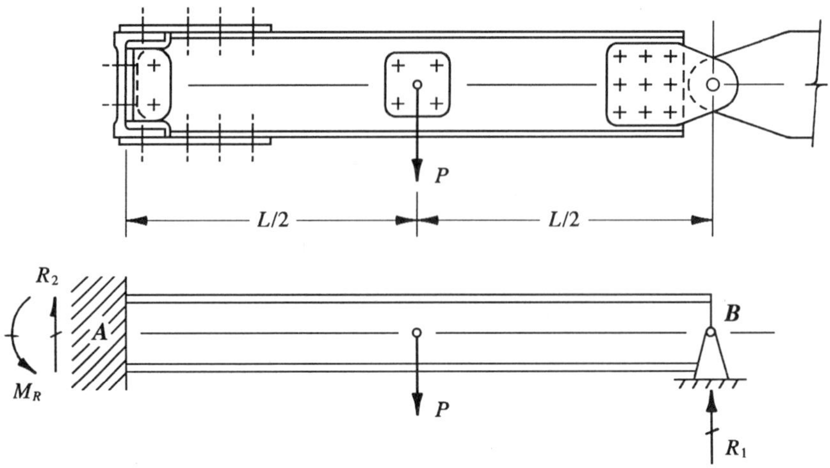

FIGURE 5-17 Beam shows that by changing the support conditions at A to a fixed support structure will also change the magnitude of the support reactions.

Failures are then predicted in the usual way:

(1) shearing failure of the transverse beam rivets,
(2) bearing failure of the transverse beam web, and
(3) bearing failure of the upstanding leg (web) of the tee clip.

In some design cases, instead of a simply-supported structure a fixed support structure is desired for aircraft production use, upper and lower cap straps can actually be incorporated with the simply-supported structure. Refer back to Fig. 5-2 for this particular structural arrangement of support members. The reinforcing members provide the continuity for the beam chords across the supported end of the structure. They supply the physical restraint in the horizontal direction that the shear clip supports considered thus far in this section cannot effectively provide (these support types were shown in Fig. 5-3). Indirectly, they (the reinforcing members) carry the axial and bending moment across the fixed-supported end. To analyze the reinforcing members for these loads, refer to Chapter 2, Sec. 2.5. (To complete the solution, also answer the following question: How are the rivets for the upper and lower straps sized and spaced?)

The support shear clips presented so far in this section (referring again to Fig. 5-3) have been analyzed with the same reaction shear R_1 at their supported ends. Note, however, if a fixed restraint is used, more reactive shear will actually be drawn (or beamed out) to the fixed-supported end. The increase in moment of inertia (or stiffness) across the supported end is another way of physically describing this structural behavior. For example, let us look at such a special case, where instead of a simply-supported restraint we provide full fixity (or cap splices) for the support structure (refer to Fig. 5-17). The reactions for this structure are determined from the equations given in Appendix D (Reference Beam Formula Solutions, Case 15):

$$(1)\ R_1 = \frac{5P}{16},\ (2)\ R_2 = \frac{11P}{16},\ \text{and}\ (3)\ M_R = \frac{3PL}{16}.$$

Note, in particular, that the reaction shear R_2 in this case is $11P/16$, instead of $P/2$ that would normally be obtained for a simply-supported structure with a concentrated load at center span. This is an important consideration sometimes overlooked by inexperienced engineers: basically, if you change the support conditions, the magnitude of the support reactions will also change. In fact, the entire loading structure used to design the basic beam structure will change. Therefore, if a fixed-support should actually be contemplated in a beam design, it must also be properly analyzed and its structural behavior predicted accordingly. Otherwise, serious design consequences or weight penalties may invariably result: (1) this could occur during structural testing, or possibly, (2) during actual production, or (3) in actual aircraft service. This concludes our discussion of shear clip supports. In Sec. 5.3, our discussions will also include the subject of tension clips and their related applications to basic aircraft structural designs. The remainder of this section will be spent solving three example problems. Each problem corresponding to the specific support types described in this section: (1) single angle clips, (2) back-to-back angle clips, and (3) tee clips.

Example 5-1 Several stiffeners constructed of channel sections are used to reinforce the air-inlet duct surface due to cabin pressurization. If the most critical stiffener reacts a load of 400 lb at its supported end, as shown in Fig. 5-18, what size rivets would be required for the shear clip support? Also write the appropriate bearing failure of the shear clip and all joined members. The bearing properties of the materials used in the analysis of this support member are listed below:

Member	Material	Mechanical Properties
Shear Clip	2024-T3 Clad QQ-A-250/5	F_{bru} = 121 ksi (e/D = 2.0) F_{bry} = 82 ksi (e/D = 2.0)
Longitudinal Member	7075-T73 QQ-A-250/12	F_{bru} = 134 ksi (e/D = 2.0) F_{bry} = 102 ksi (e/D = 2.0)
Stiffener	2024-T3510 Extr. QQ-A-200/3	F_{bru} = 108 ksi (e/D = 2.0) F_{bry} = 71 ksi (e/D = 2.0)

SOLUTION: To establish equilibrium for the reactive shearing force of 400 lb, the shear clip is isolated in the x-z plane from the rest of the structure and the

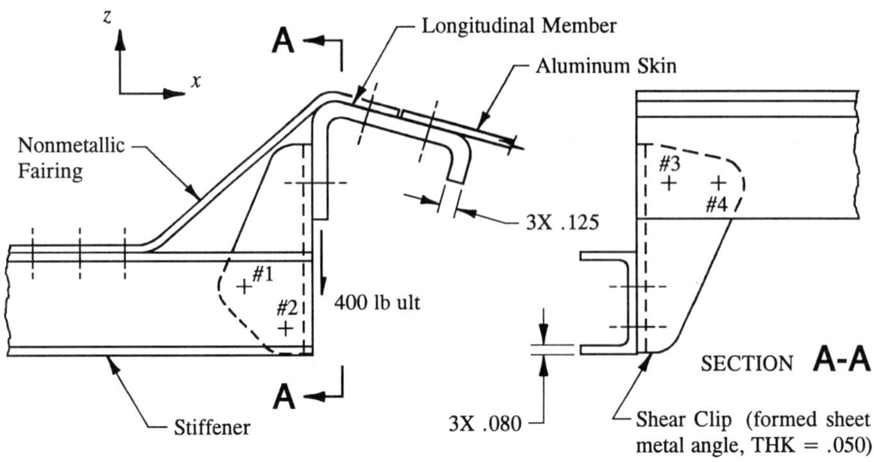

FIGURE 5-18 Support structure for the engine air-inlet duct stiffeners.

equilibrium forces V and M at the centroid of the rivet pattern determined. This is shown in Fig. 5-19(a). From statics, we obtain:

$$V = 400 \text{ lb}$$
$$M = 400(.740) = 296 \text{ in-lb.}$$

The equilibrium forces are then distributed to the fasteners as equivalent shearing forces in this same plane. The results of this distribution are given below:

$$v_1 = v_2 = \frac{V}{2} = \frac{400}{2} = 200 \text{ lb}$$
$$p_1 = p_2 = \frac{M}{H} = \frac{296}{.750} = 395 \text{ lb.}$$

Their vectorial representations are depicted in Fig. 5-19(b). It is clear from the directions indicated for the shearing forces of these fasteners that rivet #2 will be critical, i.e., highly stressed. Therefore, only the resultant shearing force of this fastener is computed. In Fig. 5-19(c), the couple-force p_2 for this fastener is replaced by its equivalent horizontal and vertical component shearing forces. Mathematically, this gives:

$$p_v = 395 \sin 45^\circ = 279 \text{ lb}$$
$$p_h = 395 \cos 45^\circ = 279 \text{ lb.}$$

Now, Fig. 5-19(d), the shearing forces are combined into one resultant force system. This is done using the Pythagorean theorem. Thus

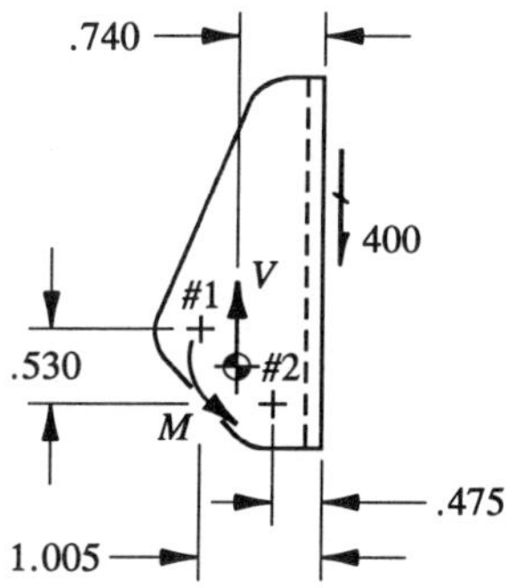

(a) Equilibrium forces V and M in the x-z plane.

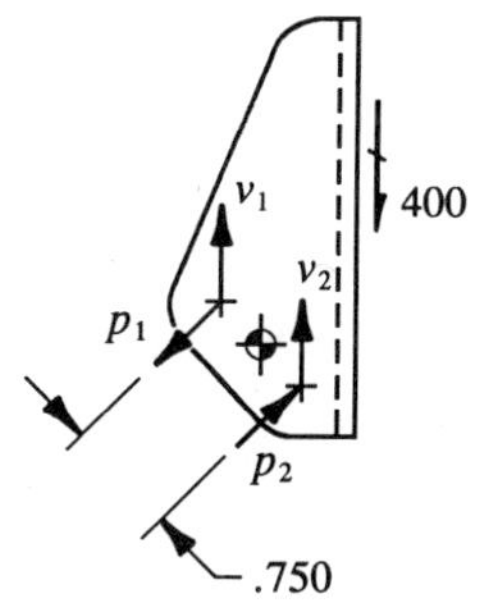

(b) Distribution of equilibrium forces to the rivets in the x-z plane.

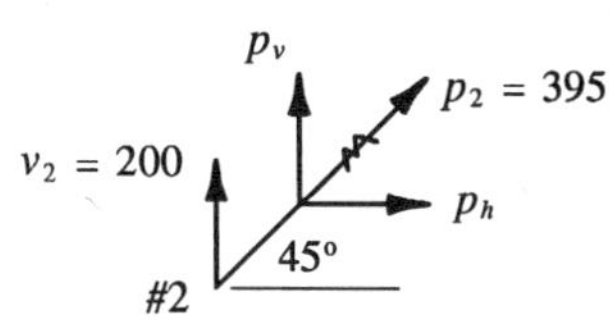

(c) Couple-force p_2 is replaced by its equivalent horizontal and vertical shearing forces.

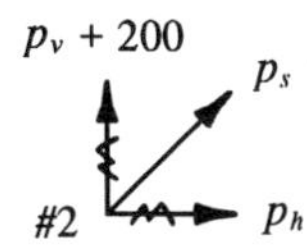

(d) Resultant force p_s is determined from the Pythagorean theorem.

FIGURE 5-19 Shear clip is isolated from its main structure and the resultant force for the critical fastener is determined.

$$p_s = (p_x{}^2 + p_z{}^2)^{1/2} = \left[(279)^2 + (479)^2\right]^{1/2} = 554 \text{ lb}$$

where: $p_x = p_h = 279$ lb

$p_z = p_v + 200 = 279 + 200 = 479$ (superposition of shearing forces).

If we choose BJ 6 rivets ($F_{su} = 30$ ksi) for our proposed rivet design, the following shearing and bearing failures are predicted:

Shearing failure of rivet #2:

$$P_{su} = F_{su} A_{shr} C_r = 862(.970) = 836 \text{ lb}$$

where: $F_{su} A_{shr} = 862$ lb (from Table 3-1)

$C_r = .970$ (from Table 3-2 in .050 in sheet thickness).

$$\text{Margin of Safety} = \text{M.S.} = \frac{P_{su}}{p_s k} - 1 = \frac{836}{554(1.15)} - 1 = +.31.$$

Bearing failure of the shear clip:

Since $F_{bru} < 1.5 F_{bry}$, Eq. 3-2 is used for this evaluation.

$$P_{bru} = F_{bru}\, t D = 121,000(.050)(.191) = 1,156 \text{ lb}$$

where: $F_{bru} = 121$ ksi $(e/D = 2.0)$
$F_{bry} = 82$ ksi $(e/D = 2.0)$
$t = .050$ in
$D = .191$ in (nominal hole diameter for a BJ 6 rivet).

$$\text{Margin of Safety} = \text{M.S.} = \frac{P_{bru}}{p_s k} - 1 = \frac{1,156}{554(1.15)} - 1 = +.81.$$

Bearing failure of the stiffener:

Here, $F_{bru} > 1.5 F_{bry}$, therefore, Eq. 3-3 is used this time.

$$P_{bru} = 1.5 F_{bry}\, t D = 1.5(71,000)(.080)(.191) = 1,627 \text{ lb}$$

where: $F_{bru} = 108$ ksi $(e/D = 2.0)$
$F_{bry} = 71$ ksi $(e/D = 2.0)$
$t = .080$ in
$D = .191$ in (nominal hole diameter for a BJ 6 rivet).

$$\text{Margin of Safety} = \text{M.S.} = \frac{P_{bru}}{p_s k} - 1 = \frac{1,627}{554(1.15)} - 1 = +1.55.$$

Now, let us rotate the shear clip into the y-z plane as diagrammed in Fig. 5-20 and determine the equilibrium forces V and M at the centroid of this rivet group. Here, this gives:

$$V = 400 \text{ lb}$$

$$M = 400(.800) = 320 \text{ in-lb}.$$

Once again, these forces are distributed to the rivets as equivalent shearing forces. The results of this distribution are shown in Fig. 5-20(b), from which we get:

$$v_3 = v_4 = \frac{V}{2} = \frac{400}{2} = 200 \text{ lb}$$

$$p_3 = p_4 = \frac{M}{H} = \frac{320}{.750} = 427 \text{ lb}.$$

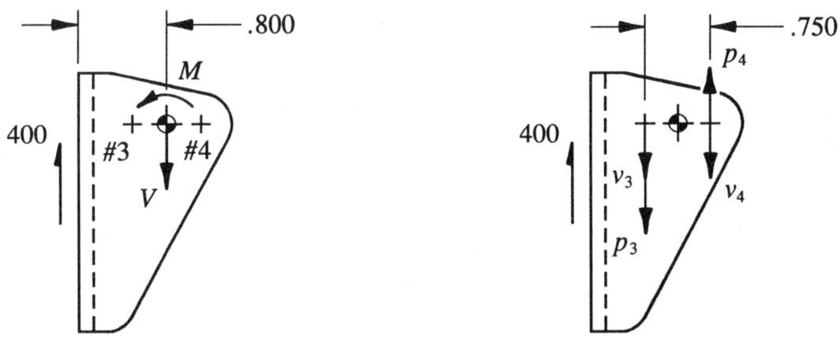

(a) Equilibrium forces V and M in the y-z plane.

(b) Distribution of equilibrium forces to the rivets in the y-z plane.

FIGURE 5-20 Resultant force for the critical fastener in the y-z plane is determined.

By inspection or by some clever reasoning, and this may usually be done in most cases, rivet #3 is critical in this plane. Its resultant shearing force (from superposition of shearing forces) is computed as follows:

$$p_s = v_3 + p_3 = 200 + 427 = 627\,\text{lb}.$$

On the other hand, the shearing forces of fastener #4, also collinear (in line), act in opposite directions to each other. For this reason, their vectorial superposition is not additive and therefore not critical enough to warrant any further examination of this fastener. The following failures are predicted:

Shearing failure of rivet #3:

$$P_{su} = F_{su} A_{shr} C_r = 862(.970) = 836 \text{ lb}$$

where: $F_{su} A_{shr} = 862$ lb (from Table 3-1)
$C_r = .970$ (from Table 3-2 in .050 in sheet thickness).

$$\text{Margin of Safety} = \text{M.S.} = \frac{P_{su}}{p_s k} - 1 = \frac{836}{627(1.15)} - 1 = +.16.$$

Bearing failure of the shear clip:

$$\text{Margin of Safety} = \text{M.S.} = \frac{P_{bru}}{p_s k} - 1 = \frac{1,156}{627(1.15)} - 1 = +.60$$

where: $P_{bru} = 1{,}156$ lb (refer back to page 306)
$p_s = 627$ lb

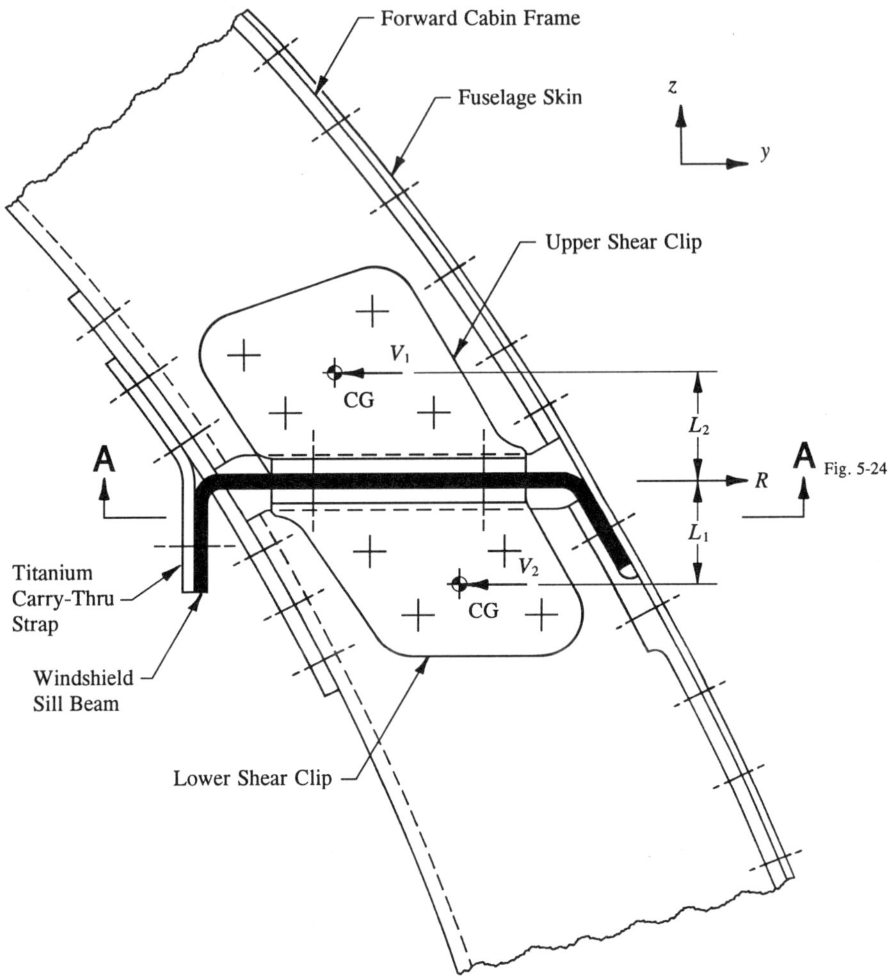

FIGURE 5-21 Windshield sill beam is attached to the forward cabin frame with back-to-back angle shear clips.

$k = 1.15$ (fitting factor used in joint and connection designs).

Bearing failure of the longitudinal member:

$$\text{Margin of Safety} = \text{M.S.} = \frac{P_{bru}}{p_s k} - 1 = \frac{3,199}{627(1.15)} - 1 = +3.44$$

where: $P_{bru} = 3,199$ lb (The engineer is encouraged to verify this value using Eq. 3-2, $P_{bru} = F_{bru} t D$.)

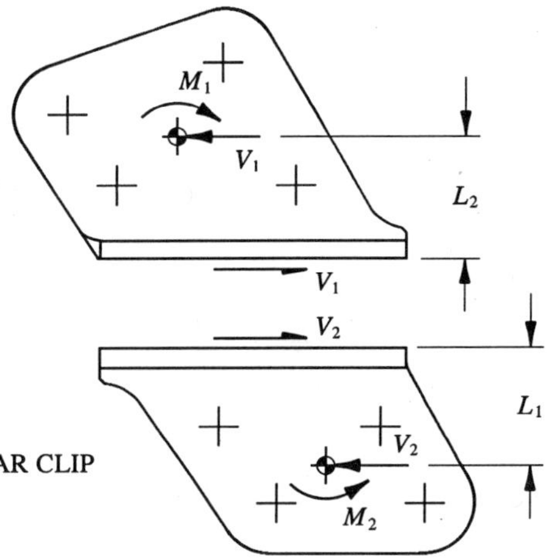

FIGURE 5-22 Equilibrium forces at the centroid of the rivet pattern in the *y-z* plane for (a) the upper shear clip and (b) the lower shear clip.

$p_s = 627$ lb
$k = 1.15$ (fitting factor used in joint and connection designs).

Example 5-2 The windshield sill beam is attached to the forward cabin frame with back-to-back angle shear clips, and the frame under maximum cabin pressurization is found to react a load R, as shown in Fig. 5-21. Discuss the analysis procedure required to substantiate the shear clips, its fasteners, and all joined members through which the reaction R is felt. Use the summary on pages 183-185 of Sec. 3.4 as a general guide to the detailed solution of this problem.

SOLUTION: A back-to-back arrangement of angle shear clips will divide the reaction R between the shear clips in proportion to the distances from their respective rivet group centroids to the line of action of the reactive force. In this problem, this refers to the distances L_1 and L_2 in Fig. 5-21. Our solution to this problem can best be followed using basic connection analysis methods: first, the equations of equilibrium are applied in the *y-z* plane to determine the distribution of load to each shear clip. In theory, let us consider the reaction R distributed to each rivet group centroid, as shown in Fig. 5-21, where the symbols V_1 and V_2 have been denoted to represent these loads. Then, from statics:

$$\Sigma F_y = 0, \qquad -V_1 + R - V_2 = 0, \quad V_2 = R - V_1$$

$$\Sigma M_{cg} = 0, \qquad (+ \quad -V_1(L_1 + L_2) + RL_1 = 0$$

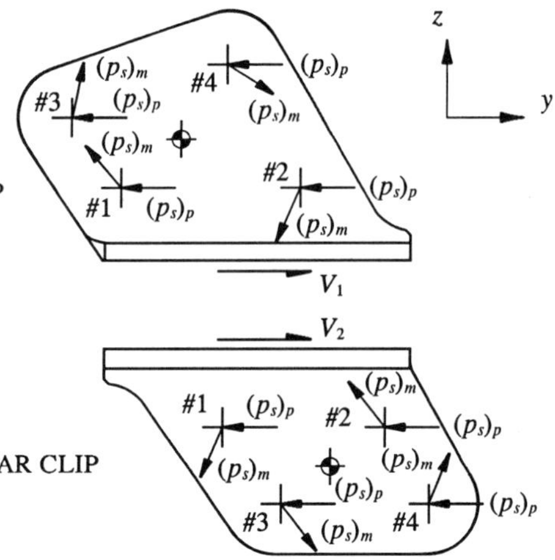

FIGURE 5-23 Distribution of equilibrium forces to the rivets of (a) the upper shear clip and (b) the lower shear clip.

$$V_1 = R\left[\frac{L_1}{L_1 + L_2}\right].$$

Now that the distribution of shears (V_1 and V_2 are known for each shear clip), the corresponding equilibrium moments occurring at each rivet group centroid can be calculated. From the principle of moments ($M = Fd$), the moments M_1 and M_2 for the upper and lower shear clips, respectively, are computed:

$$M_1 = V_1 L_2 \quad \text{(upper shear clip)}$$

$$M_2 = V_2 L_1 \quad \text{(lower shear clip)}.$$

These moments are depicted in Fig. 5-22 at the centroid of their respective rivet groups.

The rest of the solution is proceeded along as follows: the equilibrium forces V_1, M_1 and V_2, M_2 are each distributed to the rivets of their respective fastener groups in terms of equivalent shearing forces.[1] These forces are diagrammed in Fig. 5-23. From each group of rivets, the maximum stressed rivets are determined. This should be obvious from the vectorial superposition of shearing forces $(p_s)_p$ and $(p_s)_m$ at each rivet location. Two rivets from each fastener group, rivets #1 and #2, are observed to have critical combinations of potentially high shearing forces. From these forces, resultant shearing forces are computed and their values used to determine shearing and bearing failures as follows:

[1] Review, if necessary, those principles pertinent to the design and analysis of multi-riveted connection designs in Chapter 3.

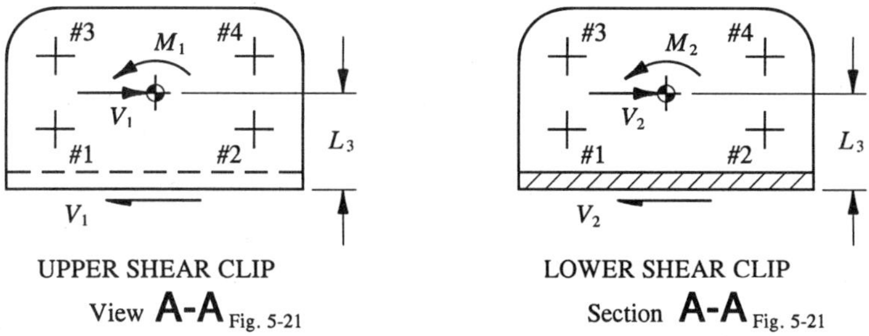

FIGURE 5-24 Equilibrium forces at the centroid of the rivet pattern in the *x-y* plane for (a) the upper shear clip and (b) the lower shear clip.

(1) Shearing failure of the maximum stressed rivets.

(2) Bearing failure of the shear clips (use the largest resultant shearing force at the location of the maximum stressed rivet).

(3) Bearing failure of the forward cabin frame (also use the largest resultant shearing force at the location of the maximum stressed rivet).

Refer back to Fig. 5-21, the shear clips are viewed riveted together in a back-to-back arrangement of their common rivet patterns. Here, the equilibrium forces V_1 and V_2 are each applied separately to their common rivet patterns in order to determine their combined rivet shearing forces. Essentially, the detailed analysis of these support members goes along the same line of reasoning as any shear clip analysis would: the shears V_1 and V_2 are each balanced separately at the centroid of their common rivet patterns and used to determine the corresponding equilibrium moments $M_1 = V_1 L_3$ and $M_2 = V_2 L_3$, Fig. 5-24. The equilibrium forces V_1, M_1 and V_2, M_2 are then each distributed to the rivets as equivalent shearing forces, Fig. 5-25. The critical rivets are found by inspection and their resultant shearing forces determined. Here, rivets #1 and #2 are critical. With the critical resultant rivet shearing forces known for each shear clip, the following failures are predicted:

(1) Shearing failure of the maximum stressed rivets (since these rivets are in double-shear, use the combined resultant shearing forces from each of the equilibrium forces V_1, M_1 and V_2, M_2).[1]

(2) Bearing failure of the shear clips (use the largest resultant shearing force from either the solution of V_1, M_1 or V_2, M_2).

(3) Bearing failure of the windshield sill beam (use the combined resultant shearing force from each of the equilibrium forces V_1, M_1 and V_2, M_2).

[1] Refer back to the analysis of back-to-back angle shear clips in this section if this point is not absolutely clear to you now (see also Fig. 5-10).

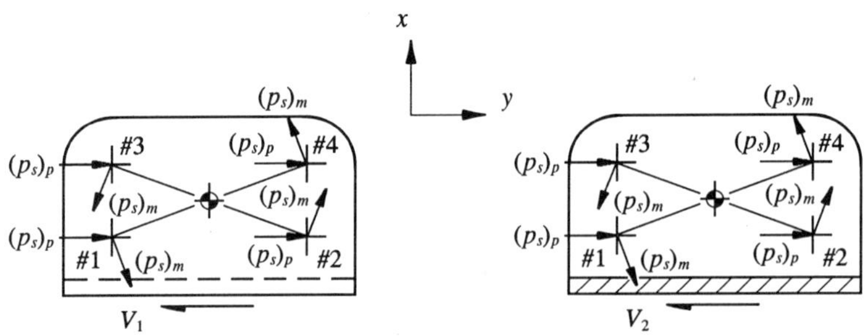

FIGURE 5-25 Distribution of equilibrium forces to the rivets of (a) the upper shear clip and (b) the lower shear clip.

Example 5-3 The intercostal loaded as shown in Fig. 5-26 reacts a maximum vertical shear of 1,400 lb and a maximum bending moment of 4,000 in-lb at its fixed-supported end. If a tee clip support is used to react the vertical shear at the fixed-supported end, determine the appropriate shearing and bearing margins of safety required for general substantiation of this particular support. (All pertinent dimensions and material properties used in the analysis solution of this problem are given in subsequent figures which follow as they are needed.)

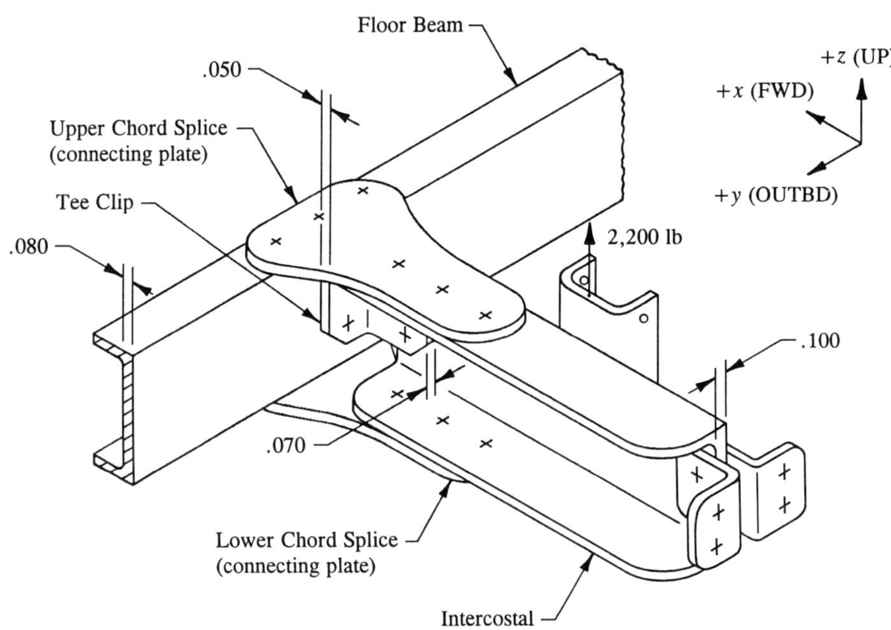

FIGURE 5-26 Tee clip support is used at the fixed-supported end of the beam.

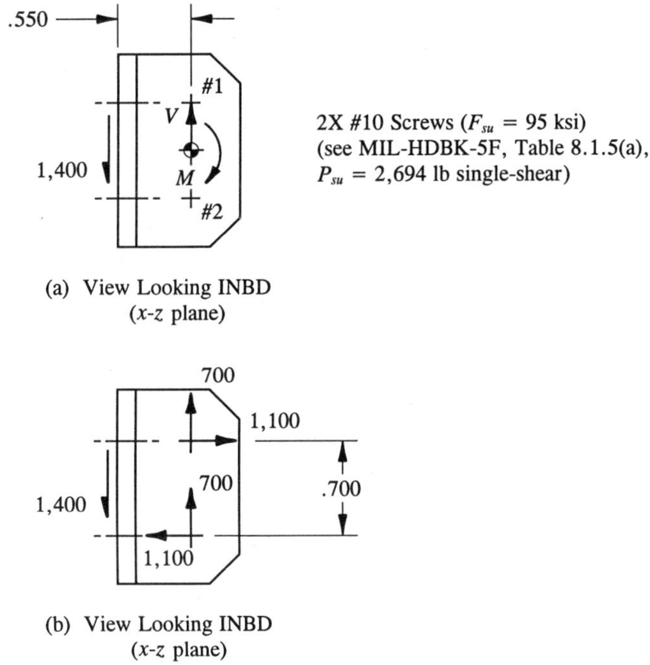

FIGURE 5-27 (a) Equilibrium forces at the centroid of the fastener pattern in the x-z plane. (b) Distribution of vertical shear to the fasteners in the x-z plane.

Member	Material	Mechanical Properties
Tee Clip	2024-T3 Aluminum Alloy Extrusion QQ-A-200/3	F_{bru} = 108 ksi, e/D = 2.0 F_{bry} = 71 ksi, e/D = 2.0
Floor Beam	7075-T73510 Aluminum Alloy Extrusion QQ-A-200/11	F_{bru} = 129 ksi, e/D = 2.0 F_{bry} = 97 ksi, e/D = 2.0
Intercostal	2024-T42 Aluminum Alloy Extrusion QQ-A-200/3	F_{bru} = 99 ksi, e/D = 2.0 F_{bry} = 69 ksi, e/D = 2.0

SOLUTION: In agreement with industry-accepted practices for the design and analysis of a fixed-supported structure, the tee clip will carry the full vertical shear of 1,400 lb while the upper and lower splice plates are assumed to carry the full bending moment of 4,000 in-lb. Their analyses are performed separately. Specifically, the tee clip is analyzed by the methods of this section and the splice plates are analyzed by the methods of Chapter 2.

Essentially, the tee clip is isolated from the main structure and the equilibrium forces V and M in the x-z plane necessary to free-body the shear clip in static equilibrium are determined. These forces are shown in Fig. 5-27(a) and their magnitudes determined from statics:

$$V = 1,400 \text{ lb} \quad (\text{from } \Sigma F_z = 0)$$
$$M = 1,400(.550) = 770 \text{ in-lb} \quad (\text{from } \Sigma M_{cg} = 0).$$

In Fig. 5-27(b), the equilibrium forces V and M are then replaced by equivalent fastener shearing forces. The following relationships are used to determine the distribution of loads to fasteners #1 and #2:

$$v_1 = v_2 = \frac{V}{2} = \frac{1,400}{2} = 700 \text{ lb}$$
$$p_1 = p_2 = \frac{M}{H} = \frac{770}{.700} = 1,100 \text{ lb}.$$

Combining these values vectorially (by the Pythagorean theorem), the resultant shearing forces of fasteners #1 and #2 are determined:

$$p_s = ({v_1}^2 + {p_1}^2)^{1/2} = ({v_2}^2 + {p_2}^2)^{1/2} = \left[(700)^2 + (1,100)^2\right]^{1/2}$$
$$p_s = 1,304 \text{ lb}.$$

From this, the shearing and bearing failures of the tee clip, its fasteners, and attached intercostal are predicted:

Shearing failure of fasteners #1 and #2:

$$\text{Margin of Safety} = \text{M.S.} = \frac{P_{su}}{p_s k} - 1 = \frac{2,694}{1,304(1.15)} - 1 = +.80$$

where: $P_{su} = 2,694$ lb (see Fig. 5-27)
$p_s = 1,304$ lb
$k = 1.15$ (fitting factor used in joint and connection designs).

Bearing failure of the tee clip:

Since $F_{bru} > 1.5F_{bry}$, Eq. 3-3 is used to determine the allowable bearing force of the material P_{bru}.

$$P_{bru} = 1.5F_{bry}tD = 1.5(71,000)(.070)(.190) = 1,416 \text{ lb}$$

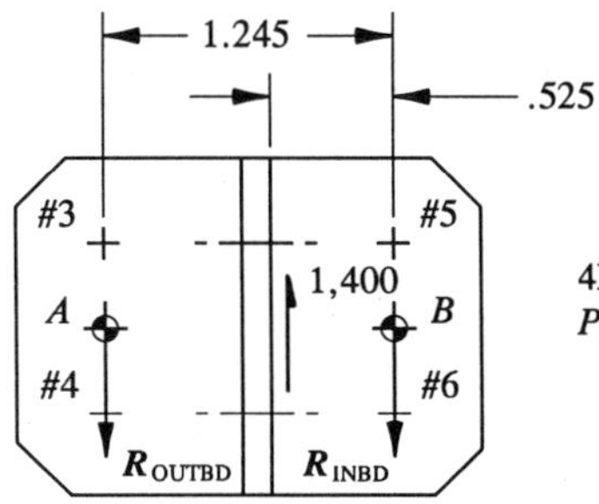

(a) View Looking FWD
(y-z plane)

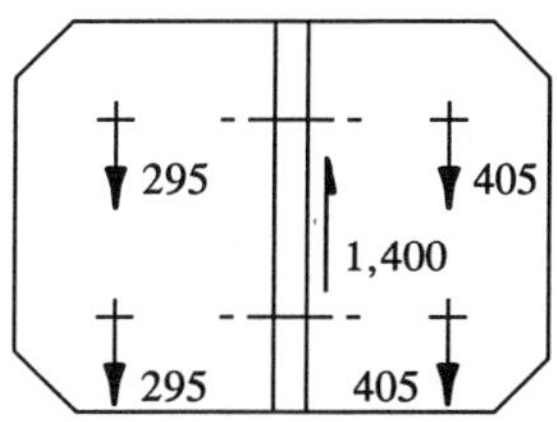

(b) View Looking FWD
(y-z plane)

FIGURE 5-28 (a) Centroid of each rivet group idealized as a point of support. (b) Distribution of vertical shear to the rivets in the y-z plane.

where: F_{bru} = 108 ksi (e/D = 2.0)
F_{bry} = 71 ksi (e/D = 2.0)
t = .070 in
D = .190 in (nominal shank diameter for a #10 diameter screw).

$$\text{Margin of Safety} = \text{M.S.} = \frac{P_{bru}}{p_s k} - 1 = \frac{1,416}{1,304(1.15)} - 1 = -.06.$$

Bearing failure of the intercostal:

This time, $F_{bru} < 1.5F_{bry}$, therefore, Eq. 3-2 is used to determine P_{bru}.

$$P_{bru} = F_{bru}tD = 99,000(.100)(.190) = 1,881 \text{ lb}$$

where: F_{bru} = 99 ksi (e/D = 2.0)
F_{bry} = 69 ksi (e/D = 2.0)
t = .100 in
D = .190 in (nominal shank diameter for a #10 diameter screw).

$$\text{Margin of Safety} = \text{M.S.} = \frac{P_{bru}}{p_s k} - 1 = \frac{1,881}{1,304(1.15)} - 1 = +.25.$$

Now, looking forward at the fixed-supported end (or y-z plane), Fig. 5-28(a), we obtain the following distribution of idealized shearing forces at the centroid of each rivet group:

$$R_{\text{OUTBD}} = 1,400\left[\frac{.525}{1.245}\right] = 590 \text{ lb} \quad (\text{from } \Sigma M_B = 0)$$

$$R_{\text{INBD}} = 1,400 - R_{\text{OUTBD}} = 1,400 - 590 = 810 \text{ lb} \quad (\text{from } \Sigma F_z = 0).$$

Distribution of these forces to the rivets of their respective rivet groups is then achieved as follows (see Fig. 5-28b):

$$v_3 = v_4 = \frac{590}{2} = 295 \text{ lb}$$

$$v_5 = v_6 = \frac{810}{2} = 405 \text{ lb}.$$

Shearing and bearing failures are then predicted for the critical rivets:

Shearing failure of rivets #5 and #6:

$$P_{su} = F_{su} A_{shr} C_r = 596(.995) = 593 \text{ lb}$$

where: $F_{su} A_{shr} = 596$ lb (from Table 3-1)
$C_r = .995$ (from Table 3-2 in .050 sheet thickness).

$$\text{Margin of Safety} = \text{M.S.} = \frac{P_{su}}{p_s k} - 1 = \frac{593}{405(1.15)} - 1 = +.27.$$

Bearing failure of the tee clip:

Here, $F_{bru} > 1.5 F_{bry}$, therefore, Eq. 3-3 is used again to determine P_{bru}.

$$P_{bru} = 1.5 F_{bry} t D = 1.5(71,000)(.050)(.159) = 847 \text{ lb}$$

where: $F_{bru} = 108,000$ psi $(e/D = 2.0)$
$F_{bry} = 71,000$ psi $(e/D = 2.0)$
$t = .050$ in
$D = .159$ in (nominal hole diameter for a BJ 5 rivet).

$$\text{Margin of Safety} = \text{M.S.} = \frac{P_{bru}}{p_s k} - 1 = \frac{847}{405(1.15)} - 1 = +.82.$$

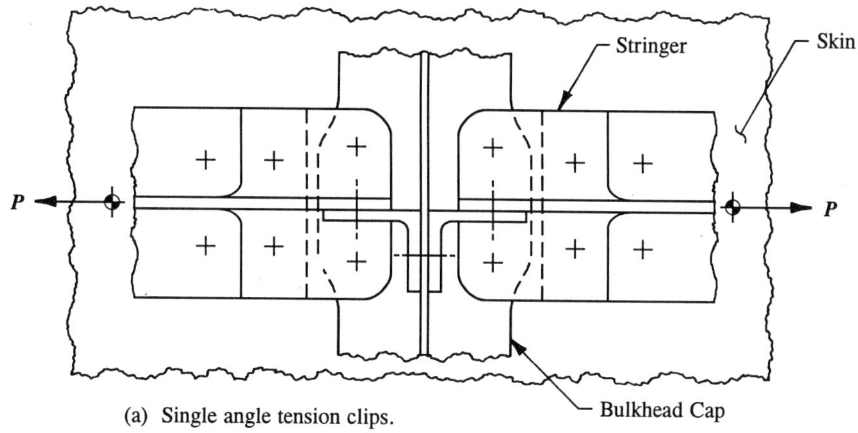

(a) Single angle tension clips.

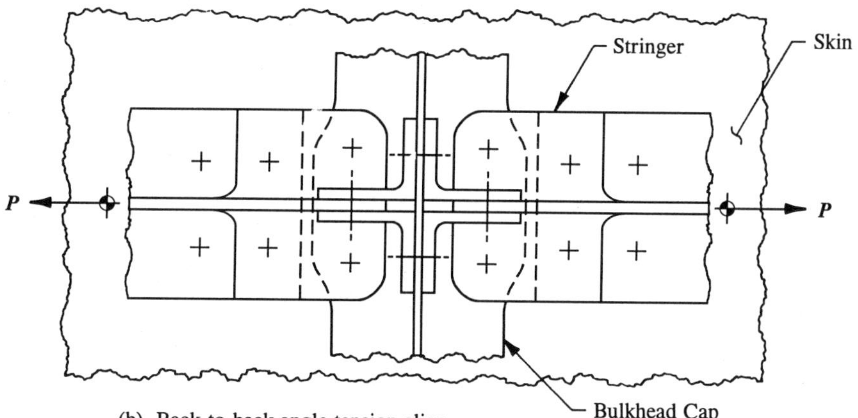

(b) Back-to-back angle tension clips.

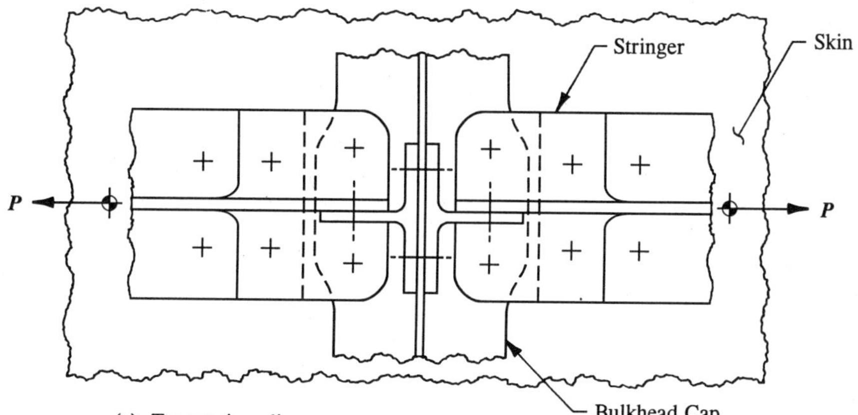

(c) Tee tension clips.

FIGURE 5-29 Tension clip supports using (a) a single angle clip, (b) back-to-back angle clips, and (c) a tee clip.

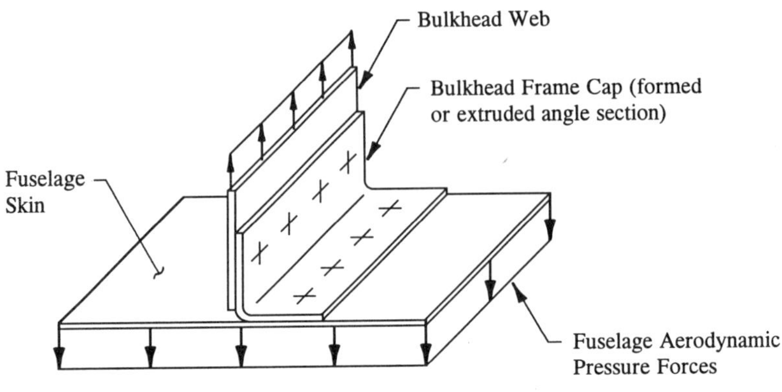

(a) Single angle tension clip.

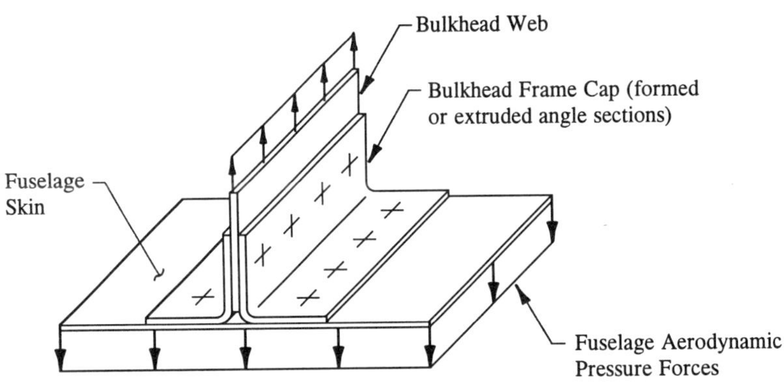

(b) Back-to-back angle tension clips.

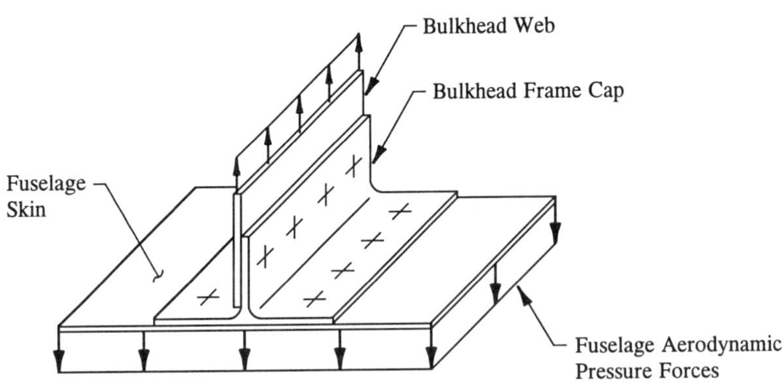

(c) Tee tension clip.

FIGURE 5-30 Continuous tension clip supports using (a) a single angle clip, (b) back-to-back angle clips, and (c) a tee clip.

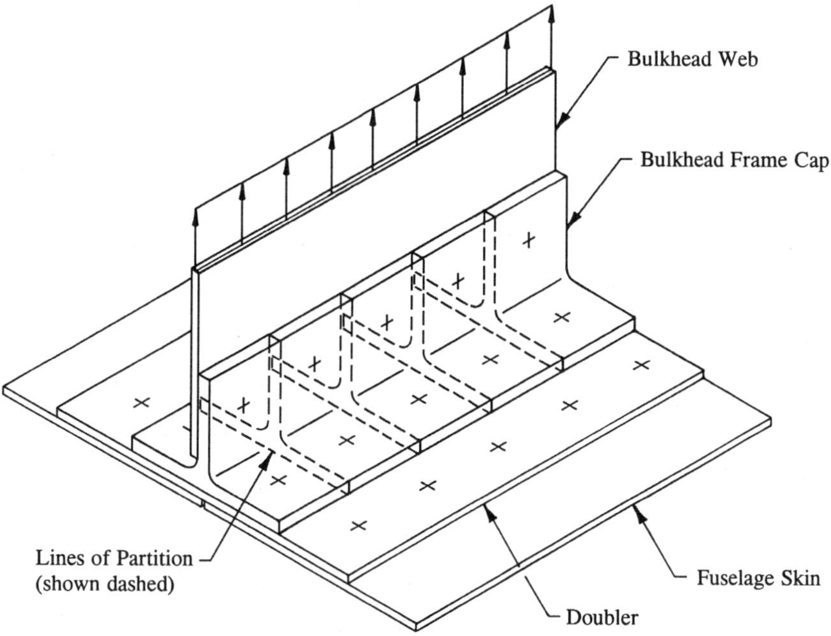

FIGURE 5-31 Bulkhead cap partitioned into tee tension clip members.

Bearing failure of the floor beam:

Inasmuch as $F_{bru} < 1.5F_{bry}$, Eq. 3-2 is used to compute P_{bru}.

$$P_{bru} = F_{bru}\,tD = 129,000(.080)(.159) = 1,641 \text{ lb}$$

where: $F_{bru} = 129,000$ psi ($e/D = 2.0$)
$F_{bry} = 97,000$ psi ($e/D = 2.0$)
$t = .080$ in
$D = .159$ in (nominal hole diameter for a BJ 5 rivet).

$$\text{Margin of Safety} = \text{M.S.} = \frac{P_{bru}}{p_s k} - 1 = \frac{1,641}{405(1.15)} - 1 = +2.52.$$

5.3 Design and Analysis of Tension Clip Supports. Tension clips may occur in many different types of aircraft structures. Three basic cross-sectional areas are considered in this section for their design: (1) single angle clips, (2) back-to-back angle clips, and (3) tee clips. Their structural applications are illustrated in Fig. 5-29. They require the same detailing as do the main structural members of a primary structure. Tension clips are primarily used to join one structural member to

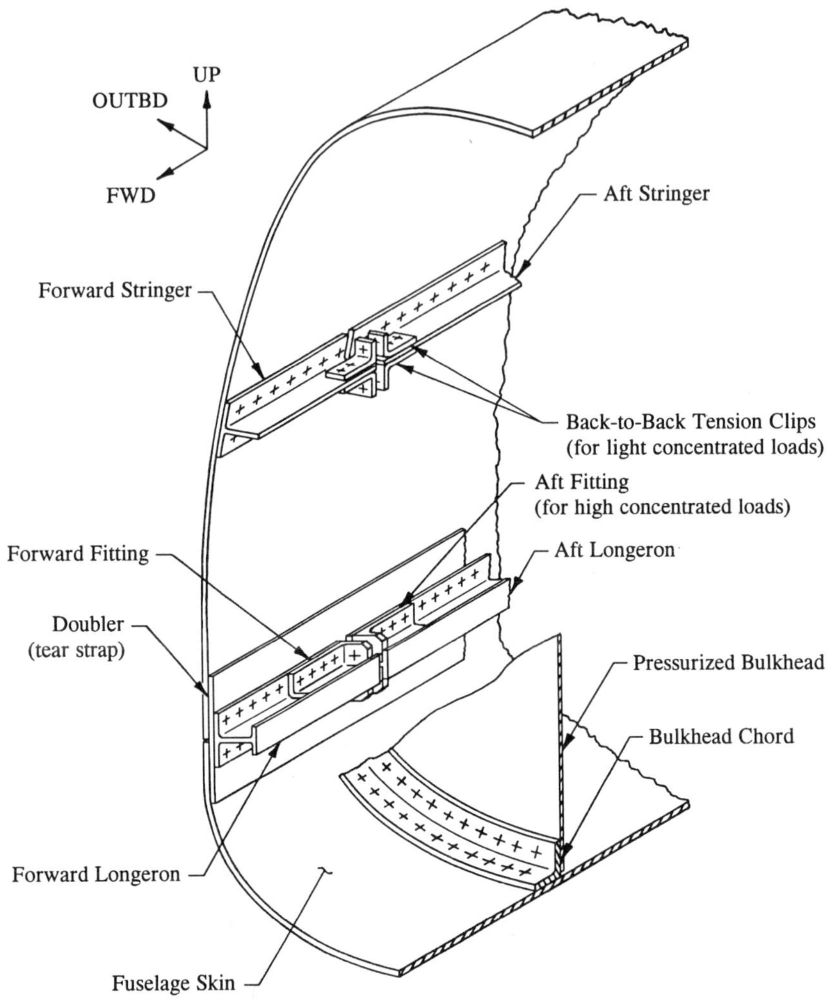

FIGURE 5-32 Diagram shows back-to-back tension clips and angle fittings used to splice members across a pressure bulkhead (simplified structure shown).

another. In so doing, they provide a continuous load path for the joined members to carry axial tension loads across their joint. Tension clips can also exist as very long continuous members. A bulkhead frame cap, for example, is just such a member, as shown in Fig. 5-30. Here the aerodynamic outward pressure forces on the surface of the fuselage skin will produce tension forces through the bulkhead frame cap. To analyze this member as a tension clip, the frame cap is partitioned into individual tension clip members as shown in Fig. 5-31.

For the most part, a tension clip is an inefficient splicing member that is primarily used in smaller load applications. For larger load applications, machined

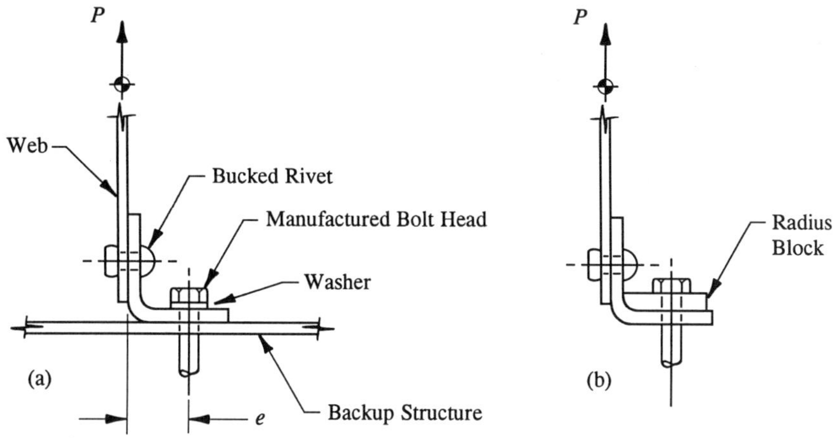

FIGURE 5-33 (a) Single angle tension clip is loaded in the plane of the web. (b) Radius block is used to reinforce the tension clip.

fittings or "bathtub" fittings are usually recommended for design. Fittings will satisfy maximum strength and stiffness requirements of the structure better at higher design loads.

If a structure, like a pressurized bulkhead, cannot be physically cut out to allow access or penetration of an axially loaded tension member, the engineer should consider back-to-back angle tension clips, or maybe heavy fittings, such as bathtub fittings, to carry the axial tension loads across the pressurized structure. This condition is illustrated in Fig. 5-32, where tension clips and bathtub fittings are used here as intermediary members to transfer axial tension loads from one side of the bulkhead to the other without having to physically cut out the bulkhead structure itself. If, however, certain design parameters do not permit the use of bathtub fittings, the following industry-accepted method of analysis for the design of tension clips is given to help illustrate their straightforward design solution.

In all applications of tension, only tension bolts rather than rivets should be used where tension clips are employed for design. Bolt heads or washer edges should be located as close as possible to the tangency points of the fillet radii of extruded angles and bend radii of formed sheet metal angles. This will reduce excessive deflections that might not otherwise be acceptable for design use. In addition, the relative stiffness of a tension clip should be made to match as close as is practically possible to its backup structure. Also, the FAA requires a fitting factor of 1.15 to be applied to each fitting (tension clip), its means of attachment, and the bearing upon the joined members when no form of structural testing has been proved for the structural members. In addition to a fitting factor of 1.15 for the members analyzed, a 20% minimum margin of safety should be maintained for each tension clip design.

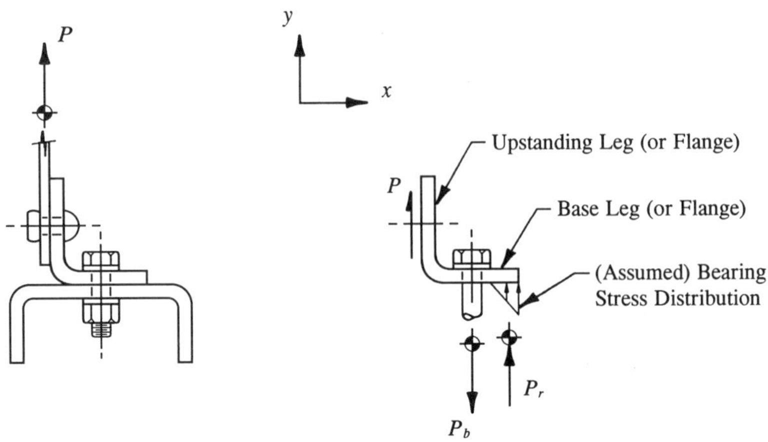

FIGURE 5-34 Equilibrium forces necessary to balance the tension clip are indicated.

In this section, our main emphasis of study will focus on the determination of the flange bending strength of basic tension clip designs. In some cases, however, if a small bolt is used with a thick tension clip design, the bolt may actually fail before flange bending failure of the base flange occurs.[1] Conversely, however, if a large bolt is used with a thin tension clip design, the clip (or base flange) may actually fail before the bolt even begins to yield, yet alone fail. The latter condition (large bolt, thin clip) will be the main focus of attention considered here in this section for the design of tension clip members.

A typical single angle tension clip is diagrammed in Fig. 5-33(a). The tension force P is applied in the plane of one flange and reacted by the base flange of the other. To prevent undue flange bending, tension bolts no smaller than a ¼-inch in diameter should be installed. To increase the overall efficiency of the tension clip, the bolt should be installed with the manufactured head on the inside of the clip. A washer under the manufactured head can also help to spread the load out over a larger surface area.

For higher load applications, a tension clip can be safely beefed up by using a radius block, as shown in Fig. 5-33(b). Rivets should not be used to carry primary tension loads. However, when rivets are unavoidably used in secondary tension load applications (such as those which may occur from panel buckling), their tension allowable strengths are based on the following design criteria:

(1) For protruding, shear-head rivets, use two-thirds (2/3) of the single-shear allowable strength of these rivets.

---

[1] See Sec. 5.4 for the analysis and design of tension bolts that may prematurely fail due to the effects of prying action in tension clip designs.

(2) For countersunk, shear-head rivets, use one-half (1/2) of the single-shear allowable strength of these rivets.

In Fig. 5-34, a single angle tension clip is isolated from its main structure and the equilibrium forces necessary to maintain equilibrium of this member are imposed. The prying load is developed from the bearing stresses that occur at the interface of the base leg of the tension clip and the backup structure. The engineer is referred specifically to Sec. 5.4, where the effects of this condition are fully treated. Until then, let us just say that the effects of prying action will always produce a bolt load that is greater than the applied load. From a statics solution of this tension clip, i.e., summing forces in the vertical direction, we can mathematically formulate an expression describing this additional effect on the bolt.

$$\Sigma F_y = 0, \qquad P - P_b + P_r = 0, \quad P_b = P + P_r$$

where: P = applied tension load
P_b = bolt tension load
P_r = prying load.

The magnitude of the prying force P_r will be investigated in the next section when our study of prying action will be incorporated with the analysis of the bolt.

Fatigue-life is always an important design consideration to the reliability and structural integrity of tension clips, not to be overlooked by the engineer. Tension clips are fatigue-sensitive members that require careful and precise planning of their designs. Where loads are cycled repeatedly from tension to compression, fatigue failure from the resulting alternating deflections of the tension clip may become critical—thus, fatigue failure may control its overall design. For such cases, the clip should be treated by designing for its life expectancy or fatigue-life rather than by its static strength. If tension clips are subjected to high repeated loads producing high deflections, the engineer should consider in these cases "bathtub" fittings.

Tension clips made from tee-shaped extruded sections, Fig. 5-29(c), are unquestionably the most efficient of the proposed tension clip designs. Maximum strength and stiffness are greatest for these types for any given thickness. Additionally, use tension bolts to increase stiffness and strength of the basic clip design. Otherwise, use monel rivets and carefully check the prying loads on the fastener while maintaining a conservative margin of safety in tension for the overall design. Aluminum rivets are definitely an inferior design alternative and should not be considered for practical design use, if possible.

The analysis of tension clip supports in this section will be determined by conventional stress analysis methods, i.e., from basic principles. This means isolating the tension clip from its main structure with all the applied and reactive loads correctly indicated. To the balanced structure, section cuts are taken to locate the critical bending section. Bending stresses across the critical section are determined using Mc/I_{na}. Next, the ultimate allowable bending stress F_{bu} of the material is determined and a margin of safety is written for the critical section. The analysis and procedure for determining the inelastic design of bending members is given in Appendix J (the engineer is encouraged to review this material before proceeding ahead with the remaining material of this chapter).

Some aerospace companies have developed from tests parametric design curves for the solution of tension clip supports. Although these design curves can provide a quick and reliable way of determining the structural integrity of a member, they do provide some limitations to the analysis of more general design cases. The engineer should consult with his stress department to verify the use of these curves for the analysis of tension clip supports. Some aerospace companies may stipulate other design methodologies to use for their design; it may therefore be prudent to personally verify their universal acceptability and inclusion before such curves are actually utilized in the design of tension clip supports. Use the approved method of analysis that has been recommended by your structural engineering department. Although parametric design curves are used throughout the aerospace industry, and are appropriate to the analysis of most tension clip designs, their acceptability to the design of tension clips must still be overseen by those in charge of determining such matters. The examples which follow will best illustrate the solution of tension clip supports by conventional stress analysis methods.

Example 5-4 Single angle clips are used to splice a stringer across a fuel-cell bulkhead as shown in Fig. 5-35. If the stringer carries an axial tension load of 392 lb limit, 549 lb ultimate, determine the bending strength of the attached angle clips. Consider the load transfer through the stringer splice with and without a wing transverse skin splice. Assume an effective width of skin of 5.5 in. Also investigate other possible failure modes that may occur for this joint. The attached angle clips are dimensioned as shown in Fig. 5-36. The stringer load, determined from a computer model analysis solution of this joint, also includes the axial tension load that is carried by the skin. For this analysis, consider a design load factor of 1.4 and a fitting factor of 1.15 for commercial aircraft design. Assume $2D$ edge distance and a bolt head of .483 for the ¼ diameter tension bolts. Mechanical properties for clad 2024-T3: F_{tu} = 59,000 psi (LT), f_0 = 50,500 psi (LT); F_{ty} = 39,000 psi (LT), f_0 = 17,500 psi (LT).

SOLUTION: First part of this solution (with a wing transverse skin splice): The solution of this problem is straightforward. The skin and stringer are discontinuous members across the bulkhead structure; therefore, the axial tension load that each member carries must be transferred through the tension clips across the bulkhead. And since, the stringer load given in this problem also includes the load carried by the skin, it is this load that corresponds to the combined axial tension load of these members or P = 549 lb ultimate. In other words, the stringer load is actually made up of two component parts; the first being carried by the skin and the second part being carried by the stringer. The basis of this reasoning is basically how the

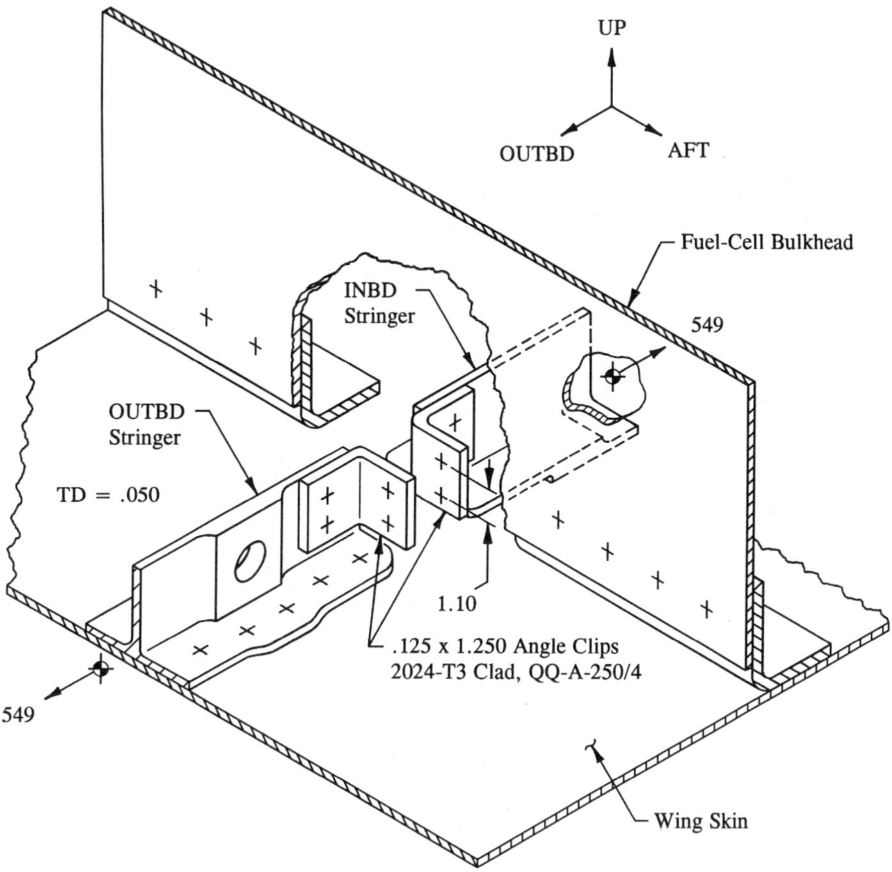

FIGURE 5-35 Single angle clips across a fuel-cell bulkhead.

analysis solution of the second part of this example will also be approached. Mathematically, this says that

$$P = P_{\text{skin}} + P_{\text{stringer}} \tag{5-1}$$

where: P = combined axial tension load (given)
P_{skin} = load carried by the skin
P_{stringer} = load carried by the stringer.

The transfer of load across the joint is shown in Fig. 5-37.

To analyze the tension clip support for bending strength, its structural configuration must first be partitioned into two identical tension clip supports. This is accomplished as was previously described in this section for continuous tension

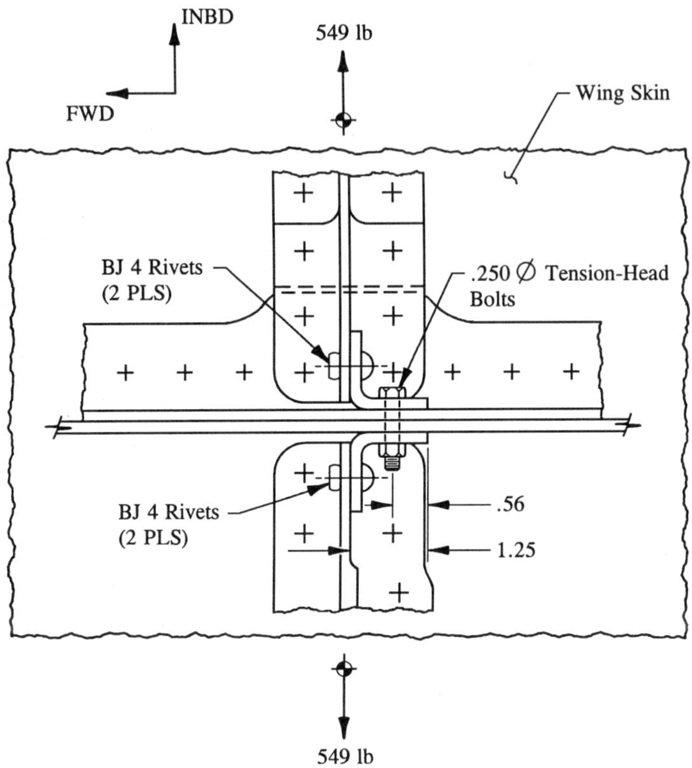

FIGURE 5-36 View looking down across the fuel-cell bulkhead.

clip supports. One of the isolated tension clips is then free-bodied with the applied and reactive forces indicated on its structure (see ahead to Fig. 5-41). The critical section of the tension clip is located at the inside edge of the bolt head where the internal bending moment along the base flange of the tension clip is a maximum. After a discussion of prying forces has been presented in the next section, the engineer is encouraged to again review the solution of this problem and verify on his own the location of this critical section. Bending stresses are calculated at the critical section as follows:

$$f_b = \frac{Mc}{I_{na}} = \frac{123(\frac{.125}{2})}{.0001709} = 44{,}982 \text{ psi ult; } 32{,}130 \text{ psi limit}$$

where: $M = 274(1.25 - .56 - \frac{.483}{2}) = 123$ in-lb ult

$$c = \frac{.125}{2} = .0625 \text{ in}$$

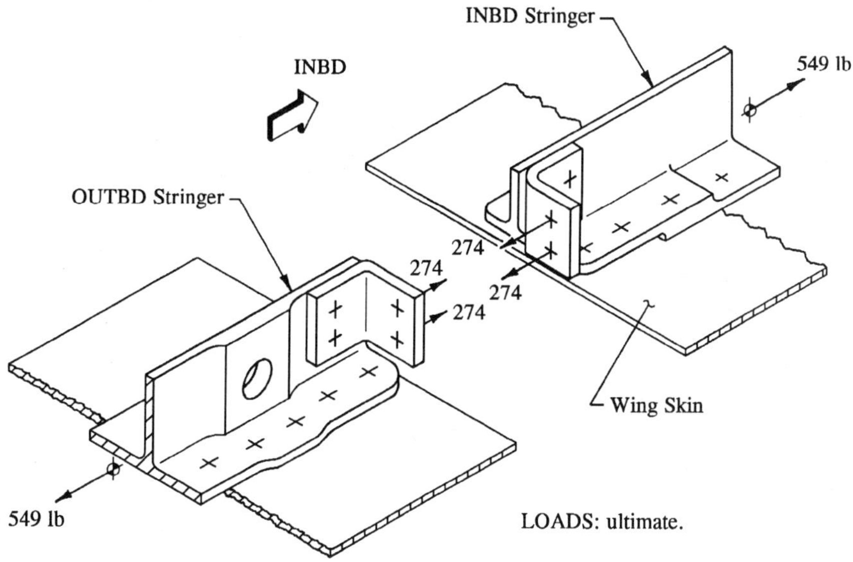

FIGURE 5-37 Distribution of stringer load to the tension bolts for a simplified wing transverse skin splice.

$$I_{na} = \frac{BH^3}{12} = \frac{1.05(.125)^3}{12} = .0001709 \text{ in}^4.$$

Precluding local instability, structural failure[1] of the tension clip will occur above the proportional limit stress of the material. For this reason, the ultimate bending stress allowable of the base flange is determined:

$$F_{bu} = f_m + f_0(K - 1) = 59,000 + 50,500(1.5 - 1) = 84,250 \text{ psi}.$$

The margin of safety for ultimate bending strength is then written as follows:

$$\text{Margin of Safety} = \text{M.S.} = \frac{F_{bu}}{f_b k} - 1 = \frac{84,250}{44,982(1.15)} - 1 = +.63.$$

Now, to meet permanent set requirements at limit load, the yield bending stress allowable of the tension clip is determined:

$$F_{by} = f_m + f_0(K - 1) = 39,000 + 17,500(1.5 - 1) = 47,750 \text{ psi}.$$

[1] Refer to Appendix J for a discussion of inelastic stress design of rectangular sections in bending.

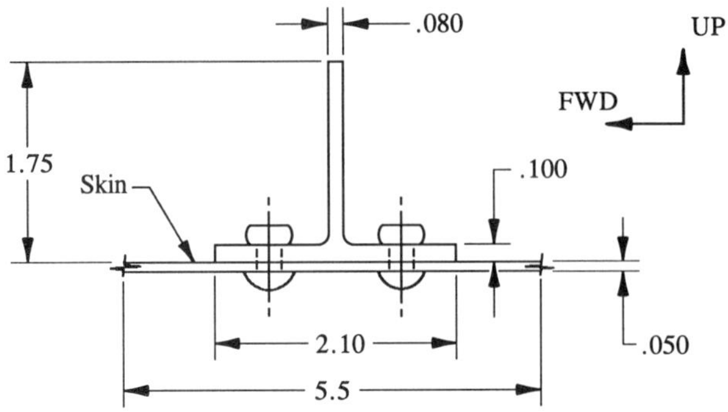

FIGURE 5-38 Stringer cross-sectional area.

Substituting this value into the margin of safety expression for the yield bending strength gives:

$$\text{Margin of Safety} = \text{M.S.} = \frac{F_{by}}{f_b k} - 1 = \frac{47,750}{32,130(1.15)} - 1 = +.29.$$

Analyzing structure from basic principles (as this problem has shown) will provide the engineer with the flexibility and increased confidence to analyze similar or related structures that one may encounter on-the-job.

Second part of this solution (without a wing transverse skin splice): In this solution, only the axial tension load that is carried by the stringer will be transferred across the bulkhead through the tension clips. The skin being a continuous member here will sustain its load across the bulkhead region. No transfer of load will occur for this member. (From axial stiffness considerations) a simple ratio of areas of the skin and stringer, Fig. 5-38, will suffice to determine the distribution of axial tension load P that is carried by each member. The axial tension load carried by the stringer is determined as follows:

$$P_{\text{stringer}} = P\left[\frac{A_{\text{stringer}}}{A_{\text{total}}}\right] = 549\left[\frac{.342}{.617}\right] = 304 \text{ lb ultimate; } 217 \text{ lb limit}$$

where: $A_{\text{stringer}} = 2.10(.100) + (1.75 - .100).080 = .342 \text{ in}^2$

$A_{\text{skin}} = 5.5(.050) = .275 \text{ in}^2$

$A_{\text{total}} = A_{\text{skin}} + A_{\text{stringer}} = .275 + .342 = .617 \text{ in}^2.$

And then, solving Eq. 5-1 for the axial tension load that is carried by the skin gives:

$$P_{\text{skin}} = P - P_{\text{stringer}} = 549 - 304 = 245 \text{ lb ultimate; } 175 \text{ lb limit.}$$

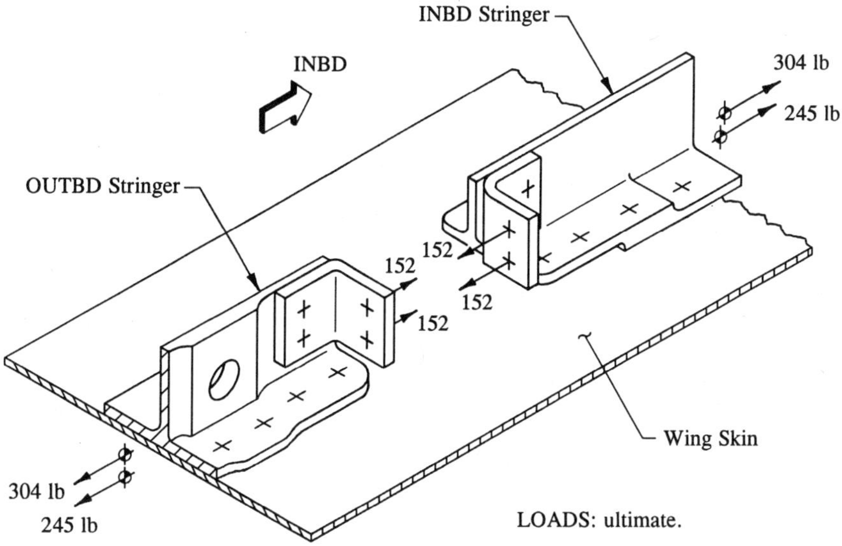

FIGURE 5-39 Distribution of stringer load to the tension bolts for a continuous wing skin.

The stringer axial tension load calculated on the previous page, as opposed to the one originally given in this problem, divides equally between the tension bolts as shown in Fig. 5-39.

$$p_t = \frac{P_{\text{stringer}}}{2} = \frac{304}{2} = 152 \text{ lb ultimate/bolt; } 109 \text{ lb limit/bolt.}$$

Comparing these loads with those of Fig. 5-37 clearly shows that the tension clip supports are now less critical. Consequently, no margins of safety need be written for flange bending failure since our previous solution would envelope our flange bending solution here. To summarize: This problem has shown that the skin is a significant load-carrying member in tension. To neglect its ability to carry load is to pay some weight penalty for the overall designed structure, in this case, the tension clip supports.

Ultimate Tension Failure of the Skin and Stringer Combination:

Here, the ultimate strength of the skin and stringer in tension will correspond to the sum of the material strengths of the individual members making up the total section area. Equation 3-6 is used to formulate a general expression for the actual computation of this quantity.

$$(P_t)_{\text{net}} = (F_{tu}A)_{\text{stringer}} + (F_{tu}A)_{\text{skin}}$$

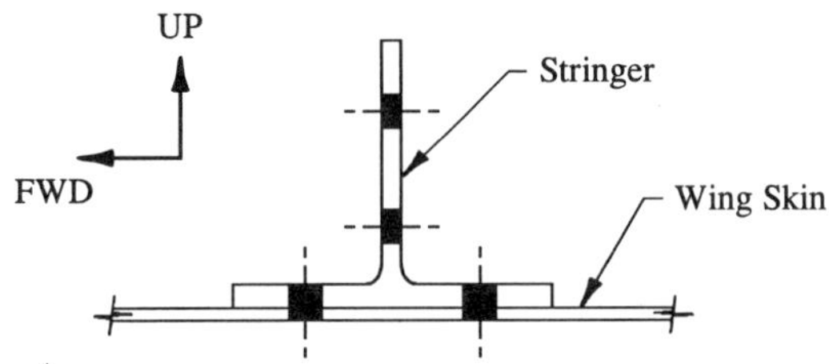

FIGURE 5-40 Tension failure of the skin and stringer combination. Shaded portions of the section area are assumed to be ineffective in carrying axial tension loads.

where: F_{tu} = ultimate allowable tension stress of the material
A_{net} = net cross-sectional area (see Fig. 5-40).

The margin of safety for tension failure of the skin and stringer (in composite) is written as follows:

$$\text{Margin of Safety} = \text{M.S.} = \frac{(P_t)_{\text{net}}}{p_t} - 1$$

where p_t = 549 lb ultimate (given).

Other structural checks required include: (1) shearing failure of the rivets, (2) bearing failure of the tension clip, (3) bearing failure of the stringer, and (4) bolt tension failure due to prying effects, see Fig. 5-41.

Example 5-5 The engine compartment is housed by an aluminum cowling as shown in Fig. 5-42. For the outward differential pressure distribution given on the surface of the cowling, determine the ultimate bending failure of the firewall beam cap. The cap is composed of formed sheet metal angles made of clad 2024-T3 aluminum alloy sheet material. See Fuselage Station 40 in Fig. 5-43 for specific drawing details. Consider a fitting factor of 1.15 for commercial aircraft design. From a general policy directive of tension clip members, also include the additional requirement that the members be able to maintain an overall margin of safety of 20%. Mechanical properties for clad 2024-T3: F_{tu} = 59,000 (LT), F_{ty} = 39,000 (LT), and F_{cy} = 42,000 (LT). Since the value of f_0 is not given in this problem for this material, the engineer can approximate this value by using the lower value of F_{ty} or F_{cy}.

SOLUTION: A simple engineering technique often used by the engineer in his approach to a mathematically complex loading solution is employed here in the solution of this problem. Although the aerodynamic pressure loading occurs

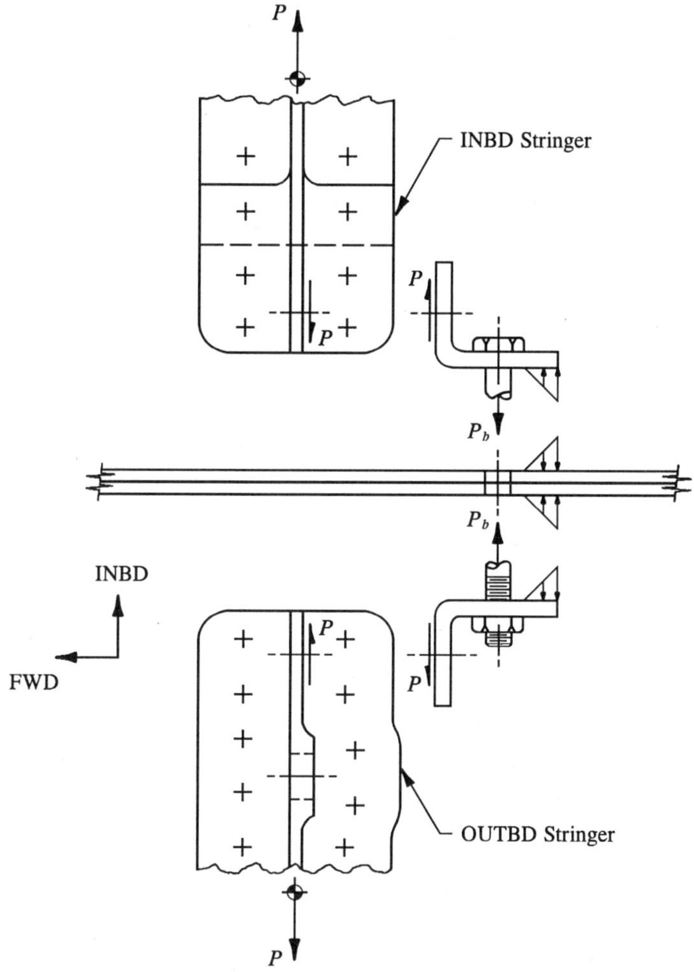

FIGURE 5-41 Bolt tension failure due to prying effects (see analysis procedure in Sec. 5.4).

completely around the cowling, the engineer only needs to consider a "finite strip of loading," usually unity in his analysis approach. Of course, any size strip of loading could be used since one particular strip of loading can always be converted to another equivalent strip of loading later in the analysis, if needed.

Let us now proceed on a logical and rational basis by taking a 1.40 in strip of pressure loading under consideration, as shown in Fig. 5-44. This is done because the fasteners (probably, airlocs) are also spaced 1.40 in apart themselves. Each strip of pressure loading will then represent the loading carried by each bolt along the boundary of the firewall structure. If the structure (beam flanges) can then be

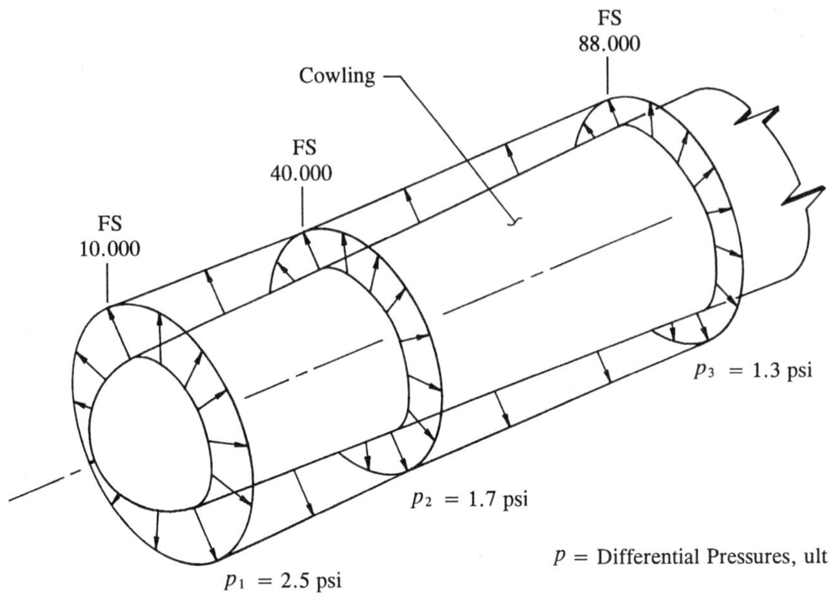

FIGURE 5-42 Cowling simplified airload distribution.

shown to be of adequate structural strength for the 1.40 in strip of loading per bolt considered, then the many other 1.40 in strips per bolt that make up the complete aerodynamic pressure loading around the fuselage structure will also be substantiated. Since the concept of pressure loading can sometimes be rather nebulous (confusing or difficult to deal with), let us instead replace such a loading by a distributed load acting along the 1.40 in strip of pressure loading. If we do this, we obtain the following peak distributions in a more convenient form:

$$w_1 = p_1(1.40) = 2.5(1.40) = 3.50 \text{ lb/in ult}$$

$$w_2 = p_2(1.40) = 1.7(1.40) = 2.38 \text{ lb/in ult}$$

$$w_3 = p_3(1.40) = 1.3(1.40) = 1.82 \text{ lb/in ult.}$$

From these loads, the reaction shears R_1, R_{fwd}, R_{aft}, and R_2 at Fuselage Stations FS 19, FS 40, FS 40 and FS 88, respectively, can be determined (refer to the loading schedule of Fig. 5-44). Next, the solution is separated into a two-part problem: (1) the strip loading between FS 10 and FS 40, or Bay #1 and (2) the strip loading between FS 40 and FS 88, or Bay #2. The trapezoidal loading that each strip carries in each bay is separated further into two convenient loading types, i.e., into triangular and rectangular loading distributions, as shown in Fig. 5-45. These distributions are then represented as equivalent concentrated loads acting at the center of pressure of their particular loading areas. This gives:

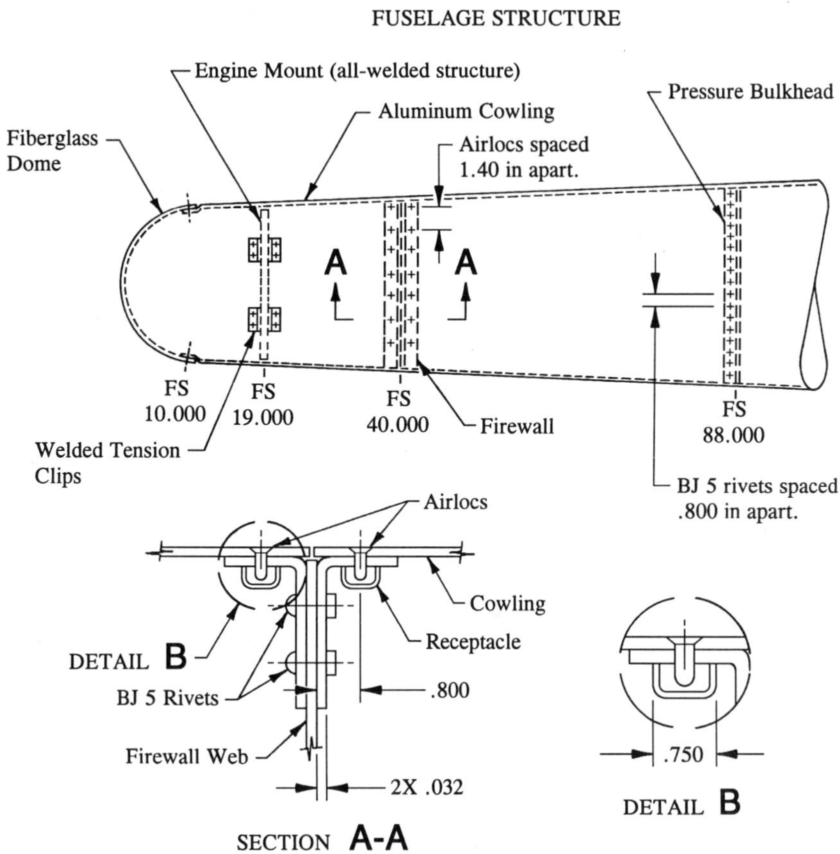

FIGURE 5-43 Engine compartment is shown housed in an aluminum cowling.

$$
\begin{aligned}
P_1 &= \tfrac{1}{2}(30)(3.50 - 2.38) = 16.8 \text{ lb} \\
P_2 &= 30(2.38) = 71.4 \text{ lb} \\
P_3 &= \tfrac{1}{2}(48)(2.38 - 1.82) = 13.4 \text{ lb} \\
P_4 &= 48(1.82) = 87.4 \text{ lb.}
\end{aligned}
$$

If we treat the 1.40 in strip of loading in each bay as a separate beam, the following shear reactions, from statics, are determined:

Shear Reactions (Bay #1):

$$
\Sigma M_A = 0, \quad (\overset{\curvearrowleft}{+}) \quad -16.8(1) - 71.4(6) + R_{fwd}(21) = 0
$$
$$
R_{fwd} = 21.2 \text{ lb/bolt}
$$

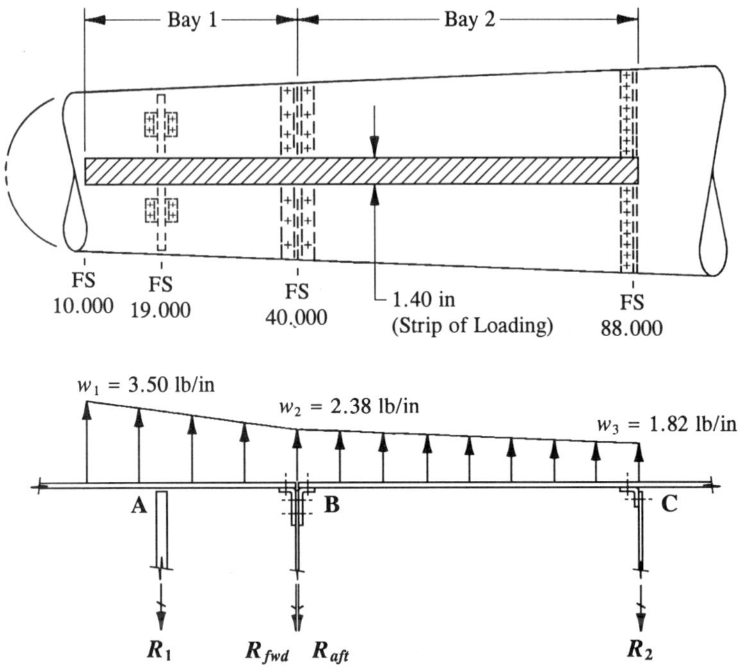

FIGURE 5-44 A strip of loading 1.40 in wide is taken to idealize the aerodynamic pressure loading around the fuselage shell.

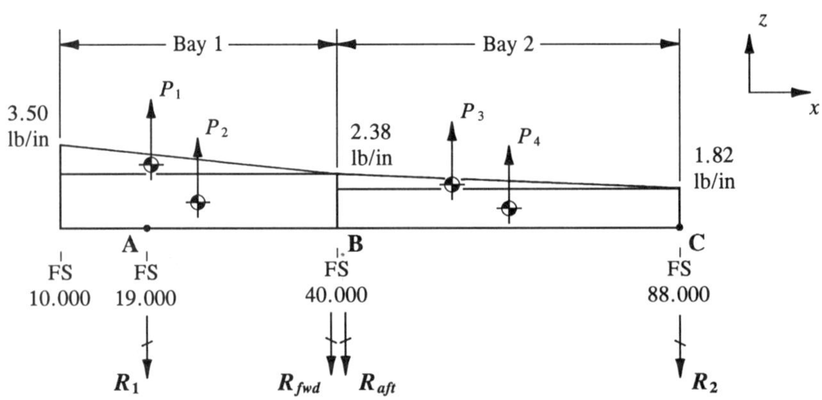

FIGURE 5-45 Separation of trapezoidal loading into two separate loading types: (a) the uniformly distributed load and (b) the uniformly varying distributed load.

and, from

$$\Sigma F_z = 0, \qquad -R_1 + 16.8 + 71.4 - R_{fwd} = 0.$$

Substituting R_{fwd} into this equation and solving for R_1 gives:

$$R_1 = 67.0 \text{ lb/bolt}.$$

Shear Reactions (Bay #2):

$$\Sigma M_C = 0, \qquad \circlearrowleft{+} \qquad -R_{aft}(48) + 13.4(32) + 87.4(24) = 0$$

$$R_{aft} = 52.6 \text{ lb/bolt}$$

and, from

$$\Sigma F_z = 0, \qquad -R_{aft} + 13.4 + 87.4 - R_2 = 0.$$

Substituting R_{aft} into this equation and solving for R_2 gives:

$$R_2 = 48.2 \text{ lb/bolt}.$$

Generally speaking, back-to-back tension clips are more efficient by virtue of their geometrically more efficient structural configuration. The reason is that the opposite tension clip provides some restraint for the other angle. The increased stiffness at their interface essentially helps to minimize the moments that develop in their base flanges. This has been verified by tests that have shown that symmetrically loaded back-to-back angle clips are actually 25% stronger than the sum of their individual strengths when these members act separately. Since $R_{fwd} \neq R_{aft}$, the angles are not loaded symmetrically. And, therefore, the unbalanced moment created by their dissimilar loads on the firewall cap is treated by analyzing each angle separately, as shown in Fig. 5-46. However, only the aft angle of the firewall cap needs to be analyzed for our solution here since the forward angle is considerably less critical and therefore, structurally, should be enveloped by the other (angle).

To predict ultimate failure, the allowable bending stress of the material is computed (see Eq. A-18 and discussion of inelastic bending in Appendix J):

$$F_{bu} = f_m + f_0(K - 1) = 59,000 + 39,000(1.5 - 1) = 78,500 \text{ psi}$$

where: $f_m = F_{tu} = 59,000$ psi
$f_0 = F_{ty} = 39,000$ psi (this value is approximated by using the value of F_{ty})
$K = 1.5$ for a rectangular section.

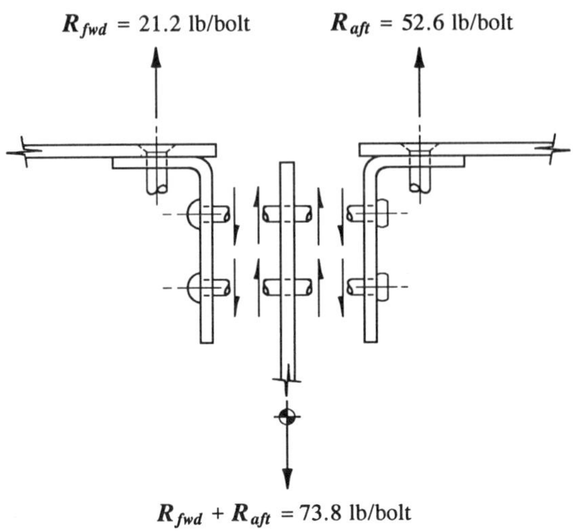

FIGURE 5-46 Unbalanced moment created by the dissimilar loads on the firewall cap is treated by analyzing each angle separately.

The flange bending stress is calculated for the critical section:

$$f_b = \frac{Mc}{I_{na}} = \frac{22.4(.016)}{.000003823} = 93,748 \text{ psi ult}$$

where: $M = R_{aft}(.800 - \frac{.750}{2}) = 52.6(.425) = 22.4$ in-lb ult

$R_{aft} = 52.6$ lb/bolt (see Fig. 5-46)

$c = \frac{.032}{2} = .016$ in

$I_{na} = \frac{bh^3}{12} = \frac{1.40(.032)^3}{12} = .000003823 \text{ in}^4.$

To predict the ultimate failure of the aft angle, the following expression is written:

$$\text{Margin of Safety} = \text{M.S.} = \frac{F_{bu}}{f_b k} - 1 = \frac{78,500}{93,748(1.15)} - 1 = -.27.$$

This is not exactly a perfect design! How then can this design be improved? Let us look at one possible solution: if the thickness of the angles are increased. How can we pinpoint the required thickness to meet the particular design requirements of this problem? The easiest and most direct way of determining the thickness dimension t is to solve for this value in the margin of safety expression for ultimate bending failure. This will avoid a trial-and-error approach to the analysis and thereby simplify the solution to this problem. All terms in this equation containing the variable t and design requirements of the problem must be included. Hence

$$\text{Margin of Safety} = \text{M.S.} = \frac{F_{bu}}{f_b(1.15)} - 1 = +.20.$$

From definitions, we have $f_b = Mc/I_{na} = 6M/bt^2$, where $c = t/2$ and $I_{na} = bt^3/12$. Now, substituting this and all known values into the above equation and solving for the required thickness, we obtain:

$$\begin{aligned} F_{bu} &= f_b(1.15)(1.20) \\ 78,500 &= \frac{6M}{bt^2}(1.15)(1.20) \\ t^2 &= .00169 \\ t &= .041 \text{ in} \end{aligned}$$

where: $F_{bu} = 78,500$ psi (from page 335)
$M = 22.4$ in-lb ult
$b = 1.40$ in.

The engineer is encouraged to investigate other possible redesign alternatives, such as changes in material, additional beef up, etc., that may also influence dramatically the acceptable design choices of this problem. For example, a material change of a higher strength in tension in the longitudinal transverse (LT) grain direction can also effectively increase the overall allowable bending strength of the firewall cap. Perhaps it would, but, in the long run, would it be less costly for production design?

5.4 Prying Action of Tension Members. Thus far in our study of tension clip supports, we have primarily concerned ourselves with flange bending failure. This was done using conventional stress analysis methods of the previous section. Also important to a successful design of a tension clip is the ultimate strength in tension of the attachment bolt, as shown in Fig. 5-47(a). Tension bolts are commonly used in the design of tension clips to prevent premature clip failure. Their usage, however, is limited to bolts equal to or greater than a ¼-inch in diameter. In some applications, steel (monel) rivets are permissible if their usage is principally limited to very light tension load applications. For example, in the case of light equipment mounting brackets, such as those used for the purpose of supporting electrical and mechanical equipment, electrical wiring harnesses, fuel lines, etc., their usage is acceptable. Steel rivets should only be used when tension bolts are uneconomical to use in production.

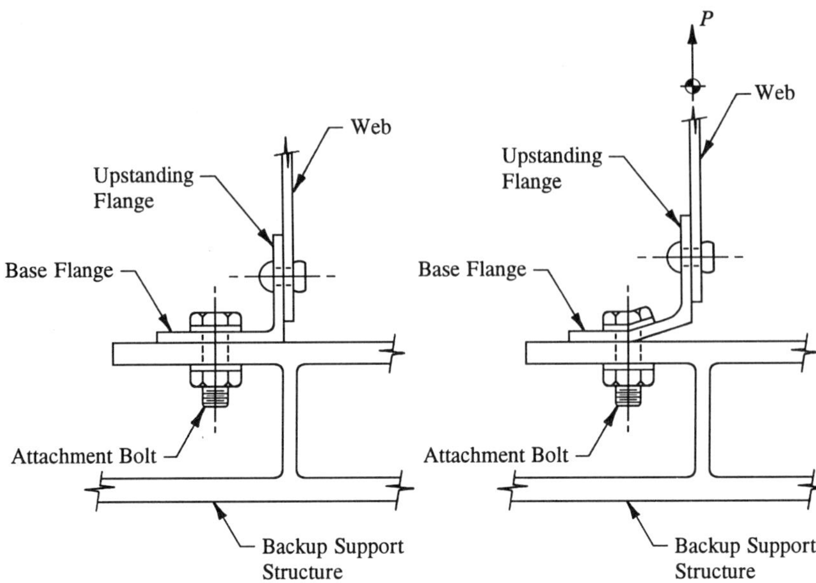

(a) Unloaded Tension Clip

(b) Deflected Shape of a Loaded Tension Clip

FIGURE 5-47 (a) Unloaded tension clip. (b) Criticality of the attachment bolt in a loaded tension clip.

Prying action, sometimes referred to as "heel-and-toe action," is a term used to describe the bearing stresses that develop between the thick base flange of an axially loaded tension clip or fitting and its backup support structure. For example, when the tension clip of Fig. 5-47(b) rotates, a prying force is produced on the base flange of the tension clip as well as on the backup support structure, as shown in Fig. 5-48. The bolt is designed for the applied load plus the prying force developed between the mating surfaces of the joined members. Here, the backup support structure to which the tension clip is attached must also sustain the prying loads applied to it. The bearing distribution from these prying effects is assumed to be linear from a peak at the end of the base flange (or toe) to zero at the edge of the washer. However, if no washer is used, the bearing distribution is assumed to bear out at the edge of the bolt head. The opening effect of the tension clip causes an increased tension load in the bolt. To view this mathematically, the tension clip is isolated and the forces necessary to balance this member are applied. Using the equations of static equilibrium, the true bolt load P_b is found:

$$\Sigma M_{CL} = 0, \quad \circlearrowleft + \quad P_r b - Pa = 0$$

$$P_r = \frac{Pa}{b}. \tag{5-2}$$

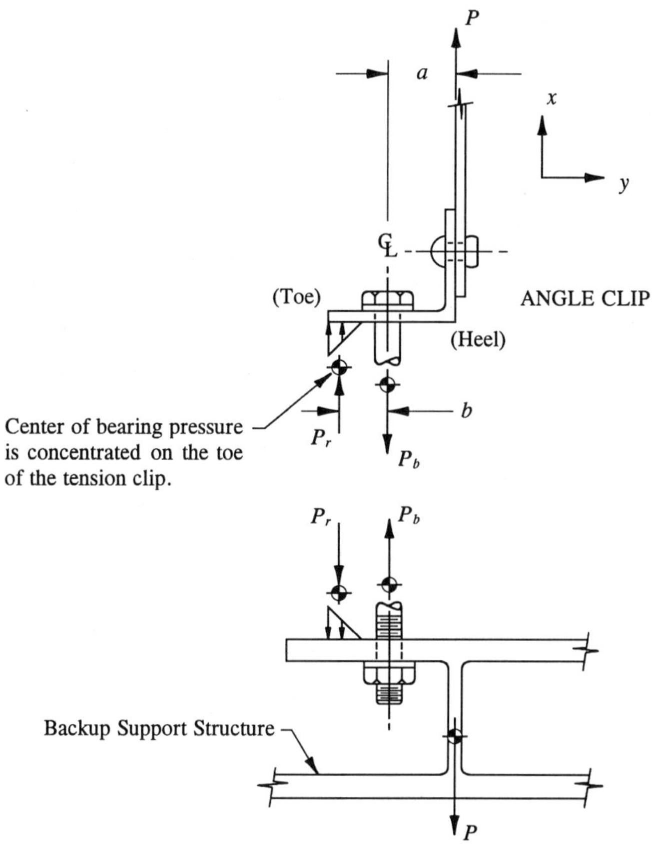

FIGURE 5-48 Prying forces are shown produced on the base flange of the tension clip and backup support structure.

$$\Sigma F_x = 0, \qquad P_r - P_b + P = 0$$

$$P_b = P + P_r. \tag{5-3}$$

Expressed in words, Eq. 5-3 states that the axial tension force in the bolt consists of two parts: namely, the applied force P and the prying force P_r due to flange bending of the base flange. Hence, the prying force will always produce a bolt load that is greater than the applied load. The additional increase in bolt load exerted by the prying force is why a small tension bolt may sometimes fail in tension before a thick tension clip will actually fail in bending of its base flange. Therefore, since the fastener may actually control the basic design of the tension clip as a result of this condition, where possible, tension attachments (or bolts) should be used. Substituting Eq. 5-2 into Eq. 5-3, we obtain:

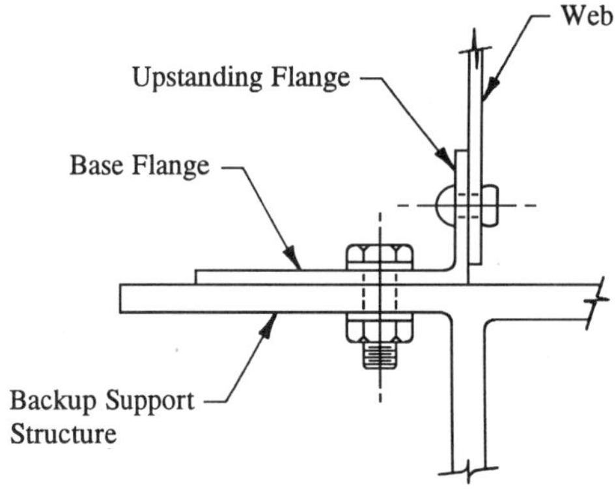

FIGURE 5-49 Exaggerated length of a base flange of a tension clip.

$$P_b = P + \frac{Pa}{b} = P\left[1 + \frac{a}{b}\right] \tag{5-4}$$

where: P_b = bolt load (this includes the prying force)
P = applied tension load
a = distance measured from the shear plane of the upstanding leg to the centerline of the base flange bolt
b = distance measured from the center of bearing pressure of the prying force distribution to the centerline of the base flange bolt.

Let us now look at a special case, where the base flange of a tension clip is made very long and thin, perhaps even to the extent of exaggerating its extended length as shown in Fig. 5-49. When a tension load P is applied, as shown in Fig. 5-50, the clip and supporting structure will simultaneously feel the increasing prying force at the interface or mating surfaces. Under very light loading, though, even this exaggerated design can produce a prying distribution that agrees reasonably well with previously observed theoretical predictions. Realistically, however, as the tension load P is increased to ultimate design levels, the picture of redistribution can radically change, as viewed in Fig. 5-51, where the center of bearing pressure of the prying force distribution actually shifts closer to the bolt location. This natural propensity to curl or lift up at higher loads is precisely why a more rational appraisal of the actual prying distribution of a thin base flange is needed. Essentially, some portion of the flange area must be considered ineffective in resisting flange bending loads. Engineering judgment based on past engineering experience will ultimately dictate the proper amount to consider for each particular design case. How much is shown shaded in this same figure.

In general, most aerospace structures are designed to be compact. Assuming they are, a tension clip design will have no more than *3D* edge distance for the

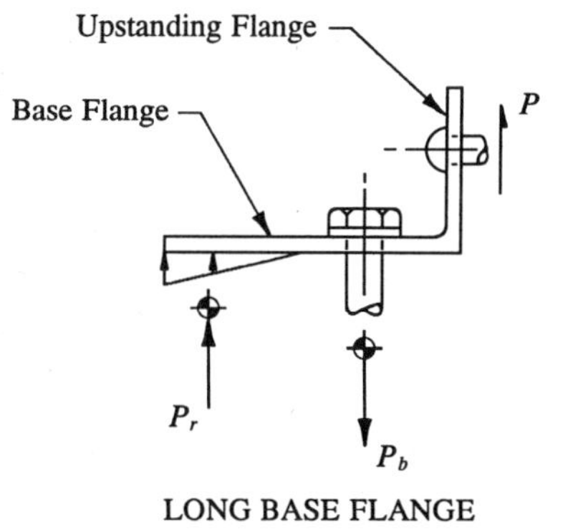

FIGURE 5-50 Tension clip under very light loading.

attachment bolt used in relatively thin base flanges, say, $t < .125$ in. For most designs, however, an edge distance of $2D$ is normally recommended and, therefore, if used, should eliminate the uncertainty and ambiguity of how actual prying (or bearing) distribution of the base flange is distributed. Failure of the bolt is predicted as follows:

$$\text{Margin of Safety} = \text{M.S.} = \frac{P_{tu}}{P_b k} - 1$$

where: P_{tu} = ultimate allowable tension strength of the bolt
P_b = bolt load (this includes the prying force)
k = 1.15 (fitting factor used in joint and connection designs).

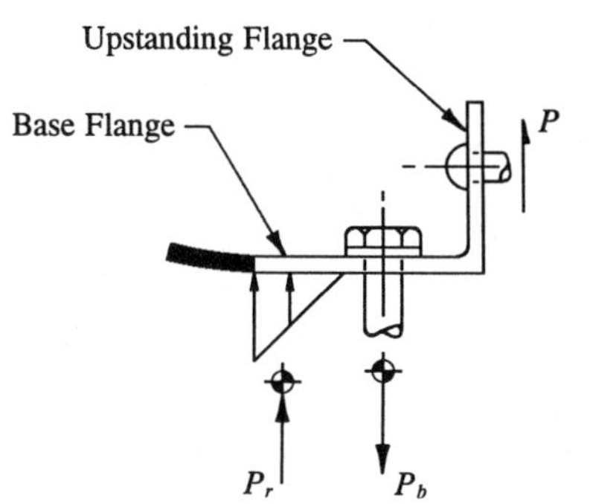

FIGURE 5-51 Reduced stiffness of a long base flange shifts the center of pressure of the prying forces closer to the bolt.

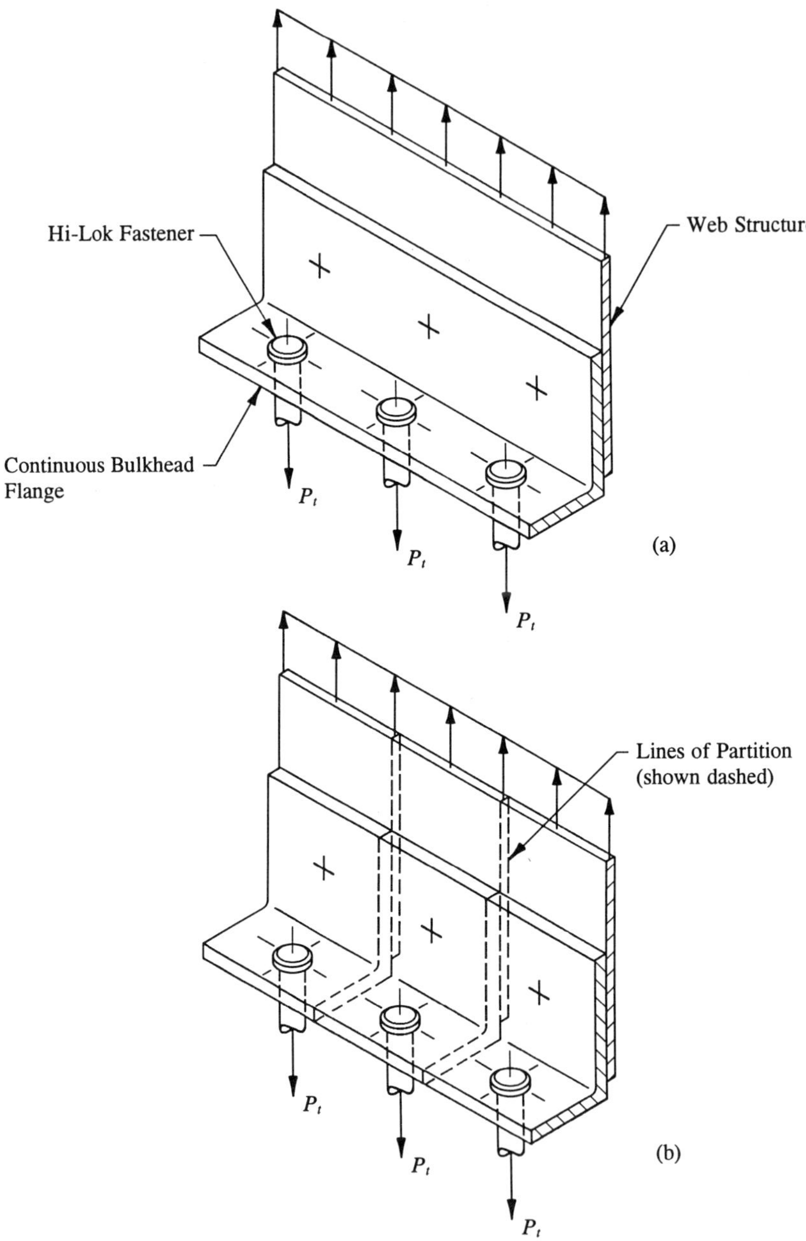

FIGURE 5-52 (a) Continuous bulkhead flange in tension. (b) Bulkhead flange is partitioned into individual tension clip supports.

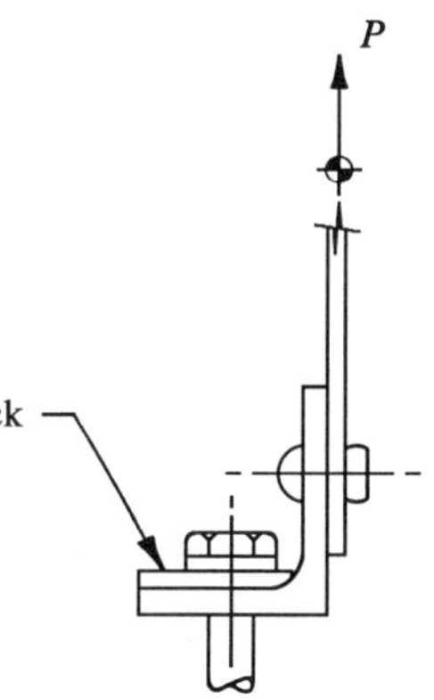

FIGURE 5-53 Radius block or fitted washer is used to increase the flange bending strength of a tension clip.

Furthermore, if the reliability and structural integrity of the tension clip as a whole is to be assured, tension bolts should also be designed for a margin of safety of 20% or greater.

To develop the maximum tensile strength of the continuous bulkhead flange shown in Fig. 5-52(a), the fastener spacing must be such as to prevent premature tension failure of the bulkhead flange, its fasteners, and the backup support structure (not shown). The bulkhead flange is partitioned into individual tension clip supports, as shown in Fig. 5-52(b), and each tension clip is analyzed according to its flange bending strength. Additionally, fasteners should be located close to the tangency points of fillets (and bend radii of formed sheet metal angles) so that excessive deflections and localized stress concentrations can be adequately minimized. If additional strength is required, a radius block or fitted washer can be used by nesting it within the tension clip, as shown in Fig. 5-53.

Prying effects are also prevalent in a tension tee clip, as viewed in Fig. 5-54. To illustrate the bearing distribution that occurs between the contact (mating) surfaces of these members, the bulkhead chord (idealized as a tee clip) and backup support structure are separated from each other and the equilibrium forces necessary to balance their particular configurations are drawn, as shown in Fig. 5-55. Summing forces in the vertical direction, we obtain from statics:

$$\Sigma F_x = 0, \qquad P + 2P_r - 2P_b = 0$$

$$P_b = \frac{P}{2} + P_r \tag{5-5}$$

where: P_b = bolt load (this includes the prying force)
P = applied tension clip load
P_r = prying force.

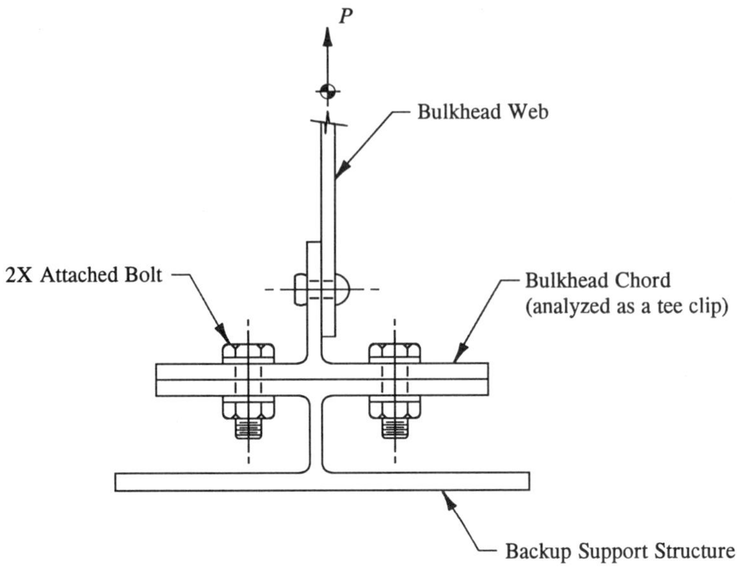

FIGURE 5-54 Bulkhead chord idealized as a tee clip.

The prying force P_r in Eq. 5-5 can be algebraically determined if the degree of restraint or fixity of the attachment bolts were known. However, for most commonly used bolts, if no prior structural testing has been done to substantiate the degree of actual bolt fixity, full fixity is generally assumed. This assumption should provide the necessary conservatism required to reliably predict an accurate detailed bolt analysis. Using the assumption of full fixity then, the center section of the tee clip is isolated and free-bodied, as shown in Fig. 5-56. The equilibrium forces are determined from existing indeterminate beam formula solutions (refer to Appendix D, "Reference Beam Formula Solutions," Case 21). The solution of these forces is shown in Fig. 5-57.[1] Now, the prying force distribution is determined by isolating and free-bodying the end section of the tee clip, as shown in Fig. 5-58.

$$\Sigma M_{CL} = 0, \quad (+ \quad \frac{PL}{8} - P_r b = 0$$

$$P_r = \frac{PL}{8b} \tag{5-6}$$

where: P_r = prying force
P = applied tension clip load

[1] Indeterminate beams cannot be solved by simple statics alone. They require more complex methods of analysis. A complete and detailed examination of their analytical solutions is not however treated in this book. The engineer is referred to an advanced college textbook on this subject.

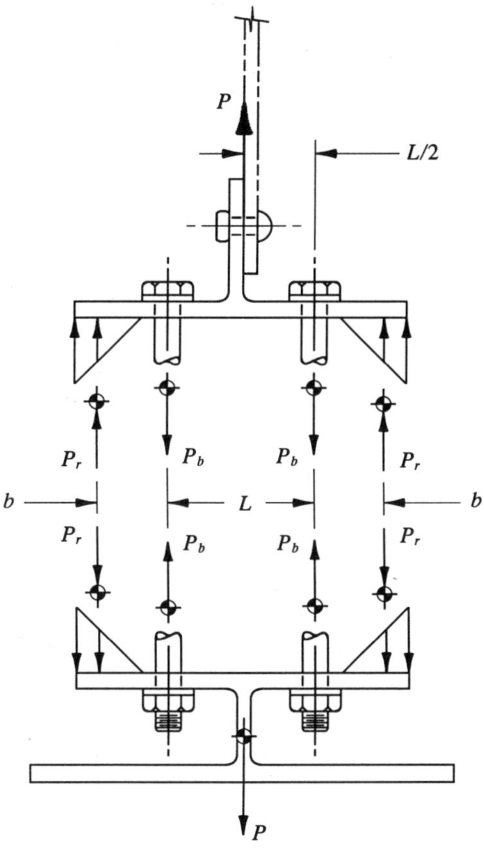

FIGURE 5-55 Distribution of load at the interface of a symmetrically loaded tee clip and its backup support structure.

L = distance measured between bolt centerlines
b = distance measured from the bolt centerline to the center of bearing pressure of the prying force distribution.

Now, substituting the value of P_r from Eq. 5-6 into the previous equation for P_b (see Eq. 5-5), we obtain:

$$P_b = \frac{P}{2} + P_r = \frac{P}{2} + \frac{PL}{8b}. \tag{5-7}$$

Up to this point in our study of support members, we have primarily concerned ourselves with (1) the in-plane loading of shear clip supports and (2) the out-of-plane loading of tension clip supports. In another case, a hypothetical force

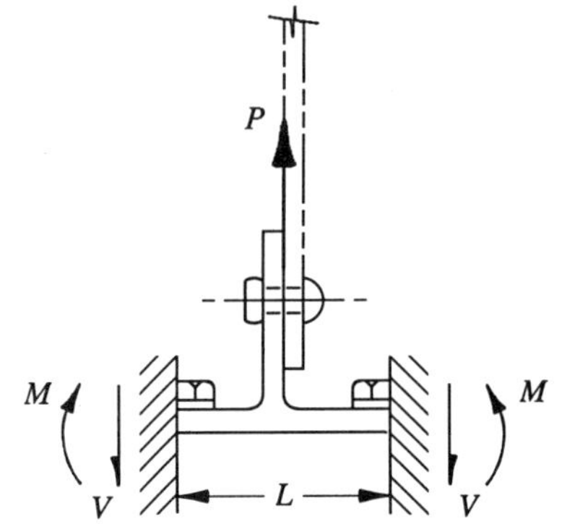

FIGURE 5-56 Center section of the tee clip is isolated and free-bodied.

system may actually produce shearing and tension forces simultaneously on the support structure. Unless these forces are developed within the plane of the attached legs of the support structure, they cannot be vectorially superimposed. Some special treatment of their combined loading effects is required. The reason is that allowable shearing and tension stresses of most materials are different, and, consequently, *different loading effects* cannot be vectorially combined into one resultant force system. Instead, interaction or failure equations, developed empirically, have been specially formulated so that different type loads can be conveniently combined together into one resultant force system. The following partial list of interaction equations for rivets and bolts has been prepared. Their corresponding margins of safety are valid only for fasteners having an $F_{tu} \leq 160$ ksi. Fasteners having an $F_{tu} > 160$ ksi must be experimentally verified based on a rational and conservative approach to their solutions.

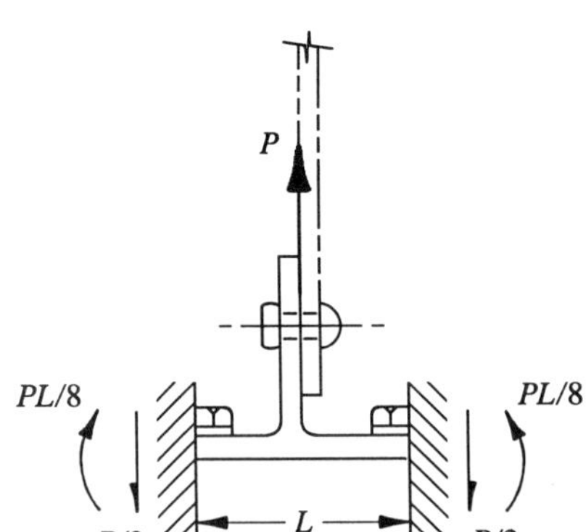

FIGURE 5-57 Beam reactions indicated on a properly drawn diagram of the center section of the tee clip.

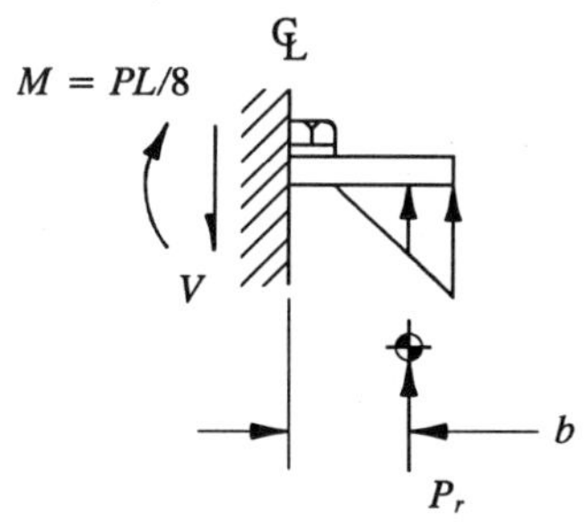

FIGURE 5-58 End section of the tee clip is isolated and free-bodied. From this, the prying force distribution is determined.

Interaction Equations[1] for Rivets and Bolts:

Aluminum and Steel Rivets:

$$R_s^2 + R_t^2 = 1. \tag{5-8}$$

Steel and Titanium Screws and Bolts:

$$R_s^3 + R_t^2 = 1. \tag{5-9}$$

Hi-Loks and Jo-Bolts:

$$R_s^{10} + R_t = 1 \tag{5-10}$$

where: $R_s = \dfrac{p_s k}{P_{su}}$ and $R_t = \dfrac{p_t k}{P_{tu}}$

p_s = ultimate shear force
P_{su} = ultimate allowable shear strength
p_t = ultimate tension force
P_{tu} = ultimate allowable tensile strength
k = fitting factor used for joint and connection designs (normally, a value of 1.15 is used for tension clip designs).

These equations may be interpreted as an indication that failure will occur when the sum of the load ratios is equal to or greater than 1.0. To determine a numerical value for the margin of safety, the following graphical method for combined shear and tension is presented:

---

[1] Interaction equations are determined by actual testing of various rivets and bolts under combined loading conditions.

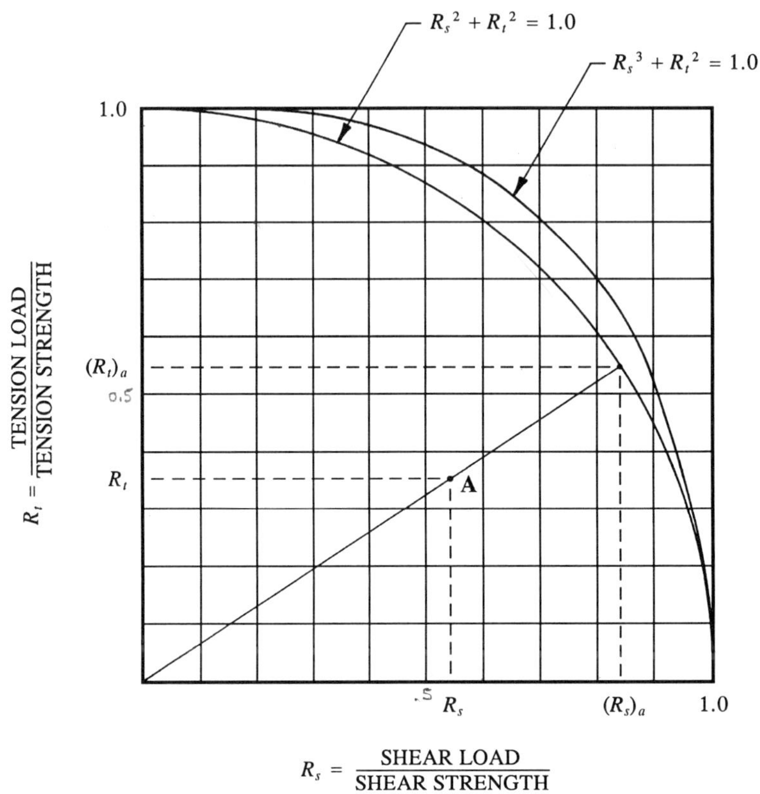

FIGURE 5-59 Interaction curves for rivets and bolts in combined shear and tension.

(1) Locate the point in Fig. 5-59 corresponding to the load ratios R_s and R_t (see point A).

(2) Draw a line from the origin through this point until it intersects the interaction equation under consideration.

(3) The point of intersection establishes the allowables $(R_s)_a$ and $(R_t)_a$.

(4) Determine the margin of safety by making one of the following comparisons:

$$\text{Margin of Safety} = \text{M.S.} = \frac{(R_s)_a}{R_s} - 1 \qquad \text{or} \qquad \text{M.S.} = \frac{(R_t)_a}{R_t} - 1.$$

The example which follows will help illustrate the practical applications of this method.

Example 5-6 A symmetrically loaded aluminum fitting made of 7075-T73 extruded material, QQ-A-200/11, is attached to the firewall bulkhead and used to

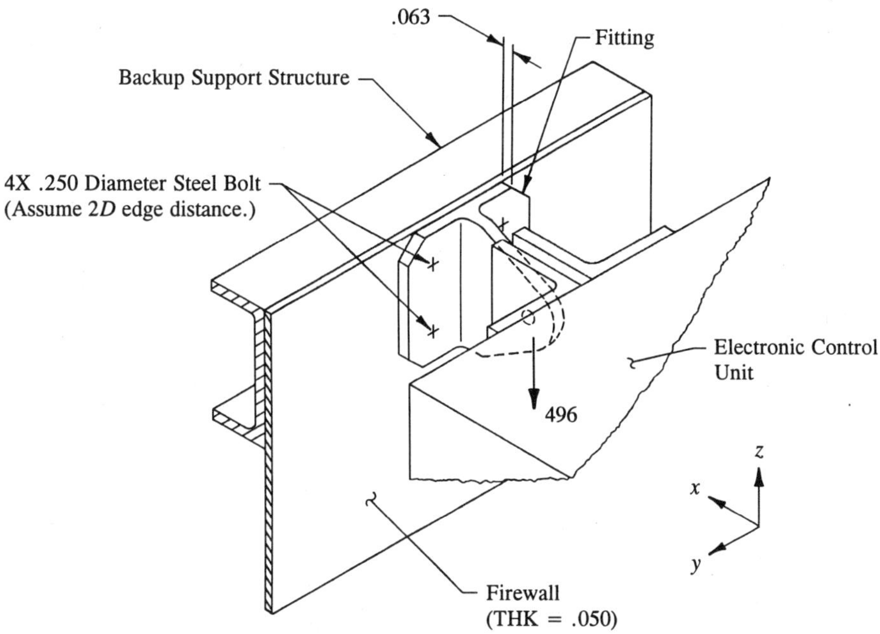

FIGURE 5-60 Symmetrically loaded aluminum fitting is attached to the firewall bulkhead and used to support an electronic control unit.

support an electronic control unit weighing 80 lb, as shown in Fig. 5-60. Design the fitting and the attachment bolts for 6.2g. Determine the margin of safety for the most critical fastener. The fastener allowables are P_{su} = 500 lb in single-shear strength and P_{tu} = 800 lb in tensile strength. The bolt head is .484 inch in diameter. To meet the FAA requirement for the strength of a fitting that has not been proven by analysis or qualification testing, consider a fitting factor of 1.15. Mechanical properties of 7075-T73 aluminum alloy extrusion: F_{tu} = 66,000 psi (LT), F_{ty} = 56,000 psi (LT), and F_{cy} = 59,000 psi (LT), THK = .062 - .249.

SOLUTION: To free-body the fitting, we must take the structure one plane at a time, as we did for a shear clip support, and apply the equations of equilibrium to obtain the overall structural balance of this member. Here the fitting is first isolated and free-bodied in the *x*-*z* plane as shown in Fig. 5-61(a). The bending moment *M* determined there (that is, at the centroid of the fastener pattern) is further distributed as a horizontal couple-force between the upper bolt attachments and the lower base flange portion of the bracket: one force acting along the centerline of the upper bolts and the other acting along the center of bearing pressure of the lower base flange, as shown in Fig. 5-61(b). The contact stresses depicted in this figure are referred to as bearing stresses, not bolt compression forces. Hence, the lower

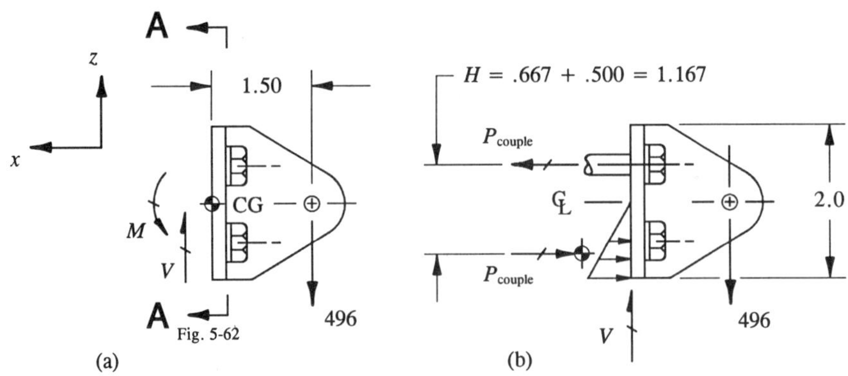

FIGURE 5-61 Aluminum fitting is isolated and free-bodied in the x-z plane: (a) equilibrium forces necessary to balance the fitting and (b) distribution of the equilibrium forces to the bolts.

bolts do not actually carry this load. Here, the bearing stresses are entirely carried by the lower base flange.

Bolt Analysis:

$$\Sigma F_z = 0, \qquad V - 496 = 0, \quad V = 496 \text{ lb}$$
$$\Sigma M_{cg} = 0, \qquad (+ \quad -M + 496(1.5) = 0, \quad M = 744 \text{ in-lb.}$$

From definitions, the moment is replaced by a couple-force as follows:

$$P_{\text{couple}} = \frac{M}{H} = \frac{744}{1.167} = 638 \text{ lb}$$

where H = distance between the centerline of the upper bolts and the center of bearing pressure of the lower base flange. Now, in the y-z plane, Fig. 5-62, the vertical shear V is distributed equally between the four fasteners, or

$$p_s = \frac{V}{4} = \frac{496}{4} = 124 \text{ lb}$$

where V = 496 lb. Using the solution provided in this section for the prying distribution of a symmetrically loaded tee clip, Eq. 5-7, we obtain the following bolt load (also refer to Fig. 5-63):

$$P_b = \frac{P}{2} + \frac{PL}{8b} = \frac{P_{\text{couple}}}{2} + \frac{P_{\text{couple}}L}{8b} = \frac{638}{2} + \frac{638(1.250)}{8(.414)}$$
$$P_b = 319 + 241 = 560 \text{ lb}$$

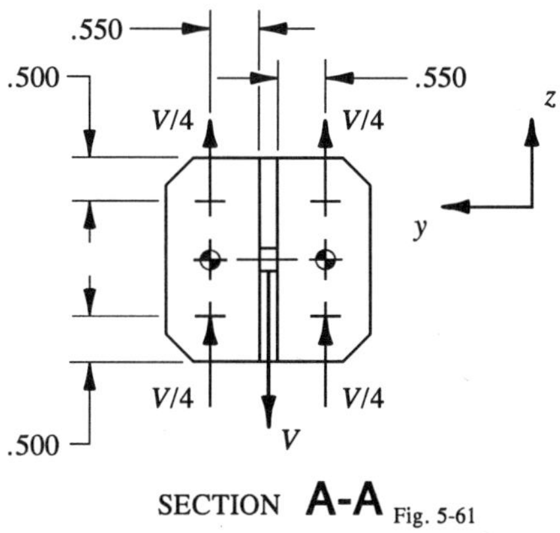

FIGURE 5-62 Distribution of vertical shear V to the bolts of the tee clip.

where the magnitude of the prying force P_r is 241 lb.

The upper bolts are more critical than the lower bolts since they react both shear and tension loads while the lower bolts react only shear (remember, the bearing forces are reacted by the base flange, not by the bolts themselves). The following interaction equation is used to verify the combined loading strength of each critical bolt.

$$R_s^{\,3} + R_t^{\,2} = 1 \quad \text{(from Eq. 5-9)}$$

where: $R_s = \dfrac{p_s k}{P_{su}} = \dfrac{124(1.15)}{500} = .285$

$R_t = \dfrac{p_t k}{P_{tu}} = \dfrac{560(1.15)}{800} = .805$

p_s = 124 lb (bolt shear load)

$p_t = P_b$ = 560 lb (bolt tension load)

P_{su} = 500 lb (given)

P_{tu} = 800 lb (given)

k = 1.15 (fitting factor used in the design of joint and connection designs).

To determine whether this meets acceptable design requirements of the fastener, the load ratios R_s and R_t are plotted using the interaction failure curve provided in Fig. 5-59, page 348. The margin of safety of the fastener for the combined loading is indicated by how close the plotted point lies to the interaction curve. For this example, a margin of safety of approximately 22% is determined. The engineer is encouraged to verify this value by performing the necessary

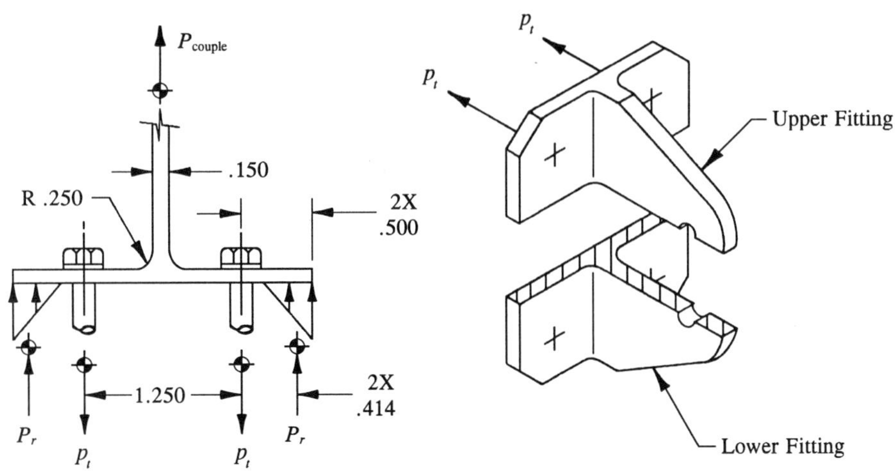

FIGURE 5-63 Upper part of the tee fitting is idealized as a tension-loaded tee clip.

computations (refer to our earlier bolt analysis requirement that at least a 20% margin of safety must be maintained for tension bolts). This then completes the bolt analysis portion of this problem.

Tee Clip Analysis: Let us now assume that the upper part of the firewall fitting acts as a tension-loaded tee clip, and determine its ultimate strength. The isometric drawing in Fig. 5-63 shows the actual method of partitioning this member. All of the forces indicated are known quantities previously determined in the analysis of this problem. The rest of this solution is to determine the critical section where bending stresses are maximum. These stresses are then compared to the ultimate allowable bending stress of the base flange (see Appendix J for the design and analysis of inelastic bending members).

5.5 Problem for Solution. For the tee fitting loaded as shown in Fig. 5-64, make the following stress checks: (a) Using conventional stress analysis methods, determine the bending strength of the base flange of the tee fitting (include a fitting factor of 1.15 while additionally maintaining a positive margin of safety of 20% at ultimate load). Assume a design load factor of 1.5. (*Hint:* The engineer is encouraged here to determine actual bolt loads by properly balancing the fitting under load. This is accomplished by redeveloping Eq. 5-7 for the geometric characteristics of an unsymmetrically loaded tee fitting.) The bolt head is .433 inch in diameter. The bolt spacing is 1.00 in. (b) Determine the required base flange thickness to meet the design requirements at ultimate. (c) Write the margin of safety in tension for the bolts (use an ultimate tension allowable of 6,980 lb for single-shear joints).

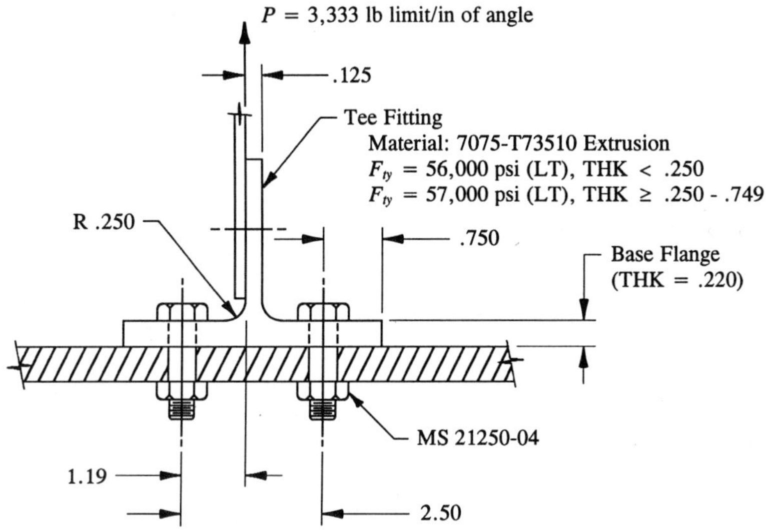

FIGURE 5-64 Tee fitting loaded in tension.

CHAPTER 6

Crippling of Compression Members

6.1 Introduction. In this chapter, we will focus our attention on the structural behavior of compression members with stable cross-sectional areas. That is, members that are sufficiently short in length to prevent column instability. The structural phenomenon of column instability will be treated in a separate chapter (refer to Chapter 7 for the design and analysis of column members). Of course, a long compression member can preclude column instability if such a member is stabilized by either an attached web, an attached skin, or both. The engineer is referred to Fig. 6-1 where the structural arrangement of a multi-spar wing structure is schematically diagrammed.

Note, in particular, how the web and skin members in compression will provide the lateral stability (restraint) to prevent column action from occurring for the main structural members (i.e., stringers and spar caps) of this mock structure. In other words, the bowing effect of the web and skin members will induce tension forces in these members which will then tend to force the compression members back to their original positions. Hence, for compression stable members, compression allowables are normally based on crippling strength, not column failure.

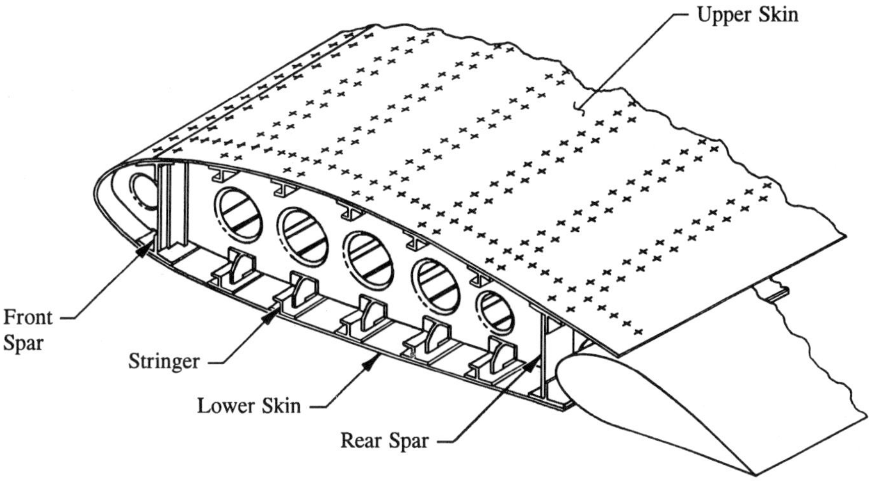

FIGURE 6-1 Structural arrangement of a multi-spar wing.

Crippling analysis of built-up compression members is presented in Sec. 6.4. However, before this subject is discussed in depth, the following related topics are presented: (1) inter-rivet buckling of compression members, Sec. 6.2; and (2) effective sheet areas of built-up sections in compression, Sec. 6.3. The engineer is encouraged to thoroughly review these intermediate sections before proceeding ahead with the material of Sec. 6.4.

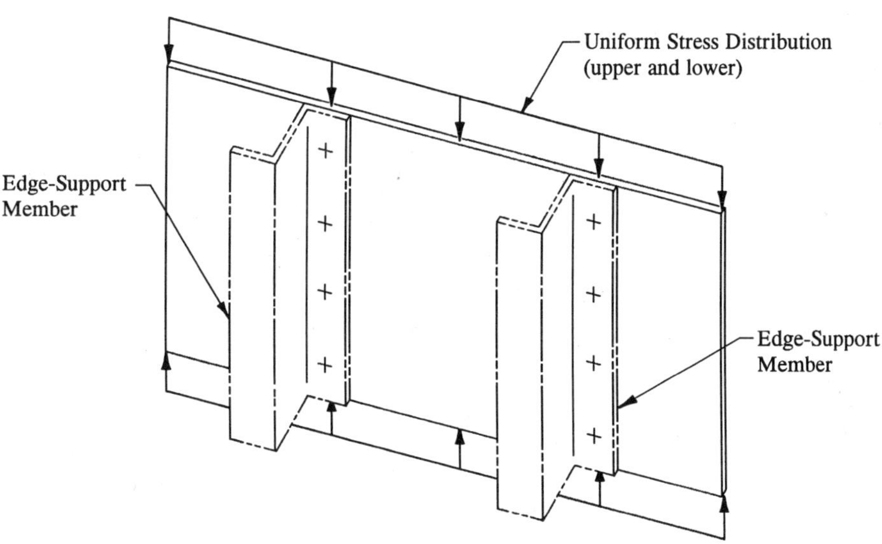

FIGURE 6-2 Compression-loaded flat plate.

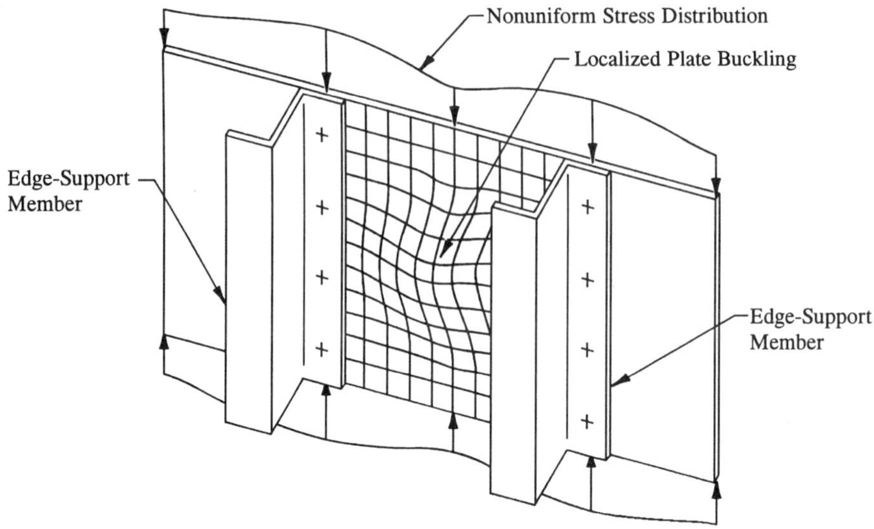

FIGURE 6-3 Localized plate buckling.

A flat sheet or plate is considered structurally inefficient and a rather poor design choice for the purpose of carrying compression loads. The allowable buckling stress[1] of such a member is rather low compared to the buckling strength of formed and extruded structural shapes (analyzed in Sec. 6.4 of this chapter). Observe the nonbuckled state of the compression-loaded plate shown in Fig. 6.2. Without the edge-support members (indicated in phantom), the plate would be laterally unstable at some critical load and would ultimately collapse (fail).

Now look at Fig. 6-3. Note, in particular, how the plate stresses are no longer uniform across the buckled plate region. For this member, localized buckling will first appear in the middle portion of the plate. However, the plate will not actually fail (or collapse) because the supported sides of the plate have the inherent ability to carry additional load. The additional increase in load is theoretically shed (transferred) by the middle portion of the plate to the much stiffer supported sides. Consider the middle portion of the plate to actually sustain the compression load which caused it to buckle. Failure of the plate is reached when the supported sides of the plate have yielded. The edges of the plate along the rivet line are assumed to be simply-supported. This condition is true if the fasteners along the supported edges of the plate have been properly sized and spaced.

Now, an analogy can be made between the edge-supported members used in this illustration and the stiffer corners (or joints) of formed and extruded shapes. That is: that edge-supported members can theoretically provide the same restraint capability that corner edges of structural shapes can. Note that no allowance (or difference) is made here between the relative stiffness between formed and

[1] Refer to Chapter 8 for the design and analysis of shear-resistant beams.

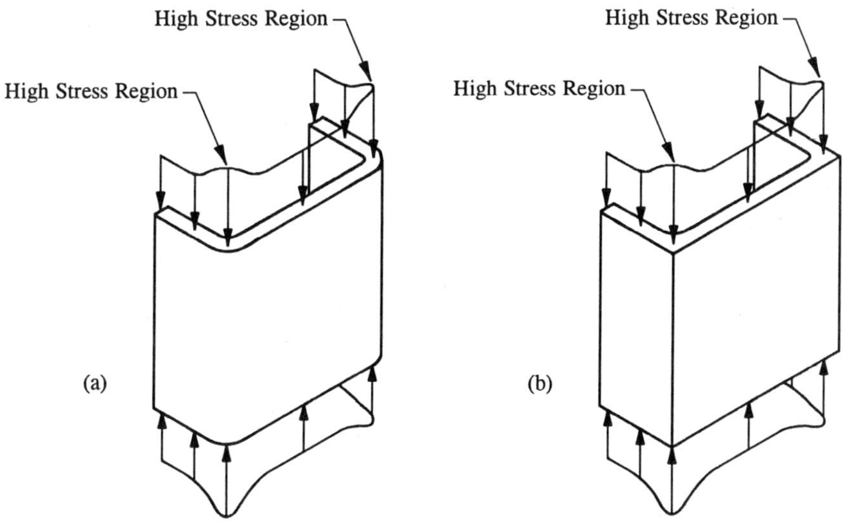

FIGURE 6-4 Stress distribution of (a) a formed sheet metal channel and (b) an extruded channel.

extruded sections. We can now use this argument to describe the state of stress of a formed (or extruded) channel section. Refer to Fig. 6-4(a) and (b). The stiffer corners of such a member are considered simply-supported (shown by the cross-hatched areas in Fig. 6-5) since they provide the restraint capability for the plate elements that make up the channel section. For instance, the included web is supported at both ends, while the flanges are only supported at one end; the other ends are unsupported (or free). For an angle section, Fig. 6-6, the flanges are supported by the corner, while the other ends are unsupported. Many other structural shapes are also possible. For example, an I-beam section, a T-beam section, an H-beam section, etc., can also have similar restraint capabilities of their flanges and included webs.

The ultimate allowable crippling stress of formed and extruded sections is reviewed in detail in Sec. 6.4. Allowable values are determined by the solution of Eqs. 6-16 and 6-17. The engineer is also referred to his company's engineering stress department for the recommended use of established reference crippling curves. If such curves are provided by aerospace companies for general design use, their incorporation should be specifically included as additional reference material to Sec. 6.4, "Crippling of Built-up Sections in Compression." Reference design curves are provided by most aerospace companies to simplify the trivial computations often required by the solution of Eq. 6-16 in the analysis of crippling members. Structural engineers needing such documents (reference design curves) should look for them in company structures manuals. They can usually be found in a crippling or column section of these manuals. These curves are provided to save engineers valuable time: the time saved can then be better used to complement a

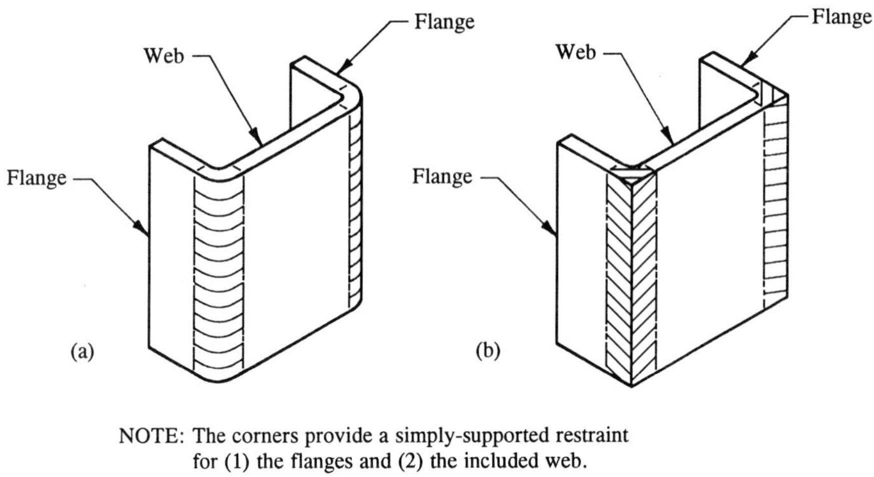

FIGURE 6-5 Edge-support conditions for (a) a formed sheet metal channel and (b) an extruded channel.

wider range of other possible design candidates. Thus, if you can minimize some of the trivial algebraic computations, the engineering time saved can then be better used for more productive and innovative design accomplishments. Several different methods of crippling analysis are currently used today by major aerospace companies. However, the most universally accepted method used by practicing engineers is called "The Needham Method," and will be the main focus of study in this chapter.

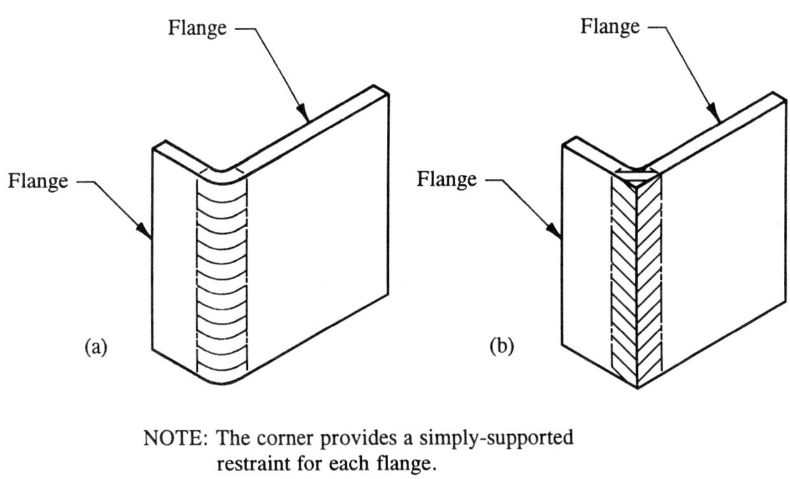

FIGURE 6-6 Edge-support conditions for (a) a formed sheet metal angle and (b) an extruded angle.

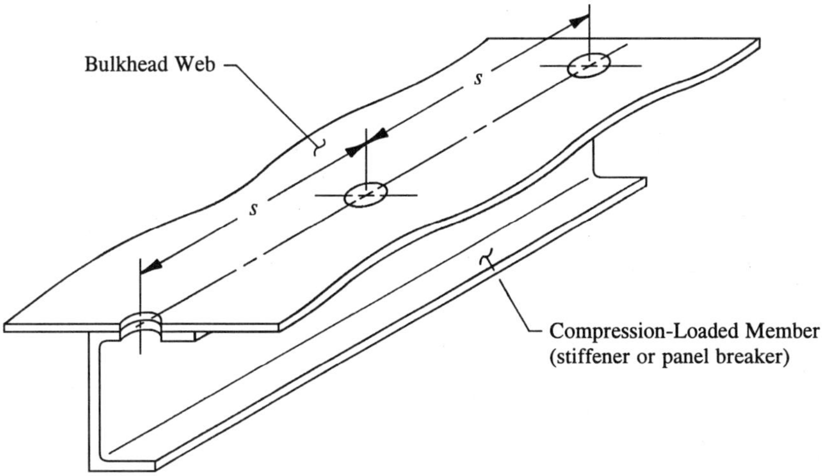

FIGURE 6-7 Bulkhead web riveted to a compression-loaded member can cause inter-rivet buckling of the sheet between rivets.

Whether or not an engineering company uses this particular method, it would still benefit most engineers who do not know it, in the long run, to learn it. A thorough knowledge and understanding of its basic principles and detailed methods of analysis now will more than compensate the engineer later for his diligence and persevering efforts to master its essential details. Engineering is not an exact science. One method of analysis may not lend itself easily to all the vagaries and peculiarities of a dependable design solution. For this reason, engineers should become thoroughly familiar with alternative methods of analysis to validate preexisting design solutions. Maybe to some this would seem redundant, but nonetheless it usually proves a very important point: knowledge is a most valuable commodity. If one plans to spend a lifetime in the aerospace industry pursuing a professional career in structural engineering, this method of analysis will eventually prove to be "stress-worthy."

6.2 Inter-Rivet Buckling of Compression Members. The wing or fuselage skin riveted to a compression-loaded member can prematurely buckle between rivets before structural failure of the compression member occurs. This type of buckling is depicted in Fig. 6-7 for a bulkhead web, and is not to be confused with actual structural failure. The word "prematurely" is used here to refer to inter-rivet buckling of the attached skin between rivets at a stress level below the compression allowable of the compression-loaded member. In fact, any riveted member subjected to compression loading can also prematurely buckle between rivets (this includes the riveted flange of the compression-loaded member itself described here in this illustration). The engineer is also referred to Fig. 6-8, where other aircraft structural members, such as stringers, a longeron, and a frame, are depicted riveted

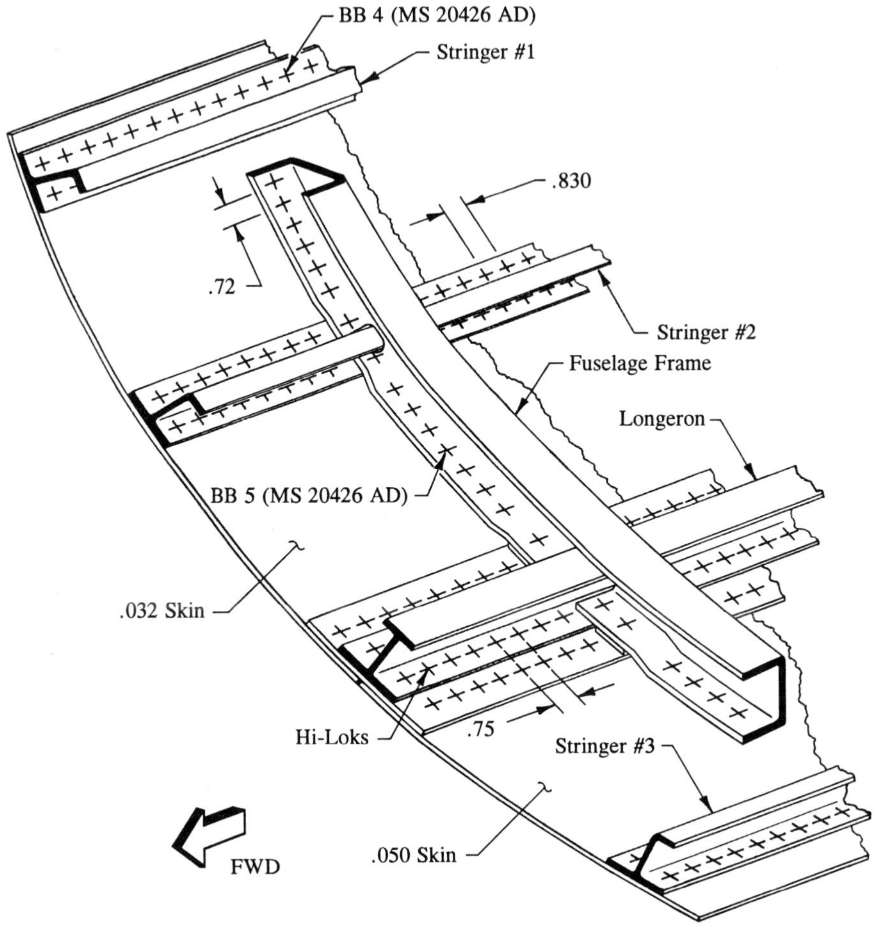

FIGURE 6-8 Fuselage skin riveted to structural members, such as stringers, longerons, and fuselage frames, that can potentially undergo compression loading.

to the fuselage skin. The flanges of these members (skin side) will undergo some form of compression loading at some time and therefore must be investigated for premature inter-rivet buckling. Of course, inter-rivet buckling does not occur for members in tension.

The buckled skin of a riveted compression member can sustain the load which produced the buckled state but no additional increase in load can be carried by this member. However, while the skin buckles and holds the load which precipitated buckling, the compression member continues to accept additional load until its compression allowable has been reached. Inter-rivet buckling is therefore a state of stress or condition which precipitates buckling of a riveted member at a stress level below the allowable compression (failure) stress of the main structural member (this member could be a stringer, a longeron, a stiffener, a frame cap, or a bulkhead cap). The effect of this condition on a compression member is fully considered in Sec. 6.4. Until then, let us mathematically interpret the basic concepts and theory of inter-rivet buckling expounded upon thus far in this section by formulating the following inequalities:

(1) If $F_{ir} \geq F_{cc}$, the structure precludes inter-rivet buckling, and the full allowable crippling stress F_{cc} is used for the structural member.

(2) If $F_{ir} < F_{cc}$, the structure prematurely buckles between rivets, and a reduction in crippling strength results.

The terms F_{ir} and F_{cc} are defined as follows: F_{ir} is the allowable inter-rivet buckling stress of the riveted structural member, i.e., flange, skin, or web (see Fig. 6-7); and F_{cc} is the allowable crippling stress of the main structural member, i.e., stringer, longeron, stiffener, frame cap, or bulkhead cap (this allowable is calculated without attached skin or web).

Since a riveted member is potentially strong enough to carry load up to the allowable compression strength of a compression-loaded member, it would be desirable to take full advantage of this additional strength by designing each riveted member to this allowable value. To optimize his designs, the engineer will prevent premature inter-rivet buckling. However, if such a design criterion cannot be realistically met for an existing design, and premature inter-rivet buckling does occur, a reduction in compression strength for the buckled member would be required. This reduction, as we will see in Sec. 6.4, will also reduce the allowable crippling strength of the compression-loaded member.

Inter-rivet buckling therefore should be avoided in all phases and aspects of structural designs. If, however, this condition cannot be totally prevented from occurring, it should nevertheless be thoroughly appraised and its structural behavior determined. Such a condition, if it should occur, can result in a slight decrease in the overall performance of the compression-loaded member. Therefore, to achieve a well-balanced design, or perhaps, better yet, to avoid a slight to moderate weight penalty of the structure being analyzed, the engineer must eliminate its occurrence. Any deviation from this prescribed criterion must be fully treated by the design engineer. This means that all structural deficiencies caused by premature inter-rivet buckling must either be substantiated by test or documented by structural analysis or theory. The most efficient design (in compression) is therefore one that can prevent premature inter-rivet buckling.[1] However, if for some reason a design should not meet this basic requirement, be that intentional or not, or possibly

[1] An aircraft structural wing is usually designed with closer fastener spacing on the upper wing surface than on its lower wing surface because compression loads are usually larger on the upper surface due to higher wing up-bending loads. Thus, to prevent premature inter-rivet buckling, the upper surface will usually have tighter fastener spacing due to the higher compression loads on that surface.

because it may just be too costly (structurally) to attain in the present structural design phase,[1] its occurrence can be treated by the analysis methods of Sec. 6.4.

Two basic methods of inter-rivet buckling (or sheet instability) analysis are presented in this chapter: (1) inelastic instability of a column in compression, Eq. 6-1; and (2) inelastic instability of a flat sheet (or plate) in compression, Eq. 6-2. The former or column instability approach will be the main and preferred method of analysis used in this chapter. The latter or flat sheet or plate instability approach, even though not specifically treated in this section, will nevertheless be briefly reviewed and discussed in Appendix I. The engineer is encouraged to study its basic principles and methodologies so that a broader perspective and overview of the nature and principles of inter-rivet buckling analysis can be had. This alternative method is widely used in the aerospace industry and for this reason the engineer should also master total familiarity with its principles and applications.

Inelastic Instability of a Column in Compression

$$F_c = \frac{c\pi^2 E_t}{(L/\rho)^2} \tag{6-1}$$

where: F_c = allowable column stress

L = actual column length (also defined by $L'\sqrt{c}$)

c = end-fixity coefficient for different attachment types (see values given in Table 6-1, page 363)

E_t = compression tangent-modulus (use a compression stress-strain curve or a compression tangent-modulus curve to obtain this value), refer to MIL-HDBK-5

ρ = radius of gyration, $\sqrt{I/A}$

L' = effective column length, $L/\sqrt{c}$.

Inelastic Instability of a Flat Sheet or Plate in Compression

$$F_{ir} = \frac{c\pi^2 E_t}{12(1-\mu^2)}\left[\frac{t}{s}\right]^2 \tag{6-2}$$

where: F_{ir} = allowable inter-rivet buckling stress

E_t = compression tangent-modulus

μ = Poisson's ratio (see mechanical-property tables for specific materials in MIL-HDBK-5)

t = skin thickness

s = fastener spacing

c = end-fixity coefficient (use values given in Table 6-1).

[1] For instance, during the structural test phase of a prototype structure, it may be entirely prohibitive (uneconomical) to actually initiate a redesign effort of a structurally deficient member.

TABLE 6-1 END-FIXITY COEFFICIENTS FOR DIFFERENT ATTACHMENT TYPES

End-Fixity Coefficient c	Type of Attachment
4.0	bolts (Hi-Loks, Jo-Bolts, etc.)
3.5	spot welds
3.0	universal (solid, protruding-head rivets)
1.5	countersunk or dimpled (flush, tension-head rivets)
1.0	countersunk or dimpled (flush, shear-head rivets)

Inter-rivet buckling analysis based on column instability of riveted members (Eq. 6-1) will be developed in the remaining paragraphs of this section. Basically, this method uses industry-established column instability curves to determine the allowable inter-rivet buckling stresses of riveted members. Such a curve is shown in Fig. 6-9, where the allowable compression column stress F_c is plotted versus the slenderness ratio L'/ρ for a given material (refer ahead to Eq. 6-3).

When a plate (or sheet) buckles at an operating stress level above the proportional limit of the material, a reduction in plate bending stiffness occurs. The effects of exceeding this limit on the buckled member are incorporated into a compression tangent-modulus term E_t. However, if column instability curves are used (F_c vs. L'/ρ), the evaluation of this term is avoided altogether since all column instability curves inherently include this term in their graphical solutions (see graphical representation of Eq. 6-3 in Fig. 6-9). The compression tangent-modulus E_t is a measure of the bending stiffness of a member in the inelastic range of compression stresses, while the more familiar term, Young's modulus E_c, is a measure of bending stiffness of a member in the elastic range of compression stresses. Below the proportional limit of the material, or elastic range, Young's modulus and the tangent modulus have the same value or $E_t = E_c$.

Column instability curves are usually obtained from the materials engineering group for different material types (the stress department should also have a current list of approved column curves available for design use). If a column curve is not available for a specific type of material, the engineer is encouraged to develop his own values necessary to establish such a curve. However, before a column instability curve for a specific type of material can be established, Eq. 6-1 must first be expressed in terms of the slenderness ratio L'/ρ. Substituting the column length $L = L'\sqrt{c}$ into Eq. 6-1, we obtain a new column expression in terms of L'/ρ:

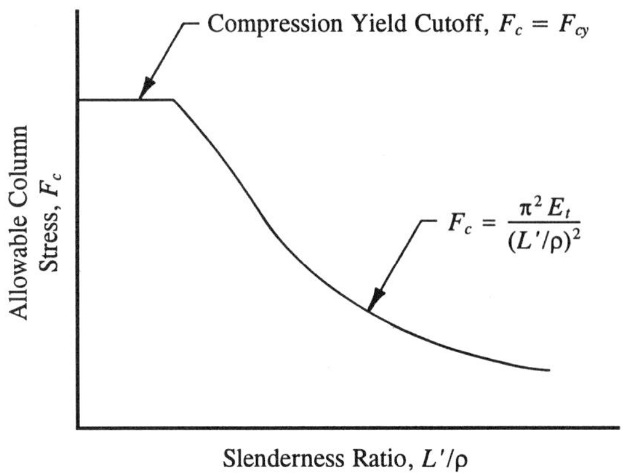

FIGURE 6-9 Column instability curve is used to determine the allowable inter-rivet buckling stress of riveted members in compression.

$$F_c = \frac{\pi^2 E_t}{(L'/\rho)^2}. \tag{6-3}$$

From this expression, the allowable column compression stress F_c versus the effective slenderness ratio L'/ρ is plotted. This is done for several different stress levels of F_c. For example, for a given stress level, say 10 ksi, 15 ksi, 20 ksi, 25 ksi, 30 ksi, etc., and corresponding values of the tangent modulus[1] E_t, the effective slenderness ratios L'/ρ are determined. The assumed values of F_c and corresponding values of L'/ρ are then plotted on graph paper and a curve drawn through these points. This then is the basic method that is used to establish column instability curves for different material types.

Let us now focus our attention on the main intent of study of this section: that is, to develop an expression for inter-rivet buckling based on inelastic column instability. To arrive at such an expression, let us make the following general assumption, that a riveted sheet in compression acts as a column. The rivets are assumed to provide the support restraint for the ends of the idealized column. This restraint capability is measured by the end-fixity coefficient of the rivet (see values in Table 6-1). If we treat such a member (between rivets) as a column, Fig. 6-10, the inter-rivet buckling stress in terms of column failure then becomes:

$$F_{ir} = \frac{\pi^2 E_t}{(L'/\rho)^2} \tag{6-4}$$

where the allowable column stress F_c in Eq. 6-3 is replaced by the allowable inter-

[1] Refer to a stress-strain curve or to MIL-HDBK-5 for an applicable compression tangent-modulus curve to use.

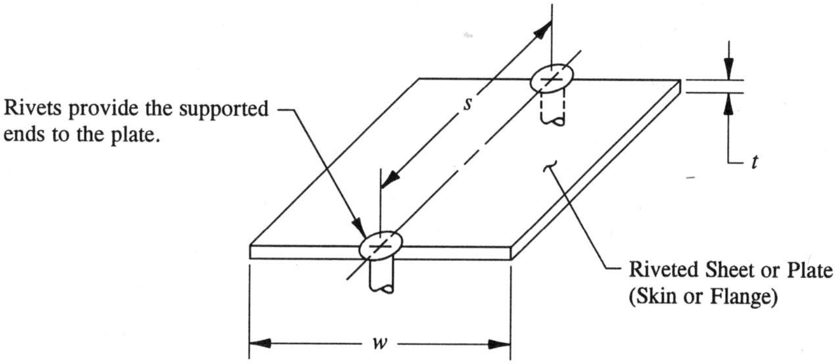

FIGURE 6-10 A riveted sheet or plate idealized as a column between rivets.

rivet buckling stress F_{ir} of the riveted compression member. Substituting the section properties L', I, and A for the idealized column in the expression for L'/ρ gives:

$$L'/\rho = \frac{L/\sqrt{c}}{\sqrt{I/A}} = \frac{2\sqrt{3}}{\sqrt{c}}\,\frac{s}{t} \tag{6-5}$$

$$\text{where: } L' = \frac{L}{\sqrt{c}} = \frac{s}{\sqrt{c}} \text{ and } I = \frac{bh^3}{12} = \frac{wt^3}{12}$$
$$\rho = \sqrt{I/A}$$
$$A = wt.$$

From this equation, the following table is constructed for different attachment types.

TABLE 6-2 EFFECTIVE SLENDERNESS RATIOS L'/ρ FOR DIFFERENT ATTACHMENT TYPES

Type of Attachment*	End-Fixity Coefficient, c	L'/ρ
Bolts (Hi-Loks, Jo-Bolts, etc.)	4.0	$\sqrt{3}\,s/t$
Universal (solid, protruding-head rivets)	3.0	$2\,s/t$
Countersunk (flush, tension-head rivets)	1.5	$2\sqrt{2}\,s/t$
Countersunk (flush, shear-head rivets)	1.0	$2\sqrt{3}\,s/t$

* Use $c = 3.5$ for spot welds not verified by structural testing. Substituting this value in Eq. 6-5, we obtain $L'/\rho = 1.852\,s/t$.

For any given rivet, knowing the values of s and t, Table 6-2 may be used to determine the slenderness ratio L'/ρ. Then, with this value and a column instability curve of a specific material (F_c vs. L'/ρ), determine the allowable inter-rivet buckling stress F_{ir}. The advantage of this method is as follows: by using established column instability curves we have completely avoided having to determine a value for the compression tangent-modulus E_t. To help illustrate further the concepts of inter-rivet buckling of riveted members, and the use of column instability curves and Table 6-2, the engineer is referred to specific example problems in Secs. 6.3 and 6.4.

6.3 Effective Sheet Areas of Built-up Sections in Compression. Most main structural members of an aircraft structure, such as stiffeners, longerons, stringers, wing spar caps, fuselage frame and bulkhead caps, have some sort of sheet or outer covering of skin material attached to them. Rarely do such members act completely alone (by themselves); some type of sheet covering is usually involved. Although a thin, flat sheet attached to a compression member has a relatively low buckling strength in compression, the attached member can still provide some ability (or capacity) to carry compression loads. To neglect the capacity of the sheet material to carry compression load can cause a slight to moderate weight penalty of the main structural member. Therefore, to avoid a weight increase as a consequence, the load-carrying ability of the sheet material must be considered. The procedure used to determine the load capacity in compression of the attached sheet is based on the effective area of the sheet at some predetermined or existing operating stress level, usually the stress corresponding to the main compression member (stringer, stiffener, longeron, etc.). In tension, it should be recalled that even the thinnest structural members are considered fully effective (refer to earlier chapters of this book). The word "effective" in stress analysis means that the effective

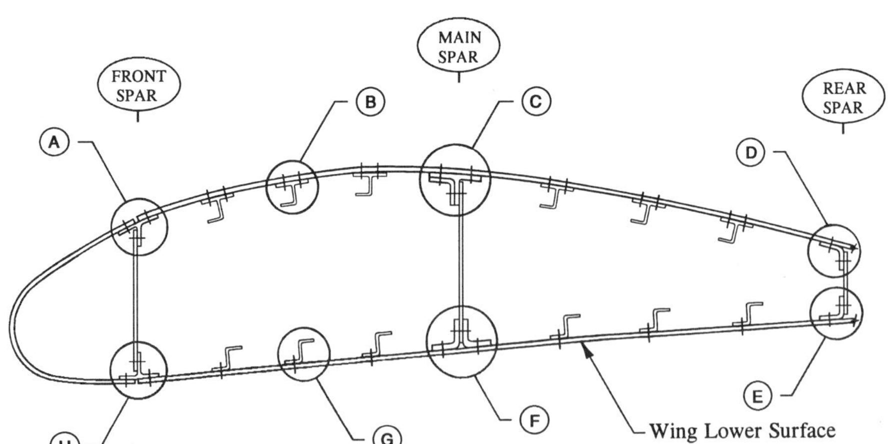

FIGURE 6-11 Wing cross-sectional area (views depicted are shown in Fig. 6-12).

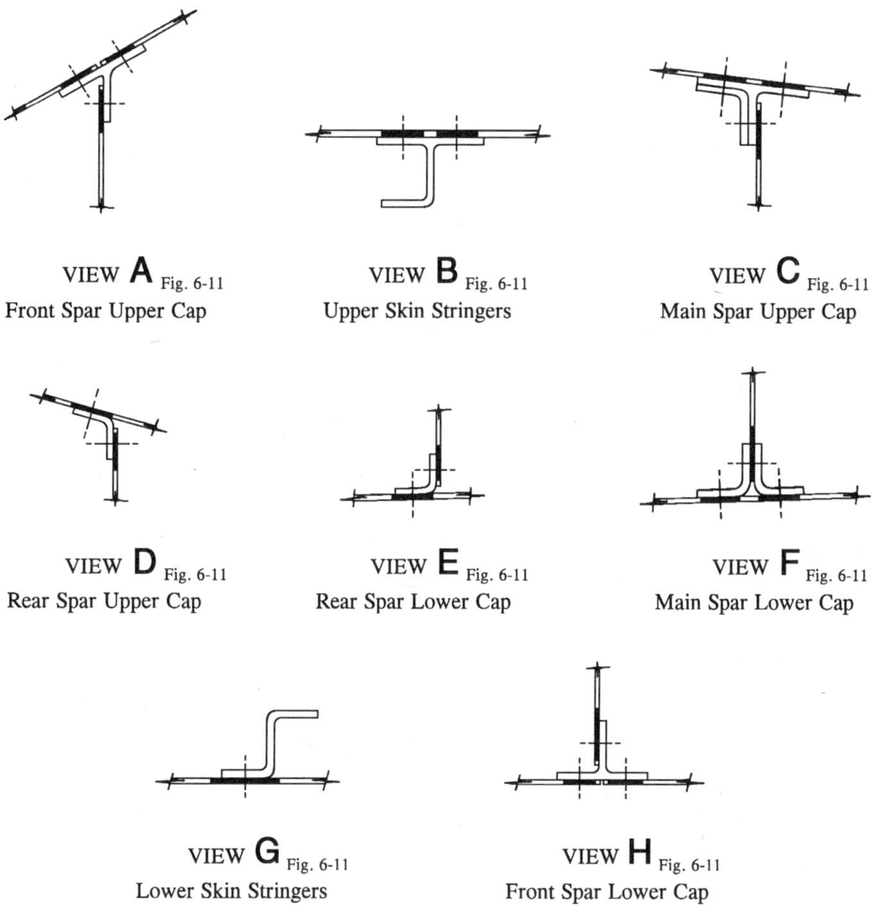

FIGURE 6-12 Section areas with effective web and skin areas shown shaded.

member is structurally able to carry a load (be that compression, tension, bending, torsion or for that matter any other type or combination of these loads).

The main emphasis of study of this section will therefore be to determine the load-carrying ability of sheet members in compression. Also included in this section will be a blend of some of the previous concepts of inter-rivet buckling (Sec. 6-2) as they specifically relate to the theory of sheet effective areas and the crippling stress of formed and extruded structural shapes (Sec. 6-4).

The engineer is now referred to Fig. 6-11 where the cross-sectional area of a typical wing structure is shown. The main members, assumed to be in compression, are shown with effective web and skin areas shaded in Fig. 6-12. The stress distribution of an attached sheet (skin or web structural member) before and after buckling has occurred is illustrated in Figs. 6-13(a) and (b). Here, the sheet and

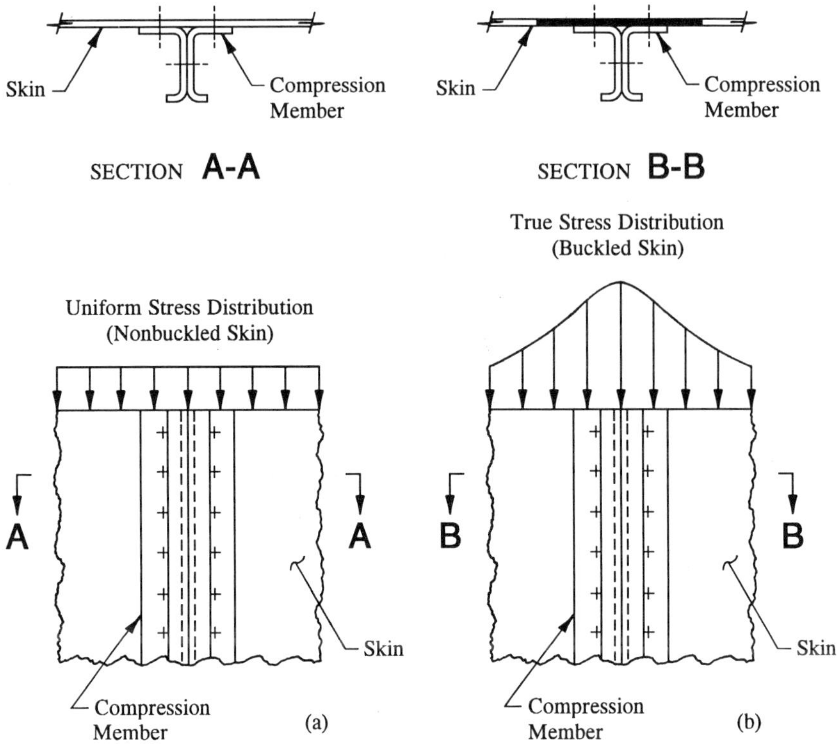

FIGURE 6-13 Stress distribution of an attached sheet: (a) before sheet buckling and (b) after sheet buckling.

compression member (in composite) shown in Fig. 6-13(a) is depicted with a uniform compression stress distribution across the total cross-sectional area of the composite structure. Such a stress distribution will normally occur for a nonbuckled, stable sheet member—in this state, the sheet is considered fully effective. The sheet and compression member will develop a uniform stress distribution until the sheet actually begins to buckle. Then, the true stress distribution is that as shown in Fig. 6-13(b). The buckled sheet maintains the stress which produced the buckled state, but it (the buckled sheet) cannot accept any additional load. The engineer should not confuse this condition with inter-rivet buckling. The latter occurs between rivets while the former occurs in an open bay, say, between stringers in an aircraft structure; both of which are a result of compression loading. In the middle portion of this open bay, specifically between the stringers, the buckling strength of the sheet is rather low. However, as the stringers are approached, the buckling strength of the sheet increases until it reaches the compression crippling strength F_{cc} of the stringer directly over this member. The attached sheet and stringer will then fail in unison.

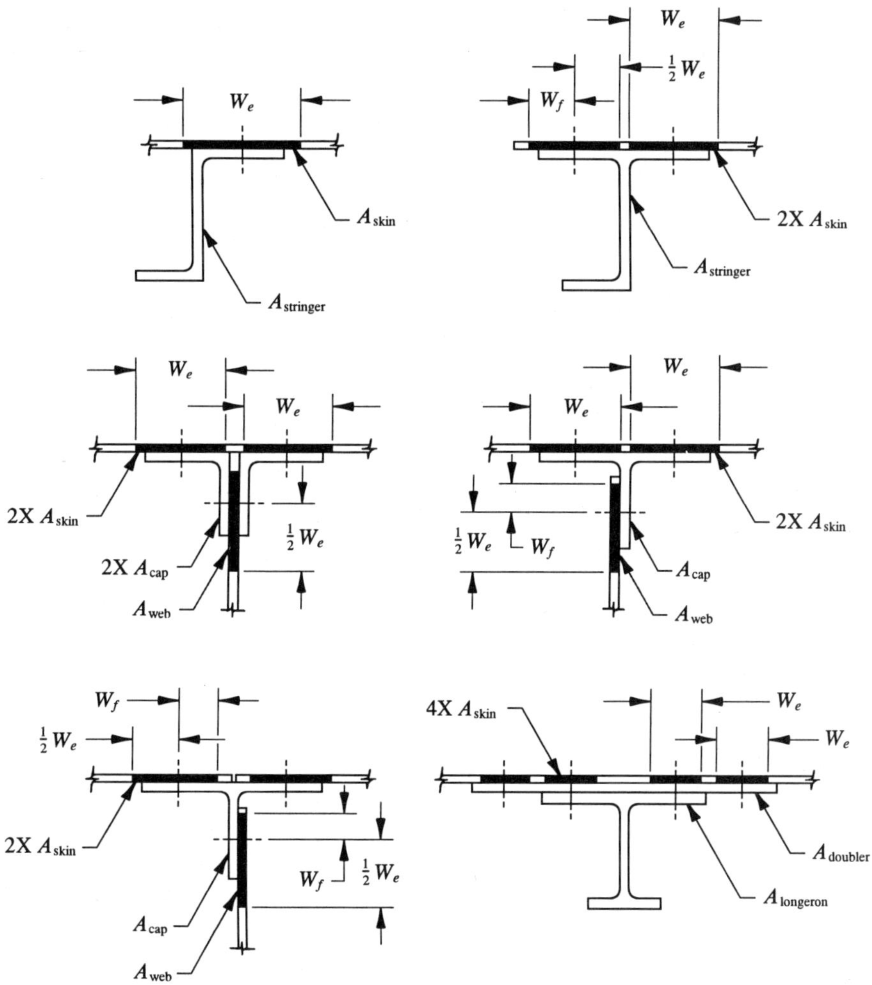

Note: Do not overlap effective sheet widths (i.e., do not use more effective area than actually exists between fasteners; verify your calculations between fasteners before using calculated values).

FIGURE 6-14 Effective sheet areas of riveted sheet members in compression.

Structural tests of buckled sheet members in compression have been correlated to the amount of sheet area considered effective for a compression-loaded member. The results provide a simple and direct method of determining this area in terms of effective sheet widths or W_e and W_f. These terms (shown shaded in Fig. 6-14) are defined for various cross-sectional areas of compression-loaded members. Their values are normally based on the operating stress level of the main compression member.[1]

Effective sheet width calculations are determined from the following equations:

$$W_e = 1.7t\sqrt{E_c/f_c} \tag{6-6}$$

$$W_f = .62t\sqrt{E_c/f_c} \tag{6-7}$$

where: W_e = effective width of sheet (boundary condition; no free edges)
W_f = effective width of sheet (boundary condition; one free edge)
f_c = operating stress level of the main compression member (compression load divided by the area of the compression member)
E_c = compression modulus of elasticity of the skin
t = thickness of the sheet material.

From the preceding equations, the effective sheet areas are then calculated as follows:

$$(\text{Area})_e = W_e t \tag{6-8}$$

and

$$(\text{Area})_f = W_f t \tag{6-9}$$

where t is the thickness of the attached sheet material.

An alternative solution is accomplished by substituting the allowable crippling stress F_{cc} for f_c in Eqs. 6-6 and 6-7. The resulting equations in this form are more convenient to use, as subsequent example problems in this section will clearly demonstrate:

$$W_e = 1.7t\sqrt{E_c/F_{cc}} \tag{6-10}$$

$$W_f = .62t\sqrt{E_c/F_{cc}} \tag{6-11}$$

where F_{cc} is the allowable crippling stress of the main compression member. The actual computations of this quantity are discussed in Sec. 6.4.

---

[1] Since the sheet and main compression member are structurally attached together with rivets, each member will experience the same strains (or deformations) along their lengths. In theory, the members must also develop the same stress levels. Assuming that the rivets provide a simply-supported restraint for the attached sheet material, which is usually the case for most commonly designed riveted sheet members of a typical aircraft structure, these stresses will correspond to the operating stress level of the main compression member.

Using the allowable crippling stress of the compression member theoretically forces the effective sheet members (web and/or skin) to fail at this same prescribed stress level. This is a reasonable assumption since a composite structure (a structure made up of several members) normally fails when all members are fully stressed. Of course, Eqs. 6-6 and 6-7 can also be used if, for example, effective sheet widths (or areas) are desired at operating stress levels.

The engineer should recall from Sec. 6-2 that the inter-rivet buckling stress F_{ir} of a riveted compression member must be greater than or equal to the allowable crippling stress F_{cc} of the main compression member to prevent premature inter-rivet buckling. However, if the value of F_{ir} is less than the value of F_{cc} (which presumes premature inter-rivet buckling), then a reduction in effective sheet strength occurs. To account for this reduction, the effective sheet widths calculated from Eqs. 6-10 and 6-11 must now be slightly modified or reduced by the following ratios:

$$(W_e)_r = W_e\left[\frac{F_{ir}}{F_{cc}}\right] \tag{6-12}$$

and

$$(W_f)_r = W_f\left[\frac{F_{ir}}{F_{cc}}\right] \tag{6-13}$$

where: F_{ir} = allowable inter-rivet buckling stress of the riveted sheet member
F_{cc} = allowable crippling stress of the main compression member
W_e = effective width of sheet (from Eq. 6-10)
W_f = effective width of sheet (from Eq. 6-11).

Reduced effective sheet areas are then recalculated as follows:

$$(\text{Area})_e = (W_e)_r\, t \tag{6-14}$$

$$(\text{Area})_f = (W_f)_r\, t. \tag{6-15}$$

Let us now summarize the previous arguments:

(1) If $F_{ir} \geq F_{cc}$, use the effective sheet widths W_e and W_f.

(2) If $F_{ir} < F_{cc}$, use the reduced effective sheet widths $(W_e)_r$ and $(W_f)_r$.

In conclusion: To derive an approximate solution for the effective sheet width of riveted sheet members, the yield compression stress allowable of the material —normally used as a maximum compression value for aircraft design—is used here as a limiting value or cutoff stress for F_{cc} in Eqs. 6-10 and 6-11. Hence, for

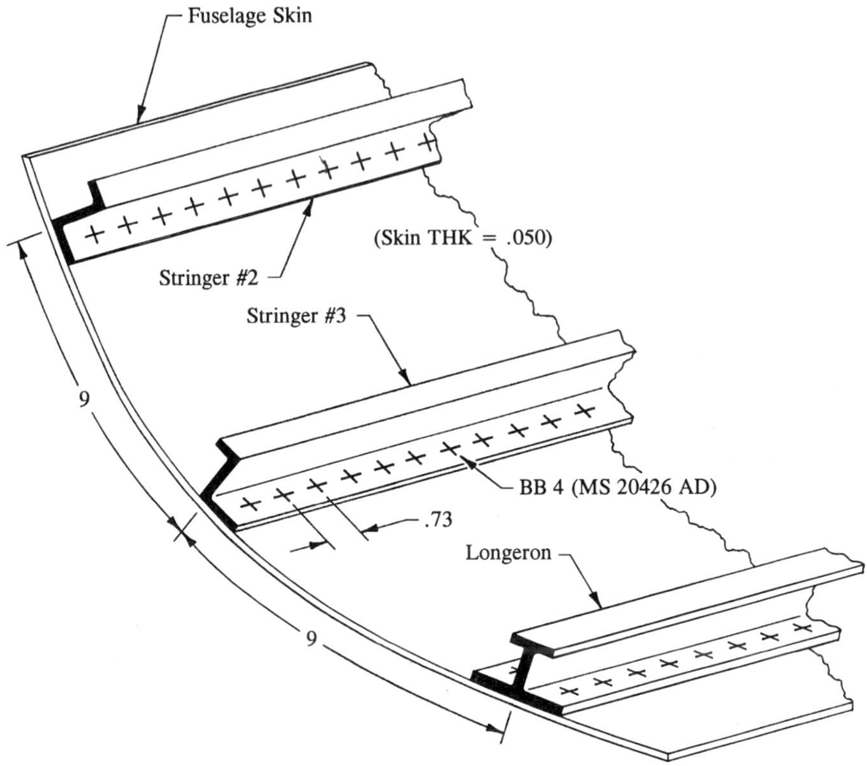

FIGURE 6-15 Fuselage shell supported by longitudinal zee stringers.

any given material, knowing the values of F_{cy} and E_c, the approximate solution for effective sheet width is determined. In a similar manner, the engineer can formulate other approximate solutions for different materials (refer to MIL-HDBK-5 for specific material types).

Example 6-1 The fuselage shell (skin panels) is supported by longitudinal (long axis) zee stringers, as shown in Fig. 6-15. For an allowable crippling stress of 30,579 psi (see ahead to Table 6-6 and calculation of this quantity on page 399), determine the effective skin area (in compression) acting with each stringer. Then use the ultimate stringer loads given from a computer model solution of these members, Fig. 6-16, to predict the following structural failures: (1) compression failure of the skin-stringer composite section, (2) tension failure of the skin-stringer composite section, and (3) shearing failure of the skin rivets. (*Hint:* Skin shear flows can be determined from stringer loads using Eq. 4-1 or $q = \Delta P/L$.) Material: skin, 2024-T3 aluminum clad, QQ-A-250/5; stringers, 2024-T3 extrusion, QQ-A-200/3. Sign convention adopted for stringer loads: a positive value (+)

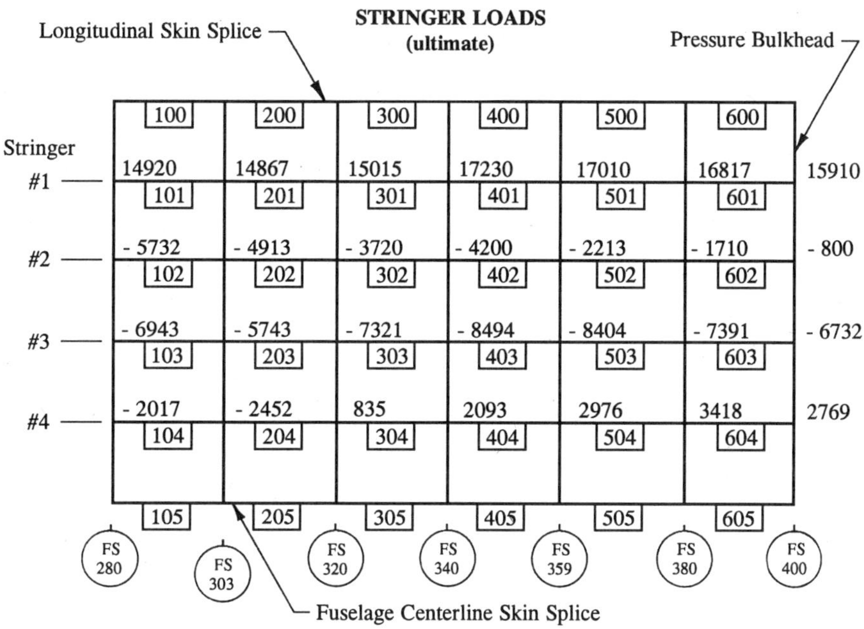

FIGURE 6-16 Ultimate stringer loads.

indicates an axial tension load and a negative value (–) indicates an axial compression load.

SOLUTION: The cross-sectional area of a typical stringer is shown in Fig. 6-17. Equation 6-10 is used to determine the amount of sheet material (i.e., width of skin) that is effective in compression with this member. The allowable crippling stress of the stringer or 30,579 psi is used for this evaluation. This will force the stringer and skin to fail simultaneously at this predetermined value:

$$W_e = 1.7t\sqrt{E_c/F_{cc}} = 1.7(.050)\sqrt{\frac{10,700,000}{30,579}} = 1.590 \text{ in.}$$

For the skin area to be fully effective at a stress level of 30,579 psi, premature inter-rivet buckling of the skin must be prevented. Inter-rivet buckling of the attached flange of the Z-section stringer must also be prevented. However, this particular evaluation is determined when the allowable crippling stress of the stringer is computed. The basic procedure used to make this particular modification is described in full detail when our study of compression members resumes in Sec. 6.4. Let us now determine a value for the inter-rivet buckling stress of the attached skin. First, the value of L'/ρ (from Table 6-2) for BB 4 rivets spaced .73 in apart is determined.

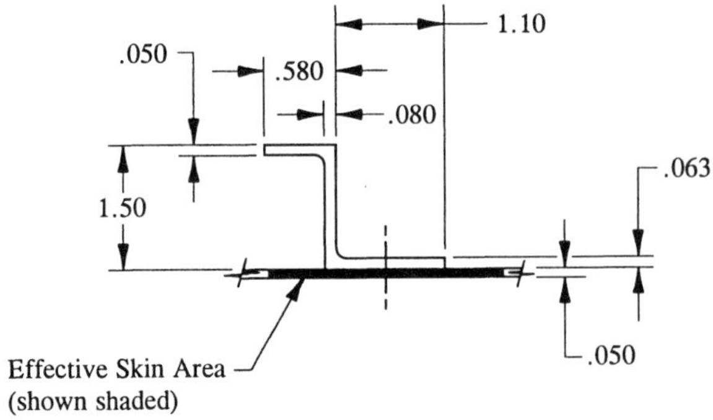

FIGURE 6-17 Cross-sectional area of a typical stringer.

$$L'/\rho = 2\sqrt{2}\ \frac{s}{t} = 2\sqrt{2}\left[\frac{.73}{.050}\right] = 41.3$$

where: $s = .73$ in
$t = .050$ in.

With the value of L'/ρ and a column instability curve for 2024-T3 aluminum clad material (QQ-A-250/5), we obtain the allowable inter-rivet buckling stress F_{ir} for the skin or 30,200 psi. But, since $F_{ir} < F_{cc}$, the effective width W_e must be further reduced to account for premature inter-rivet buckling of this member. Hence, from Eq. 6-12, we obtain:

Effective Width of Skin:

$$(W_e)_r = W_e\left[\frac{F_{ir}}{F_{cc}}\right] = 1.590\left[\frac{30,200}{30,579}\right] = 1.570 \text{ in.}$$

Area Calculations

In compression, the total effective cross-sectional area of the skin-stringer composite section is

$$A_c = A_{\text{stringer}} + A_{\text{skin}} = .214 + .078 = .292 \text{ in}^2$$

where: $A_{\text{stringer}} = (.580 - .080).050 + 1.500(.080) + 1.100(.063) = .214 \text{ in}^2$
$A_{\text{skin}} = (W_e)_r t = 1.570(.050) = .078 \text{ in}^2$ (effective skin area).

In tension, the total effective cross-sectional area of the skin-stringer composite section is

$$A_t = A_{\text{stringer}} + A_{\text{skin}} = .214 + .450 = .664 \text{ in}^2$$

where: $A_{\text{stringer}} = .214 \text{ in}^2$ (same area as that of the stringer in compression)
$A_{\text{skin}} = 9(.050) = .450 \text{ in}^2$ (the skin is fully effective in tension, see Fig. 6-18).

Compression Strength of the Skin-Stringer Composite Section:

$$P_{cc} = F_{cc} A_c = 30,579(.292) = 8,929 \text{ lb}$$

where: $F_{cc} = 30,579$ psi
$A = .292 \text{ in}^2$.

Compression failure is predicted by:

$$\text{Margin of Safety} = \text{M.S.} = \frac{P_{cc}}{p_c} - 1 = \frac{8,929}{8,494} - 1 = +.05$$

where: $P_{cc} = 8,929$ lb
$p_c = 8,494$ lb ultimate (see Fig. 6-16, Stringer #3, Bar No. 403).

Tension Strength of the Skin-Stringer Composite Section:

$$P_t = F_{tu} A_t = (F_{tu})_{\text{skin}} A_{\text{skin}} + (F_{tu})_{\text{stringer}} A_{\text{stringer}}$$
$$P_t = 59,000(.450) + 57,000(.214) = 38,748 \text{ lb}$$

where: $(F_{tu})_{\text{skin}}$ = ultimate allowable tension stress of the skin, see Table A-4
$(F_{tu})_{\text{stringer}}$ = ultimate allowable tension stress of the stringer, see Table A-2
A_{skin} = effective skin area in tension (Fig. 6-18)
A_{stringer} = stringer cross-sectional area.

Tension failure is predicted by:

$$\text{Margin of Safety} = \text{M.S.} = \frac{P_t}{p_t} - 1 = \frac{38,748}{17,230} - 1 = +1.25$$

where: $P_t = 38,748$ lb
$p_t = 17,230$ lb ultimate (see Fig. 6-16, Stringer #1, Bar No. 401).

Shear Strength of the Skin Rivets:

To determine the shear strength of the skin rivets, fastener shearing forces or skin shear flows must be known along the stringers. Shear flows can be obtained

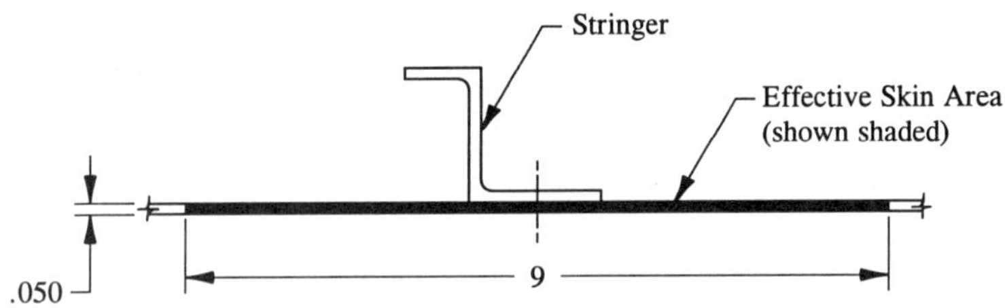

FIGURE 6-18 Effective skin area in tension.

directly from stringer loads, and then from these, fastener shearing forces can be determined. The following will help illustrate this procedure:

$$q = \frac{\Delta P}{L} \quad \text{(refer back to Eq. 4-1, page 226)}$$

where: q = applied shear flow

ΔP = change in load between the axial forces at the ends of the stringer

L = distance measured between axial forces at the ends of the stringer.

Physically, this equation can be described as follows: the change in load between axial forces at the ends of the stringer is what the skin rivets must actually develop to maintain static equilibrium of this member. To determine a maximum design value, the following stringers are isolated and free-bodied, as shown in Fig. 6-19:

STRINGER #1 (Bar No. 301)

$$\Sigma F_x = 0, \qquad -15{,}015 - \Delta P + 17{,}230 = 0, \quad \Delta P = 2{,}215 \text{ lb}$$

$$q = \frac{\Delta P}{L} = \frac{2{,}215}{20} = 111 \text{ lb/in.}$$

STRINGER #2 (Bar No. 402)

$$\Sigma F_x = 0, \qquad 4{,}200 - \Delta P - 2{,}213 = 0, \quad \Delta P = 1{,}987 \text{ lb}$$

$$q = \frac{\Delta P}{L} = \frac{1{,}987}{19} = 105 \text{ lb/in.}$$

STRINGER #4 (Bar No. 204)

$$\Sigma F_x = 0, \qquad 2{,}452 - \Delta P + 835 = 0, \quad \Delta P = 3{,}287 \text{ lb}$$

$$q = \frac{\Delta P}{L} = \frac{3{,}287}{17} = 193 \text{ lb/in} \quad \text{(maximum value).}$$

STRINGER #1 (Bar No. 301)

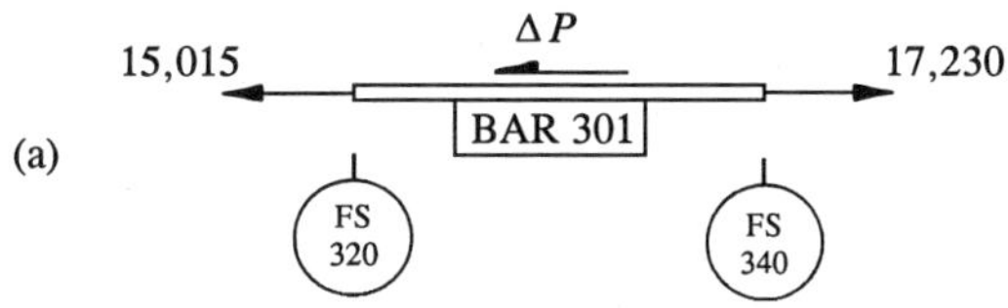

STRINGER #2 (Bar No. 402)

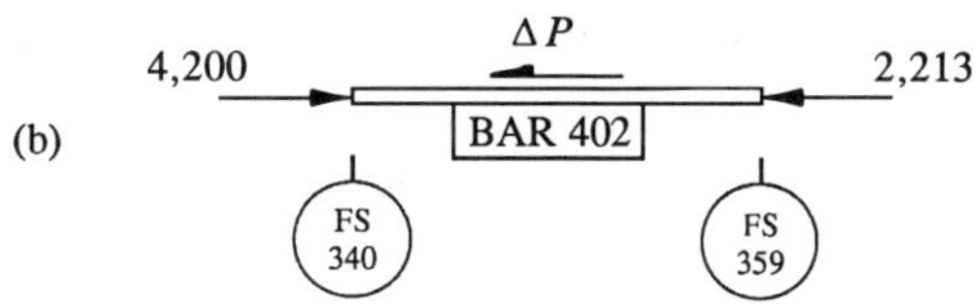

STRINGER #4 (Bar No. 204)

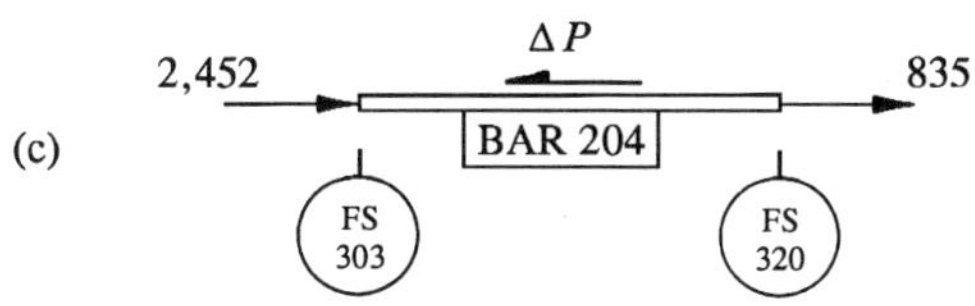

FIGURE 6-19 Stringers are isolated and free-bodied.

To obtain rivet shearing forces, the following equation is applied:

$$p_s = qs = 193(.73) = 141 \text{ lb ultimate (refer back to Eq. 4-10, page 254)}$$

where: p_s = fastener shearing forces
q = applied shear flow
s = fastener spacing.

Ultimate Allowable Shear Strength of the Skin Rivets:

The static joint strength for BB 4 rivets (MS 20426 AD) installed in machine-countersunk .050 aluminum skin is 340 lb (see Table 8.1.2.2(f) in MIL-HDBK-5F for this value). It is recalled that joint rivet allowables for machine-countersunk rivets are based on prescribed government agency specifications.[1]

---

[1] Rivet shear allowables calculated using Equation 3-1 of Chapter 3 are valid only for solid, protruding-head rivets.

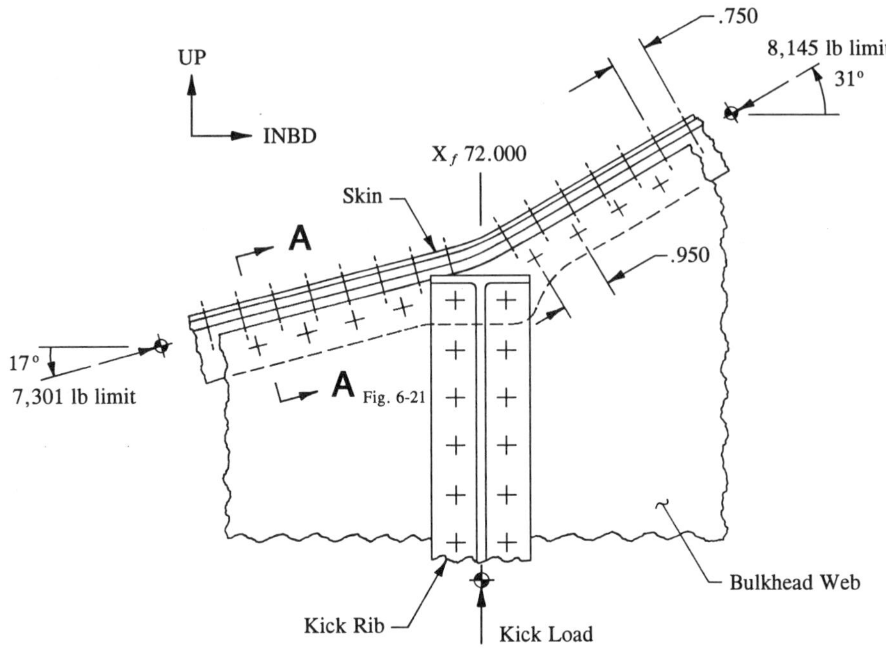

FIGURE 6-20 Vertical unbalance of this joint is reacted by the kick rib.

Shearing failure is predicted as follows:

$$\text{Margin of Safety} = \text{M.S.} = \frac{P_{su}}{p_s k} - 1 = \frac{340}{141(1.15)} - 1 = +1.10$$

where: $P_{su} = 340$ lb

$p_s = 141$ lb ultimate

$k = 1.15$ (fitting factor for joint or connection design).

Bearing failure of the skin and stringer flange is left as a supplementary exercise for the engineer to complete. Refer to Sec. 3.2 for the analysis details and procedure to determine this particular failure mode. This evaluation should however yield very high margins of safety for both the skin and riveted flange members.

Example 6-2 The Y_f 847 bulkhead is joined to the X_f 72 kick rib of the wing carry-through structure, as shown in Fig. 6-20. The vertical unbalance of this joint is reacted by the kick rib. Determine this unbalance for the compression loads indicated. Is the kick load compression or tension on the rib? If the bulkhead cap (Section A-A) is constructed of members as shown in Fig. 6-21, determine the effective

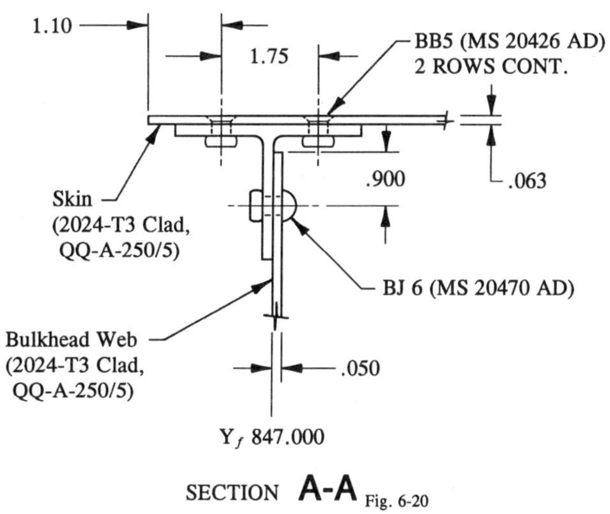

FIGURE 6-21 Bulkhead cap cross-sectional area.

areas of skin and web in compression. Assume an allowable crippling stress of 21,700 psi for the T-section (Area = .400 in^2). After the effective areas of the skin and web are determined, calculate the compression allowable load of the bulkhead cap—this includes the T-section and skin and web members acting in composite.

SOLUTION: Since the main cap member (T-section) is stabilized by web and skin members, the compression cap is physically prevented from actually failing as a column. Instead, compression failure will occur by crippling of the composite section. This means that the T-section, effective skin and web members will all undergo or reach collapsing failure simultaneously (this should occur at the same stress level for each member of the same type material). For members of different material types, a few additional comments are necessary.[1] The kick load (or reaction R in Fig. 6-22) is obtained by a vertical balance of loads at the joint intersection. From statics, the kick load R is obtained:

$$\Sigma F_y = 0, \qquad 7,301 \sin 17^\circ - 8,145 \sin 31^\circ + R = 0$$

$$R = 2,060 \text{ lb limit}.$$

Notice how the line of action of each load meets at a common point of intersection. This eliminates unbalanced moments produced by joint eccentricities and thus produces a good overall joint design. The design engineer should always

[1] The engineer is referred to Elmer F. Bruhn, *Analysis and Design of Flight Vehicle Structures*, Sec. C7.13, "Effective Width When Sheet and Stiffener Have Different Material Properties," p. C7.12, Tri-State Offset Company, Cincinnati, Ohio, 1965.

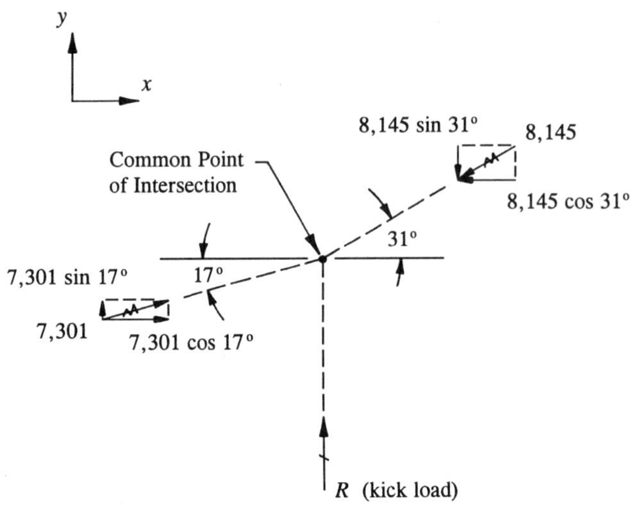

FIGURE 6-22 Vertical balance of loads at the joint intersection.

strive to minimize joint eccentricities, especially in the preliminary design phase of a structure where most designs are conceptualized. To neglect their occurrence will only lead to and produce unnecessary complications and weight penalties later that might otherwise be avoided now.

The effective widths of skin and web (shown shaded in Fig. 6-23(a)) are defined according to Eqs. 6-10 and 6-11. Use this figure as a general guide to the solution of effective areas of these members.

Effective Sheet Widths of Skin:

$$(1)\quad W_e = 1.7t\sqrt{E_c/F_{cc}} = 1.7(.063)\sqrt{\frac{10,700,000}{21,700}} = 2.378 \text{ in}$$

$$\tfrac{1}{2}W_e = \tfrac{1}{2}(2.378) = 1.189 \text{ in.}$$

$$(2)\quad W_f = .62t\sqrt{E_c/F_{cc}} = .62(.063)\sqrt{\frac{10,700,000}{21,700}} = .867 \text{ in}$$

where: $F_{cc} = 21,700$ psi (given)
$E_c = 10,700,000$ psi (see Table A-4 in Appendix E)
$t = .063$ in.

For the skin areas to be fully effective (as calculated) at a stress level of 21,700 psi, premature inter-rivet buckling of the skin must be prevented. To do this, $F_{ir} \geq F_{cc}$ must be maintained for this member (the engineer should refer back

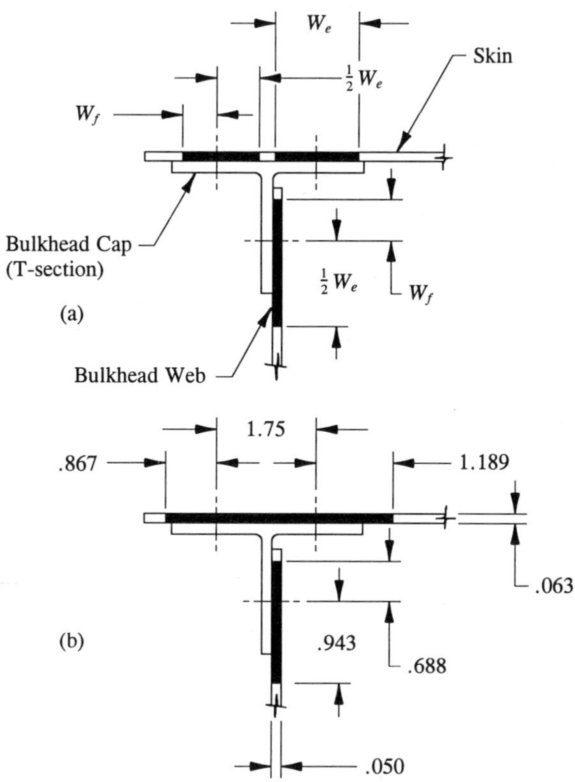

FIGURE 6-23 Cross-sectional area of the bulkhead cap, (a) defined for the skin and web areas and (b) calculated values for the skin and web areas.

to the arguments given at the beginning of this section if this criterion is not clearly understood). For BB 5 rivets, the end-fixity coefficient c is 1.5. From Table 6-2, the corresponding effective slenderness ratio is

$$L'/\rho = 2\sqrt{2}\,\frac{s}{t} = 2\sqrt{2}\left[\frac{.750}{.063}\right] = 33.7$$

where: $s = .750$ in (see Fig. 6-20)
$t = .063$ in.

Now, using a column curve for clad 2024-T3 aluminum alloy material, with a value of $L'/\rho = 33.7$, we obtain the allowable inter-rivet buckling stress F_{ir} of the skin or 32,300 psi. Since this value is greater than F_{cc}, the effective sheet widths are not corrected. Their values are shown in Fig. 6-23(b). Observe from this figure that no more than 1.75 in of effective skin material can be used between skin rivet lines, even though our effective width calculations would have indicated more ($1/2\,W_e + 1/2\,W_e = W_e = 2.378$). In other words, the effective area of the skin is bounded by the material existing between skin rivets or 1.75 in.

Effective Sheet Widths of Web:

$$(1)\quad W_e = 1.7t\sqrt{E_c/F_{cc}} = 1.7(.050)\sqrt{\frac{10,700,000}{21,700}} = 1.887 \text{ in}$$

$$\tfrac{1}{2}W_e = \tfrac{1}{2}(1.887) = .943 \text{ in.}$$

$$(2)\quad W_f = .62t\sqrt{E_c/F_{cc}} = .62(.050)\sqrt{\frac{10,700,000}{21,700}} = .688 \text{ in}$$

where: $F_{cc} = 21,700$ psi (given)
$E_c = 10,700,000$ psi (see Table A-4 in Appendix E)
$t = .050$ in.

If the web is completely effective (that is, based on effective sheet area calculations) at a stress level of 21,700 psi, this member must also prevent premature inter-rivet buckling ($F_{ir} \geq F_{cc}$). For BJ 6 rivets, the end-fixity coefficient c is 3.0. And from Table 6-2, the corresponding effective slenderness ratio is

$$L'/\rho = 2\frac{s}{t} = 2\left[\frac{.950}{.050}\right] = 38.0$$

where: $s = .950$ in (see Fig. 6-20)
$t = .050$ in.

Again, using a column curve for clad 2024-T3 aluminum alloy material, with a value of $L'/\rho = 38.0$, we obtain the allowable inter-rivet buckling stress F_{ir} of the web or 31,200 psi. At this value, premature inter-rivet buckling is avoided and the web is considered fully effective (based, that is, on the effective width calculations above). These values are also shown in Fig. 6-23(b). The total effective area of the bulkhead cap section in compression is

$$A_c = A_{\text{cap}} + A_{\text{skin}} + A_{\text{web}} = .400 + .240 + .082 = .722 \text{ in}^2$$

where: $A_{\text{cap}} = .400$ in (given)
$A_{\text{skin}} = (.867 + 1.750 + 1.189)(.063) = .240 \text{ in}^2$
$A_{\text{web}} = (.688 + .943)(.050) = .082 \text{ in}^2$.

The compression allowable load of the composite bulkhead cap section is

$$P_{cc} = F_{cc} A_c = 21,700(.722) = 15,667 \text{ lb}.$$

Crippling failure is then predicted as follows:

$$\text{Margin of Safety} = \text{M.S.} = \frac{P_{cc}}{p_c} - 1 = \frac{15,667}{12,217} - 1 = +.28$$

where: $P_{cc} = 15,667$ lb
$p_c = -8,145$ lb limit (see Fig. 6-20); $-12,217$ lb ultimate.

6.4 Crippling of Built-up Sections in Compression. In this section, the subject of crippling of built-up sections in compression is presented. However, before the engineer actually proceeds ahead with the study of this material, the following related topics and their applications should be thoroughly understood: (1) inter-rivet buckling of compression members and (2) effective sheet areas of built-up sections in compression. The engineer is referred to Secs. 6.2 and 6.3, respectively, for their review and general study. Some fundamental background and understanding of these subjects are essential to our study and basic understanding of crippling of built-up sections in compression in this section.

When referring to compression failures, three general categories should immediately come to mind:

(1) Column failures - where the allowable compression stress of a structural member is based on column instability (see Chapter 7, "Column Members").

(2) Crippling failures - where the allowable compression stress of a structural member is based on the structural shape (or geometry) of the cross-sectional area of the member.[1]

(3) Block-compression failures - where the allowable compression stress of a structural member is based on a maximum stress cutoff corresponding to the magnitude of the ultimate allowable tension stress of the material or F_{tu}, again refer to Chapter 7.[2]

If a flat sheet or plate is formed into a structural shape, as shown in Fig. 6-24, the formed sheet metal member inherently becomes stiffer. This follows from the physical nature of the geometrically more efficient structural shape of this member.

---

[1] In addition, the allowable compression stress of such a member is based on a maximum stress (or cutoff value) corresponding to the yield compression stress of the material or F_{cy}.

[2] The engineer is cautioned here not to place any undue emphasis or importance (structurally) on the word "tension," since the actual structural member considered will always physically be loaded in "compression." The ultimate allowable tension stress of the material is only used here as an indication of an ideal maximum or acceptable cutoff value for the allowable compression stress permissible for the design of members undergoing this type of failure.

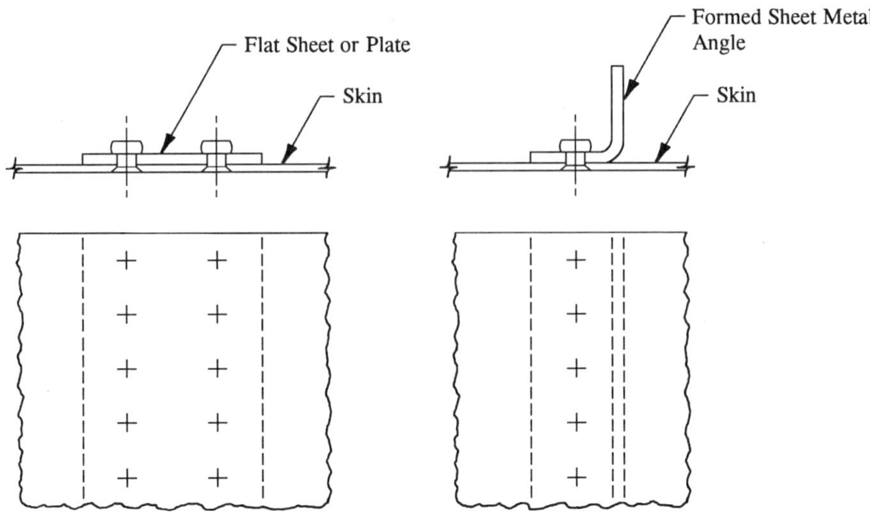

FIGURE 6-24 Flat sheet formed into a geometrically more efficient shape.

Theoretically what happens is that the stiffer corner provides the ability (or increased capacity) to accept additional load that the rather inefficient (low buckling) sheet or plate by itself cannot. Basically, after the plate elements have buckled, the increasing load on the section is transferred to the stiffer corners. Therefore, a formed section has the ability to carry a higher compression load before ultimate failure or collapse of the total section occurs, even though the plate-like elements theoretically have buckled. In other words, the formed section is made up of plate-like elements that theoretically buckle at relatively low stress values. Even so, as the section is continued to be loaded, the plate-like elements that buckled have not actually failed in the strict sense of the word "failure." That is, this form of buckling implies or refers to the inherent ability of such members to sustain load. The higher stress build-up of the structural shape is identified here as

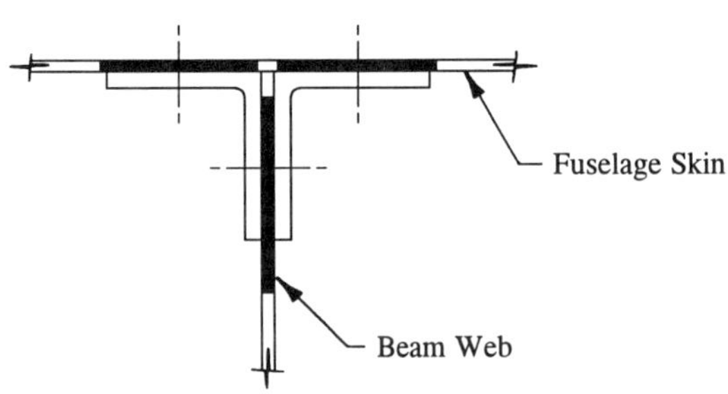

FIGURE 6-25 Compression cap stabilized by web and skin members.

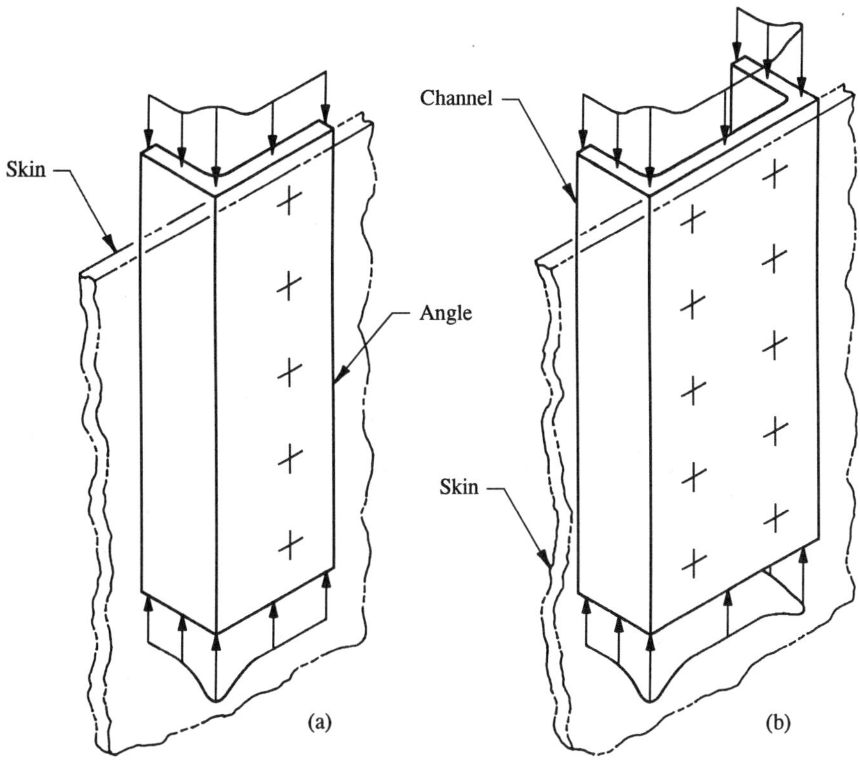

FIGURE 6-26 Nonuniform stress distribution for (a) an extruded angle and (b) an extruded channel in compression.

"crippling" failure. When crippling failure of a structural member occurs, all structural components of that member will fail simultaneously (including the plate-like elements) at one prescribed (allowable) stress level.

Now, refer to Fig. 6-25. If the compression cap of this beam structure is stabilized by web and skin members, the compression cap no longer behaves as a true column. In this case, the compression allowable of the cap is based on the crippling stress F_{cc} of the composite section (this should include all members that make up the total cross-sectional area of the compression cap: skin, web, and main members). Simply put, this means that crippling is not influenced directly by the effects of column instability. This of course assumes the structure is laterally stable under load: no sideways motion of the structure can occur which can precipitate the ultimate collapse (or failure) of the structural member as a column. Also, the structural member is sufficiently short in length to prevent column instability. Hence, if these conditions are met, one can safely say that the allowable crippling strength of such a member (or noncolumn) is principally governed by the geometric dimensions (or shape) of the cross-sectional area of the member.

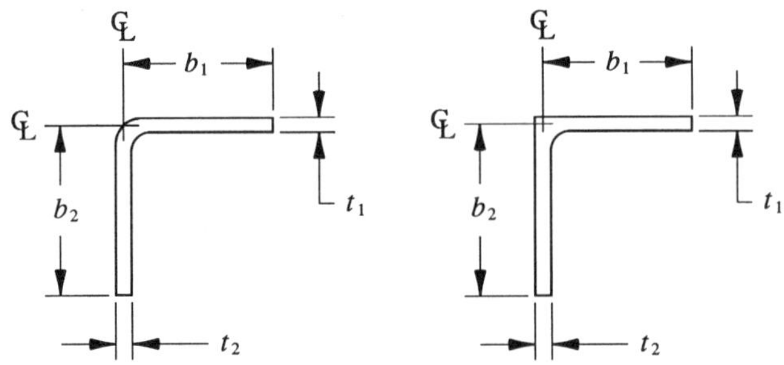

Formed Sheet Metal Angle

Extruded Angle

$$\frac{b'}{t} = \frac{b_1 + b_2}{t_1 + t_2}$$

FIGURE 6-27 Dimensions of b and t for formed and extruded angle sections.

When a beam (formed or extruded structural shape) is loaded in compression, the plate-like elements that make up the structural shape of the beam will begin to buckle. As the load is increased however, the stiffer corners of these elements will accept the higher stress build-up. Failure is reached at a stress level corresponding to the local crippling (failure) stress F_{cc} of the composite section (this includes all structural members that make up the total cross-sectional area). From this description, one can deduce the following conclusion: that the crippling stress of a structural shape will always be higher than the buckling stress of the individual plate-like elements forming the structural shape. The stress distribution in Fig. 6-26 shows how the higher stress build-up (or intensity) at the corner of an angle section can occur. In theory, the crippling stress is assumed to be uniformly distributed over the structural shape, but in reality, the actual stress varies considerably along the cross-sectional area as shown in this figure. Consequently, the crippling stress of individual members can actually be greater than the composite crippling stress of the total cross-sectional area.

Although the plate-like elements of a formed or extruded section have buckled (commonly referred to as local buckling), the structural shape as a whole can still assume additional load until failure. Local buckling refers to a state of stress in which the buckled plate-like elements of the structural shape do not actually fail. This condition results because deformations have not been sufficient to cause such failure. Crippling of compression members, however, presumes total and catastrophic (permanent) failure. Therefore, compression members must be carefully studied to ensure their reliability and structural integrity in production designs.

The allowable crippling stress of a formed or extruded angle section, Fig. 6-27, is given by the following general formula:[1]

$$F_{cc} = \frac{C_e \sqrt{F_{cy} E_c}}{(b'/t)^{3/4}} \tag{6-16}$$

where: F_{cc} = allowable crippling stress
F_{cy} = yield compression stress allowable of the material
E_c = elastic modulus of the material in compression
C_e = material and edge-support coefficient (see Table 6-3, page 390)
b'/t = equivalent b/t ratio, as defined in Fig. 6-27 for formed and extruded angle sections.

In general, the corner (or fillet area) of an extruded angle section is usually neglected by the analyst. The reason is that the actual restraint capability of most structural shapes is usually unknown. Specifically, the distribution of stresses in the corners of extruded structural shapes have not been theoretically verified nor well-defined enough to justify the corner area of the extruded member to be considered effective or included in the analysis of compression members. The method of analysis presented thus far in this section is based on tests and some empirical data; however, the method is sufficiently accurate for aircraft design. Whether or not the fillet area is considered effective in the crippling strength of compression members is left entirely up to the discretion of the proper agency or governing body in charge of overseeing such matters.

Nondimensional crippling curves are sometimes provided by structural engineering departments for design engineering use. The basic approach, if applied successfully, can usually save the engineer invaluable time by avoiding repeat computations necessary in the solution of Eq. 6-16 for crippling calculations. If such curves are available, they should be used unless specific material design curves are instead provided; in which case these curves are instead used. Either curve will save the engineer considerable time to warrant their specific inclusion in the material of this section. Empirical data have shown that the bend radii of formed sections and fillet radii of extruded sections have a negligible effect on the crippling strengths of these structural forms. Also, the crippling strength of an angle section is not very sensitive to variations of included angle. Generally, included angles ranging from 70° to 120° are permissible without any structural loss (decrease in allowable crippling strength), and therefore, Eq. 6-16 is also applicable for these special structural shapes.

---

[1] The following references are recommended: (1) Heimerl, G.J., "Determination of Plate Compressive Strengths," *NACA TN No. 1480*, December 1948; and (2) Needham, R.A., "The Ultimate Strength of Aluminum Alloy Formed Structural Shapes in Compression," *Journal of the Aeronautical Sciences*, Vol. 21, No. 4, p. 224, April 1954.

When the allowable crippling stress of a member exceeds the proportional limit of the material, a reduction in overall stiffness occurs. This causes the structural member to buckle at a stress below the actual calculated value indicated by the solution of Eq. 6-16. The problem of inelastic stresses (stresses occurring above the proportional limit of the material) can however be resolved by limiting the maximum value of the allowable crippling stress to the yield compression stress allowable of the material F_{cy}. Above the proportional limit of the material, Hooke's Law is no longer valid, but varies depending upon operating stress levels on a stress-strain diagram.

The application of Eq. 6-16 applies to both formed and extruded angle sections; no difference is made between the allowable crippling stress solutions of their alternative structural design forms. Most fillet areas of extruded structural shapes are neglected in crippling calculations—their omission should generally produce slightly conservative results for the compression members. However, the actual area of a formed structural shape must be considered; otherwise, the analysis results of that member will be (slightly) unconservative. Since most commonly used aircraft structural members (H-sections, I-sections, T-sections, and other structural shapes) can be theoretically duplicated or identified in terms of a series of angle sections, these more complex structural shapes can also be analyzed by this method. Mathematically, this is done by determining the weighted-average allowable crippling stress of the structural shape based on the individual angle sections describing the entire geometrical shape. To predict the weighted-average allowable crippling stress of these structural shapes, the following equation is presented:[1]

$$(F_{cc})_{\text{average}} = \frac{\Sigma(F_{cc}A)}{\Sigma A} \qquad \textbf{(6-17)}$$

where: $(F_{cc})_{\text{average}}$ = weighted-average allowable crippling stress of the structural shape

$\Sigma(F_{cc}A) = (F_{cc}A)_1 + (F_{cc}A)_2 + (F_{cc}A)_3 + \ldots + (F_{cc}A)_n$

$\Sigma A = A_1 + A_2 + A_3 + \ldots + A_n$

F_{cc} = allowable crippling stress of a formed or extruded angle section

A = area of a formed or extruded angle section.

The structural shapes shown in Fig. 6-28 can be used as standards of comparison against which to check the crippling of other similar and related structural shapes often encountered in actual engineering designs. The structural shapes given can be defined in terms of either formed or extruded angle sections since no difference is made between their structural forms in the analysis of crippling members used in this section. The angle sections of a structural shape will accept load

[1] For an extruded T-section, this method is slightly conservative. Test values have shown that the allowable crippling stress for such a section is actually 4% higher.

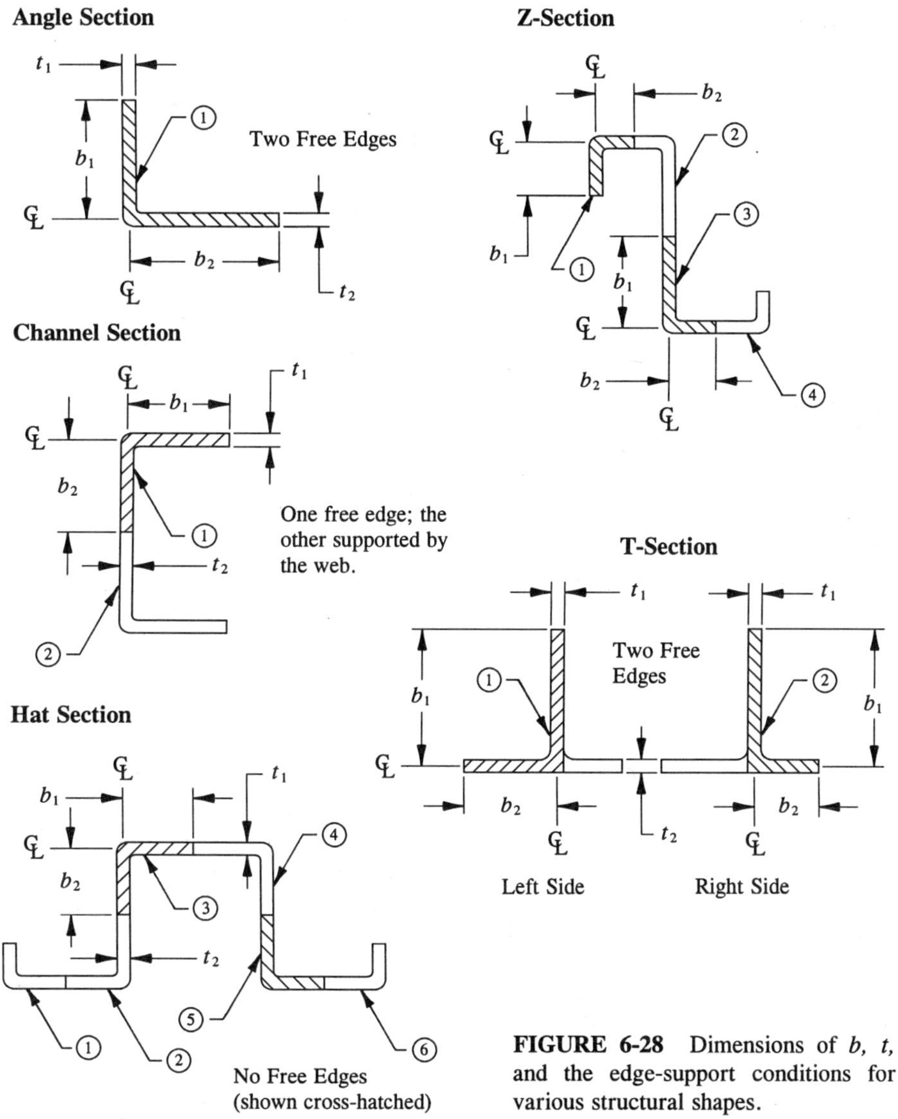

FIGURE 6-28 Dimensions of b, t, and the edge-support conditions for various structural shapes.

until all sections of that structural shape are fully loaded. Then, the structural shape will reach its maximum load capacity at failure.[1] This maximum is measured by the allowable crippling stress of the member, and is limited by the yield

[1] This does not necessarily mean that the elements of the structural shape have actually yielded. On the contrary, from earlier discussions of this subject, the plate-like elements of the structural shape have buckled, not yielded. The structural shape actually deforms as a unit until the ultimate collapsing stress of the entire section has been reached. Crippling is therefore the concept of total combined failure.

compression stress allowable of the material. This limitation also helps to establish and control the design of fatigue-sensitive structural members. Higher values are permissible if the particular section in question has been substantiated by structural test.

The crippling strength of a compression member is also a function of the degree of edge-restraint of the web and flange elements that make up the cross-sectional area of the member. An angle section, for instance, provides a simply-supported edge (or corner) for each of its plate-like (flange) elements, as shown in Fig. 6-29. The stiffer corners (shown cross-hatched in this figure) represent simply-supported edges for the flange and included web elements of these structural shapes. A channel section also provides simply-supported edges for its flange elements, while additionally providing simply-supported edges for the included web. Table 6-3 lists the support restraint capabilities possible for various materials in terms of edge-support coefficients C_e.[1]

TABLE 6-3 MATERIAL AND EDGE-SUPPORT COEFFICIENTS*

Material	Edge-Condition	C_e
Aluminum	2 free edges	0.295
	1 free edge	0.317
	no free edges	0.339†
Steel	2 free edges	0.274
	1 free edge	0.318
	no free edges	0.362†
Titanium	2 free edges	0.272
	1 free edge	0.307
	no free edges	0.342†

* In this table, a free edge refers to the unsupported edge of a structural member.

† These values were linearly extrapolated from the previous test values given in this table for that material.

The solution of Eq. 6-17 for the allowable crippling stress of various structural shapes is best arrived at in tabular form, as shown in Table 6-4. In general, beam caps are constructed of combinations of formed and extruded sections joined together by attachment rivets. The allowable crippling stress of these riveted members should be compared to the allowable inter-rivet buckling stress F_{ir} between

[1] The coefficients listed in this table are based on nominal values (refer specifically to a company structures manual).

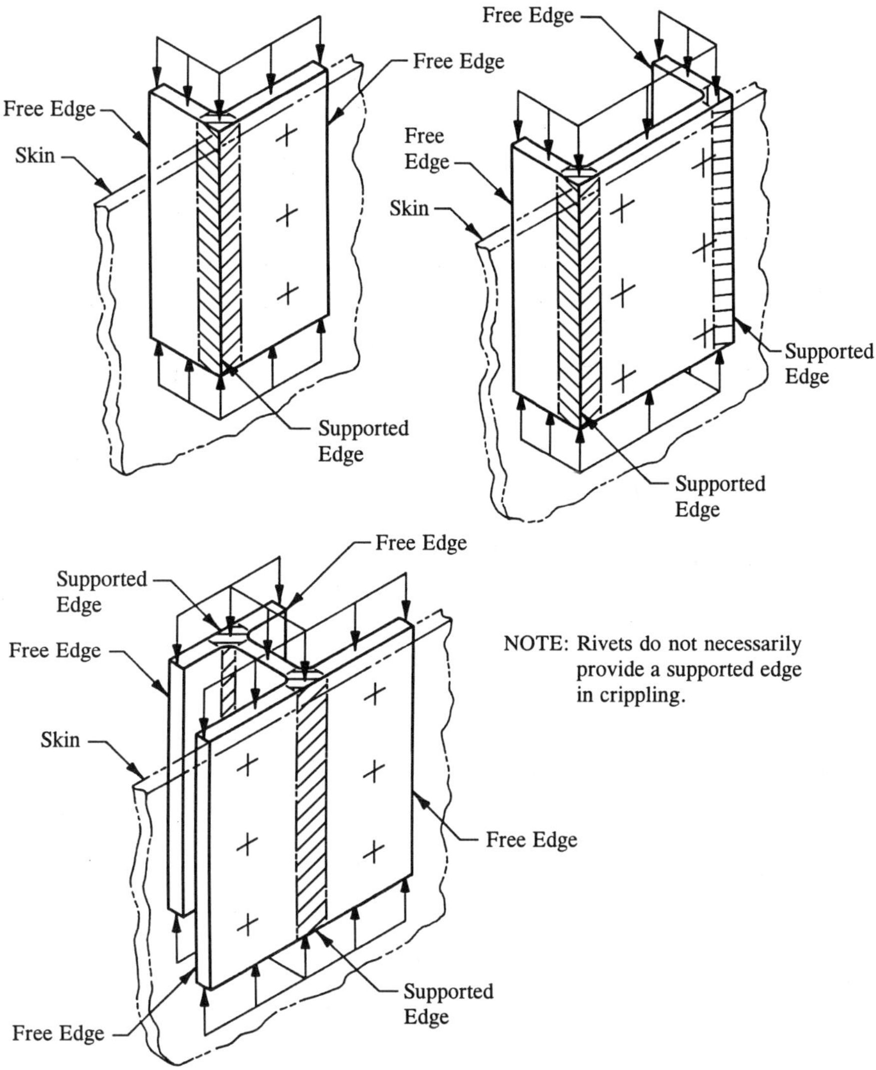

FIGURE 6-29 Edge-restraints of web and flange elements.

rivets so that any reduction in effective sheet area necessary can be made for these members. For instance, if the inter-rivet buckling stress F_{ir} between rivets of a compression member occurs prematurely (is lower than the crippling stress of the main member), the value of F_{ir} then becomes the limiting value of F_{cc} in computing the crippling stress of that member. Written as an inequality, if $F_{ir} < F_{cc}$, then the value of F_{ir} instead of F_{cc} is used for that particular member in Table 6-4.

TABLE 6-4 CRIPPLING CALCULATIONS

ELEMENT	b'/t	C_e	F_{cc}*	A	$F_{cc}A$
1					
2					
3					
n					
			Total	ΣA	$\Sigma F_{cc}A$

* If $F_{ir} < F_{cc}$, use the value of F_{ir} instead of F_{cc} for that element in this table. Otherwise, use the following equations to complete this table:

$$F_{cc} = \frac{C_e \sqrt{F_{cy} E_c}}{(b'/t)^{3/4}} \qquad \text{where: } b'/t = \frac{b_1 + b_2}{t_1 + t_2}.$$

The allowable compression strength (compression force measured in pounds) of a composite section (cross-sectional area composed of a main member, web, and skin) is expressed mathematically by the following equation:

$$P_{cc} = F_{cc}(A_{\text{main}} + A_{\text{skin}} + A_{\text{web}}) \tag{6-18}$$

$$P_{cc} = F_{cc} A_c \tag{6-19}$$

where: P_{cc} = allowable compression force of the composite section
F_{cc} = crippling stress allowable of the main compression member (use Table 6-4 to compute this value)
A_{main} = cross-sectional area of the main compression member
A_{skin} = effective sheet area of skin in compression
A_{web} = effective sheet area of web in compression
$A_c = A_{\text{main}} + A_{\text{skin}} + A_{\text{web}}$.

Failure is predicted by the following equation:

$$\text{Margin of Safety} = \text{M.S.} = \frac{P_{cc}}{p_c} - 1 \tag{6-20}$$

where: P_{cc} = allowable compression strength of the composite section, lb
p_c = applied load of the main compression member, lb.

Crippling is therefore defined as an average stress at failure of a structural shape. The length of which is assumed to be small to prevent column instability

TABLE 6-5 CRIPPLING OF STRUCTURAL SHAPES IN BENDING

Bending Member	Effective b'/t	Boundary Condition
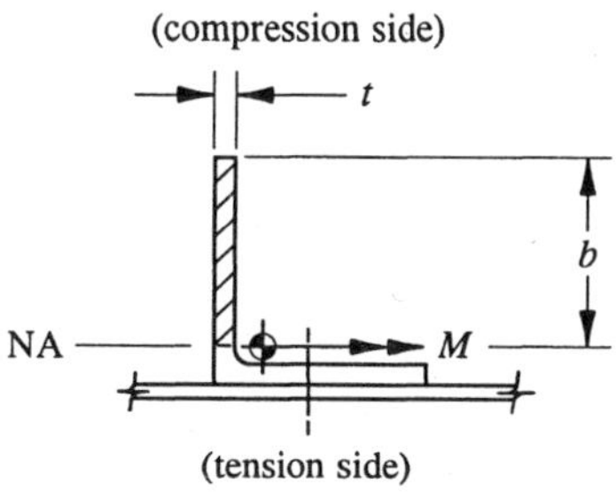	$\frac{b'}{t} = \frac{\frac{2}{3}b}{t} = \frac{2}{3}\frac{b}{t}$	One free edge; the other edge supported (refer to Table 6-3, p. 390).
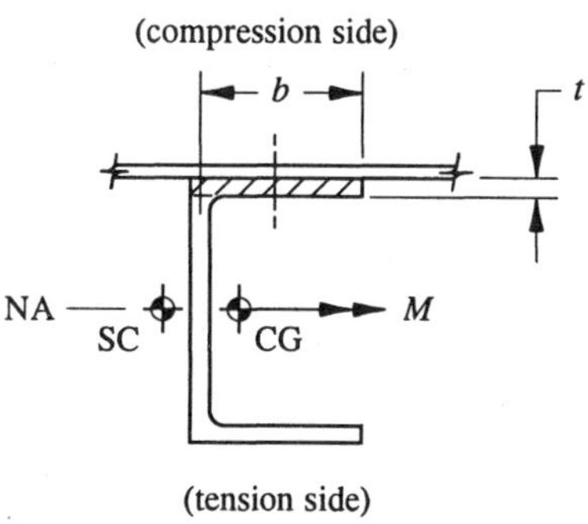	$\frac{b'}{t} = \frac{b}{t}$	One free edge; the other edge supported (refer to Table 6-3, p. 390).
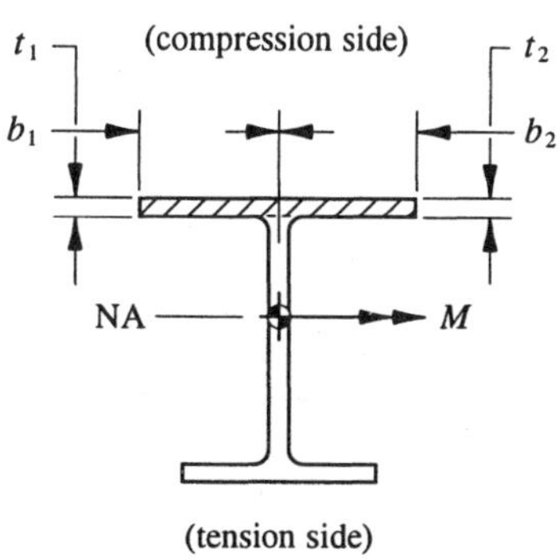	$\frac{b'}{t} = \frac{b_1 + b_2}{t_1 + t_2}$	One free edge; the other edge supported (refer to Table 6-3, p. 390).

from occurring for that member. Although the actual stresses may vary across the structural shape, and may be somewhat higher at the corners than the average crippling stress computed for the total section considered, the structural shape is still assumed to fail at this average stress value. The main member by itself (excluding the web and skin members) controls the overall design of the composite section for crippling. What this means is that the web and skin members, if they exist, are

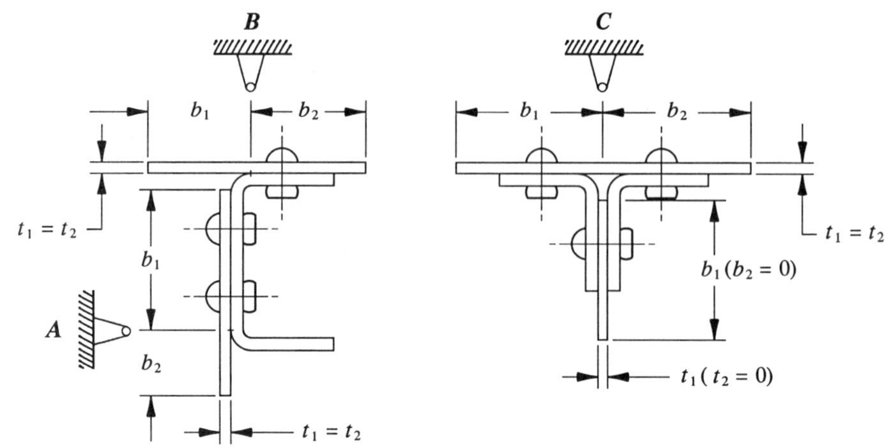

FIGURE 6-30 Reinforcing plates (straps or doublers) attached to built-up sections in compression provide theoretical points of support for the plates. Imaginary supports at *A* and *B* are indicated at the tangency points of the bend radiuses.

considered effective compression members so long as their failures are forced to occur at the allowable crippling stress of the main structural member. This point should be clear from our discussions of crippling failure of composite sections presented earlier in this section.

Crippling Failure of Structural Shapes in Bending

A structural shape in bending is handled a little differently than a member under uniform compression load. The latter is of course the basis of the analysis of most crippling members in this section. The former, or bending member, produces maximum stresses (compression and tension) at the outermost fibers of the section and lower stresses as the centroid of the cross-sectional area is approached. To represent the crippling strength of this member in bending, the compression flange, by itself more representative of a uniform stress distribution, is taken for the value of b'/t. These values are described in Table 6-5 for several different structural shapes in bending. Two points are worth noting about this table. First, the angle section: here, a 2/3 factor is used as a purely subjective guideline to account for the nonuniform stress distribution on the compression side of this bending member. Second, the channel section: for this structural arrangement of members, the effective skin area is based on the crippling allowable stress of the compression flange, not the angle sections that make up the total section area of this member. For each structural arrangement of members in this table, crippling failure is predicted by comparing the allowable crippling stress F_{cc} to the maximum extreme fiber stress on the compression side of each flange. Example 6-5 (see page 419) will help to illustrate the practical applications of this table.

Reinforcing Plates (or Straps) Attached to Built-up Sections in Compression

Formed sheet metal angles, such as those shown in Fig. 6-30, can provide an edge of support for reinforcing plates (or straps). Refer to the (imaginary) supports indicated for these members at *A*, *B*, and *C* in this figure. Structural tests have shown conclusively that the rivets or bolts attaching these members together themselves do not necessarily provide an edge of support as far as crippling failure of these members is concerned. Specific support capabilities of other combinations of built-up sections in compression for the most part have been quite limited. In those cases where high stress intensities at the corners of complex structural shapes have not been clearly understood, the structural engineer must rely on his past engineering experience and know-how for their solutions. And therefore, it is recommended that a conservative approach to the analysis of their designs be taken in areas not specifically substantiated by structural test.

Allowable Crippling Stress of Round Tubes in Compression

The equation below represents the allowable crippling stress of round tubes in compression:

$$F_{cc} = \frac{0.5\sqrt{E_c E_t}}{D/t} \qquad \textbf{(6-21)}$$

where: F_{cc} = allowable crippling stress of a round tube
E_c = modulus of elasticity in compression
E_t = tangent modulus of elasticity in compression
D = outside diameter of the tube
t = wall thickness of the tube.

This equation should only be used if structural test data are not available to substantiate existing designs.

Temperature Correction Effects for Built-up Sections in Compression

The effects of temperature must also be considered in the design of stable compression members. Here, the elastic modulus of elasticity in compression and the yield compression stress allowable of the material are used to make this evaluation. The allowable crippling stress, Eq. 6-16, due to elevated temperatures is modified as follows:

$$(F_{cc})_{\text{temp}} = F_{cc}\frac{\sqrt{(F_{cy}E_c)_{\text{temp}}}}{\sqrt{(F_{cy}E_c)_{\text{room temp}}}} \qquad \textbf{(6-22)}$$

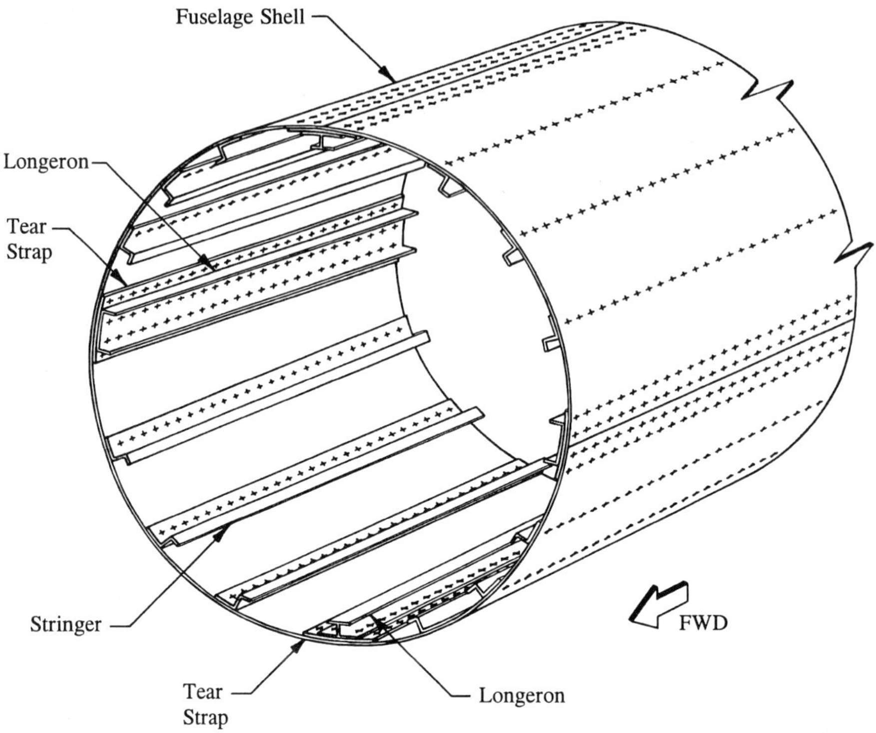

FIGURE 6-31 Fuselage barrel section supported by longitudinal members (frames removed for clarity).

where: $(F_{cc})_{\text{temp}}$ = allowable crippling stress at elevated temperatures
F_{cc} = allowable crippling stress at room-temperature (see Eq. 6-16)
F_{cy} = yield compression stress allowable of the material
E_c = elastic modulus of elasticity in compression.

Example 6-3 The fuselage shell is supported by longitudinal members as shown in Fig. 6-31. Using the method of crippling analysis of this section, determine the allowable crippling stress of the zee stringers (assume that all of the stringers are of typical construction and material). Then, with the allowable crippling stress known for these members, determine the allowable compression strength of the stringers with and without attached skin. The stringers are constructed of 2024-T3 aluminum alloy extrusion, QQ-A-200/3, and the skin is constructed of clad 2024-T3 aluminum alloy material, QQ-A-250/5. The fuselage skin is countersunk with BB 5 rivets spaced .73 in apart. When calculating the effective area of the zee stringer, also consider the fillet area of this member.

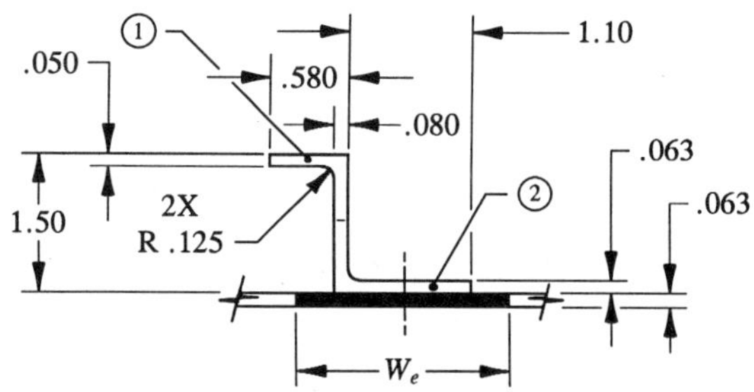

FIGURE 6-32 Cross-sectional area of the zee stringer with effective skin area.

SOLUTION: The longerons and stringers are riveted to the fuselage outer shell longitudinally to meet aviation strength and bending stiffness requirements of the fuselage structure. The way these members are physically restrained will determine their structural behavior to carry different types of loads. In general, fuselage stringers are designed for axial compression or tension, while longeron members carry both axial and bending loads. Both members are primarily used to support and reinforce the outer shell of the fuselage. The cross-sectional area of a typical zee stringer (with effective skin) is shown in Fig. 6-32. The allowable crippling stress of this member is determined by isolating the stringer from the skin into two angle sections, as shown in Fig. 6-33, and computing the values of b'/t and F_{cc} for each angle. Use values of $E_c = 11.0 \text{ x } 10^6 \text{ psi}$ and $F_{cy} = 34{,}000 \text{ psi}$ for the stringer material (refer to the mechanical-property tables in MIL-HDBK-5F for 2024-T3 aluminum alloy extrusion or to Table A-2 in Appendix E).

ELEMENT ①

From Fig. 6-27,

$$b'/t = \frac{b_1 + b_2}{t_1 + t_2} = \frac{.540 + .718}{.050 + .080} = 9.7.$$

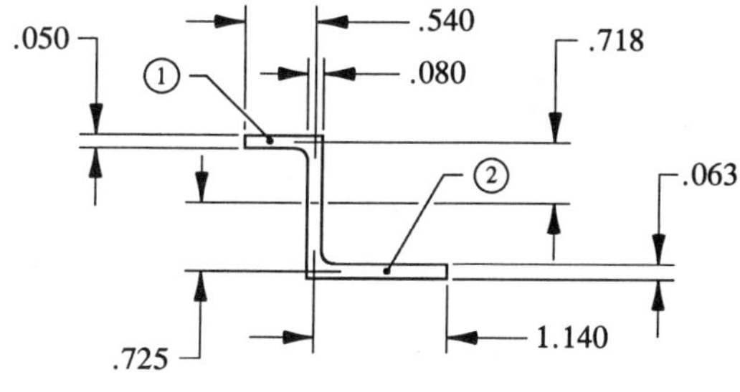

FIGURE 6-33 Stringer is isolated from the skin and divided into two angle sections.

Substituting this value into Eq. 6-16 gives:

$$F_{cc} = \frac{C_e\sqrt{F_{cy}E_c}}{(b'/t)^{3/4}} = \frac{.317\sqrt{34,000(11.0 \text{ x } 10^6)}}{(9.7)^{3/4}} = 35,271 \text{ psi}.$$

ELEMENT ②

$$b'/t = \frac{b_1 + b_2}{t_1 + t_2} = \frac{.725 + 1.140}{.063 + .080} = 13.0.$$

Substituting this value into Eq. 6-16 gives:

$$F_{cc} = \frac{C_e\sqrt{F_{cy}E_c}}{(b'/t)^{3/4}} = \frac{.317\sqrt{34,000(11.0 \text{ x } 10^6)}}{(13.0)^{3/4}} = 28,316 \text{ psi}.$$

Next, Table 6-6 is constructed using the general column headings set up in Table 6-4 for crippling calculations.

TABLE 6-6 STRINGER ALLOWABLE CRIPPLING STRESS

Element	b'/t (Fig. 6-27)	C_e (Table 6-3)	F_{cc} (Eq. 6-16)	A*	$F_{cc}A$
1	9.7	.317	34,000†	.088	2,992
2	13.0	.317	28,316	.133	3,766
			Total	.221	6,758

* The stringer area is calculated as follows (refer to Table 6-7 for the exact formula used to compute the area of a fillet):

$$A_1 = .050(.540 + .040) + .080(.718 - .025) + .215(.125)^2 = .088 \text{ in}^2$$

$$A_2 = .080(.725 + .031) + .063(1.140 - .040) + .215(.125)^2 = .133 \text{ in}^2.$$

† The calculated value of F_{cc} for this element is actually 35,271 psi. However, since this value exceeds the yield allowable compression stress of the material, the cutoff stress for F_{cy} or 34,000 psi is used instead.

TABLE 6-7 FILLET AREA OF AN EXTRUDED ANGLE AND BENT AREA OF A FORMED ANGLE

FILLET AREA: $A = .215R^2$

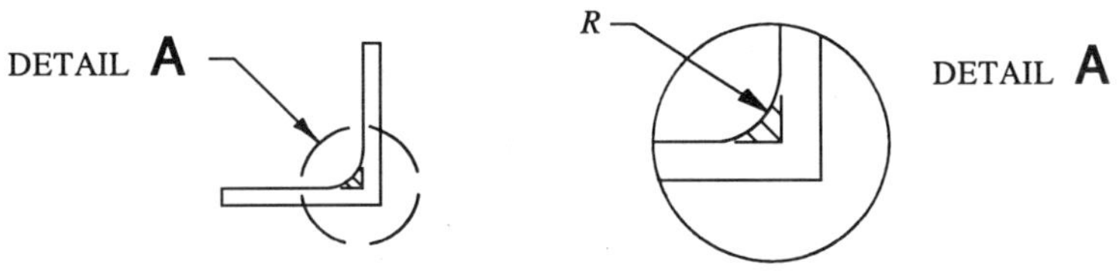

BENT AREA: $A = \frac{\pi}{4}(R_0^2 - R_1^2)$

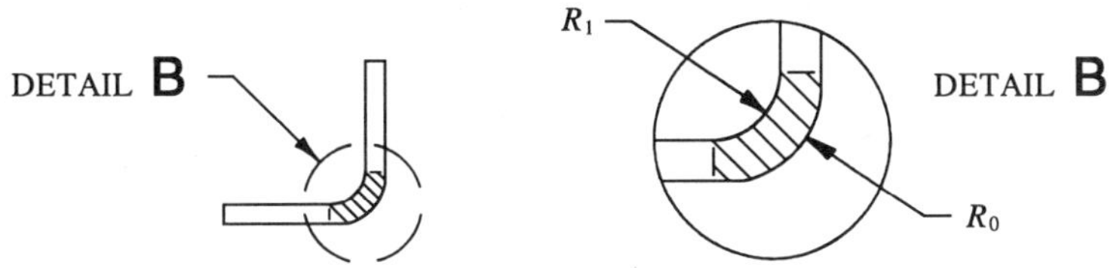

$$(F_{cc})_{\text{stringer}} = \frac{\Sigma(F_{cc}A)}{\Sigma A} = \frac{6,758}{.221} = 30,579 \text{ psi.}$$

Since the flange of the stringer (refer back to Fig. 6-32) is riveted to the fuselage skin, for this member to be fully effective at a stress level of 30,579 psi, premature inter-rivet buckling of this member must be prevented (that is, such that $F_{ir} \geq F_{cc}$). From Table 6-2 (see page 365), the effective slenderness ratio L'/ρ is determined. For a machine-countersunk, tension-head rivet in the fuselage skin, the end-fixity coefficient $c = 1.5$. However, since the flange of the stringer is not actually countersunk, the equation corresponding to $c = 3.0$ is more appropriately used for this computation.

$$L'/\rho = 2\frac{s}{t} = 2\left[\frac{.730}{.063}\right] = 23.2$$

where: $s = .730$ in (given)
$t = .063$ in (thickness of the stringer flange).

With the value of $L'/\rho = 23.2$, enter a column curve for 2024-T3 aluminum alloy extrusion material, and determine the allowable inter-rivet buckling stress F_{ir} of the flange or 34,000 psi (this value corresponds to the cutoff stress for F_{cy}). Since $F_{ir} > F_{cc}$, no correction is made for premature inter-rivet buckling.

Allowable Crippling Strength of the Z-Stringer (without effective skin area):

The allowable crippling strength of the zee stringer without the effective skin area is obtained by multiplying the allowable crippling stress of the stringer by the actual area of the stringer alone. Here the basic stress equation for axial members ($f = P/A$) is used for this computation.

$$(P_{cc})_{\text{stringer}} = (F_{cc})_{\text{stringer}} A_{\text{stringer}} = 30,579(.221) = 6,758 \text{ lb}$$

where: $(F_{cc})_{\text{stringer}} = 30,579$ psi (as calculated from page 399)
$A_{\text{stringer}} = .221 \text{ in}^2$ (from Table 6-6).

Allowable Crippling Strength of the Composite Z-Stringer (including the effective skin area):

The allowable crippling strength of the composite stringer—that is, stringer plus effective skin—is obtained by multiplying the allowable crippling stress of the stringer by the total area of the stringer plus effective skin.

$$(P_{cc})_{\text{composite}} = (F_{cc})_{\text{composite}} A_{\text{composite}} = 30,579(.347) = 10,611 \text{ lb}$$

where: $(F_{cc})_{\text{composite}} = 30,579$ psi (from page 399)
$A_{\text{composite}} = .347 \text{ in}^2$ (see ahead to page 401).

Effective Width and Area of Skin:

Width of Skin:

$$W_e = 1.7\, t \sqrt{E_c / F_{cc}} = 1.7(.063)\sqrt{\frac{10,700,000}{30,579}} = 2.003 \text{ in}$$

where: $F_{cc} = 30,579$ psi (from page 399)
$E_c = 10.7 \text{ x } 10^6$ psi (see Table A-4 in Appendix E)
$t = .063$ in (skin thickness).

Area of Skin:

$$A_{\text{skin}} = W_e t = 2.003(.063) = .126 \text{ in}^2$$

where: $W_e = 2.003$ in
$t = .063$ in (skin thickness).

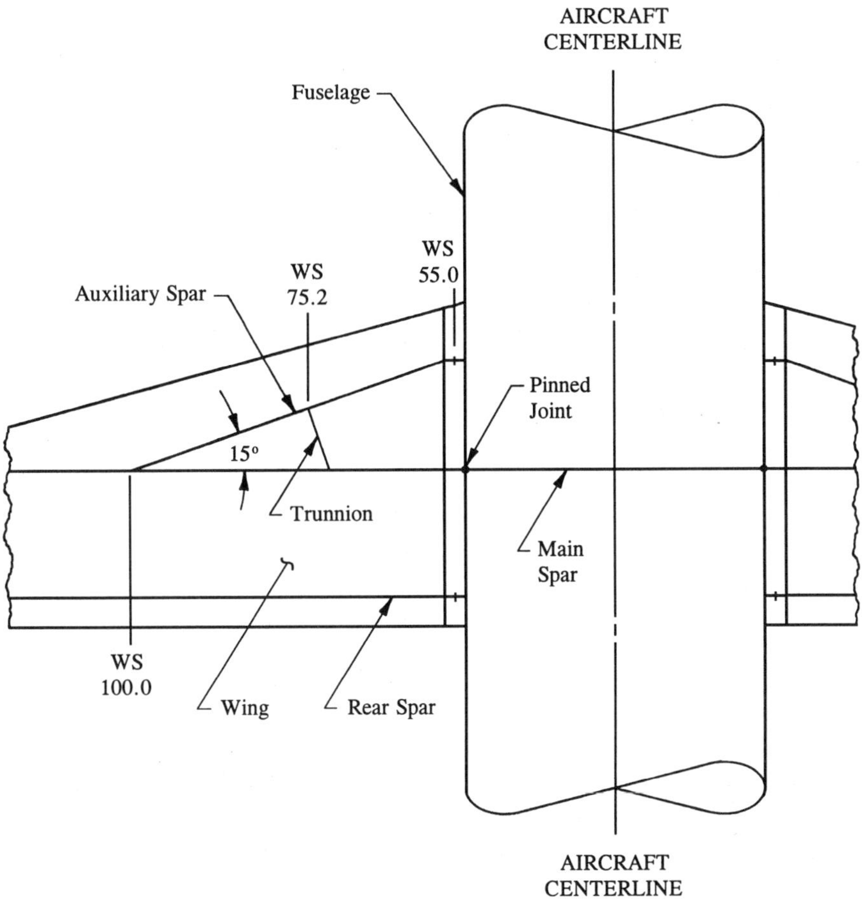

FIGURE 6-34 Plan view of wing and fuselage structures.

The effective area of the composite section is computed as follows:

$$A_{\text{composite}} = A_{\text{skin}} + A_{\text{stringer}} = .126 + .221 = .347 \text{ in}^2$$

where: $A_{\text{skin}} = .126 \text{ in}^2$
$A_{\text{stringer}} = .221 \text{ in}^2$ (from Table 6-6 on page 398).

If the effective area of skin W_e is fully effective at a stress level of 30,579 psi, premature inter-rivet buckling of the skin must be prevented below the allowable crippling stress of the stringer (that is, such that $F_{ir} \geq F_{cc}$). From Table 6-2 on page 365, the effective slenderness ratio L'/ρ for a BB 5 rivet (machine-countersunk, tension-head rivet, end-fixity coefficient $c = 1.5$) is

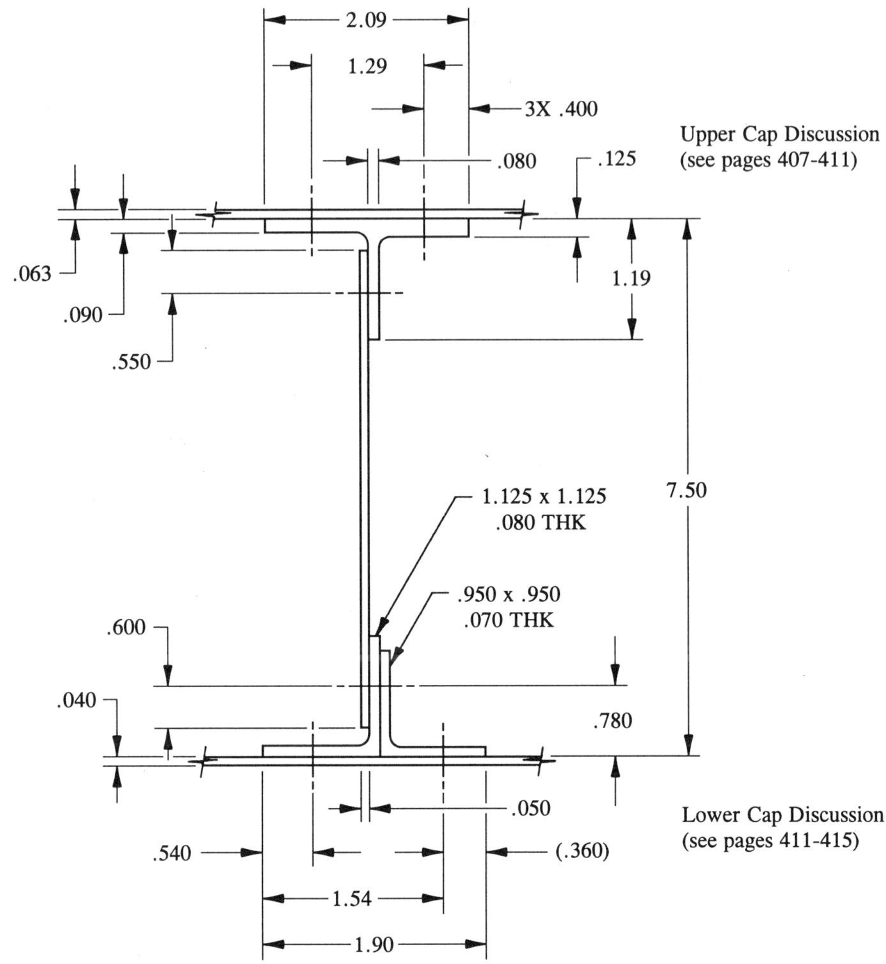

FIGURE 6-35 Auxiliary wing spar cross-sectional area. (Dimensions that are pertinent to the analysis are shown.)

$$L'/\rho = 2\sqrt{2}\,\frac{s}{t} = 2\sqrt{2}\left[\frac{.730}{.063}\right] = 32.8$$

where: s = .730 in (given)
t = .063 in (skin thickness).

With this value and a column curve for clad 2024-T3 aluminum alloy material, we obtain the allowable inter-rivet buckling stress F_{ir} or 32,800 psi. Therefore, since $F_{ir} > F_{cc}$, no correction is necessary for the skin due to premature inter-rivet buckling.

In conclusion, the allowable crippling strength of the stringer is 57.0% greater with skin than without skin. This can have a rather significant impact on production model designs if much emphasis at all is placed on weight reduction and cost-savings. Compare the values of 10,611 lb and 6,758 lb in our preceding solution. To neglect the combined capabilities of the skin and stringer would indeed be a high weight penalty for the fuselage structure to pay.

Example 6-4 The auxiliary wing spar (or gear beam) of a high-performance, single-engine aircraft is critical for 2-point brake roll. Refer to the plan view of the wing and fuselage structures in Fig. 6-34. The trunnion reaction for the gear beam is 7,000 lb ultimate acting at Wing Station 75.2. The auxiliary spar is built-in like a fixed-support at the main spar and simply-supported at the wing root where the auxiliary wing spar attaches to the fuselage structure. Determine the compression allowables for the beam cap cross-sectional areas shown in Fig. 6-35. Then, with these allowable values, write the compression margins of safety for each cap. To simplify the solution of this problem, neglect the fillet areas of the extruded members. Also assume that inter-rivet buckling along the web rivet lines is precluded for both web and extruded members. Use BB 5 rivets (MS 20426 AD) spaced .980 in apart for the upper and lower wing skins and BJ 5 rivets (MS 20470 AD) spaced .750 in apart for the web.

List of Materials

Member	Material	Material Code
upper wing skin	clad 2024-T3 aluminum alloy sheet	QQ-A-250/5
lower wing skin	clad 2024-T3 aluminum alloy sheet	QQ-A-250/5
upper extruded tee	2024-T3 aluminum alloy extrusion	QQ-A-200/3
web	clad 2024-T3 aluminum alloy sheet	QQ-A-250/5
lower left extruded angle	2024-T3 aluminum alloy extrusion	QQ-A-200/3
lower right extruded angle	2024-T3 aluminum alloy extrusion	QQ-A-200/3

SOLUTION: From basic trigonometry, the actual length of the auxiliary wing spar is determined. See Fig. 6-36.

$$b = \frac{24.8}{\cos 15^\circ} = 25.7 \text{ in}$$

$$a = \frac{20.2}{\cos 15^\circ} = 20.9 \text{ in.}$$

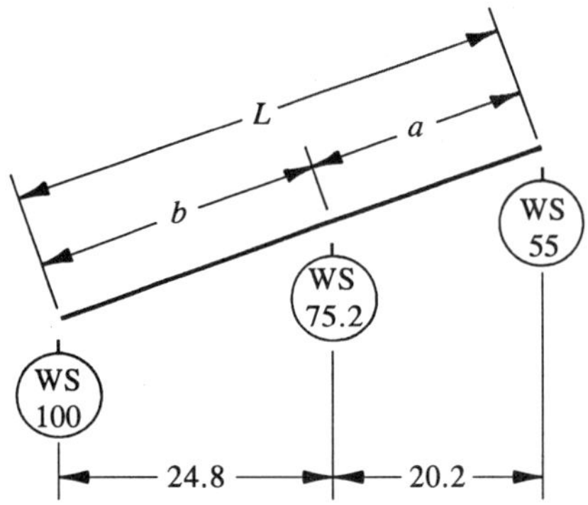

FIGURE 6-36 From geometry, the length of the auxiliary wing spar is determined.

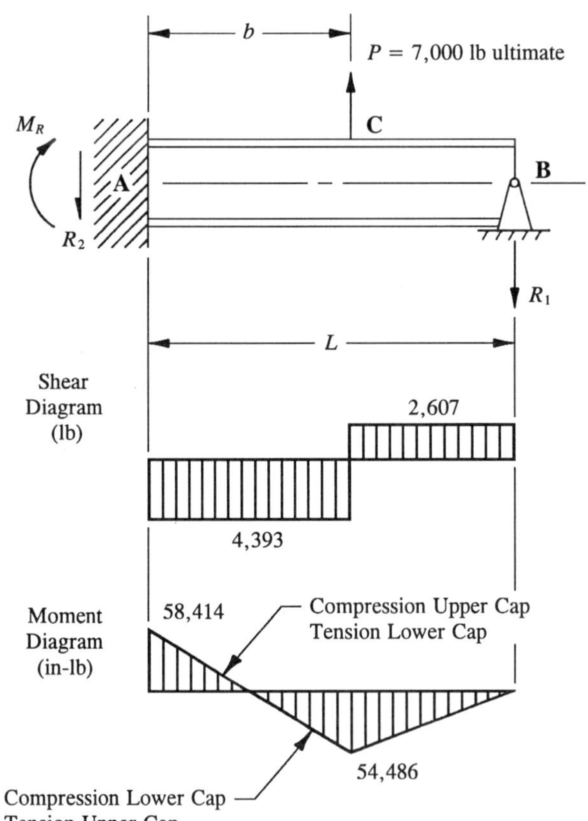

FIGURE 6-37 Auxiliary wing spar is isolated and free-bodied with accompanying shear and bending moment diagrams constructed.

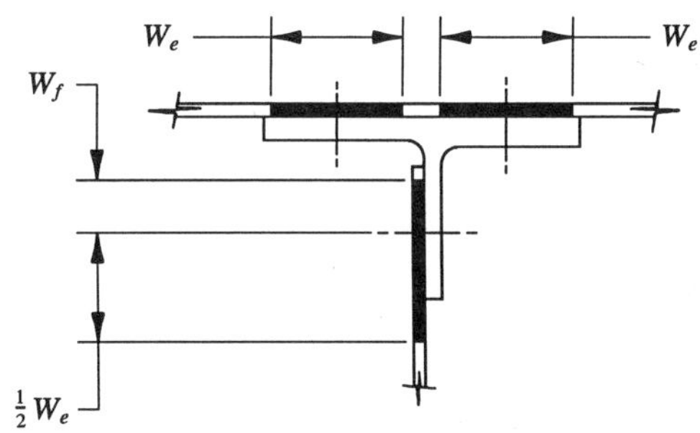

FIGURE 6-38 Auxiliary wing spar upper compression cap with effective skin and web areas shown shaded (see Fig. 6-35).

The total length of the auxiliary spar is therefore

$$L = b + a = 25.7 + 20.9 = 46.6 \text{ in.}$$

The auxiliary wing spar is isolated from the wing structure and the beam reactions necessary to free-body diagram (or balance) this structure are drawn, as shown in Fig. 6-37. Since the beam is statically indeterminate, one or more of the reactive forces are superfluous. Theoretically, if a reaction or support can be removed without affecting the overall stability of the structure as a whole, that reaction or support is redundant. Essentially, this means that the redundant member is not needed or necessary to establish overall equilibrium of the structure. This redundancy is known as the static indeterminacy of beams. The reactions for such a beam cannot normally be determined from the equations of static equilibrium alone. For this reason, the beam formula solutions provided in Appendix D have been formulated to help us arrive at their values. The engineer is referred to Case 16 of this appendix for the solutions to the unknown reactions R_1, R_2, and M_R. The first of these equations for R_1 is solved:

$$R_1 = \frac{P}{2}\left[\frac{3b^2L - b^3}{L^3}\right] = \frac{7,000}{2}\left[\frac{3(25.7)^2(46.6) - (25.7)^3}{(46.6)^3}\right]$$

$$R_1 = 2,607 \text{ lb ult.}$$

With the value of R_1 known, the rest of our solution for reactions, that is, for R_2 and M_R, reduces to a simple case of statics. Taking this basic approach, we obtain the values of R_2 and M_R as follows:

$$\Sigma F_z = 0, \qquad R_2 = 7,000 - R_1$$

$$R_2 = 7,000 - 2,607 = 4,393 \text{ lb ult}$$

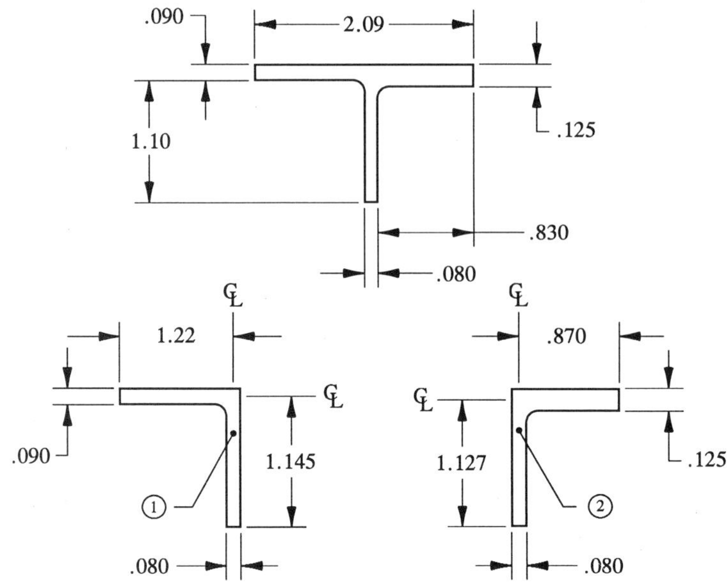

FIGURE 6-39 Extruded T-section is divided into two angle sections.

$$\Sigma M_A = 0, \quad \circlearrowleft + \quad M_R - 7{,}000b + R_1 L = 0$$
$$M_R = 7{,}000b - R_1 L.$$

Now, substituting R_1 into this equation gives:

$$M_R = 7{,}000(25.7) - 2{,}607(46.6) = 58{,}414 \text{ in-lb ult.}$$

Alternatively, the cookbook beam formula solutions, referring to the straightforward solution of reaction equations provided in Appendix D, could also have been used if that systematic way of solving this problem was instead preferred by the engineer. The engineer is encouraged to use these standard equation solutions here by comparing them to our statics solution approach. The reason for performing a statics solution in the first place was simply to point out an important concept or approach to the basic structural theory of statically indeterminate beams: that a statically indeterminate beam can be reduced to a statically determinate one, and then from this determinacy the remaining beam reactions can be found from the equations of static equilibrium. With these reactions and the general knowledge of internal loads analysis of beams, the shear and bending moment diagrams of the auxiliary wing spar are drawn. Refer to Fig. 6-37 for their graphical representations.[1] Next, the wing spar is analyzed for that portion of its structure carrying the

[1] A review of the basic principles of their construction are found and discussed in Chapter 1, in particular, the engineer is referred to Sec. 1.6.

maximum shear. This occurs along the beam from A to C in this figure, where the value of shear is 4,393 lb ultimate. Using this value, the spar is analyzed for (1) the basic web thickness and (2) the sizing and spacing requirements of web rivets along the upper and lower beam caps. The engineer should review Chapter 4, "Shearing Stresses," for specific analysis details and guidelines to their design substantiation. On the other hand, the maximum bending moments will design the upper and lower beam caps for compression and tension failures.

Upper Cap Crippling Analysis

The upper cap of the auxiliary wing spar is isolated with effective skin and web areas, as shown in Fig. 6-38. The main structural member (extruded T-section) of this cap is then isolated from the rest of the structure and the allowable crippling stress of this member is computed. However, before this value can actually be determined, the extruded T-section must be divided into two angle sections, as shown in Fig. 6-39. The crippling allowable stress of each angle is then averaged together to obtain the weighted-average allowable crippling stress of the T-section as a whole. Specifically, the sum of the crippling allowable loads of the individual angle sections that make up the T-section is divided by the gross area of the angle sections (see Eq. 6-17). From earlier discussions, that is, the application of this equation and specific column headings used in setting up Table 6-4 for crippling computations, this will be the basic approach used here in our solution of crippling stresses. Use values of $E_c = 11.0 \text{ x } 10^6$ psi and $F_{cy} = 34{,}000$ psi for the T-section (refer to the mechanical-property tables in MIL-HDBK-5F for 2024-T3 aluminum alloy extrusion material).

Crippling computations are performed as follows:

ELEMENT ①

$$b'/t = \frac{b_1 + b_2}{t_1 + t_2} = \frac{1.220 + 1.145}{.090 + .080} = 13.9.$$

Substituting this value into Eq. 6-16 gives:

$$F_{cc} = \frac{C_e\sqrt{F_{cy}E_c}}{(b'/t)^{3/4}} = \frac{.295\sqrt{34{,}000(11.0 \text{ x } 10^6)}}{(13.9)^{3/4}} = 25{,}061 \text{ psi}.$$

ELEMENT ②

$$b'/t = \frac{b_1 + b_2}{t_1 + t_2} = \frac{.870 + 1.127}{.125 + .080} = 9.7.$$

Substituting this value into Eq. 6-16 gives:

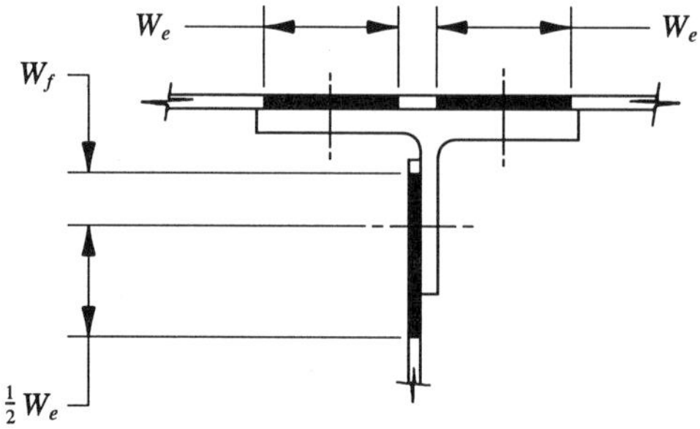

FIGURE 6-40 Auxiliary wing spar upper compression cap with effective skin and web areas shown shaded (Repeated).

$$F_{cc} = \frac{C_e\sqrt{F_{cy}E_c}}{(b'/t)^{3/4}} = \frac{.295\sqrt{34,000(11.0 \text{ x } 10^6)}}{(9.7)^{3/4}} = 32,823 \text{ psi.}$$

These values are listed in Table 6-8.

TABLE 6-8 UPPER CAP (T-SECTION) ALLOWABLE CRIPPLING STRESS

Element	b'/t (Fig. 6-27)	C_e (Table 6-3)	F_{cc} (Eq. 6-16)	A*	$F_{cc}A$
1	13.9	.295	25,061	.201	5,037
2	9.7	.295	32,823	.199	6,532
			Total	.400	11,569

* $A_1 = 1.26(.090) + 1.100(.080) = .201 \text{ in}^2$
$A_2 = .910(.125) + 1.065(.080) = .199 \text{ in}^2$.

The appropriate column totals are then substituted into Eq. 6-17 to find the weighted-average allowable crippling stress.

$$(F_{cc})_{\text{upper cap}} = \frac{\Sigma(F_{cc}A)}{\Sigma A} = \frac{11,569}{.400} = 28,922 \text{ psi.}$$

The allowable compression strength (or force) of the upper cap will now be determined with attached effective skin and web areas, as shown in Fig. 6-40. Omitting these members from consideration, even in high compression load

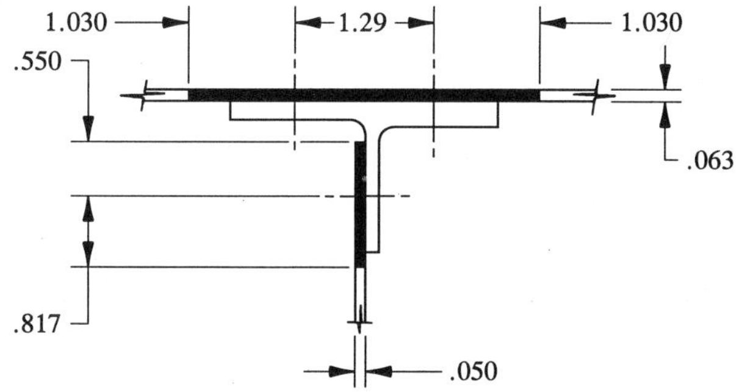

FIGURE 6-41 Effective skin and web areas defined for the auxiliary wing spar upper compression cap.

applications, can often lead to overweight structure and costly overdesigns. Refer to the previous example problem where the compression strength of the main structural member (stringer) was compared with and without effective skin areas. The results were quite dramatic for the particular structural members used in that analysis.

Effective Skin and Web Areas:

Upper Skin:

$$W_e = 1.7t\sqrt{E_c/F_{cc}} = 1.7(.063)\sqrt{\frac{10,700,000}{28,922}} = 2.060 \text{ in}$$

$$\tfrac{1}{2}W_e = \tfrac{1}{2}(2.060) = 1.030 \text{ in.}$$

Web:

$$(1)\quad W_e = 1.7t\sqrt{E_c/F_{cc}} = 1.7(.050)\sqrt{\frac{10,700,000}{28,922}} = 1.635 \text{ in}$$

$$\tfrac{1}{2}W_e = \tfrac{1}{2}(1.635) = .817 \text{ in}$$

$$(2)\quad W_f = .62t\sqrt{E_c/F_{cc}} = .62(.050)\sqrt{\frac{10,700,000}{28,922}} = .596 \text{ in}$$

where: $F_{cc} = 28,922$ psi
$E_c = 10,700,000$ psi
$t = .063$ in (upper skin thickness)
$t = .050$ in (web thickness).

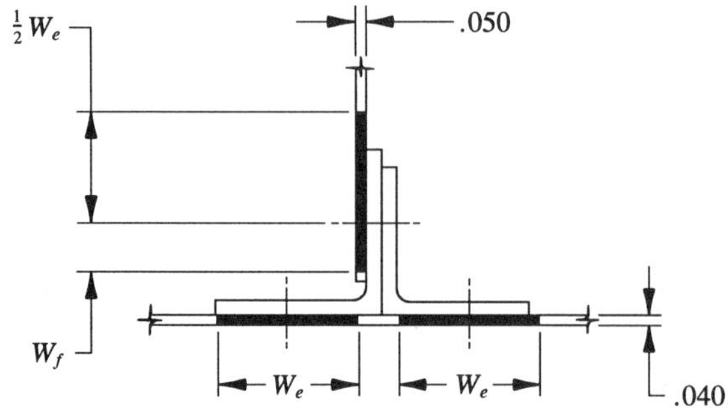

FIGURE 6-42 Auxiliary wing spar lower compression cap with effective skin and web areas shown shaded (see Fig. 6-35).

For the upper skin area to be fully effective (as calculated) at a stress level of 28,922 psi, premature inter-rivet buckling of this member must be prevented. For this to occur, it must be shown that $F_{ir} \geq F_{cc}$. From Table 6-2, the effective slenderness ratio L'/ρ for a BB 5 rivet (machine-countersunk, tension-head rivet, end-fixity coefficient $c = 1.5$) is

$$L'/\rho = 2\sqrt{2}\,\frac{s}{t} = 2\sqrt{2}\left[\frac{.980}{.063}\right] = 44.0$$

where: $s = .980$ in (given)
$t = .063$ in (upper skin thickness).

Now, with a value of $L'/\rho = 44.0$ and a column curve for clad 2024-T3 aluminum alloy material, we obtain the allowable inter-rivet buckling stress F_{ir} of the skin or 29,600 psi. Since this value is greater than F_{cc} (see page 408), the effective width of skin as previously calculated is not corrected. The effective areas of web and skin are shown shaded in Fig. 6-41. Note, in particular, that no more than 1.29 in of effective skin material can actually be taken between skin rivet lines, even

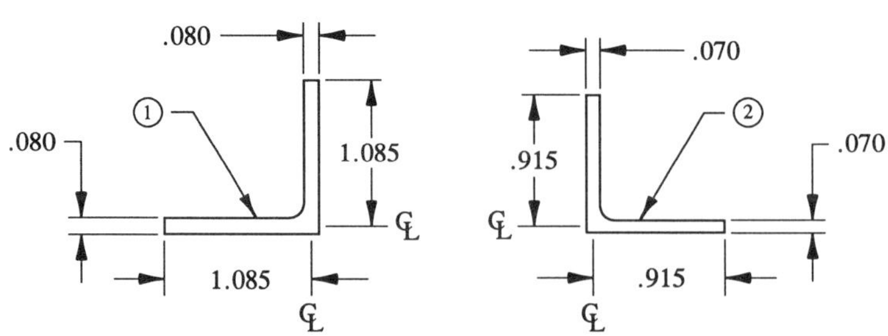

FIGURE 6-43 Extruded angle sections are separated from the auxiliary wing spar lower compression cap.

though our previous effective width calculations have indicated more. The effective area of the skin is physically bound by the material existing between the two rows of skin rivets or 1.29 in. The effective cap area in compression is

$$A_c = A_{\text{main}} + A_{\text{skin}} + A_{\text{web}} = .305 + .211 + .068 = .584 \text{ in}^2$$

where: $A_{\text{main}} = (1.26)(.090) + (.830)(.125) + (1.10)(.080)$
$A_{\text{main}} = .305 \text{ in}^2$ (actual area excluding fillets)
$A_{\text{skin}} = (1.030 + 1.030 + 1.29)(.063) = .211 \text{ in}^2$
$A_{\text{web}} = (.550 + .817)(.050) = .068 \text{ in}^2$.

Now, using Eq. 6-19, the allowable compression load of the upper beam cap is found:

$$P_{cc} = F_{cc} A_c = 28,922(.584) = 16,890 \text{ lb}$$

where F_{cc} is 28,922 psi (see page 408) and A_c is .584 in^2.

Lower Cap Crippling Analysis

The lower cap of the auxiliary wing spar is isolated with effective skin and web areas, as shown in Fig. 6-42. The main structural members of this cap, Fig. 6-43, are then isolated from the rest of the structure and the allowable crippling stress of these members is determined. From Eq. 6-16, the crippling allowable stress of each angle section is computed separately. Their values are then averaged together to obtain the weighted-average allowable crippling stress of their combined sections. The application of Eq. 6-17 and the crippling computations used in setting up Table 6-4 for the upper beam cap are again used here in our solution of crippling strength of the lower beam cap. Use values of $E_c = 11.0 \times 10^6$ psi and $F_{cy} = 34,000$ psi for the angle sections (refer to the mechanical-property tables in MIL-HDBK-5F for 2024-T3 aluminum alloy extrusion).

Crippling computations are performed as follows:

ELEMENT ①

$$b'/t = \frac{b_1 + b_2}{t_1 + t_2} = \frac{1.085 + 1.085}{.080 + .080} = 13.6.$$

Substituting this value into Eq. 6-16 gives:

$$F_{cc} = \frac{C_e \sqrt{F_{cy} E_c}}{(b'/t)^{3/4}} = \frac{.295 \sqrt{34,000(11.0 \times 10^6)}}{(13.6)^{3/4}} = 25,474 \text{ psi}.$$

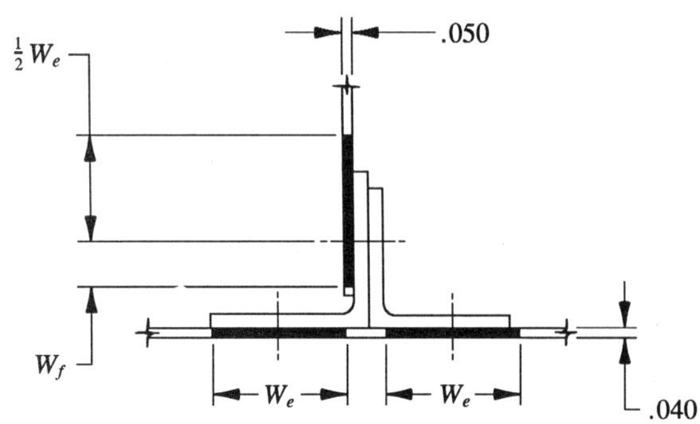

FIGURE 6-44 Auxiliary wing spar lower compression cap with effective skin and web areas shown shaded (Repeated).

These values are listed in Table 6-9.

ELEMENT (2)

$$b'/t = \frac{b_1 + b_2}{t_1 + t_2} = \frac{.915 + .915}{.070 + .070} = 13.1.$$

Substituting this value into Eq. 6-16 gives:

$$F_{cc} = \frac{C_e\sqrt{F_{cy}E_c}}{(b'/t)^{3/4}} = \frac{.295\sqrt{34,000(11.0 \times 10^6)}}{(13.1)^{3/4}} = 26,200 \text{ psi}.$$

TABLE 6-9 LOWER CAP (BACK-TO-BACK ANGLES) ALLOWABLE CRIPPLING STRESS

Element	b'/t (Fig. 6-27)	C_e (Table 6-3)	F_{cc} (Eq. 6-16)	A*	$F_{cc}A$
1	13.6	.295	25,474	.174	4,432
2	13.1	.295	26,200	.128	3,354
			Total	.302	7,786

* $A_1 = 1.125(.080) + 1.045(.080) = .174 \text{ in}^2$
$A_2 = .950(.070) + .880(.070) = .128 \text{ in}^2$.

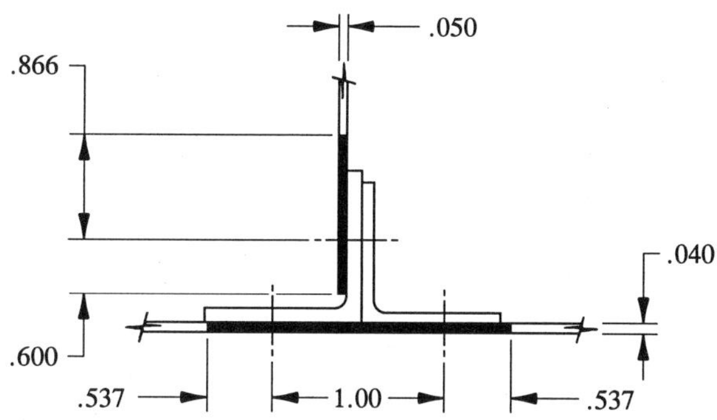

FIGURE 6-45 Effective skin and web areas defined for the auxiliary wing spar lower compression cap.

The appropriate column totals are then substituted into Eq. 6-17 to find the weighted-average allowable crippling stress.

$$(F_{cc})_{\text{lower cap}} = \frac{\Sigma(F_{cc}A)}{\Sigma A} = \frac{7,786}{.302} = 25,781 \text{ psi.}$$

The allowable compression strength (or force) of the lower cap is also determined with attached effective skin and web areas. Effective areas are shown in Fig. 6-44.

Effective Skin and Web Areas:

Lower Skin:

$$W_e = 1.7t\sqrt{E_c/F_{cc}} = 1.7(.040)\sqrt{\frac{10,700,000}{25,781}} = 1.385 \text{ in}$$

$$\tfrac{1}{2}W_e = \tfrac{1}{2}(1.385) = .692 \text{ in.}$$

Web:

$$(1)\quad W_e = 1.7t\sqrt{E_c/F_{cc}} = 1.7(.050)\sqrt{\frac{10,700,000}{25,781}} = 1.732 \text{ in}$$

$$\tfrac{1}{2}W_e = \tfrac{1}{2}(1.732) = .866 \text{ in}$$

$$(2)\quad W_f = .62t\sqrt{E_c/F_{cc}} = .62(.050)\sqrt{\frac{10,700,000}{25,781}} = .632 \text{ in}$$

where: $F_{cc} = 25,781$ psi (from above)
$E_c = 10,700,000$ psi

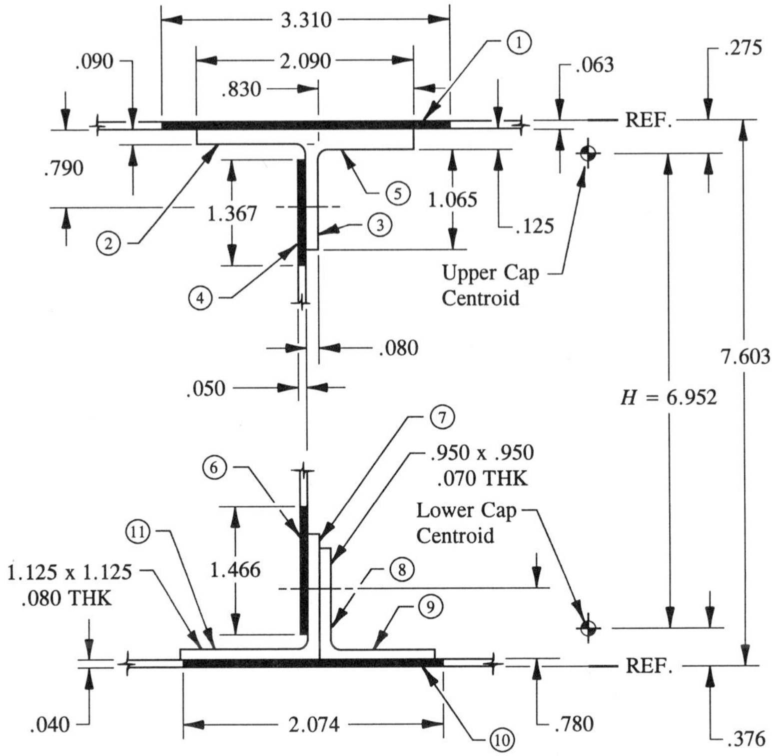

FIGURE 6-46 Upper and lower compression cap areas for the auxiliary wing spar.

t = .040 in (lower skin thickness)
t = .050 in (web thickness).

For the lower skin area to be fully effective (as calculated) at a stress level of 25,781 psi, premature inter-rivet buckling of this member must also be prevented. Therefore, it must be shown that $F_{ir} \geq F_{cc}$. Since the same rivets and corresponding spacing of rivets are used for the lower skin rivets as the upper, will the same allowable inter-rivet buckling stress F_{ir} occur for this member? This notion on the surface seems correct, however, it is absolutely wrong! Inter-rivet buckling, it is recalled, is also a function of material thickness, and since these members have different thicknesses their allowable inter-rivet buckling stresses will also be different. To verify this, consider Table 6-2 and determine the effective slenderness ratio L'/ρ for a BB 5 rivet (machine-countersunk, tension-head, end-fixity coefficient $c = 1.5$). Hence

$$L'/\rho = 2\sqrt{2}\,\frac{s}{t} = 2\sqrt{2}\left[\frac{.980}{.040}\right] = 69.3$$

where: $s = .980$ in (given)
$t = .040$ in (lower skin thickness).

Now, with a value of $L'/\rho = 69.3$ and a column curve for clad 2024-T3 aluminum alloy material, we obtain the allowable inter-rivet buckling stress F_{ir} of the skin or 20,000 psi. Since this value is less than F_{cc}, the effective width of skin (from the previous calculations on page 413) is reduced to account for premature inter-rivet buckling of this member. Hence, from Eq. 6-12, we obtain:

$$(W_e)_r = W_e\left[\frac{F_{ir}}{F_{cc}}\right] = 1.385\left[\frac{20,000}{25,781}\right] = 1.074 \text{ in}$$

$$\tfrac{1}{2}(W_e)_r = \tfrac{1}{2}(1.074) = .537 \text{ in.}$$

The effective skin and web areas are shown shaded in Fig. 6-45. The effective cap area in compression is therefore

$$A_c = A_{\text{main}} + A_{\text{skin}} + A_{\text{web}} = .302 + .083 + .073 = .458 \text{ in}^2$$

where: $A_{\text{main}} = (1.125)(.080) + (1.045)(.080) + (.950)(.070) + (.880)(.070)$
$A_{\text{main}} = .302 \text{ in}^2$
$A_{\text{skin}} = (.537 + 1.00 + .537)(.040) = .083 \text{ in}^2$
$A_{\text{web}} = (.866 + .600)(.050) = .073 \text{ in}^2$.

Now, using Eq. 6-19, the allowable compression load of the lower beam cap is found:

$$P_{cc} = F_{cc}A_c = 25,781(.458) = 11,808 \text{ lb}$$

where: $F_{cc} = 25,781$ psi
$A_c = .458 \text{ in}^2$.

Beam Cap Loads for the Auxiliary Wing Spar

Let us now refer to the bending moment diagram of the auxiliary wing spar, Fig. 6-37, page 404, and determine the maximum applied compression loads for the upper and lower beam caps of this structural member. From theory and a general understanding of internal loads analysis, it can be reasoned that maximum bending moments of a structure will also produce maximum compression and tension loads for the beam cap members of that structure. For the auxiliary wing spar, these maximum values will occur at two different points: The first, at the fixed-supported end at A or 58,414 in-lb, and the second, at the applied loading point at C or 54,486 in-lb. The sign conventions for these bending moments are indicated as shown in this same figure. To arrive at beam cap loads, each maximum applied bending moment is replaced by its equivalent couple-force acting between the upper and lower cap centroids of the beam (refer to Appendix B for specific details of this loading representation). Upper and lower cap centroids are determined from effective compression cap areas and their values computed in tabular form (see Tables 6-10 and 6-11). Also refer to Fig. 6-46 for the actual dimensions used in this table.

TABLE 6-10 UPPER CAP CENTROID

Element	b	h	y	A	Ay
1	3.310	0.063	0.031	0.209	0.006
2	1.260	0.090	0.108	0.113	0.012
3	0.080	1.100	0.703	0.088	0.062
4	0.050	1.367	0.986	0.068	0.067
5	0.830	0.125	0.125	0.104	0.013
			Total	0.582	0.160

$$Y_{cg} = \frac{\Sigma\, Ay}{\Sigma\, A} = \frac{.160}{.582} = .275 \text{ in.}$$

TABLE 6-11 LOWER CAP CENTROID

Element	b	h	y	A	Ay
6	0.050	1.466	0.953	0.073	0.070
7	0.080	1.045	0.642	0.084	0.054
8	0.070	0.880	0.550	0.062	0.034
9	0.950	0.070	0.075	0.066	0.005
10	2.074	0.040	0.020	0.083	0.002
11	1.125	0.080	0.080	0.090	0.007
			Total	0.458	0.172

$$Y_{cg} = \frac{\Sigma\, Ay}{\Sigma\, A} = \frac{.172}{.458} = .376 \text{ in.}$$

LOADING CASE #1:

$$P_{\text{couple}} = \frac{M}{H} \quad \text{(Appendix B, see Eq. A-7)}$$

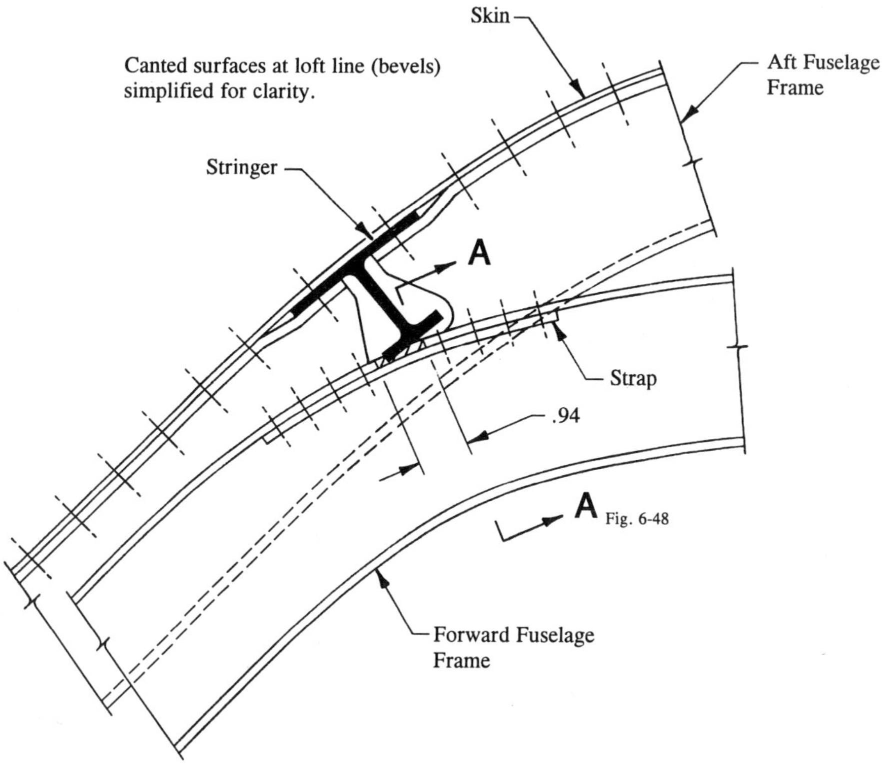

FIGURE 6-47 Flange portion of fuselage frame is cut away to allow stringer clearance.

$$P_{\text{couple}} = \frac{58,414}{6.952} = 8,402 \text{ lb} \quad \text{(compression upper, tension lower)}$$

where: M = 58,414 in-lb (from page 406)
H = 6.952 in (distance between cap centroids, see Fig. 6-46).

LOADING CASE #2:

$$P_{\text{couple}} = \frac{M}{H} \quad \text{(Appendix B, see Eq. A-7)}$$

$$P_{\text{couple}} = \frac{54,486}{6.952} = 7,837 \text{ lb} \quad \text{(compression lower, tension upper)}$$

where: M = 54,486 in-lb (from Fig. 6-37, page 404)
H = 6.952 in (distance between cap centroids, see Fig. 6-46).

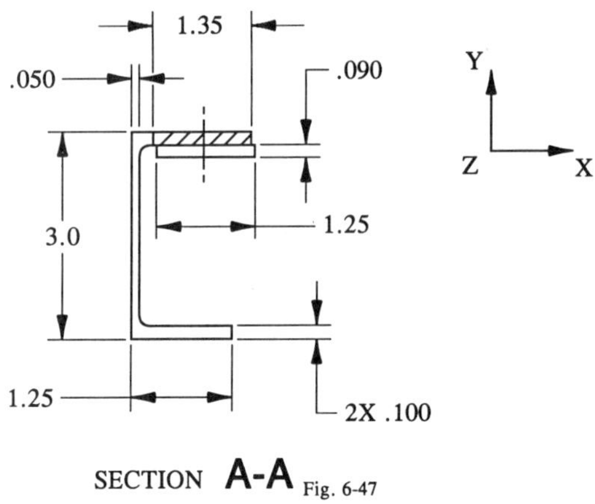

FIGURE 6-48 Cross-sectional area of fuselage frame (portion removed shown cross-hatched).

Crippling failure of the upper beam cap is predicted by:

$$\text{Margin of Safety} = \text{M.S.} = \frac{P_{cc}}{P_{\text{couple}}} - 1 = \frac{16,890}{8,402} - 1 = +1.01$$

where: P_{cc} = 16,890 lb (upper cap crippling strength from page 411)
P_{couple} = 8,402 lb (this load was derived from the reactive bending moment M_R = 58,414 in-lb acting at support A of the auxiliary wing spar).

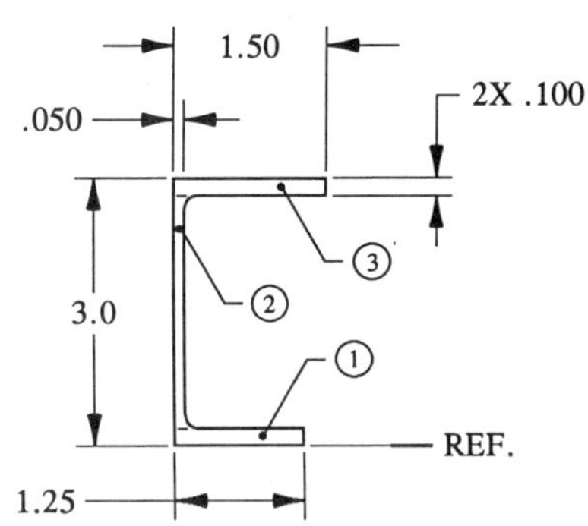

FIGURE 6-49 Original frame section is partitioned into rectangular element areas.

Crippling failure of the lower beam cap is predicted by:

$$\text{Margin of Safety} = \text{M.S.} = \frac{P_{cc}}{P_{\text{couple}}} - 1 = \frac{11,808}{7,837} - 1 = +.51$$

where: $P_{cc} = 11,808$ lb (lower cap crippling strength from page 415)
$P_{\text{couple}} = 7,837$ lb (this load was derived from the internal bending moment $M = 54,486$ in-lb acting at point C of the auxiliary wing spar).

Example 6-5 The flange of the forward fuselage frame was cut away to allow clearance for a longitudinal (long axis) stringer, as shown cross-hatched in Fig. 6-47. What size strap and how many fasteners would be required to substantiate conformity to the original frame structure for production aircraft, given the following maximum frame internal loads at this critical section?

$$M_x = -5,000 \text{ in-lb ultimate}$$
$$P_z = -3,000 \text{ lb ultimate}$$
$$V_y = 0.$$

Consider these loads acting at the centroid of the basic frame section and their proper orientation on the structure based on the sign convention adopted for right-hand-rule. The local coordinate system used for this section is shown in Fig. 6-48. The frame structure is a channel section made of 2024-T3 aluminum alloy extrusion (QQ-A-200/3). The engineer is referred to MIL-HDBK-5F for the values of F_{cy} and E_c for this material.

SOLUTION: The cross-sectional area of the forward fuselage frame through the cutaway portion of the frame flange is shown in Fig. 6-48. A strap (1.25 x .090) made of clad 2024-T3 aluminum alloy sheet, QQ-A-250/5, across the weakened section of the frame is used to reinforce the structure. To substantiate the basic frame structure (or channel section) for production aircraft, the repaired structure (or strap design proposal) must be designed of a weaker strength than the actual frame structure used for production. This is done mathematically by comparing the margins of safety of the proposed structural repair to the margins of safety of the original production model design. Since compression will control the design of the basic frame structure, crippling failures will be compared in our study.

Production Model Design (original frame structure):

Here, the compression flange of the original frame structure (channel section, see Fig. 6-49) is used to determine the value of b'/t, not the series of angle sections that make up the structural shape of the channel section. This gives:

$$b'/t = \frac{1.500 - .025}{.100} = 14.75.$$

From Table 6-3 (see page 390), with one free edge and the material 2024-T3 aluminum alloy extrusion, QQ-A-200/3, we find C_e = .317. In addition, from MIL-HDBK-5F, the values of F_{cy} = 34,000 psi and E_c = 11.0 x 10^6 psi are also found for this material. Substituting these values into Eq. 6-16, we obtain the allowable crippling stress of the compression flange, or

$$F_{cc} = \frac{C_e\sqrt{F_{cy}E_c}}{(b'/t)^{3/4}} = \frac{.317\sqrt{34,000(11.0 \text{ x } 10^6)}}{(14.75)^{3/4}} = 25,757 \text{ psi}.$$

The basic section properties of the forward fuselage frame structure are tabulated as shown in Table 6-12. Their values are needed to determine the combined axial and bending stresses of the compression flange of the basic channel section. The channel section is partitioned into three elements as shown in Fig. 6-49.

TABLE 6-12 SECTION PROPERTIES OF THE FORWARD FUSELAGE FRAME STRUCTURE (CHANNEL SECTION ONLY)

Element	b	h	y	A	Ay	Ay^2	I_o
1	1.250	0.100	0.050	0.125	0.006	0.000	0.000
2	0.050	2.800	1.500	0.140	0.210	0.315	0.091
3	1.500	0.100	2.950	0.150	0.442	1.305	0.000
			Total	0.415	0.658	1.620	0.091

$$Y_{cg} = \frac{\Sigma Ay}{\Sigma A} = \frac{.658}{.415} = 1.586 \text{ in}$$

$$I_{cg} = \Sigma I_o + \Sigma Ay^2 - Y_{cg}(\Sigma Ay)$$
$$I_{cg} = .091 + 1.620 - 1.586(.658) = .667 \text{ in}^4.$$

Assuming that calculated stresses are elastic, as well as they should be for compression design, this further implies the following:

$$Y_{na} = Y_{cg} = 1.586 \text{ in}$$

and

$$I_{na} = I_{cg} = .667 \text{ in}^4.$$

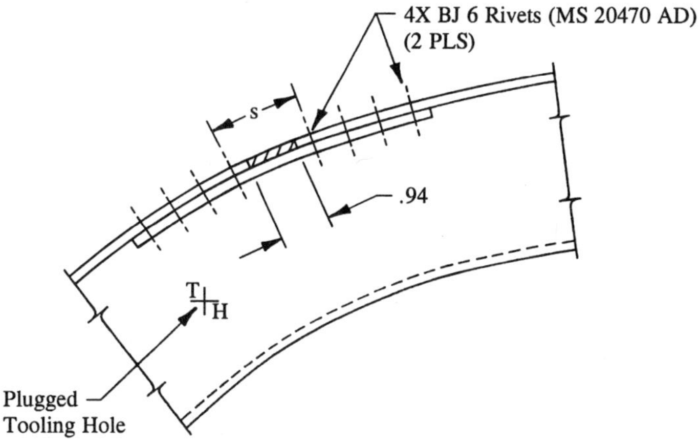

FIGURE 6-50 Critical spacing of rivets is indicated across the cut out region.

From Chapter 2, Eq. 2-9, combined axial and bending stresses are computed for the upper flange (at the midpoint of element #3). This location is chosen arbitrarily to establish an average stress level across the flange for this structural member.

Compression stress of the upper flange:

$$f_c = \pm \frac{P}{A} \pm \frac{Mc}{I_{na}}$$

$$= -\frac{3,000}{.415} - \frac{5,000(2.95 - 1.586)}{.667} = -7,229 - 10,225$$

$$f_c = -17,454 \text{ psi} \quad \text{(compression stress at the midpoint of element \#3).}$$

Then, with this stress and the allowable crippling stress of the compression flange, crippling failure of the production model design (based on the original frame section) is predicted.

$$\text{Margin of Safety} = \text{M.S.} = \frac{F_{cc}}{f_c} - 1 = \frac{25,757}{17,454} - 1 = +.48.$$

Proposed Strap Design:

The load carried by the cutaway portion of the channel is easily found by multiplying the operating stress level of this member by that portion of flange area that was cut away. Hence, we have for this member:

$$P_{\text{cut}} = f_c A_{\text{cut}} = 17,454(.135) = 2,356 \text{ lb} \quad \text{(compression load)}$$

where: $f_c = -17,454$ psi
$A_{\text{cut}} = 1.35(.100) = .135 \text{ in}^2$ (refer to Fig. 6-48).

Now, let us force this load to be carried by the proposed strap design. If we do this, the following stress is obtained for this member:

$$f_{\text{strap}} = \frac{P_{\text{cut}}}{A_{\text{strap}}} = \frac{2,356}{1.25(.090)} = -20,942 \text{ psi} \quad \text{(compression stress)}.$$

This stress is then compared to the allowable crippling stress of the strap. Its value, or F_{cc}, is computed from Eq. 6-16. Here, the full width of the unsupported strap is used for the value of b', where $b'/t = 1.25/.090 = 13.9$. (The attached members do not provide an edge of restraint for the strap in this position.) Therefore, from Table 6-3, with two free edges and the material clad 2024-T3 aluminum alloy sheet, the coefficient of edge-restraint $C_e = .295$. And, from MIL-HDBK-5F, the following additional properties of this material are found: $F_{cy} = 37{,}000$ psi and $E_c = 10.7 \times 10^6$ psi. Substituting these values into Eq. 6-16, we obtain the allowable crippling stress of the proposed strap design, or

$$F_{cc} = \frac{C_e \sqrt{F_{cy} E_c}}{(b'/t)^{3/4}} = \frac{.295\sqrt{37,000(10.7 \times 10^6)}}{(13.9)^{3/4}} = 25,784 \text{ psi}.$$

Before this value can be used, however, inter-rivet buckling of the strap must be prevented. To meet this criterion, it must be shown that $F_{ir} \geq F_{cc}$ for this member. The critical spacing of BJ 6 rivets is seen as the distance s in Fig. 6-50 (use a nominal hole diameter of .191 for this rivet).

$$s = (2D + .030) + (2D + .030) + .94 = 1.76 \text{ in}$$

$$L'/\rho = 2\frac{s}{t} = 2\left[\frac{1.76}{.090}\right] = 39.1\,.$$

With a value of $L'/\rho = 39.1$ and a column curve for clad 2024-T3 aluminum alloy material, we obtain the allowable inter-rivet buckling stress F_{ir} of the strap or 30,800 psi.

Then, comparing stresses, it is apparent that the strap will not prematurely buckle; therefore, the full allowable crippling stress of 25,784 psi will limit the design of this member in compression, not the limitation imposed by the inter-rivet buckling stress of 30,800 psi. Essentially the strap will cripple with the channel extrusion since the fasteners are spaced close enough together to prevent premature inter-rivet buckling of this member.

Crippling failure of the strap is predicted as follows:

$$\text{Margin of Safety} = \text{M.S.} = \frac{F_{cc}}{f_{\text{strap}}} - 1 = \frac{25,784}{20,942} - 1 = +.23.$$

Comparing crippling margins of safety, we find that the strap (M.S. = + .23) is slightly weaker than the production model structure (M.S. = + .48). This means that if the strap design proposal can be successfully structurally tested, the higher strength probability of the production model structure will also be assured (structurally substantiated). The foregoing discussion has described what is referred to as "the method of comparative analysis."

Shearing failure of the strap rivets:

If eight (8) BJ 6 rivets ($p_s = 862$ lb) are used for the attachment rivets of the strap design, the following shear loads are carried by each rivet:

$$p_s = \frac{2,356}{4} = 589 \text{ lb/rivet}.$$

A BJ 6 rivet develops its full shear strength in .063 in thick material; therefore, no correction is made for high bearing stresses that occur when this rivet is installed in the much thicker strap—or even in the frame flange member. From Eq. 3-1,

$$P_{su} = F_{su} A_{shr} C_r = 862(1.0) = 862 \text{ lb}$$

where: $F_{su} A_{shr} = 862$ lb (from Table 3-1)
$C_r = 1.0$ (from Table 3-2 in .090 in sheet thickness).

$$\text{Margin of Safety} = \text{M.S.} = \frac{P_{su}}{p_s k} - 1 = \frac{862}{589(1.15)} - 1 = +.27.$$

Bearing failure of the frame flange:

Since $F_{bru} > 1.5 F_{bry}$, Eq. 3-3 is used to determine the allowable bearing strength of this member.

$$P_{bru} = 1.5 F_{bry} t D = 1.5(71,000)(.100)(.191) = 2,034 \text{ lb}$$

where: $F_{bru} = 108,000$ psi ($e/D = 2.0$)
$F_{bry} = 71,000$ psi ($e/D = 2.0$)
$t = .100$ in (thickness of the flange)
$D = .191$ in (nominal hole diameter for a BJ 6 rivet).

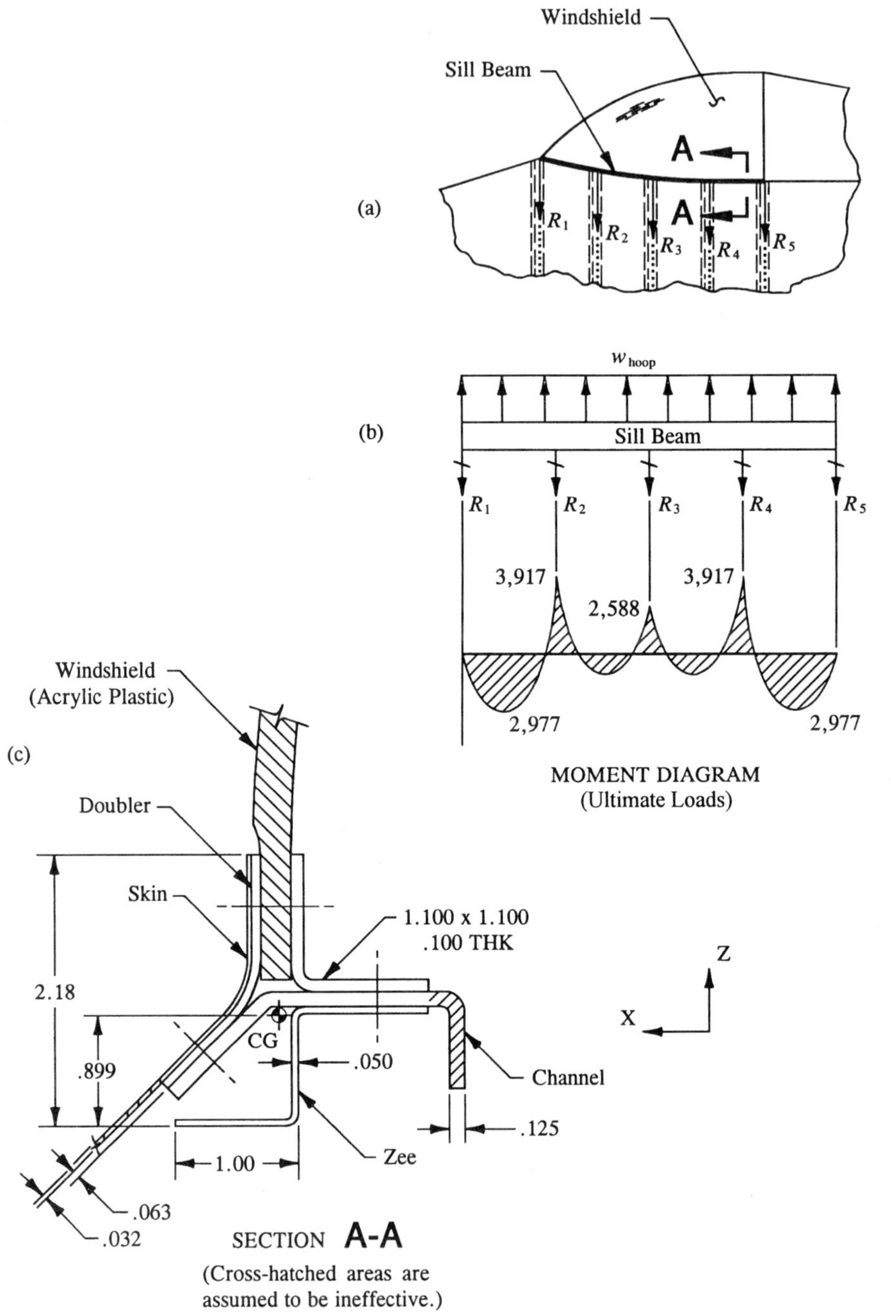

FIGURE 6-51 (a) Windshield supported along its boundary structure by a sill beam. (b) Isolated sill beam and accompanying moment diagram. (c) Sill beam cross-sectional area.

$$\text{Margin of Safety} = \text{M.S.} = \frac{P_{bru}}{p_s k} - 1 = \frac{2,034}{589(1.15)} - 1 = +2.00.$$

Bearing failure of the strap:

Since $F_{bru} < 1.5F_{bry}$, Eq. 3-2 is used to determine the allowable bearing strength of this member.

$$P_{bru} = F_{bru}\,tD = 125,000(.090)(.191) = 2,149 \text{ lb}$$

where: $F_{bru} = 125,000$ psi $(e/D = 2.0)$
$F_{bry} = 84,000$ psi $(e/D = 2.0)$
$t = .090$ in (thickness of the strap)
$D = .191$ in (nominal hole diameter for a BJ 6 rivet).

$$\text{Margin of Safety} = \text{M.S.} = \frac{P_{bru}}{p_s k} - 1 = \frac{2,149}{589(1.15)} - 1 = +2.17.$$

6.5 Problem for Solution. The windshield shown in Fig. 6-51 is supported along its boundary structure by a sill beam. Hoop loading (resulting from cabin pressurization) is carried along the sill beam and reacted by fuselage stub frames. Given the resulting bending moment diagram for the sill beam, determine margins of safety for critical compression members. Assume tension stresses are less critical. The effective cross-sectional area (Section A-A) precludes inter-rivet buckling. The moment of inertia for this section about the x-axis is .233 in^4 (which also includes the effectivity of the skin). The sill beam material is clad 2024-T3 aluminum alloy sheet and plate material, $E_c = 10.7 \times 10^6$ psi, $F_{cy} = 36,000$ psi (THK = .010 - .062), and $F_{cy} = 37,000$ psi (THK = .063 - .128).

CHAPTER 7

Column Members

7.1 Introduction. This chapter differs from the traditional treatment of column analysis by emphasizing more fundamentals and giving less emphasis and attention to the theoretical derivations and vagaries of mathematically complex column solutions normally given in advanced textbooks on this subject. The difference between columns and other structural members, those of noncolumns, specifically crippling members loaded in compression, must be clearly differentiated if the correct structural approaches and limitations imposed in this chapter on column designs are to be fully understood. Noncolumns, even though these members are compressed, do not fail as real column members. They are usually stabilized by some external covering of wing or fuselage skin material, and thus prevented from sideways motion to cause them to fail as columns. These special column types or noncolumns were studied in detail in the previous chapter on "Crippling."

Column design, in which "stability" principally determines the "ultimate compression strength" of a column member, will be the main focus of study in this chapter. However, only torsionally stable columns will be considered. Torsional instability of column members is not specifically treated nor included in this chapter; this remains an advanced topic beyond the main intent and scope of practical column design to warrant their inclusion here in this text. The following types of columns will be investigated in subsequent sections of this chapter: (1) Euler columns, Sec. 7.4; (2) Johnson-Euler columns, Sec. 7.5; and (3) sheet-stiffened, built-up column sections, also in Secs. 7.4 and 7.5. Columns are of special importance to airframe and missile design, and therefore should merit particular attention when they occur. Since their structural behavior in actual structure are generally not well understood, their designs should be carefully treated and include some expected degree of conservatism in their analyses.

Columns generally fail suddenly and quite dramatically. For this reason, some degree of conservatism in their analyses is usually considered, even essential in their designs. When a flat sheet or plate buckles, the buckled member can sustain its load while the increasing load simply shifts to the surrounding structure, usually to members that are considerably stiffer. Columns are not so fortunate or forgiving; but fail catastrophically without warning. Such failures are why columns must be carefully designed to meet the particular design conditions and requirements in which they occur in actual structure. Before a column is physically included in actual structure, it must be theoretically and experimentally verified. Essentially, a column is loaded to its maximum value, and if its design is structurally proved by these tests, the column can then be incorporated in actual structure. Generally speaking, the correct method of attack is of the utmost importance to the basic success or failure of efficient, trouble-free column designs. The engineer must be able to recognize when and if column members occur, and take the appropriate action to remedy, correct or repair them if these members are found structurally deficient. Compact structures, such as closed sections, make the very best designed columns. Open sections, such as angles, channels, I-sections, H-sections, and T-sections, are torsionally unstable and therefore their competency as columns should be carefully checked to prevent column twisting. In some cases, even structural testing may be required to establish their structural integrity before drawing releases.

The simplest form of a column is described as a structural member that is concentrically loaded in compression, and physically restrained at its column ends. Concentrically refers to the manner in which the column axial load is applied to the column. Here, the column axial load is applied along the longitudinal centroidal axis of the column member. Observe the simple column structure of Fig. 7-l(a), where the member is uniformly compressed by the axial force P that is applied to the column and simply-supported (pinned) at its ends. Under this applied load the column will compress but will remain essentially straight throughout its length. The material will strain rapidly in the direction of the applied compression load until the column actually buckles. At this point, the column becomes unsafe, even dangerous, and unpredictable.[1] Column buckling refers to actual structural failure of the column member (here, the column experiences large deflections immediately). Structural failure occurs when the column reaches its critical column load. This type of failure corresponds to the ultimate carrying capacity of the column member. Another way of describing this is: The column is stable if its stiffness EI can carry the ever-increasing compression load.[2]

[1] Such a member, if actually contemplated in actual structure, should be carefully monitored during structural testing.

[2] The stress at which buckling is said to occur is principally a function of the relative stiffness EI of the material, instead of the strength properties of its material. The ultimate carrying capacity of a column is therefore dependent on the physical constants of the material—this is measured by the stiffness or compression elastic modulus of the column material and the moment of inertia of the column section. This will become apparent when we present the Euler column equation in Sec. 7.4.

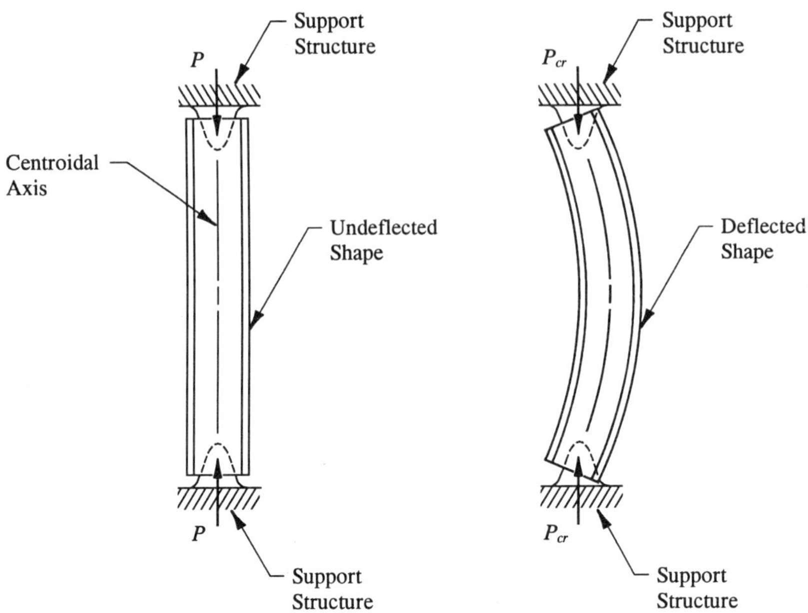

(a) Before Buckling (b) After Buckling

FIGURE 7-1 Concentrically loaded column physically restrained at its ends.

In effect, what happens to the column at failure is that the rate of deflection in the direction of the applied load becomes considerably greater after buckling than with the simple stress-strain relationship that occurred before failure. The deflected shape of the column now looks something like the shape shown in Fig. 7-l(b). In theory, buckled columns can undergo several different modes of failure; however, the higher modes, as shown in Fig. 7-2, can only be achieved if they are physically restrained from moving laterally. Lateral supports establish points of inflection where internal bending moments are zero for the buckled shape of the column. Without lateral restraints to prevent this motion, a column will always deflect in accordance with the first theoretical mode of failure.

Column failures are governed by one of the following forms of instability: (1) primary failures, where column stresses are either elastic or plastic; and (2) secondary failures, where column stresses are usually limited to elastic design. Primary or general instability failures may result from flexural instability, torsional instability, or by simultaneous occurrence of both. Secondary or local instability failures produce distortion (or crippling) of the column section, but the element section areas of the column are not themselves translated or rotated. Columns in actual structure normally occur as a combination of these types. Such columns, subjected to both primary and secondary failures, are considered in Sec. 7.5. Flexural (or bending) instability refers to column translation, while torsional instability refers to

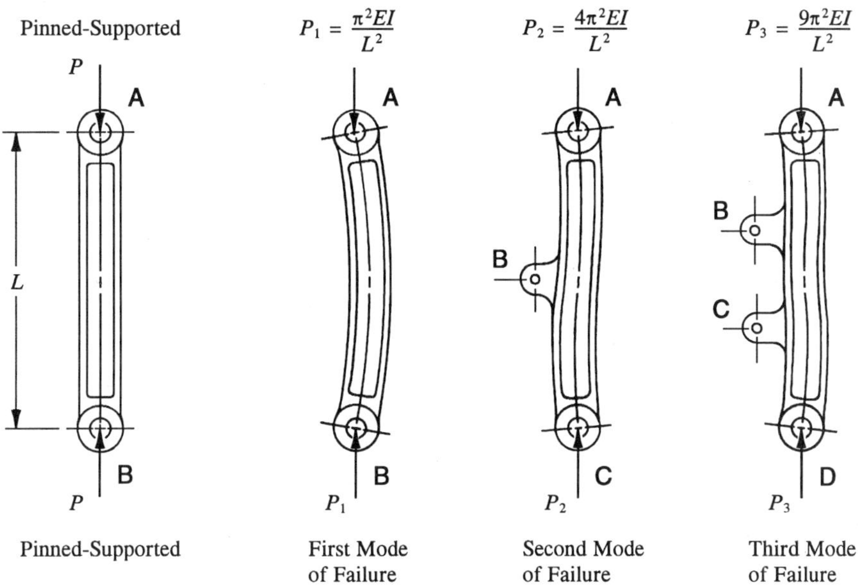

FIGURE 7-2 Theoretical column failure modes.

actual twisting (or warping) of the column. Both types of failures can also physically occur by combined action. In the design and analysis of compression members, none of the above failures should be ignored. Essentially, the structure is designed by the least allowable value obtained from the failures described. Figures 7-3, 7-4, and 7-5 illustrate quite dramatically the difference between distortion, translation, and rotation, respectively, of actual column members. The distinction made here between these failures is however only theoretical since most column failures are a combination of these types.

In Sec. 7.3, combined distortion (local buckling) and flexural instability of torsionally stable columns are reviewed. Torsional instability can occur by twisting about an axis parallel to the longitudinal axis of the column passing through the shear center of the column section. Shear center refers to the elastic axis[1] of a beam or column about which the member will physically twist. Column buckling from torsional instability, in its purest form, occurs by twisting, no distortion or translation occurs before or after structural failure. If, however, torsional instability is suspected in an actual design case, and the true structural behavior of the torsion member is not absolutely certain, the structural performance of this member might be better achieved through some form of structural testing than to approach the problem analytically.

[1] Restricted to aeronautical engineering, the elastic axis of an aircraft wing is a theoretical line (or axis) to which transverse loads must be applied to prevent the wing from physically twisting. The engineer is referred to a college textbook for a more detailed explanation of this subject.

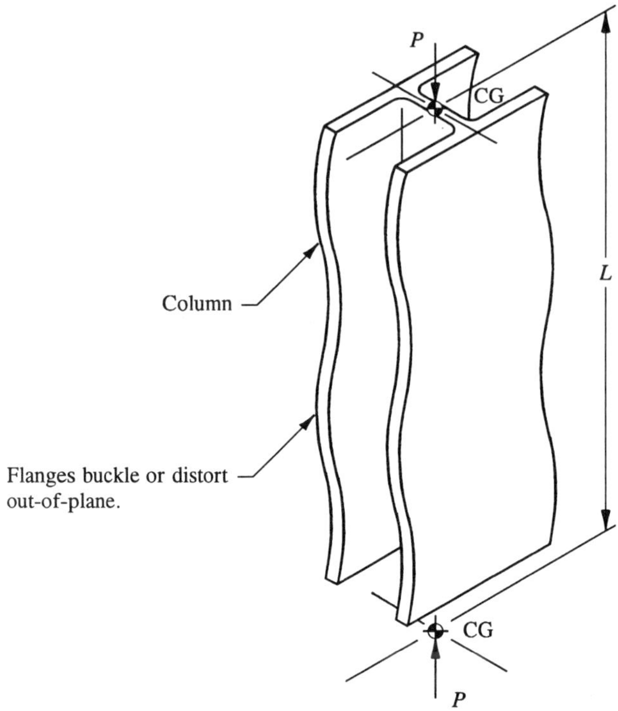

FIGURE 7-3 Diagram shows a column in distortional instability (local buckling).

7.2 **Support End-Conditions and Standard Loading Types.** Column end-conditions and manner of loading can largely determine the relative stiffness or bending rigidity of a column member. If not properly designed for, each factor can severely and detrimentally impact the overall structural performance and behavior of the column. Column end-conditions are important factors necessary to the overall performance of the column, and if their values are correctly perceived, the true performance appraisal of the compression member will be satisfied. The influence of column loading, also an important design consideration of columns, is described pictorially in Table 7-1. From this table, it is quite apparent that different loading types can cause a marked difference in column behavior—compare the large differences in end-fixity coefficients given in this table for columns having the same end-conditions. For example, compare Cases 1, 3, 5, and 7 with Cases 2, 4, 6, and 8, respectively, and then realize that these factors can also influence strength and stiffness of the column structure. The constant c is theoretically predicted and correlated with tested data for any given material in terms of end-conditions and manner of loading of a column at or near impending failure. And since failure, by definition, represents the critical stress or allowable of a column, by simple reasoning, the end-fixity coefficient also influences column strength.

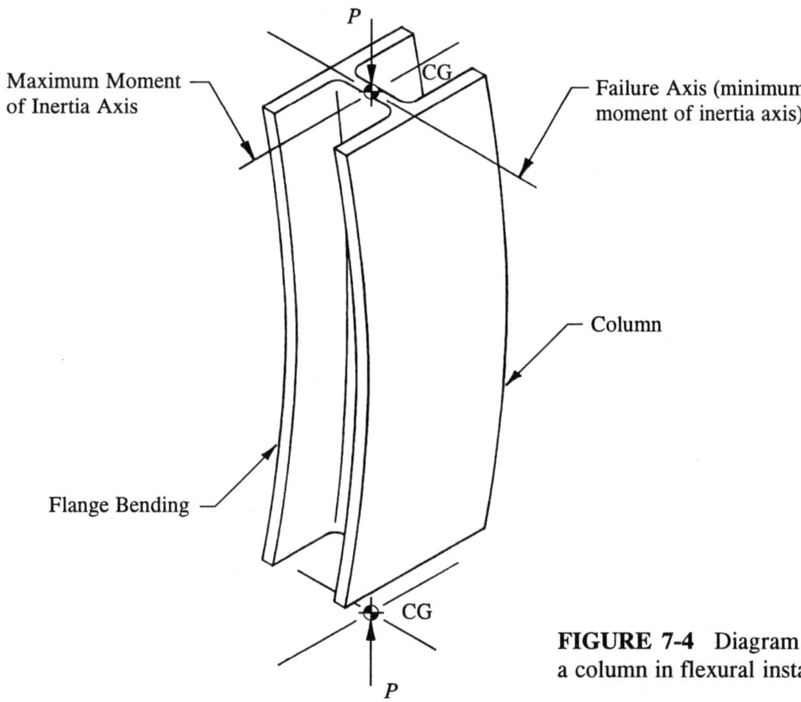

FIGURE 7-4 Diagram shows a column in flexural instability.

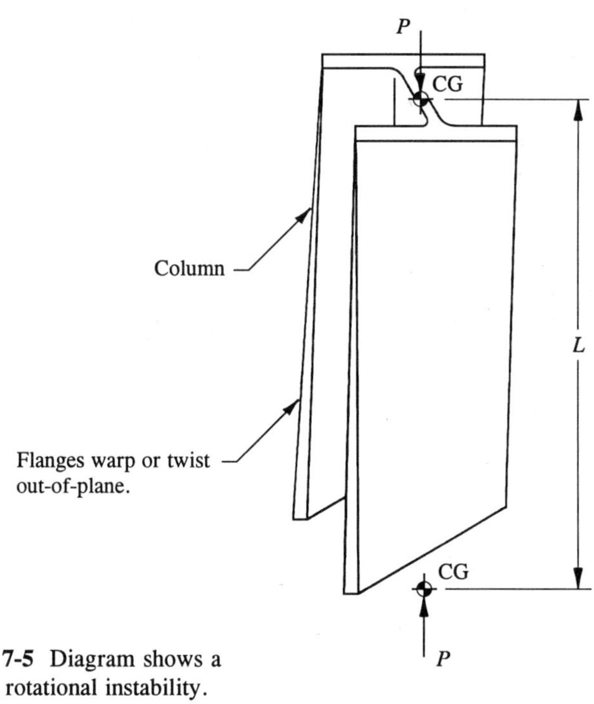

FIGURE 7-5 Diagram shows a column in rotational instability.

TABLE 7-1 COLUMN END-FIXITY COEFFICIENTS

Column Description	Loading Condition	End-Condition	End-Fixity Coefficient, c
Case 1 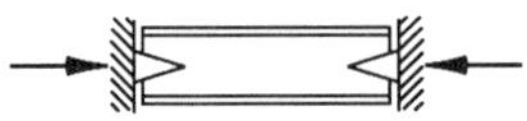	Concentrated Axial Load	Both Ends Pinned	1.0
Case 2 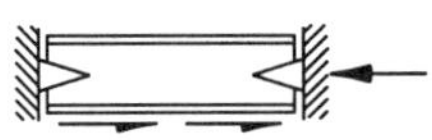	Distributed Axial Load	Both Ends Pinned	1.87
Case 3 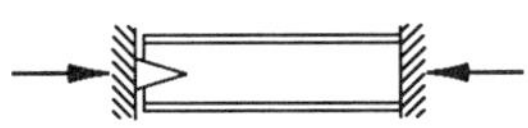	Concentrated Axial Load	One End Pinned; the Other Fixed	2.05
Case 4 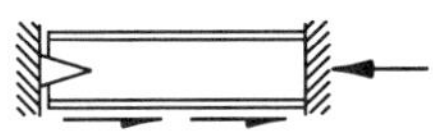	Distributed Axial Load	One End Pinned; the Other Fixed	3.55
Case 5 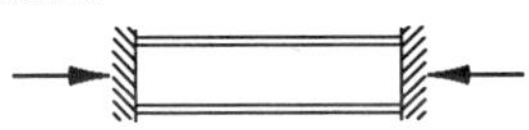	Concentrated Axial Load	Both Ends Fixed	4.0
Case 6 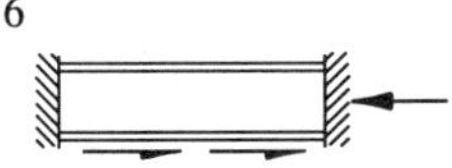	Distributed Axial Load	Both Ends Fixed	7.5
Case 7 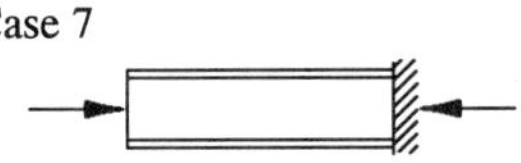	Concentrated Axial Load	One End Free; the Other Fixed	.25
Case 8 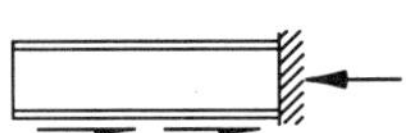	Distributed Axial Load	One End Free; the Other Fixed	.794

Although an infinite number of support types are physically possible, only two standard types are usually considered in column analysis: for example, the column is either assumed to be pinned-ended or fixed-ended. The following schematic representations, Fig. 7-6, will help to illustrate the physical characteristics of these end-conditions in actual structure for both standard types. A pinned-ended support is free to rotate or pivot about the centerline of the supported end. The best way to describe this type of support is by considering a frictionless pin, where the bending restraint or resistance offered at the supported end (or pin) is zero. On the other hand, since a fixed-ended support is physically restrained from any rotational movement, this type of support, by its very nature of being restrained, intrinsically

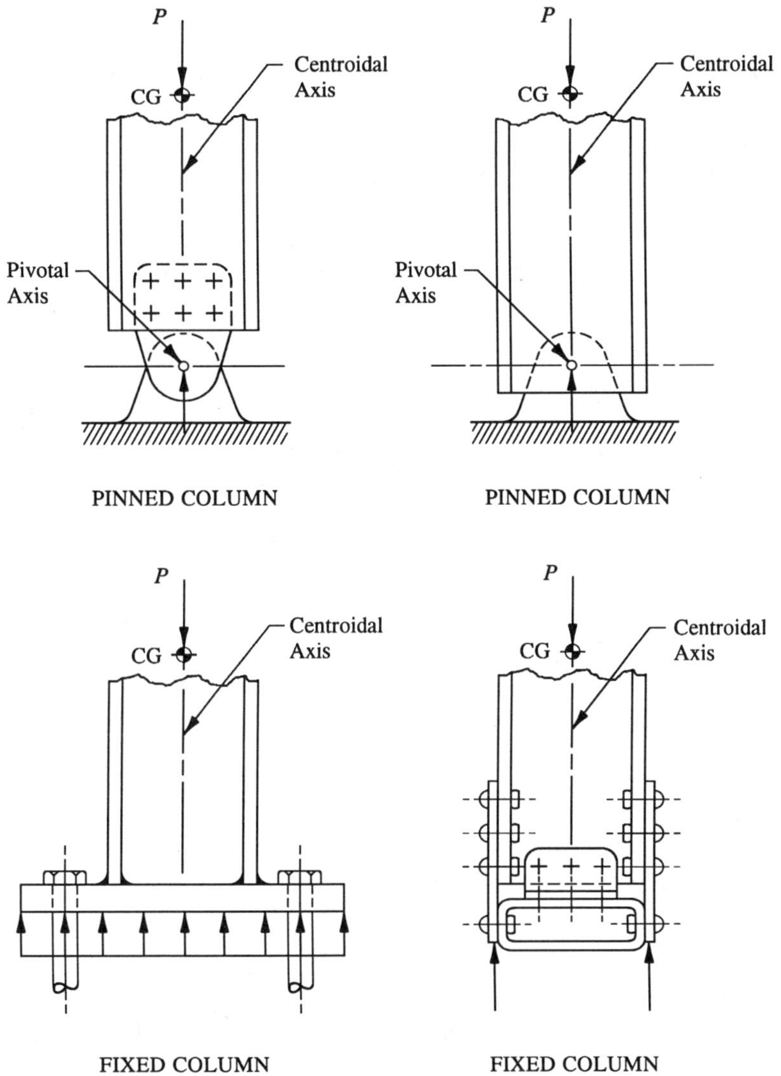

FIGURE 7-6 Types of column supports.

develops a fixed-end moment.

Other intermediate supports are also physically possible, but these supports, not so clearly defined as to warrant their specific inclusion as a standard support, must be independently investigated for their physical restraints offered. In other words, if some uncertainty and doubt exists as to the actual support restraint being offered by a column support, such columns should be carefully thought out, their evaluations approximated, and maybe in some cases even demonstrated by structural testing. In such cases, conservatism is essential to the safe and reliable performance of these members as compression columns. In some circles of engineering, without reliable structural test data to substantiate engineering judgment, a column is simply designed as if it were pinned-ended. This assumption should prove conservative since a pinned-ended support will always yield the least allowable value for the critical column stress. This limitation is generally acceptable with widespread use throughout the aerospace community and should be seriously contemplated when questionable column supports exist.

The critical column stress which causes buckling of a column depends upon many factors: the type of loading which caused that member to buckle, the support conditions at the ends of the column, the geometric properties of the column section, the material properties used, and even the effects of elevated temperatures on the material. Derived from the differential equation for beams or from test results in the lab, the first two factors, the type of loading and the support conditions of a column, are conveniently described in terms of an "effective column length." The constant c, or "end-fixity coefficient," is used here to describe these contributing factors to column failure. These coefficients are summarized in Table 7-1 for several different column types by their manner of loading and end-conditions. And in the next section, their values will be used in column equations to determine critical column stresses or allowables. The relationship between the effective length of a column and its actual length is expressed by the following equation:

$$L' = \frac{L}{\sqrt{c}} \tag{7-1}$$

where: L' = effective column length

L = actual column length

c = end-fixity coefficient (refer to Table 7-1, page 432).

From this expression and the above discussions which preceded it, the manner of loading and end-conditions, described by the column end-fixity coefficient c, accounts for these factors by modifying, in effect, the actual length of the column. For instance, from Table 7-1, a fixed-ended column, $c = 4$, is, by substituting values into Eq. 7-1, shown to be half as long as a pinned-ended column, $c = 1$. Other column comparisons could also be made, but this is left as an exercise for the engineer to investigate. When analyzing a column, be sure to use the unsupported length of the column for the actual column length L. For instance, looking ahead to Fig. 7-11, this corresponds to the column length shown.

Sometimes irregularities caused by manufacturing tolerance build-ups and unforeseen fabrication errors can also occur, but such minimal incidentals in construction are usually ignored by the analyst. However, if the manner of attaching the column ends to an adjacent structure should introduce gross blunders in measurement or significant deviations from conformity design into the structure, the column must in those cases be structurally tested. Eccentricities can however be foreseen and therefore their occurrences eliminated by forcing the applied load to occur concentric with the longitudinal (centroidal) axis of the column.

7.3 Flexural Instability Behavior of Columns. It was shown in Chapter 2, "Axial and Bending Members," that the effects of bending of a beam, of any type cross-sectional configuration, symmetrical or not, will induce or cause that member to bend around the principal bending axes of its cross-sectional area. From our previous study of complex bending stresses, we found these bending axes to be mutually perpendicular.[1] These axes were described in terms of the maximum moment of inertia and the minimum moment of inertia of the section and therefore also corresponded to the maximum and minimum principal axes passing through the centroid of area of the total section area, respectively. The resulting complex bending stresses, those computed from bending moments around the minimum and maximum principal axes, would then occur in these planes. Principal moments of inertia of a cross-sectional area are described in full detail in Appendix G (also refer to Example 2-7 in Sec. 2.9 for their specific applications to complex bending of beams).

For columns, a slightly different situation occurs altogether: Failure of these members, it can be said, occurs suddenly and without warning about the weakest bending axis of the column. For example, if a column section does not have equal stiffness or rigidity in all directions, such as the Z-section or L-section shown in Fig. 7-7, the compression member by its very nature or by its inherent behavior (to act as a column) will buckle in one specified plane: that plane results from a bending moment around the minimum moment of inertia axis (this refers to the $Y_P - Y_P$ axes of both section areas indicated in this figure).[2] For such cases, the member buckles to either side of the minimum moment of inertia axis through which the centroidal axis of the cross-sectional area passes. Another way of describing this phenomenon is by referring to the basic symmetry of the section. For example, for a symmetrical section, this includes those sections with at least one axis of symmetry, the principal axes are obvious—essentially, their locations are determined by inspection. This makes the whole problem of principal moment of inertia calculations (from Appendix G) rather academic; the same calculations would be made for these sections as regular beam sections would be for conventional moments of inertia (see Appendix F, Tables A-6 and A-7, for the general format of column headings used to set up these computations). However, if a column cross-sectional area has no axis of symmetry, the column will deflect, bend, and eventually fail, if unrestrained, around the minimum principal bending axis of its section area.

This general rule or inference applies to all column failures, and is the fundamental basis by which these particular failures are predicted, as given by the critical column stress or allowable of the column member. In subsequent sections of

---

[1] A review of these fundamentals can be found in Sec. 2.9, "Axial and Bending Stresses of Beams That Bend in Two Different Planes."

[2] A tubular or circular section may buckle sideways in any direction.

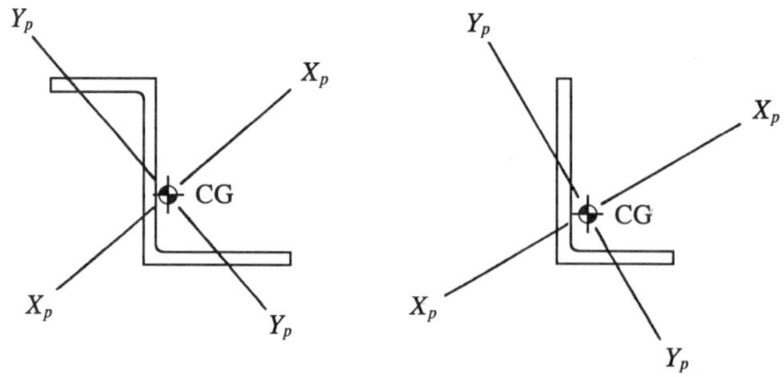

FIGURE 7-7 Maximum and minimum principal axes.

this chapter, column equations will be presented to determine these critical stresses. The minimum principal moment of inertia, a geometric property of the column cross-sectional area, not to be confused with horizontal or vertical moments of inertia, is taken as an indication or measure of the degree of resistance to column buckling—or failure. In general, most column members in an actual structure, such as longerons, fuselage frames, or floor support beams, have some sort of outer covering of sheet material attached along their column lengths, e.g., the skin of an airplane wing or fuselage (or even the web of a deep beam). For this reason, rarely do these members act completely alone.

Let us now look at the compression built-up beam caps depicted in Fig. 7-8. Such a composition or arrangement of attached members must be connected so that structurally they form an integral column. To satisfy this condition, the attached members must preclude premature inter-rivet buckling. To meet this requirement, the following criterion from Sec. 6.2 was established for riveted members: To prevent inter-rivet buckling of a riveted member, it must be shown that $F_{ir} \geq F_{cc}$. In all cases, premature inter-rivet buckling should be avoided; its occurrence simply limits the amount of effective skin area acting with the main structural member, and thus, is not particularly recommended for efficiently designed structures.

In Case a, the compression cap is free to bend about its minimum moment of inertia axis. Cases b and c are shown with their bending axes oriented such that column failure for these members will occur around their minimum and maximum principal axes, respectively. Note, in particular, how the orientation of the nested angle of Case b has not influenced column failure from that of Case a which preceded it. However, if the angle is instead oriented as shown in Case c, suppressing column failure about the minimum moment of inertia axis, the column will then appropriately fail about the maximum moment of inertia axis (or vertical axis of the member). From a design standpoint, based on deductive reasoning, Case c is a

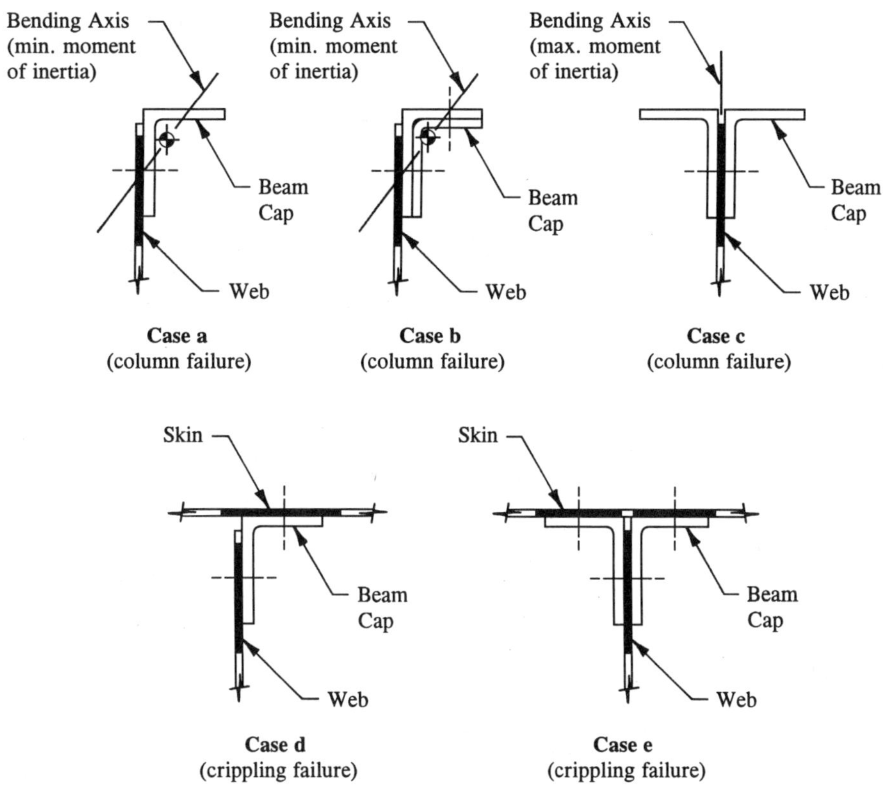

FIGURE 7-8 Compression built-up beam caps.

more efficient design, and is preferred over the nested angle configuration of Case b. The engineer is encouraged to compare moments of inertia for each column; for example, from basic principles of bending or Mc/I, we find that the operating bending stress of a simple beam is inversely proportional to its moment of inertia. The same analogy can be drawn for columns, since columns also fail by bending. Hence, this observation leads to the following conclusion: that the cross-sectional area of Case c is far more efficient by forcing column failure to occur about the strongest bending axis of the member. Nesting an angle would also help strengthen the column, but the increased benefit from this structural arrangement would be small compared to the greater advantage the structural arrangement proposed by back-to-back angles would have.

If a sheet or outer covering of skin material were attached to the cross-sectional areas of Cases a and c, the compression caps of these members would then be physically restrained from column action (by both the web and skin members)—thus making each compression cap no longer behave as a true column. The structural arrangement of these members are shown in Cases d and e. For such

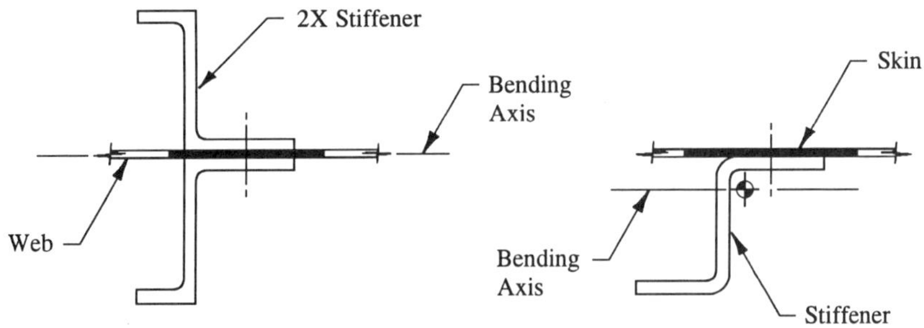

(a) Back-to-back stiffeners, $L' = L$. (b) Single stiffener, $L' = \frac{L}{2}$.

FIGURE 7-9 Column failure for stiffener-and-sheet combinations.

members, the compression allowables of each cap would be based on local crippling of their sections rather than on column instability.

The stiffener-and-sheet combinations shown in Fig. 7-9 do not act in accordance with theoretical column failures. The compression members here will bend around their composite sections parallel to the plane of their attached sheets (as indicated by the skin and web members in this figure). In either case, the tensile stresses in the sheets, in effect, produce normal stress components which tend to force the sheets and stiffeners back into their original configurations. This is shown in Fig. 7-10. This natural tendency, relatively speaking, helps to stiffen their column sections considerably by prolonging the actual failure of these members as columns. The attached sheets, being continuous members, prevent these members from classical column failures in which failure without the attached sheets presumably would have occurred around their minimum moment of inertia axes. The increased stiffness associated with this condition for a single stiffener is correlated from column test data and the results presented in terms of a reduced effective column length or $L' = L/2$. For back-to-back stiffeners, no appreciable benefit is derived from the attached sheet, therefore, no reduction in effective column length is indicated, hence $L' = L$.

Example 7-1 The structural arrangement of members shown in Fig. 7-11 is taken from an actual test fixture that was used to determine wheel spin-up loads for a nosewheel landing-gear structure. The internal forces in the members of this joint are defined from an internal loads analysis of the test fixture acting as a truss[1] under maximum loading conditions. Since compression members of a truss normally involve the selection of members based on column strength, find the principal moments of inertia for the compression member of this joint. Use the cross-sectional area shown in Fig. 7-12 to make these computations.

[1] A factor of safety of 3 is a standard value recommended by the Air Force, Navy, Army, and the Federal Aviation Administration for the design and analysis of test structures.

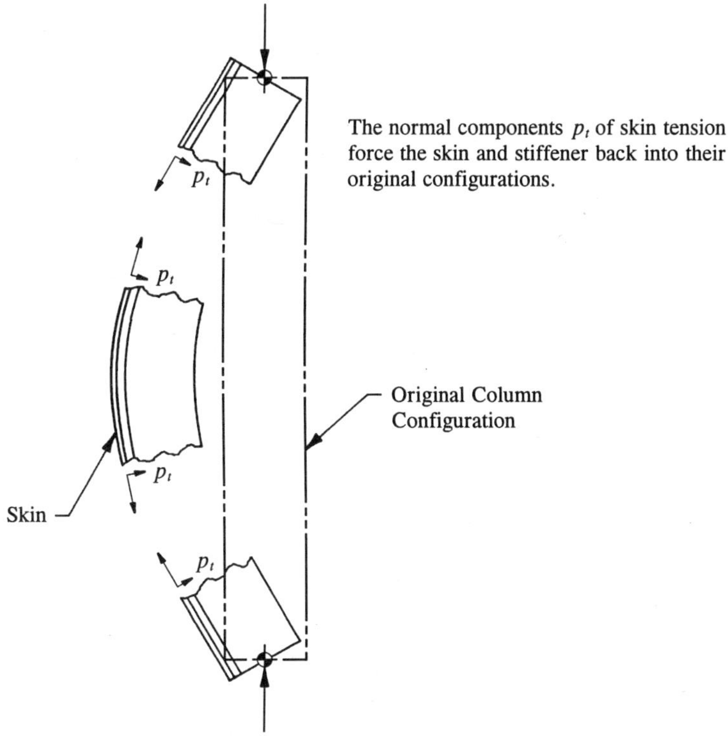

FIGURE 7-10 Normal components p_t of skin tension.

SOLUTION: It was shown in Sec. 1.10, "Method of Joints Approach to Internal Loads Analysis," that the members of a truss are either in pure axial tension or pure axial compression. Axial compression members are analyzed as columns (see design and analysis of Euler columns in Sec. 7.4), while axial tension members are analyzed from the tensile strength properties of the material (see analysis of tension members in Sec. 2.2). Further, it should be noted that pure axial members occur in this form only because the centroidal axes of the structural members riveted to the joint are concurrent (because the longitudinal axes of these members all line up at one common point on the joint). This refers to point A in Fig. 7-11. Hence, if joint eccentricities can be avoided, the joint and the attached members will not develop internal bending moments or shears. For such cases, at least as far as the analysis of compression members are concerned, the end-conditions of the column are sufficient to assume the column pinned-ended, or $c = 1.0$.

Since the axial compression member of our joint is not stabilized by any web or skin, column failure (predictably) will occur about the weakest bending axis of this member. Such an axis will correspond to the minimum moment of inertia of the cross-sectional area. Since principal axes X_p and Y_p are axes of bending about

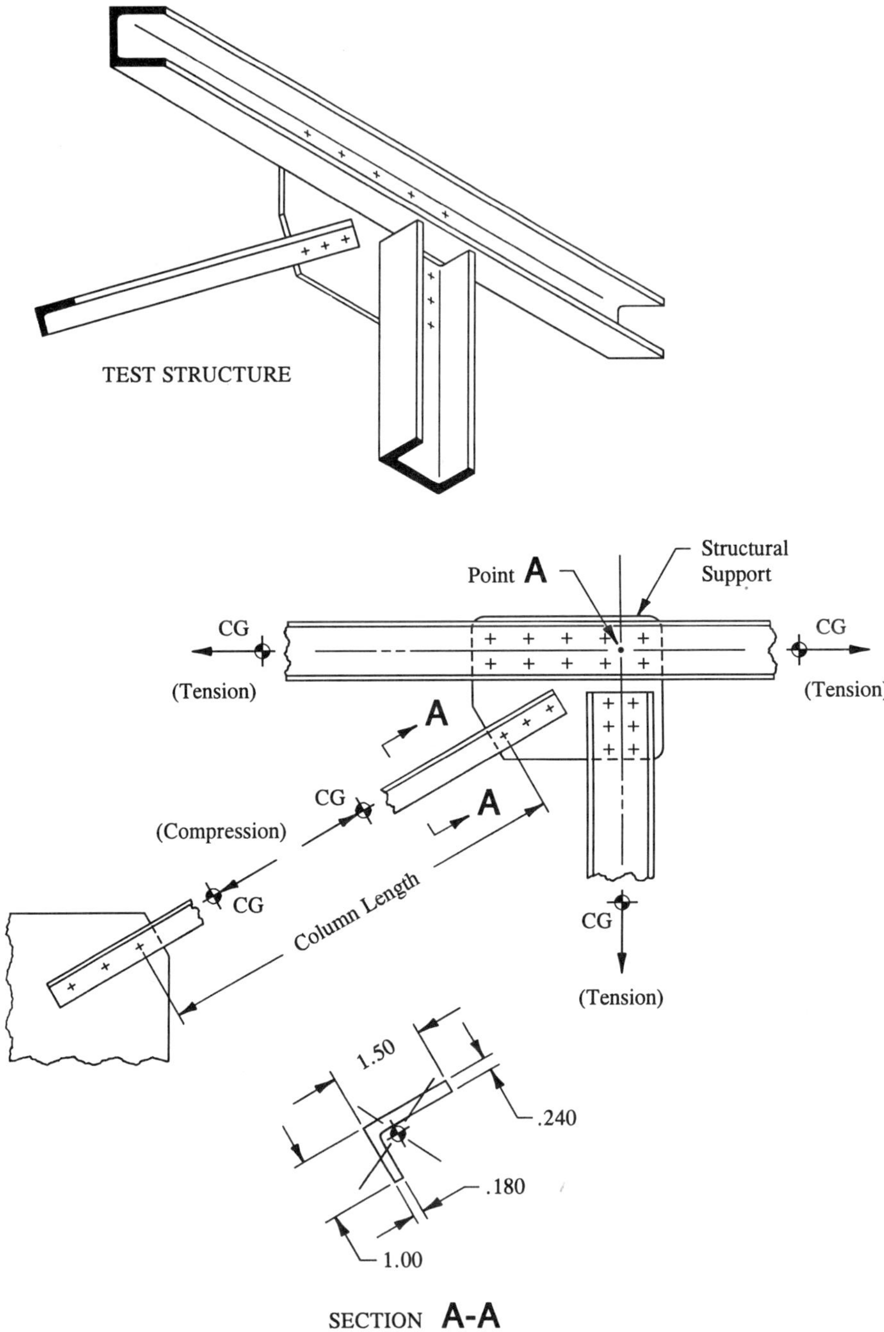

FIGURE 7-11 Structural members riveted to a common structural support.

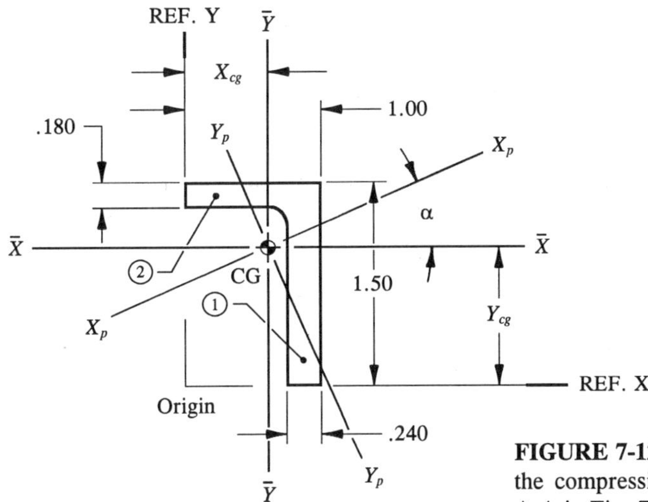

FIGURE 7-12 Cross-sectional area of the compression member (see Section A-A in Fig. 7-11).

which maximum and minimum moments of inertia occur, respectively, let us determine these values for our compression member. The following equations taken from Appendix G are used for this determination:

$$I_{xy} = \Sigma Axy - AX_{cg}Y_{cg} \quad \text{(from Eq. A-14)}$$

$$\tan 2\alpha = \frac{2I_{xy}}{I_y - I_x} \quad \text{(from Eq. A-15)}$$

$$I_{x_p} = I_x \cos^2\alpha + I_y \sin^2\alpha - I_{xy} \sin 2\alpha \quad \text{(from Eq. A-16)}$$

$$I_{y_p} = I_x \sin^2\alpha + I_y \cos^2\alpha + I_{xy} \sin 2\alpha \quad \text{(from Eq. A-17)}$$

where: $\Sigma Axy = A_1x_1y_1 + A_2x_2y_2 + A_3x_3y_3 + \ldots + A_nx_ny_n$

A = total cross-sectional area

x = distance measured perpendicular from the rectangular coordinate axis Y to the centroid of an element area

y = distance measured perpendicular from the rectangular coordinate axis X to the centroid of an element area

α = angle measured between the centroidal and principal axes (a positive angle is measured counterclockwise)

I_{xy} = product of inertia with respect to a set of parallel centroidal axes

I_y = moment of inertia around the conventional rectangular coordinate axis y passing through the centroid of the total area

I_x = moment of inertia around the conventional rectangular coordinate axis x passing through the centroid of the total area

I_{x_p} = moment of inertia around the principal axis x_p passing through the centroid of the total area

I_{y_p} = moment of inertia around the principal axis y_p passing through the centroid of the total area

X_{cg} = distance measured perpendicular from the rectangular coordinate axis Y to the centroid of the total cross-sectional area

Y_{cg} = distance measured perpendicular from the rectangular coordinate axis X to the centroid of the total cross-sectional area.

The basic approach to solve these equations is straightforward. First, determine the conventional moments of inertia I_x and I_y around a set of horizontal and vertical axes $\overline{X}$ and $\overline{Y}$, respectively. Then, using these results, solve for the principal moments of inertia I_{x_p} and I_{y_p} around the principal bending axes X_p and Y_p, respectively. Hence, starting with the computation of conventional moments of inertia I_x and I_y, we obtain the following tabulations for Section A-A (see Fig. 7-12):

MOMENT OF INERTIA I_x AROUND THE $\overline{X}-\overline{X}$ AXIS

Element	b	h	y	A	Ay	Ay^2	I_o
1	0.240	1.320	0.660	0.317	0.209	0.138	0.046
2	1.000	0.180	1.410	0.180	0.254	0.358	0.000
			Total	0.497	0.463	0.496	0.046

$$Y_{cg} = \frac{\Sigma\, Ay}{\Sigma\, A} = .932 \text{ in} \quad \text{(measured from the reference X-axis)}$$

$$I_x = \Sigma\, I_o + \Sigma\, Ay^2 - Y_{cg}(\Sigma\, Ay) = .046 + .496 - .932(.463) = .110 \text{ in}^4.$$

MOMENT OF INERTIA I_y AROUND THE $\overline{Y}-\overline{Y}$ AXIS

Element	b	h	x	A	Ax	Ax^2	I_o
1	1.320	0.240	0.880	0.317	0.279	0.245	0.002
2	0.180	1.000	0.500	0.180	0.090	0.045	0.015
			Total	0.497	0.369	0.290	0.017

$$X_{cg} = \frac{\Sigma\, Ax}{\Sigma\, A} = .742 \text{ in} \quad \text{(measured from the reference Y-axis)}$$

$$I_y = \Sigma\, I_o + \Sigma\, Ax^2 - X_{cg}(\Sigma\, Ax) = .017 + .290 - .742(.369) = .033 \text{ in}^4.$$

Next, from Eqs. A-14 and A-15, determine the position (or angle α) of the principal bending axes X_p and Y_p. The angle α is measured between the centroidal and principal axes of the section area.

$$\Sigma\, Axy = .317(.880)(.660) + .180(.500)(1.410) = .311 \text{ in}^4$$

$$I_{xy} = \Sigma\, Axy - AX_{cg}Y_{cg} = .311 - .497(.742)(.932) = -.033 \text{ in}^4$$

$$\tan 2\alpha = \frac{2I_{xy}}{I_y - I_x} = \frac{2(-.033)}{.033 - .110} = .857$$

$$2\alpha = \tan^{-1} .857$$

$$\alpha = 20^\circ\, 18'$$ (from Fig. 7-12, this angle is measured counterclockwise from the rectangular coordinate axes $\bar{X}$ and $\bar{Y}$).

The final step in our solution is to determine the principal moments of inertia I_{x_p} and I_{y_p}. From Eqs. A-16 and A-17, the following computations are made:

Maximum Moment of Inertia I_{x_p} Around the $X_p - X_p$ Axis

$$I_{x_p} = I_x \cos^2\alpha + I_y \sin^2\alpha - I_{xy}\sin 2\alpha$$

$$= .110(.93789)^2 + .033(.34694)^2 - (-.033).65077$$

$$I_{x_p} = .122 \text{ in}^4$$ (this value reflects the strongest bending axis of the column)

where: $I_x = .110 \text{ in}^4$
$I_y = .033 \text{ in}^4$
$I_{xy} = -.033 \text{ in}^4$
$\sin\alpha = .34694$
$\cos\alpha = .93789$
$\sin 2\alpha = .65077$.

Minimum Moment of Inertia I_{y_p} Around the $Y_p - Y_p$ Axis

$$I_{y_p} = I_x \sin^2\alpha + I_y \cos^2\alpha + I_{xy}\sin 2\alpha$$

$$= .110(.34694)^2 + .033(.93789)^2 + (-.033).65077$$

$$I_{y_p} = .021 \text{ in}^4$$ (this value reflects the weakest bending axis of the column)

where: $I_x = .110 \text{ in}^4$
$I_y = .033 \text{ in}^4$
$I_{xy} = -.033 \text{ in}^4$
$\sin\alpha = .34694$
$\cos\alpha = .93789$
$\sin 2\alpha = .65077$.

From the arguments given in this section, column failure of the compression member will occur about the weakest axis or $Y_p - Y_p$ principal axis, as shown in Fig. 7-13. Its value (minimum principal moment of inertia I_{y_p}) can be said to physically represent the bending stiffness of a buckled column at failure. And from its critical value, the proper sizing of the compression member based on column strength can be determined. In the next section, this minimum value will be used to determine the critical column stress of an Euler column.

7.4 Euler Columns. In this section, only column members composed of stable (nonbuckled) flange elements of a cross-sectional area are considered for column designs. Such columns consist of two basic types: Euler and Modified Euler columns. Euler columns fail by elastic instability and are sometimes referred to as "long columns," while Modified Euler columns are termed "short columns" that fail in the plastic or inelastic range of stresses. In general, short columns are more common in aircraft structures than long columns. Inelastic column behavior of short columns can be explained as follows: When a column becomes plastic (i.e., exceeds the proportional limit of the material), it will no longer return to its original configuration, instead it permanently deforms. However, elastic buckling of long columns can occur without any permanent damage to the column structure or to the surrounding structure.

Euler columns of both the elastic and inelastic column types must be torsionally stable, that is, free from rotational effects caused by actual twisting of the column. These members, or more specifically their column sections, must be translated; no distortion or rotation of these sections in their planes must occur (see Figs. 7-3, 7-4, and 7-5 of Sec. 7.1 for the actual physical descriptions of these failures). Column design of members composed of thin (buckled) flange elements of a built-up section will be reviewed in Sec. 7.5. These particular columns are called Johnson-Euler columns and form the basis for the evaluation of columns subjected to both crippling and primary column failures. It will be shown in Sec. 7.5 that crippling of unstable sections, in effect, tends to lower the critical column stress of the column as a whole from those values normally predicted by general column failure theory.

Column designs, including both elastic and inelastic failures, must closely follow the general guidelines listed below:

(1) The cross-sectional area of the column must be homogeneous—that is, having the same composition, structure, or character throughout (uniformity and consistency).

(2) The column must be straight; no initial curvature of the column is allowed.

(3) The column must be loaded longitudinally along the centroidal axis of the member; no eccentrically applied loads, either in compression or tension, must be applied to the member.

(4) Compression axial loads must only be applied at the column ends. Intermediate loaded columns are beyond the scope and main intent of this

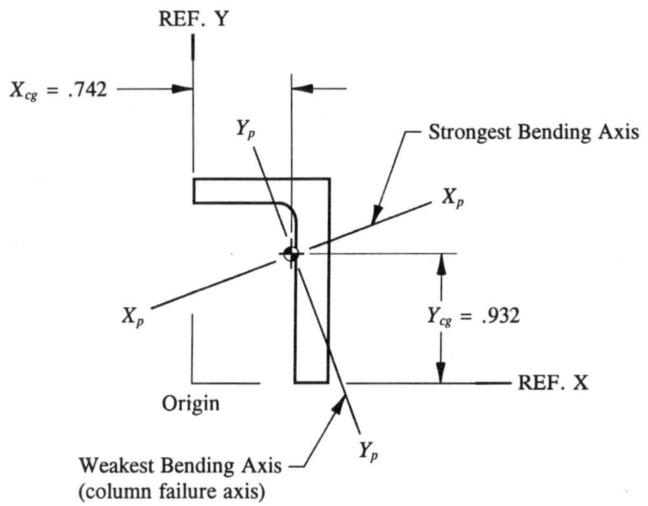

FIGURE 7-13 Column failure will occur about the weakest bending axis of the section area.

chapter—their designs fortunately do not occur very often in practice.

(5) Transverse loads must not be applied to the column (they produce beam-columns and are discussed only briefly in Sec. 2.9).

Columns which deviate from these prerequisites must be carefully analyzed though, even structurally tested, to insure their acceptability in actual structure; in particular, to meet existing design requirements which can prevent premature instability of real column designs. Any reduction in column strength for irregularities and accidentals of column design, those columns deviating from the above recommended column design requirements, would be completely justified in these particular instances. To justify some conservatism of their designs, the design engineer must rely on his better judgment and discretion for their solutions. Essentially, the engineer must give his "best shot" when analyzing irregular column designs until these members can be appropriately field-tested for their general substantiation. In the next section, column members, particularly those elements of a built-up column made from thin material, are investigated for the effects of local crippling on their designs.

The Euler column represents a structural member loaded in compression, has a stable cross-sectional area, and fails elastically. The allowable stress of a column in the elastic range is obtained from the following equation:

The "Euler" or termed "elastic instability" column is

$$F_c = \frac{c\pi^2 E_c}{(L/\rho)^2} \tag{7-2}$$

where: F_c = critical column stress or allowable

E_c = compression modulus of elasticity or Young's modulus

L = actual column length

c = end-fixity coefficient (see Table 7-1)

$\rho = \sqrt{I/A}$ = radius of gyration

I = moment of inertia about the failure axis of the column

A = column cross-sectional area.[1]

From this equation, it can be seen that the strength of an Euler column is dependent upon several factors: (1) the geometric properties of the section, I and A; (2) the material properties, E_c; (3) the length, L; and (4) the end-fixity coefficient, c (this constant refers to the type of loading which caused the member to buckle and the support conditions at the ends of the column). Also, the Euler column is valid for stresses in the long-column range, where stresses are elastic, more specifically, where structural failure of the member occurs below the proportional limit of the material. Also note from this equation that its solution is independent of the strength properties of the material, such as F_{cy}, F_{tu}, etc.

Metal aircraft structures of today have precipitated the design of columns at levels exceeding the proportional limit of the material, specifically, at inelastic stress levels. The high resulting strain deformations are typical of these members. In effect, the aircraft industry changed its restriction of elastic design of columns by allowing these members to fail in the plastic or inelastic range of stresses of the material. The higher strength capability of columns designed in the inelastic range thus gave way to the design of columns based on ultimate strength of the material. To obtain the ultimate strength of a column in the inelastic range, it was necessary to modify the Euler equation slightly—by substituting the tangent-modulus term E_t for Young's modulus E_c in the Euler expression. In this form, the ultimate allowable stress of a column could then be obtained, even if the column developed stresses in the inelastic range. The elastic Euler column was thus generalized to include inelastic or plastic design of column members. The "Modified Euler" column—or inelastic instability column—was thus created:[2]

$$F_c = \frac{c\pi^2 E_t}{(L/\rho)^2}. \tag{7-3}$$

Substituting for L from Eq. 7-1 into Eq. 7-3, we obtain:

$$F_c = \frac{\pi^2 E_t}{(L'/\rho)^2} \tag{7-4}$$

[1] Effective sheet area of web or skin that is attached to the main column structure is also analyzed in this section (in particular, see ahead to p. 452, "Column Analysis of Sheet-Stiffened, Built-up Column Sections").

[2] Also referred to as the "Tangent-Modulus formula" for the design of columns.

where: F_c = critical column stress or allowable
E_t = compression tangent-modulus
$L' = L/\sqrt{c}$ = effective column length
L = actual column length
c = end-fixity coefficient (from Table 7-1)
$\rho = \sqrt{I/A}$ = radius of gyration
I = moment of inertia about the failure axis of the column
A = column cross-sectional area.[1]

When using the Modified Euler equation, either Eq. 7-3 or 7-4, no distinction needs to be made between either a short or a long column since the compression tangent-modulus E_t for metallic materials equals the compression modulus of elasticity E_c when stresses occur in the elastic or long-column range of stresses (Euler-type column). The application of the Euler or the Modified Euler column equation precludes these members from local crippling and torsional instability. Here, the column section should be sufficiently thick (that is, where $F_{cc} \geq F_{cy}$) to prevent these types of instability failures from occurring. In summary, a Modified Euler column is either a long or short column, stresses are either elastic or inelastic, and structural failure will occur either above or below the proportional limit of the material. Also, as it will be shown in subsequent paragraphs of this section, inelastic stresses are limited to the compression yield stress of the material or F_{cy}. This upper limit for column design is also what basically controls the design of fatigue-sensitive column members.

From either Eq. 7-3 or 7-4, one can generalize the end-conditions of a column by making this general observation: A fixed-ended column is 4 times as stiff as a pinned-ended column and its effective length is one-half as long. Its ultimate allowable strength as measured by its critical column stress is therefore four times as great. These comparisons are arrived at by examining critical column stresses for a pinned-ended column, $c = 1.0$, and a fixed-ended column, $c = 4.0$, of the same material in Eq. 7-3 or 7-4. In the short-column range, however, this difference becomes less pronounced—thus eliminating most of the benefit derived by fixing the column ends in the long-column range. Essentially, it makes very little difference whether the column is pinned-ended or fixed-ended in the short-column range. To prove this point, the engineer is encouraged to compare critical column stresses for a pinned-ended and a fixed-ended column of the same material.

Up to this point, we have primarily described the structural behavior of a column by a sudden buckling at or near the critical stress of the column. (Prior to this stress the column remains essentially straight.) A column can also be described in terms of its critical column load P_c. From $f = P/A$, the critical load is obtained by

[1] Effective sheet area of web or skin that is attached to the main column structure is also analyzed in this section (in particular, see ahead to p. 452, "Column Analysis of Sheet-Stiffened, Built-up Column Sections").

multiplying each side of the Modified Euler equation, Eq. 7-4, by the cross-sectional area of the column.[1]

$$P_c = F_c A = \frac{\pi^2 E_t}{(L'/\rho)^2} A. \tag{7-5}$$

Rearranging terms in Eq. 7-5, we obtain:

$$P_c = \frac{\pi^2 E_t I}{(L')^2} \tag{7-6}$$

where: F_c = critical column stress or allowable (refer to Eq. 7-4, the Modified Euler column)
E_t = compression tangent-modulus
$L' = L/\sqrt{c}$ = effective column length
L = actual column length
c = end-fixity coefficient (use values from Table 7-1)
$\rho = \sqrt{I/A}$ = radius of gyration
I = moment of inertia about the failure axis of the column
A = column cross-sectional area.

Column Curves Established from the Modified Euler Column

The generalized or Modified Euler column, Eq. 7-4, is plotted in Figure 7-14 as a function of the critical column stress or allowable F_c versus the slenderness ratio L'/ρ (ratio of the effective length of the column to the radius of gyration of the section). The procedure which follows should help the engineer develop, if needed, his own column curves. First, this is done by rearranging terms in Eq. 7-4, and the results of these computations then establish the Modified Euler equation in a slightly different but convenient form:

$$L'/\rho = \pi\sqrt{E_t/F_c} \tag{7-7}$$

where: E_t = compression tangent-modulus (see MIL-HDBK-5 for specific values)
F_c = critical column stress or allowable
L'/ρ = slenderness ratio.

Now, assuming different values of F_c (say, 10, 20, 30, 40 ksi, etc.) in this equation, and corresponding values of E_t (refer to a stress-strain curve or tangent-

[1] If a web or skin member is attached to the main column structure, skip ahead to p. 452, "Column Analysis of Sheet-Stiffened, Built-up Column Sections," where a different procedure is outlined for their inclusion.

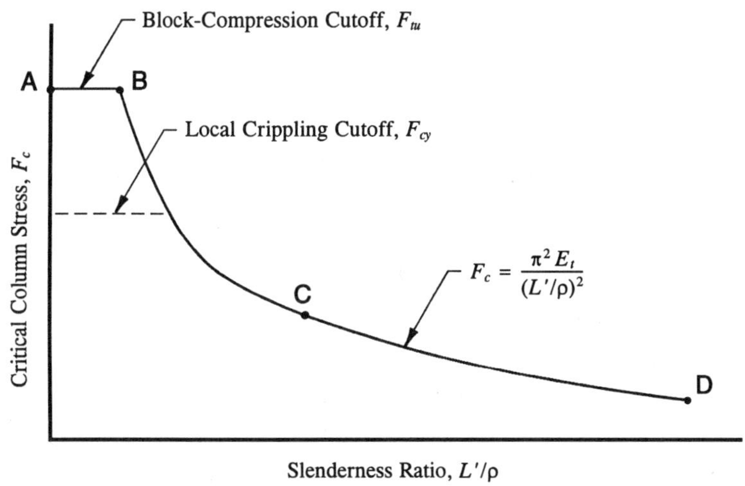

Region	Type
A-B	Block-Compression Columns
B-C	Short (inelastic) Columns
C-D	Long (elastic) Columns

FIGURE 7-14 Column instability curve is used to determine the critical column stress.

modulus curve for specific materials), we obtain the slenderness ratios L'/ρ. Plotting values of F_c versus L'/ρ, we can then, if need be, establish specific column curves for different materials. Such a curve is presented in Fig. 7-15 for clad 7075-T6 aluminum alloy sheet. For any given value of L'/ρ, column failure can be predicted—as determined by the critical column stress. As is the normal design practice of analyzing column structures, maximum inelastic column stresses (stresses above the proportional limit) are limited by the allowable compression yield strength of the material or F_{cy}. This limitation should help to control structural failures due to other design criteria—such as fatigue, creep, excessive deformations, etc., by meeting or enveloping their critical design stresses. In this regard, the engineer must thoroughly consider all possible failure modes, unless, of course, one can recognize that one particular structural failure is definitely more critical than the others. In our case, the lower allowable (assumed to be the critical column stress here) takes precedence over the other lesser, diminutive failures.

Column curves are a convenient and practical way of determining the allowable stress of a column without having to repetitiously evaluate Eq. 7-3 or 7-4 over and over again for each column member analyzed. *Design curves* are also very important for the evaluation and general substantiation of other structural

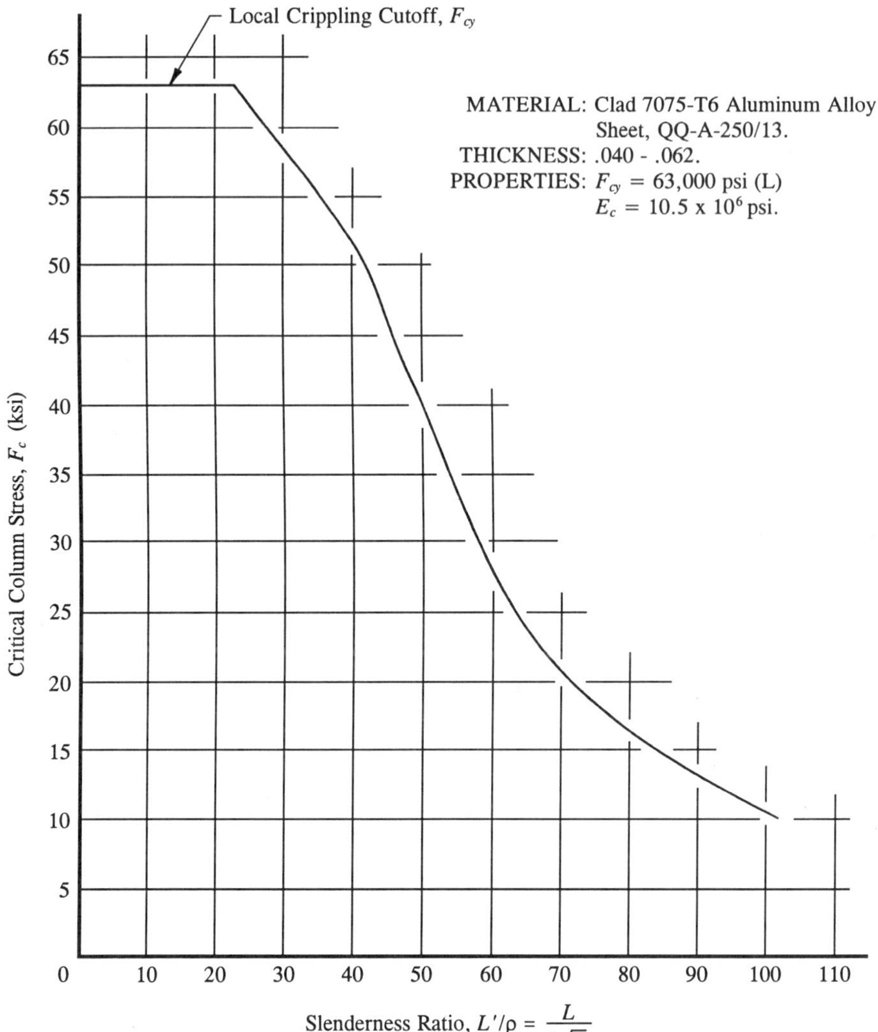

FIGURE 7-15 Column instability curve for clad 7075-T6 aluminum alloy sheet.

conditions also imposed on the design of compression-loaded members, such as inter-rivet buckling (Sec. 6.2) and crippling (Sec. 6.4).[1]

Above the proportional limit of the material, an inelastic column behaves, it could be said, like a column of an entirely different material. It should be recalled by the engineer that stiffness is measured by the tangent to the stress-strain curve of the material, and since the tangent modulus E_t constantly changes values at

[1] Refer to an aerospace company structures manual for the availability of these curves.

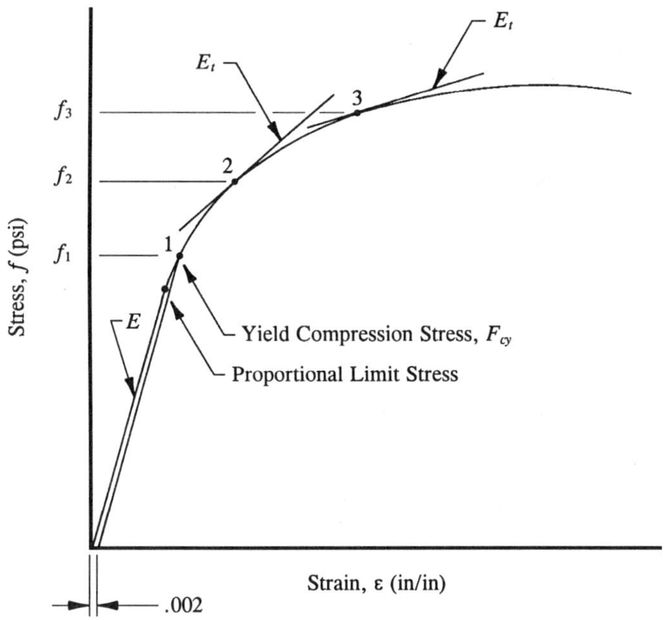

FIGURE 7-16 Typical compression stress-strain diagram.

different values of stresses above the proportional limit, the different values of E_t could actually be said to represent columns of different materials. The engineer is referred to Fig. 7-16 for a graphical description and interpretation of this somewhat abstract concept. Here, the proportional limit stress of the material, not clearly defined by this curve, is more specifically determined at point 1. For example, for this material, the general procedure used to establish a value is taken by a .2% offset strain parallel to the elastic portion of the curve. Where this line intersects the stress-strain curve establishes the proportional limit stress of the material or f_1 in this figure. At higher stress levels, the column becomes, in effect, "less stiff." This is observed from the lower sloping lines of the tangents to the stress-strain curve or tangent modulus E_t at points 2 and 3.

Column curves (F_c vs. L'/ρ) are normally presented for different materials used in conjunction with the solution of column design problems. A complete list of curves, those for each material commonly used in aircraft design, have been published by the aerospace industry. The engineer should consult with the appropriate engineering group in charge of issuing such documents, or copies of these curves can usually be obtained from an aerospace structures manual for different column materials. If, however, for some reason, specific material column curves are not provided, the engineer is encouraged to develop his own. Use Eq. 7-7 and follow the simple steps outlined previously to establish their curves.

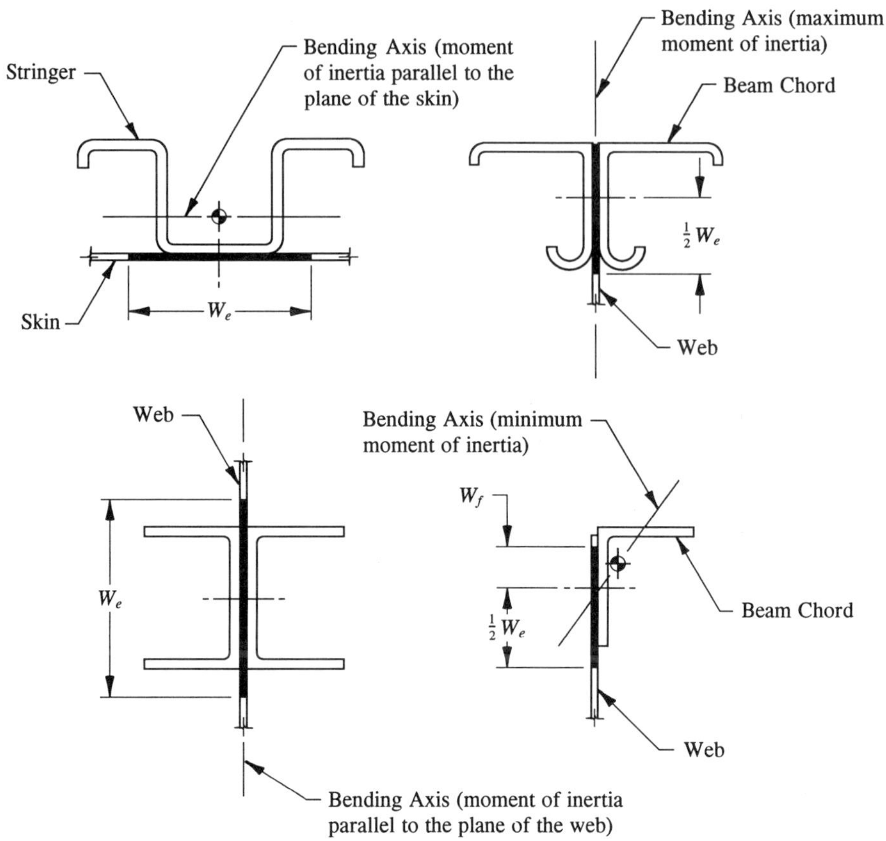

FIGURE 7-17 Sheet-stiffened, built-up column sections.

Column Analysis of Sheet-Stiffened, Built-up Column Sections

Many engineering problems encountered in actual structure deal with columns that are supported by an outer covering of fuselage or wing skin or maybe an included web of a deep beam structure. Such sections, as shown in Fig. 7-17, are commonly referred to as "sheet-stiffened, built-up column sections." Column failure of these sections, specifically of the Euler or Modified Euler type—columns which preclude local instability—are described in the following few paragraphs of this section.

Although the web and skin members of these sections essentially buckle at relatively low stress levels compared to general column failures, failure of these members is not immediate. Their buckled states do not actually represent structural failure in the strictest or purest sense of the word. Actually, a buckled sheet, even in its deformed configuration, and no matter how thin it may be, can still carry or sustain "some load" up to actual column failure. That ability and their capacity to carry part of the critical column load at failure is why we generally study and consider these members in column designs. Their importance to a well-designed, cost-effective column structure cannot be emphasized too strongly. To exclude these members from design consideration can ultimately lead to erroneous miscalculations of the basic column structure altogether.

In general, failure of most structural members occurs immediately after buckling, especially when the buckling stresses of the members are well above the proportional limit of the material (inelastic buckling). The attached sheet members of a built-up column section do not fail so dramatically. However, when they do fail, they fail when the column is fully stressed. This general tendency of buckled sheets to sustain load up to column failure should help to explain the general principles of ultimate strength developed by sheet-stiffened, built-up column sections. Although the attached sheet members of a column structure may buckle prematurely (below general column stress levels), these members do not actually cause primary column failure. From Sec. 6.3, the concept of effective sheet areas is used in our analysis here to correlate buckling of these members with the failure of the column at prescribed critical column stresses. Sheet buckling is therefore analyzed as if these members failed at column failure levels, even though buckling of these members occurs long before the column has actually developed its full strength.

The following steps are summarized to help the engineer systematically determine the critical column load P_c for sheet-stiffened, built-up sections of the Modified Euler column:

(1) Compute the effective slenderness ratio L'/ρ for the main members of the basic column section (for now, temporarily exclude the effective sheet areas attached to the main column structure).

(2) With the value of L'/ρ, enter a Modified Euler column curve for a specific material (see Fig. 7-15) and determine the critical column stress F_c, or use Eq. 7-4 for this computation.

(3) Calculate the effective sheet area of attached skin or web at a value corresponding to the critical column stress F_c obtained in step 2. (For a review of effective sheet area calculations, the engineer is referred to Sec. 6.3.)

$$W_e = 1.7t\sqrt{E_c/F_c}$$

$$W_f = .62t\sqrt{E_c/F_c}\,.$$

From these values, the corresponding effective sheet areas become:

$$A_e = W_e t$$

$$A_f = W_f t.$$

(4) Again determine the effective slenderness ratio L'/ρ, but this time, include

the effective sheet areas obtained in step 3.

(5) With the new value of L'/ρ, determine a new value for the critical column stress F_c (again use either the Modified Euler column curve or Eq. 7-4).

(6) With the critical column stress F_c obtained from step 5, repeat steps 3, 4, and 5 once again until convergence is satisfactorily achieved within acceptable bounds. (Use good engineering judgment to make this determination.)

(7) After convergence has been reached (from step 6), determine the critical column load P_c. Use Eq. 7-5 ($P_c = F_c A$) and base your computations on the composite area of the column section (that is, also include the attached effective sheet areas).

Although the above procedure involves an iterative method of analysis to find the critical column load P_c—Try it and see how time-consuming this procedure can be!—convergence is usually quite rapid. The engineer will become more familiar and mathematically more fluent with its particular details after a thorough examination of its detailed steps has been walked-through.

To simplify the computations above, base the effective sheet area of the sheet-stiffened, built-up column section on the maximum column allowable stress possible, i.e., using the compression yield stress of the material F_{cy} for the value of F_c in step 3. Convergence is then immediate (try it and see!). This approach should then avoid the necessity of having to repeat steps 3, 4, and 5 twice in the iteration procedure above. This is the most direct way of precipitating convergence of column members of this kind without having to perform the tedious iteration process itself. For most column sections, this approach should yield conservative results, essentially producing a less than 1% difference in critical column stresses. If, however, a more detailed, accurate investigation (or fine-tuning) of column failure is required, then the above iteration method should be a guide to their solution. Either method should prove satisfactory.

A final note: The attached sheet members of a column structure must be fastened so that premature inter-rivet buckling between the rivets of these compression members is prevented (inter-rivet buckling of thick, built-up sections is automatically precluded by the very nature of their relative size). To avoid their occurrence, the attached sheets should be designed so that $F_{ir} \geq F_c$, where F_{ir} is the allowable inter-rivet buckling stress of the attached sheets and F_c is the critical column stress of the main column structure at failure.

Block-Compression Failures

Columns that do not fracture in compression are commonly referred to as "compression-yielding columns" or "block-compression columns." These members are stressed beyond the proportional limit of the material and, because of their thicker cross-sectional areas, preclude local crippling. As the material of a block-compression column begins to yield (i.e., exceed the proportional limit of the material) and swell out under load, the column section continues to support the increasing applied load. Such columns act more like blocks or noncolumns than conventional column types. The theory of block-compression basically assumes columns can carry huge loads without theoretically failing. For instance, even at low values of L'/ρ (region A-B of Fig. 7-14), the ultimate compression strength (or critical column stress) of a block-compression column can theoretically approach infinity. Though rarely, if ever, would these types of column members actually be contemplated in aerospace structures. The ability of these members to enlarge in bulk under compression loads is characteristic of the general behavior of ductile metallic materials.[1] The classification of these members is purely hypothetical and conjecturable and therefore classical block-compression columns should also meet or preclude other design requirements and criteria, such as fatigue performance, excessive deformations, creep, crack-growth propagation, etc.

Before block-compression columns are considered for design, the engineer must thoroughly perceive and evaluate all other critical design aspects of the column design. Generally, for these type members, even though all design considerations and requirements of the column have been fully met, the ultimate allowable tension stress of the material or F_{tu} is chosen as the numerical equivalent limit or range of their designs.[2] This allowable value is used to establish a maximum cutoff stress for the critical column stress permissible for block-compression failures. This arbitrary criterion is necessary to prevent other structural failures from occurring unexpectedly. This practice is commonly used throughout the aerospace industry, and its strict adherence in design of block-compression columns is essential to trouble-free and cost-effective designs for long-life vehicle structures. To efficiently design these members, the engineer should try to reduce the column section so that crippling and inelastic column bending occur simultaneously. This means reducing the allowable crippling stress F_{cc} of the section to match the full column strength or critical column stress F_c of the column.

7.5 Johnson-Euler Columns. A column may fail either by flexural instability[3] (primary instability) when large lateral deflections of the column are produced; by crippling (local instability) when small localized deflections of the column section are produced; or by a combination or interaction of both types. The latter or combination type of failure is by far the more critical, causing column failure to occur long before the Euler or Modified Euler columns would have been reached. Crippling is therefore what precipitates to a large extent the premature failure of the "interaction column." From this general observation, it can then be argued that interaction failures actually represent "premature column failures." From this line of reasoning, such columns, particularly those members made from relatively thin

[1] Ductility is the ability of metals to plastically deform without actually failing the material in the process.

[2] The engineer is cautioned not to place much emphasis or importance (structurally) on the word "tension" here, since a true column is always physically loaded in "compression," not in tension.

[3] This is also sometimes referred to as translational or bending instability.

material, will actually force failure of the column to occur at a much lower stress level than would normally be expected for columns precluding this condition. Any reduction in column strength should be avoided, if possible, since their occurrence would only serve to weight penalize their designs. Such columns would then fail normally, that is, as Euler or Modified Euler columns, and thereby be far superior in strength and design than interaction columns. However, if thin outstanding flange members of a column section are used, and the section does cripple, their structural behavior can be predicted by the methods and procedures that follow in this section.

Structural shapes, those made from thin material, may fail through their compression flanges by deforming their shapes out-of-plane. The allowable stress for this type of localized failure is commonly referred to as the crushing or crippling stress of the section and is designated by the symbol F_{cc}. Its occurrence in actual column structures will usually dictate some special attention for their designs. The effect of crippling of unstable sections of a column can significantly lower the failure stress of the column from that predicted by the Euler or Modified Euler column. It was found in Chapter 6 that the maximum allowable crippling stress at which local instability failures were described were limited to the allowable compression yield stress of the material. And therefore, this limitation, by aerospace industry standards, reflects the severity of these type failures, at least to the extent that critical column stresses are reduced by the effects of crippling.

In general, columns should be designed so that crippling and general column failure occur simultaneously—at approximately the same failing stress levels. That is, such that $F_c = F_{cc}$, where F_c is the critical column stress and F_{cc} is the crippling allowable stress of the column section. This then maintains optimum column design when column members are subjected to local instability failures of this kind. When premature local instability failures do occur (where the elements of a column section are thin), mathematically, this corresponds to $F_{cc} < F_{cy}$, the well-known Johnson-Euler equation is applicable. It can also be shown that if the flanges of an I-beam section, H-beam section, T-beam section, or for that matter any thin-walled member like that, are too thin, they will deflect by crippling (where the thin outstanding flanges of these sections cripple or deform their shapes out-of-plane) before the Euler buckling stress of the column is reached. To resolve these structural differences mathematically, the interaction equation to determine combined flexural instability and crippling of columns was developed. Without proof,[1] the following equations are now presented:

$$F_c = F_{cc} - \frac{F_{cc}^2 \left[\frac{L}{\rho \sqrt{c}} \right]^2}{4 \pi^2 E_c}. \tag{7-8}$$

---

[1] These equations can be verified from an aerospace company structures manual on the subject of column instability, or from a college textbook on mechanics of materials.

Substituting for L from Eq. 7-1 ($L = L' \sqrt{c}$) into Eq. 7-8, we obtain:

$$F_c = F_{cc} - \frac{F_{cc}^2 (L'/\rho)^2}{4\pi^2 E_c} \tag{7-9}$$

where: F_c = critical column stress or allowable
F_{cc} = crippling allowable stress (refer to Sec. 6.4 for specific details to determine this value)
E_c = compression modulus of elasticity or Young's modulus
$L' = L/\sqrt{c}$ = effective column length
L = actual column length
c = end-fixity coefficient (use values from Table 7-1, p. 432)
$\rho = \sqrt{I/A}$ = radius of gyration
I = moment of inertia about the failure axis of the column
A = column cross-sectional area (this area should also include the effective sheet area of skin or web, if either of these members are attached to the main column structure).[1]

A graphical solution of this equation is conveniently plotted as a function of the critical column stress F_c versus the slenderness ratio L'/ρ. This is left as an exercise for the engineer to complete. The resulting family of design curves drawn will represent the interaction effects between flexural instability and crippling for specified values of crippling stress. Essentially, this means that the crippling stress F_{cc} of a column section determines the applicable column curve to use for each particular design case investigated. For any given values of L'/ρ and F_{cc}, interaction column failure for members subjected to premature local instability can thus be expediently predicted. Local instability or crippling can lower column strength, and for this reason, its occurrence should be limited in all aspects and applications of basic column designs. To avoid crippling in column designs and thus maximize column strength of interaction columns, it is recommended that the engineer try to force crippling failure of thin outstanding flange elements of a column section at prescribed levels of critical column stress: These stresses should correspond to the Euler or Modified Euler column (column failures for these types were discussed earlier in Sec. 7.4). If, however, premature crippling of a column should occur, Eq. 7-9 should prove invaluable in the solution of their structural competency.

Column Analysis of Sheet-Stiffened, Built-up Column Sections

Column failure of sheet-stiffened, built-up column sections are again reviewed in this section. This time, however, their designs will be based on the interaction

---

[1] For the analysis procedure required to determine the effectivity of these members, the engineer is referred ahead to pages 457-459, "Column Analysis of Sheet-Stiffened, Built-up Column Sections."

of primary column failures and local instability failures as determined by their ultimate column strengths or critical column loads. Column failures of these kind are particularly important to aerospace structures since their influence on column behavior can significantly lower critical column stresses or allowables when they occur. If such columns are actually contemplated in aircraft designs, their individual merits should be compared and carefully considered by analysis. The engineer is referred to Fig. 7-17, where the main structural members in this figure are perceived as thin structural members, and thus allowed to cripple as Johnson-Euler columns (i.e., interaction columns). Crippling should not be regarded as a condition precipitating column failure; instead, such members should be construed as structurally weakening the column structure and thereby reducing the critical column stress. Theoretically, crippling does not occur (prematurely) until the column has reached its full strength or critical column load.

Failure of a sheet-stiffened, built-up column section usually begins by web or skin buckling at relatively low values of compression stress—these members will buckle first because they are usually thinner and their allowable buckling stresses are much lower than the main members of the column section. Although sheet members buckle at relatively low values of compression stress, they can still sustain some column load in their buckled, deformed state. When such members prematurely buckle, they do not actually cause primary column failure. From basic principles of stress, where $P = fA$, the critical column load is obtained by multiplying each side of the Johnson-Euler column equation by the effective cross-sectional area of the column. This gives:

$$P_c = F_c A = \left[F_{cc} - \frac{F_{cc}^2 (L'/\rho)^2}{4\pi^2 E_c} \right] A \tag{7-10}$$

where: F_c = critical column stress or allowable (see Eq. 7-9, Johnson-Euler column)

F_{cc} = crippling allowable stress (refer to Sec. 6.4 for specific details to determine this value)

E_c = compression modulus of elasticity or Young's modulus

$L' = L/\sqrt{c}$ = effective column length

L = actual column length

c = end-fixity coefficient (use values from Table 7-1)

$\rho = \sqrt{I/A}$ = radius of gyration

I = moment of inertia about the failure axis of the column

A = column cross-sectional area (also include the effective sheet area of either skin or web).

The following steps are summarized for the analysis of sheet-stiffened, built-up column sections. In particular, this procedure should be used to determine the critical column load P_c for columns of the Johnson-Euler type (see Eq. 7-10).

(1) Compute the effective slenderness ratio L'/ρ for the main member of the basic column section (for now, temporarily exclude the effective sheet areas attached to the column main structure).

(2) Calculate the allowable crippling stress F_{cc} for the same main compression member used in step 1. (For a review of the principles and fundamentals of crippling calculations, the engineer is referred to Sec. 6.4.)

(3) With the values of L'/ρ and F_{cc}, enter a Johnson-Euler column curve of a specific material and determine the critical column stress F_c, or use Eq. 7-9 for this computation.

(4) Calculate the effective sheet area of attached skin or web at a value corresponding to the critical column stress F_c obtained in step 3. (For a review of effective sheet area calculations, the engineer is referred to Sec. 6.3.)

$$W_e = 1.7t\sqrt{E_c/F_c}$$

$$W_f = .62t\sqrt{E_c/F_c}\ .$$

From these values, the corresponding effective sheet areas become:

$$A_e = W_e t$$

$$A_f = W_f t.$$

(5) Again determine the effective slenderness ratio L'/ρ, but this time, include the effective sheet areas obtained in step 4.

(6) With the new value of L'/ρ and the same value of F_{cc}, determine a new value for the critical column stress F_c (again use either the Johnson-Euler column curve (if available) or Eq. 7-9).

(7) With the critical column stress F_c obtained from step 6, repeat steps 4, 5, and 6 once again until convergence is satisfactorily achieved within acceptable bounds.

(8) After convergence has been reached (from step 7), determine the critical column load P_c. Use Eq. 7-10 and base your computations on the composite area of the column section (include the effective sheet area).

Although the above procedure involves an iterative method of analysis to find the critical column load P_c, convergence of these members is usually quite rapid. The engineer is referred to the next paragraph and to Example 7-2, where the application and solution of a specific example problem is demonstrated using a slightly simplified approach to this step-by-step procedure.

In short, to simplify our computations of sheet-stiffened, built-up column sections, base the effective sheet area on the maximum column allowable stress possible using the allowable crippling stress of the section F_{cc} for the value of F_c in

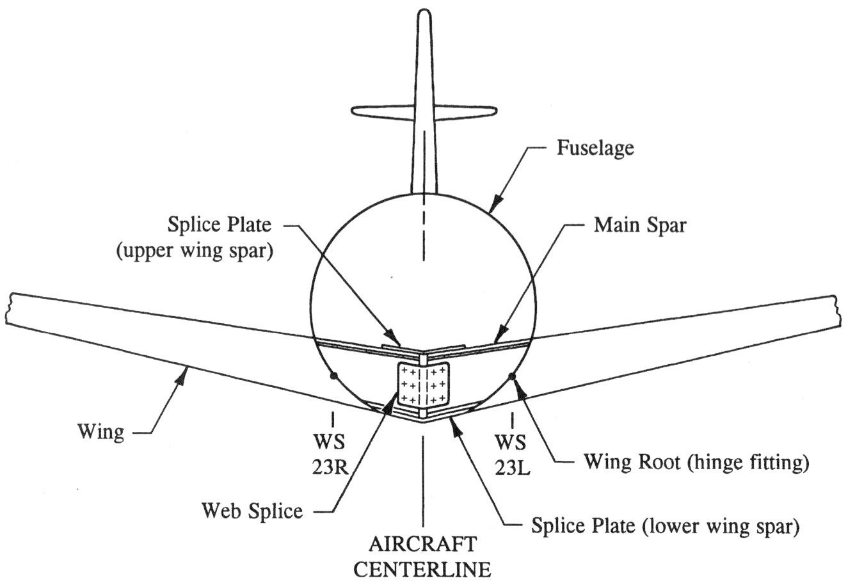

FIGURE 7-18 Main wing spars joined together at the centerline of the aircraft.

step 4 above. Convergence is then immediate (try it and see!). This approach should then avoid the necessity of having to repeat steps 4, 5, and 6 twice in the iteration procedure above. This is the most direct way of precipitating convergence of column members of this kind without actually having to perform the tedious iteration itself. For most column sections, this approach should yield conservative results, essentially producing a less than 1% difference in critical column stresses. If, however, a more detailed, accurate investigation (or fine-tuning) of column failure is required, then the above iteration method should be a guide to their solution. Either method should prove satisfactory.

Even if a column is constructed of several different members, the individual members making up the column structure must be connected to the column in such a way as to cause the column to act as an integral unit. This premise also includes the attached sheet members of the basic column structure. Structurally, this means that inter-rivet buckling must be precluded for all riveted members of the column structure if the column design is to fully develop its full column strength. To prevent inter-rivet buckling, the attached members must be designed so that $F_{ir} \geq F_c$, where F_{ir} is the allowable inter-rivet buckling stress of the attached members and F_c is the critical column stress or allowable of the composite column structure at failure. Otherwise, some reduction in critical column stress would be required for the built-up column section. Since there are no reliable and foolproof methods of analysis available to measure this behavior when it occurs, the simplest way of

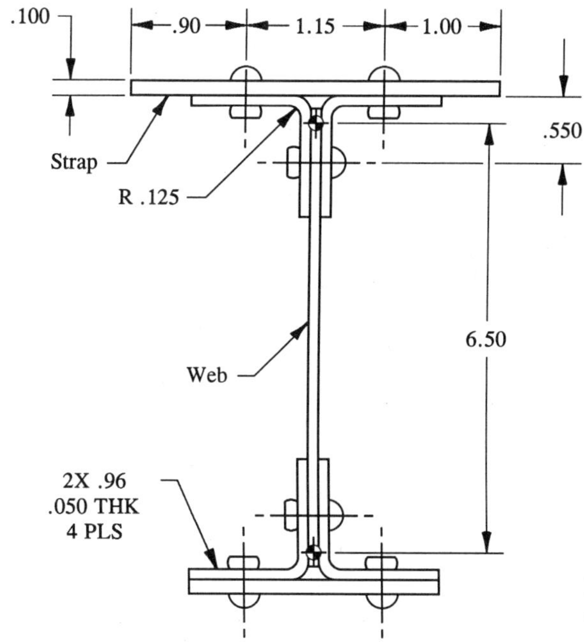

FIGURE 7-19 Main wing spar cross-sectional area.

preventing such a reduction in column strength is to avoid premature inter-rivet buckling of column members altogether.

Example 7-2 The main wing spars extend through the sides of the fuselage structure and are joined at the centerline of the aircraft by splice plates attaching their caps and webs together. The structural arrangement of these members is illustrated in Fig. 7-18. If the wing spars are critical for wing up-bending, determine the column margin of safety of the upper spar cap for a maximum bending moment of 79,665 in-lb ultimate at the wing root. Use the cross-sectional area shown in Fig. 7-19 to make your stress computations. To simplify the analysis of that section, consider the following conditions: (1) the distance between cap centroids is estimated from previous analysis to be 6.50 in apart, (2) lower cap tension stresses were computed and found not to be critical, (3) the end-fixity coefficient of the upper cap, based on company policy and some engineering judgment, is predicted to be 2.0, (4) the allowable crippling stress of the upper spar cap precludes inter-rivet buckling, and (5) the entire cross-sectional area of the spar is composed of clad 2024-T3 aluminum alloy sheet and plate material, QQ-A-250/5 (see Table A-4 in Appendix E). From the mechanical-property tables in MIL-HDBK-5F for this material, we find: $E_c = 10.7 \times 10^6$ psi, $F_{cy} = 36{,}000$ psi (THK = .010 - .062), and $F_{cy} = 37{,}000$ psi (THK = .063 - .128).

SOLUTION: Since the upper spar cap is made up of thin structural elements, column failure of this member is predicted by the general solution of the Johnson-

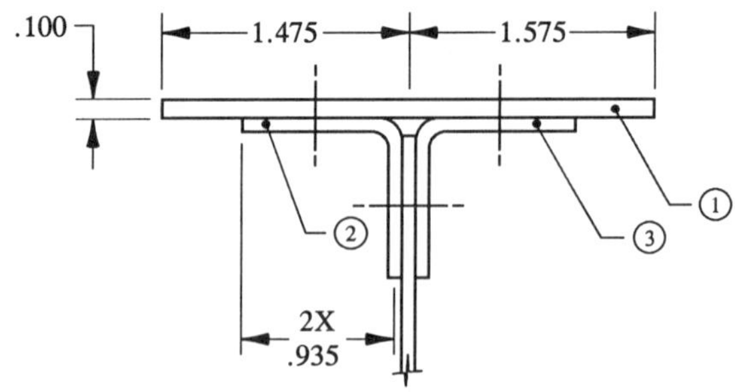

FIGURE 7-20 Upper spar cap is partitioned into angle element areas.

Euler column equation. The first step in the solution of this example is to determine the allowable crippling stress F_{cc} of the upper spar cap. The spar cap is isolated using three elements, as shown in Fig. 7-20, and the values of b'/t and F_{cc} determined for each. Also review those principles found in Chapter 6 for specific details and information pertinent to this procedure. As a brief review of that section, it should be recalled that crippling computations, at least as far as actual crippling computations go, are performed only for the main structural members of the cross-sectional area (this is done in Table 7-2). Although the web structure is not purposely included in this computation now, the crippling strength of this member will however be considered later.

$$F_{cc} = \frac{C_e\sqrt{F_{cy}E_c}}{(b'/t)^{3/4}} \qquad \text{where: } b'/t = \frac{b_1 + b_2}{t_1 + t_2}.$$

TABLE 7-2 CRIPPLING CALCULATIONS

Element	b'/t (Fig. 6-27)	C_e (Table 6-3)	F_{cc} (Eq. 6-16)	A^*	$F_{cc}A$
1	15.2	0.295	24,112	0.305	7,354
2	18.7	0.295	20,360	0.090	1,832
3	18.7	0.295	20,360	0.090	1,832
			Total	0.485	11,018

* The areas of elements 2 and 3 in this table are calculated as follows (also refer to Fig. 7-21 for the specific formula used to compute the bent areas of these members:

$$A_2 = A_3 = .785(.050) + .785(.050) + \frac{\pi}{4}[(.175)^2 - (.125)^2] = .090 \text{ in}^2.$$

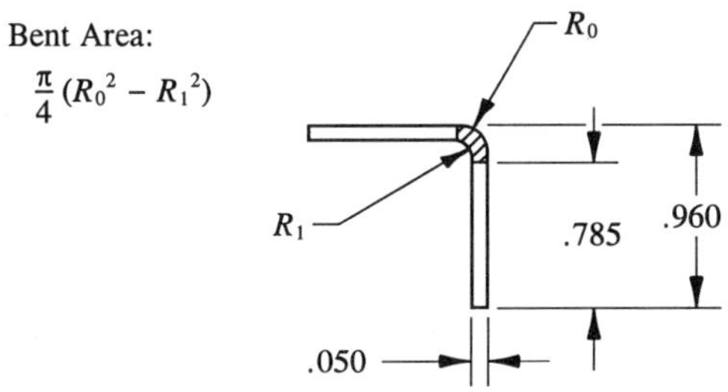

FIGURE 7-21 Formed sheet metal angle (bent area shown cross-hatched).

The appropriate column totals are then substituted into Eq. 6-17 to find the weighted-average allowable crippling stress.

$$F_{cc} = \frac{\Sigma(F_{cc}A)}{\Sigma A} = \frac{11,018}{.485} = 22,718 \text{ psi.}$$

Effective Sheet Area Calculations:

The following equations are used to calculate the effective sheet area of the web:

$W_e = 1.7t\sqrt{E_c/F_c}$ (from Eq. 6-6 as it applies to sheet-stiffened, built-up column sections)

$W_f = .62t\sqrt{E_c/F_c}$ (from Eq. 6-7 as it applies to sheet-stiffened, built-up column sections).

Let us simplify our computations of effective sheet area by using the allowable crippling stress F_{cc} instead of the critical column stress F_c in the solution of these equations. Thus avoiding the more complex iterative procedure normally required for the solution of sheet-stiffened, built-up column sections. Substituting $F_{cc} = 22,718$ psi (from above) and all other known values for the web structure in these equations gives:

$$W_e = 1.7t\sqrt{E_c/F_{cc}} = 1.7(.050)\sqrt{\frac{10.7 \text{ x } 10^6}{22,718}} = 1.845 \text{ in}$$

$$\tfrac{1}{2}W_e = \tfrac{1}{2}(1.845) = .922 \text{ in}$$

and

$$W_f = .62t\sqrt{E_c/F_{cc}} = .62(.050)\sqrt{\frac{10.7 \text{ x } 10^6}{22,718}} = .673 \text{ in}$$

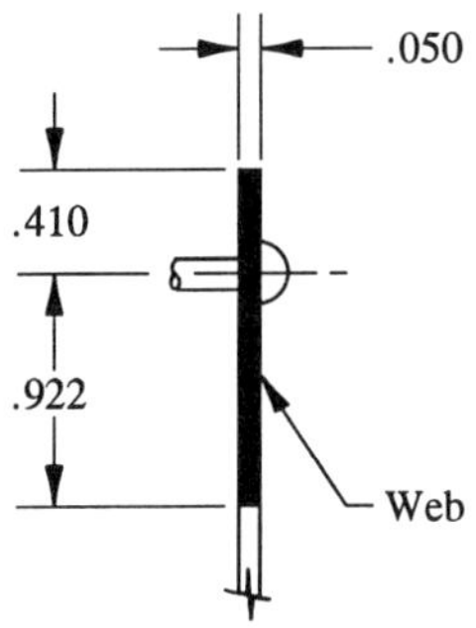

FIGURE 7-22 Effective sheet area of web.

where: t = .050 in (web thickness)
$E_c = 10.7 \times 10^6$ psi
$F_{cc} = 22{,}718$ psi.

Instead of basing failure on the critical column stress F_c, the compression strength of the web is now based on the crippling strength F_{cc} of the upper cap. The effective sheet area of the web is shown shaded in Fig. 7-22.

Johnson-Euler Column:

The next step in the solution of this problem is to calculate the moment of inertia of the upper spar cap about its failure or bending axis. This is tabulated in Table 7-3. With a vertical axis of symmetry, column failure occurs about a vertical axis of bending. This axis is shown in Fig. 7-23.

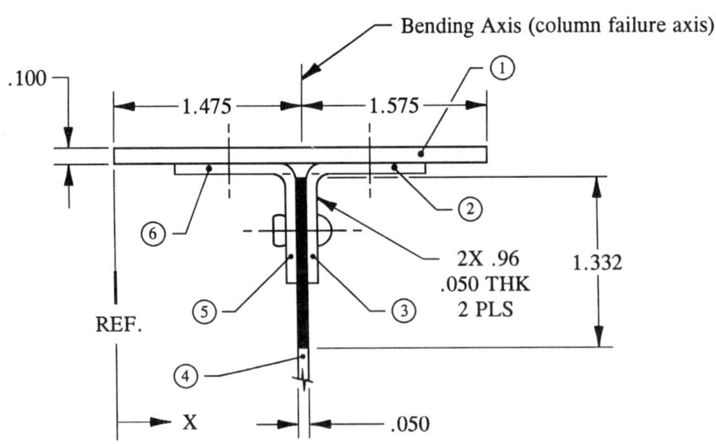

FIGURE 7-23 Upper spar cap is partitioned into rectangular element areas.

TABLE 7-3 MOMENT OF INERTIA CALCULATION

Element	b	h	x	A*	Ax	Ax^2	I_o
1	0.100	3.050	1.525	0.305	0.465	0.709	0.236
2	0.050	0.960	1.980	0.048	0.095	0.188	0.004
3	0.910	0.050	1.525	0.045	0.069	0.106	0.000
4	1.332	0.050	1.475	0.067	0.098	0.145	0.000
5	0.910	0.050	1.425	0.045	0.065	0.092	0.000
6	0.050	0.960	0.970	0.048	0.047	0.045	0.004
			Total	0.558	0.839	1.285	0.244

* Rectangular element areas are used for all member areas of the spar cap considered for the computation of moment of inertia.

$$X_{cg} = \frac{\Sigma\, Ax}{\Sigma\, A} = \frac{.839}{.558} = 1.504 \text{ in}$$

$$I_{cg} = I_y = \Sigma\, I_o + \Sigma\, Ax^2 - X_{cg}\,(\Sigma\, Ax)$$
$$I_{cg} = I_y = .244 + 1.285 - 1.504(.839) = .267 \text{ in}^4.$$

An end-fixity coefficient of 2.0 may be a rather high value to consider for such an important structural member, not to mention the uncertainties and manufacturing accidentals that are sometimes prevalent in such designs. Substituting all known values into the expression for F_c (indicated below) gives:

$$F_c = F_{cc} - \frac{F_{cc}^2\,(L'/\rho)^2}{4\pi^2 E_c}$$

$$= 22,718 - \frac{(22,718)^2\left[\dfrac{16.263}{.692}\right]^2}{4\pi^2\,(10.7 \text{ x } 10^6)}$$

$$F_c = 22,718 - 675 = 22,043 \text{ psi}$$

where: $F_{cc} = 22,718$ psi (from Table 7-2, see also page 463)
$E_c = 10.7 \text{ x } 10^6$ psi (given)
$L = 23.0$ in (unsupported length of column, see Fig. 7-18)
$L' = L/\sqrt{c} = 23.0/\sqrt{2} = 16.263$ in
$\rho = \sqrt{I/A} = (.267/.558)^{1/2} = .692$ in
$I = .267 \text{ in}^4$
$A = .558 \text{ in}^2$
$c = 2.0$ (given).

From Eq. 7-10, we obtain the allowable column load of the upper spar cap as follows:

$$P_c = F_c A = 22,043(.558) = 12,300 \text{ lb}$$

where: $F_c = 22,043$ psi (allowable column stress)
$A = .558 \text{ in}^2$ (effective area of the upper spar cap, see Table 7-3).

From Eq. A-7, Appendix B, the compression load of the upper spar cap is determined by replacing the moment M by an equivalent couple-force acting between the cap centroids of the main spar cross-sectional area. Hence, in the example considered this gives:

$$P_{\text{couple}} = \frac{M}{H} = \frac{79,665}{6.50} = 12,256 \text{ lb ultimate}$$

where: $M = 79,665$ in-lb ultimate (maximum bending moment given in this example problem, see page 461)
$H = 6.50$ in (distance between cap centroids, see Fig. 7-19).

Substituting the appropriate values into the margin of safety expression for column failure gives:

$$\text{Margin of Safety} = \text{M.S.} = \frac{P_c}{P_{\text{couple}}} - 1 = \frac{12,300}{12,256} - 1 = +.00$$

where: $P_{\text{couple}} = 12,256$ lb (upper spar cap column load)
$P_c = 12,300$ lb (allowable column load, see calculation this page).

This particular problem was taken from the actual test structure of an existing aircraft. The aircraft was structurally tested and was found to have prematurely buckled the main wing spar—column failure of the upper spar cap was observed. The total vertical wing shear at failure, as determined by strain-gauge measurements (indicated by the final reading on a load-cell indicator), was verified. The results of that test were published and will now serve as a basis for the solution of Example 7-3 which follows.

Example 7-3 During the Model 100 wing up-bending structural test, the main wing upper spar cap, analyzed as a column member in Example 7-2, failed at 147% of limit load. A whiffle-tree arrangement was used to load the wing structure to ultimate load, as shown in Fig. 7-24. The following hardware was used for the test apparatus of this structural test: (1) a load-cell indicator to monitor wing loads during structural testing, (2) wing cradles to apply torque to the wing structure, (3) fuselage straps and the nose landing-gear structure to react wing loads, and (4) a

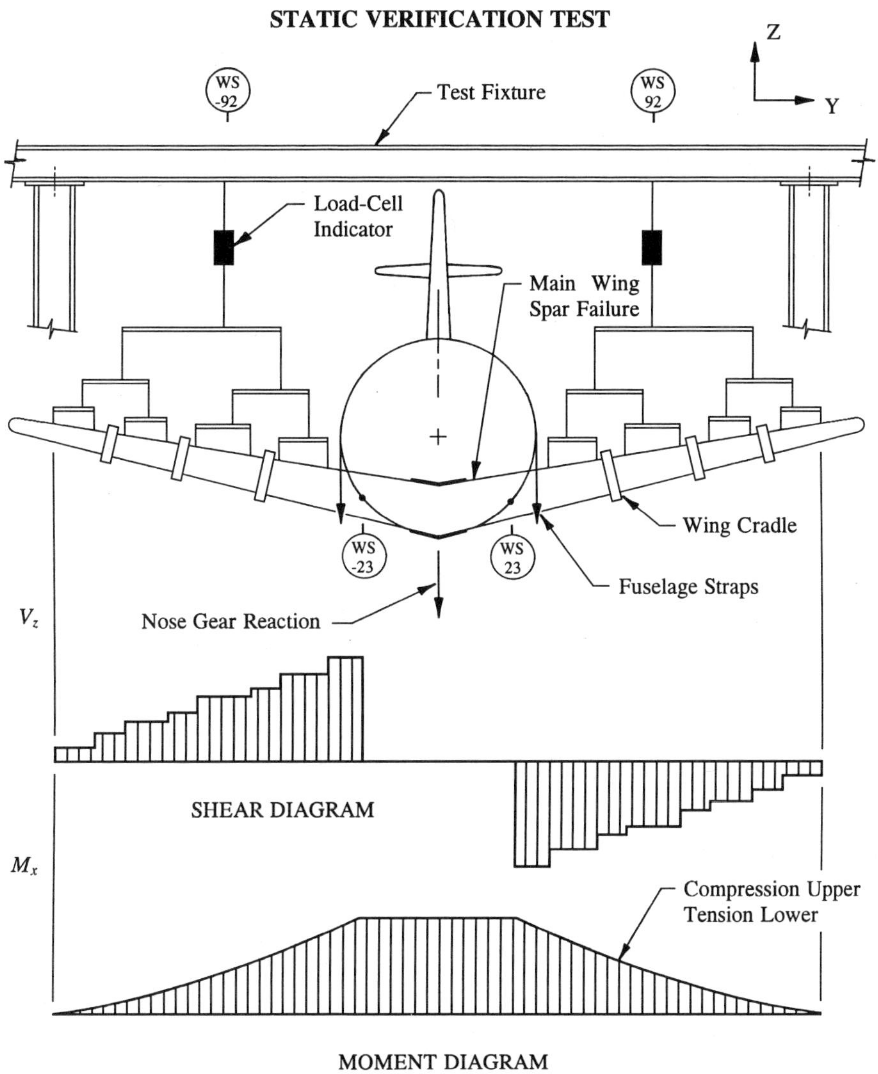

FIGURE 7-24 Wing up-bending structural test.

test fixture to support applied and reactive test loads. The load-cell indicator read a vertical wing shear of 1,136 lb at the time of failure. If the wing spar had been properly analyzed, why then did this member fail prematurely before reaching its ultimate design bending moment of 79,665 in-lb ultimate (this value corresponds to the maximum bending moment at the wing root in Example 7-2, p. 461)? Was the assumption predicted for the end-fixity coefficient $c = 2.0$ realistic for the column end-conditions of the upper spar cap? Or was the assumption actually "too high" for safe and practical column design? And if it was, could this condition or oversight have caused the reduction in structural integrity of the basic column structure that could have lead to or initiated the premature failure of this member? These questions will be subsequently answered in the following solution to this example problem.

SOLUTION: Before solving this example, let us make some general observations and practical considerations from which to establish some basic guidelines to determine the support end-conditions of a column structure. Theoretically, a pinned-ended column, $c = 1.0$, and a fixed-ended column, $c = 4.0$, do rarely occur in these idealized forms in an actual structure, the true end-conditions of a column are generally too complex to be so precisely defined or perceived as to be able to label or specify their behavior exactly as one or the other of these support kinds. The uncertainties and unknowns which are prevalent in most column designs generally preclude an accurate determination of these supported members. Although we study pinned-ended columns and fixed-ended columns as standard supports, rarely, if ever, do these types actually occur as we (like to) perceive them in actual structure.

In real structure, end-conditions are usually "intermediate," that is, they physically behave and characterize certain elements and aspects of both standard support types. When intermediate support types are suspected in an actual column structure, and no form of structural testing has been performed to verify their end-conditions, the engineer must consider in these cases some alternative judgment or evaluation of the column supports to substantiate the true column behavior.

One such approach, based to a certain extent on theoretical observations, assumes that the end-conditions of the column are pinned-ended. A pinned-ended column is said to provide no bending resistance at its supported ends. Such conservatism is essential where column end-conditions have not been substantiated by structural test. A general feeling of confidence generally prevails if intermediate support types are approached carefully and on a logical basis. This deliberate attempt to find a plausible and acceptable column solution is founded on the basic premise that the end-conditions of the questionable column member are "pinned-ended."

This approach is fundamental to basic column design. And its application, even though it would seem on the surface to lack good judgment, should not pose unnecessary conservatism on the column structure as a whole. This reasoning is true because in the short-column range of stresses most of the benefit derived by fixing the column ends has essentially been eliminated. Since most columns are of the short-column type, this conservatism is of negligible importance and impact on conventional column designs. Mathematically, this means that the critical column stress F_c is only slightly affected by the end-conditions of the column in the short-column range. Thus, satisfactory column design is assured by strict adherence to this basic design assumption.

Before we contemplate reinforcing or beefing up the failed column structure of Example 7-2, let us first determine the true end-fixity coefficient of the upper spar cap. If the load-cell indicator (at 147% limit load) read 1,136 lb at failure, the bending moment at the wing root would correspond to

$$M = 1,136(92 - 23) = 78,384 \text{ in-lb}.$$

Since this moment represents the column structure at failure, its value will also correspond to the critical column stress or allowable F_c of the upper spar cap. To arrive at this value, substitute the values of M (from above) and H (from Example 7-2) into the couple-force relationship for moments.

$$P_{\text{couple}} = \frac{M}{H} = \frac{78,384}{6.50} = 12,059 \text{ lb}.$$

The critical column stress is then found by dividing this allowable value by the effective column area.

$$F_c = \frac{P_{\text{couple}}}{A} = \frac{12,059}{.558} = 21,611 \text{ psi}$$

where: $P_{\text{couple}} = 12,059$ lb
$A = .558 \text{ in}^2$ (this value was computed in Table 7-3).

To determine why the wing spar failed before reaching its ultimate design load may be revealed by looking at the true end-fixity coefficient of the member. Its true value may give us some insight into whether the column was analyzed correctly or not; that is, whether the end-conditions of the column were correctly assumed in Example 7-2. The true end-fixity coefficient of the upper spar cap is determined at column failure, and is found by substituting all known values of the basic column section used in Example 7-2 into the Johnson-Euler column equation and solving for c. For easy reference, these values are again listed below following the computation of this quantity.

$$F_c = F_{cc} - \frac{F_{cc}^2\left[\dfrac{L}{\rho\sqrt{c}}\right]^2}{4\pi^2 E_c} \quad \text{(refer to Eq. 7-8 on page 456)}$$

$$21,611 = 22,718 - \frac{(22,718)^2\left[\dfrac{23.0}{.692\sqrt{c}}\right]^2}{4\pi^2(10.7 \text{ x } 10^6)}$$

$$-1,107 = -\frac{1,350}{c}$$

$$c = 1.22 \text{ (true end-fixity coefficient of the upper spar cap)}$$

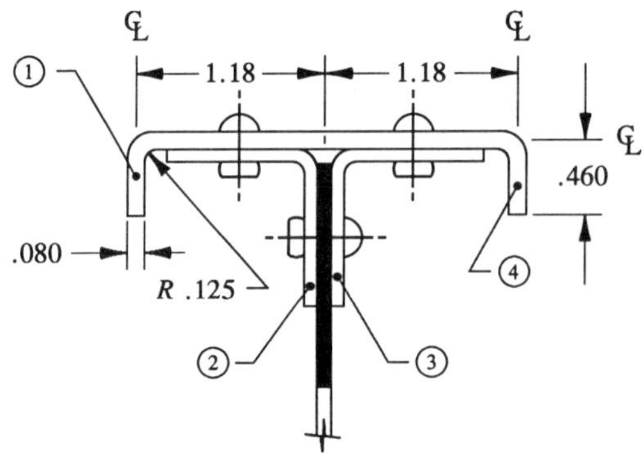

FIGURE 7-25 Upper spar cap redesigned and partitioned into angle element areas.

where: F_{cc} = 22,718 psi
E_c = 10.7 x 10^6 psi
L = 23.0 in
$\rho = \sqrt{I/A} = (.267/.558)^{1/2} = .692$ in
I = .267 in^4
A = .558 in^2.

Since the true end-fixity coefficient of the spar cap differs (is actually lower) from the value assumed in our earlier computations of critical column stress, where c was equal to 2.0, the column strength should have been reduced to account for this conflicting variation or divergence of the column end-conditions. The influence of end-conditions on column behavior can be explained analytically, simply by substituting different values of end-fixity coefficients into the Johnson-Euler equation and observing the changes in allowable strength. Furthermore, since the spar cap was marginally designed (M.S. = + .00), this reduction in column strength must have led to the premature failure of the spar cap. To account for this deficiency now, the original strap design, Fig. 7-19, will be redesigned (hopefully, more efficiently this time).

By taking full advantage of the axis of symmetry about which bending occurs for the upper spar cap; that is, from the knowledge that most efficient sections locate their material as far as possible from the neutral axis of the section area, the original strap design (a plate member) is modified slightly using return flanges, as shown by the structure of Fig. 7-25. This new strap design produces a section with the greatest moment of inertia and thus the stiffest section possible to prevent column instability. An excellent design choice, the reduction in weight and cost-savings of the new design can be realized without major modifications or reductions in column strength to the existing structure. This alternative strap design should not be construed to otherwise exhaust all alternative redesign choices possible for this structure. However, our proposal is by far the most effective way of correcting the structural flaw or deficiency of the spar cap. And, if this proposal is carefully incorporated into the basic column structure, the new strap design can have some extended benefits not realized by the former strap design.

Allowable crippling stress computations for the new strap design are again performed by the tabulation method of Sec. 6.4, Table 6-4. These computations are shown in Table 7-4. Since the same material is used for this new design as was used for the original spar cap (Example 7-2), the former values for this section are again appropriate to use here in the computations of crippling stress for our new column design. These values are indicated as follows: E_c = 10.7 x 10^6 psi, F_{cy} = 36,000 psi (THK = .010 - .062), and F_{cy} = 37,000 psi (THK = .063 - .128). (Refer to the mechanical-property tables in MIL-HDBK-5F for clad 2024-T3 aluminum alloy material.)

$$F_{cc} = \frac{C_e \sqrt{F_{cy} E_c}}{(b'/t)^{3/4}} \qquad \text{where: } b'/t = \frac{b_1 + b_2}{t_1 + t_2}.$$

TABLE 7-4 CRIPPLING CALCULATIONS

Element	b'/t (Fig. 6-27)	C_e (Table 6-3)	F_{cc} (Eq. 6-16)	A*	$F_{cc}A$
1	10.2	0.317†	34,946	0.126	4,403
2	18.7	0.295	20,360	0.090	1,832
3	18.7	0.295	20,360	0.090	1,832
4	10.2	0.317†	34,946	0.126	4,403
			Total	0.432	12,470

* The areas of elements 1, 2, 3, and 4 in this table are calculated as follows (also refer to Fig. 7-26 for the specific formula used to compute the bent areas of these members):

$$A_2 = A_3 = .785(.050) + .785(.050) + \frac{\pi}{4}[(.175)^2 - (.125)^2]$$
$$A_2 = A_3 = .039 + .039 + .012 = .090 \text{ in}^2$$

$$A_1 = A_4 = .295(.080) + 1.015(.080) + \frac{\pi}{4}[(.205)^2 - (.125)^2]$$
$$A_1 = A_4 = .024 + .081 + .021 = .126 \text{ in}^2.$$

† Assumes the effectivity of the return flanges.

The appropriate column totals are then substituted into Eq. 6-17 to find the weighted-average allowable crippling stress.

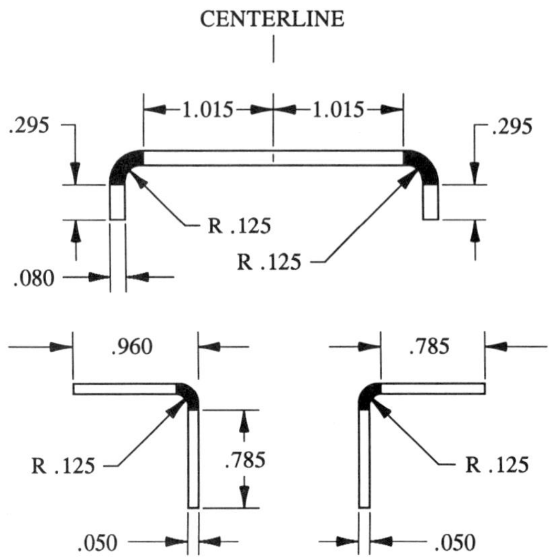

Bent Area = $\frac{\pi}{4}(R_0^2 - R_1^2)$, refer to the shaded areas above.

FIGURE 7-26 Upper spar cap is separated into three element areas. Bent areas are shown shaded.

$$F_{cc} = \frac{\Sigma(F_{cc}A)}{\Sigma A} = \frac{12,470}{.432} = 28,866 \text{ psi}.$$

Effective Sheet Area Calculations:

The following equations are used to calculate the effective sheet area of the web:

$W_e = 1.7t\sqrt{E_c/F_c}$ (from Eq. 6-6 as it applies to sheet-stiffened, built-up column sections)

$W_f = .62t\sqrt{E_c/F_c}$ (from Eq. 6-7 as it applies to sheet-stiffened, built-up column sections).

Let us simplify our computations of effective sheet area here by using the allowable crippling stress F_{cc} instead of the critical column stress F_c in the solution of these equations. Thus the iterative procedure normally required for the solution of sheet-stiffened, built-up column sections will be avoided. Substituting $F_{cc} = 28,866$ psi (from above) and all other known values for the web structure in these equations gives:

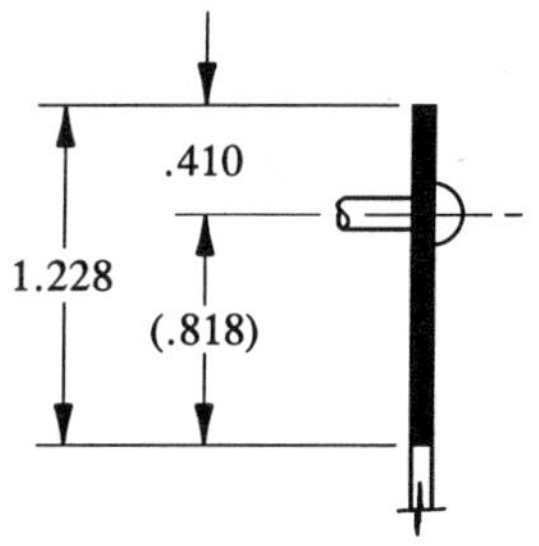

FIGURE 7-27 Effective sheet area of web.

$$W_e = 1.7t\sqrt{E_c/F_{cc}} = 1.7(.050)\sqrt{\frac{10.7 \text{ x } 10^6}{28,866}} = 1.637 \text{ in}$$

$$\tfrac{1}{2}W_e = \tfrac{1}{2}(1.637) = .818 \text{ in}$$

and

$$W_f = .62t\sqrt{E_c/F_{cc}} = .62(.050)\sqrt{\frac{10.7 \text{ x } 10^6}{28,866}} = .597 \text{ in}$$

where: $t = .050$ in (web thickness)
$E_c = 10.7 \text{ x } 10^6$ psi (given)
$F_{cc} = 28,866$ psi.

Instead of basing failure on the critical column stress F_c, the compression strength of the web is now based on the crippling strength F_{cc} of the upper cap. The effective sheet area of the web is shown shaded in Fig. 7-27.

TABLE 7-5 MOMENT OF INERTIA CALCULATION (see Fig. 7-28)

Element	b	h	x	A*	Ax	Ax^2	I_o
1	0.420	0.080	0.040	0.034	0.001	0.000	0.000
2	0.080	2.440	1.220	0.195	0.238	0.291	0.097
3	0.050	0.960	0.715	0.048	0.034	0.025	0.004
4	0.910	0.050	1.170	0.045	0.053	0.062	0.000
5	1.228	0.050	1.220	0.061	0.075	0.091	0.000
6	0.910	0.050	1.270	0.045	0.058	0.073	0.000
7	0.050	0.960	1.725	0.048	0.083	0.143	0.004
8	0.420	0.080	2.400	0.034	0.081	0.194	0.000
			Total	0.510	0.623	0.879	0.105

* Rectangular element areas are used for all member areas of the new strap design considered for the computation of moment of inertia.

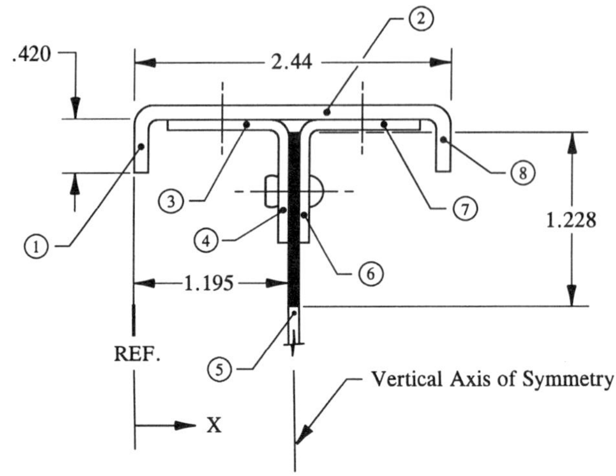

FIGURE 7-28 For this section, column failure occurs about the vertical axis of symmetry of the column.

$$X_{cg} = \frac{\Sigma Ax}{\Sigma A} = \frac{.623}{.510} = 1.222 \text{ in}$$

$$I_y = \Sigma I_o + \Sigma Ax^2 - X_{cg}(\Sigma Ax) = .105 + .879 - 1.222(.623) = .223 \text{ in}^4.$$

Johnson-Euler Column:

Before we can solve for the critical column stress in the Johnson-Euler equation, the moment of inertia of the new proposed upper spar cap about its failure or bending axis must first be calculated. This is tabulated as shown in Table 7-5. Column failure occurs again about the vertical axis of symmetry of the column section. This axis is shown in Fig. 7-28.

The true end-fixity coefficient of the spar cap is used in the column analysis of the new strap design. No better proof of structural performance and reliability of a member can be made than through actual structural testing. Therefore, since the true end-fixity coefficient of the spar cap is known, it would be of no practical benefit to assume a pinned-ended column for this member. Hence, substituting all known values into the general expression for F_c (shown below) gives:

$$F_c = F_{cc} - \frac{F_{cc}^2\left[\dfrac{L}{\rho\sqrt{c}}\right]^2}{4\pi^2 E_c}$$

$$= 28,866 - \frac{(28,866)^2 \left[\dfrac{23.0}{.661\sqrt{1.22}} \right]^2}{4\pi^2 (10.7 \times 10^6)}$$

$$F_c = 28,866 - 1,958 = 26,908 \text{ psi}$$

where: $F_{cc} = 28,866$ psi
$E_c = 10.7 \times 10^6$ psi
$L = 23.0$ in
$\rho = \sqrt{I/A} = (.223/.510)^{1/2} = .661$ in
$I = .223 \text{ in}^4$
$A = .510 \text{ in}^2$
$c = 1.22$ (true end-fixity coefficient, see page 469).

From Eq. 7-10, we obtain the following allowable column load of the new strap design:

$$P_c = F_c A = 26,908(.510) = 13,723 \text{ lb}$$

where: $F_c = 26,908$ psi
$A = .510 \text{ in}^2$ (see Table 7-5).

From Eq. A-7, Appendix B, the compression load of the upper spar cap is determined by replacing the bending moment M by an equivalent couple-force acting between the cap centroids of the main spar cross-sectional area. Hence, in the example considered this gives:

$$P_{\text{couple}} = \frac{M}{H} = \frac{79,665}{6.5} = 12,256 \text{ lb ultimate}$$

where $H \approx 6.5$ (to simplify our solution, let us assume that the distance between cap centroids of the main spar cross-sectional area remains the same for the new strap design).

Predicted Column Failure:

$$\text{Margin of Safety} = \text{M.S.} = \frac{P_c}{P_{\text{couple}}} - 1 = \frac{13,723}{12,256} - 1 = +.12.$$

Let us now compare the original flat strap design (Example 7-2) with that of the redesigned strap design (this example) as far as weight and strength considerations of these members are concerned. Critical column stresses and effective column areas are required to make these comparisons. These values are summarized in the following table:

Member	Cap Area A, in^2	Allowable Column Load P_c, lb	Ref.
Original Strap	.558	12,059	(see Table 7-3, p. 465)
Redesigned Strap	.510	13,723	(see Table 7-5, p. 473)

Strength Comparison:

$$\% \text{ Change in load} = \frac{13,723 - 12,059}{12,059}(100) = 13.8\% \text{ stronger}.$$

Weight Comparison:

$$\% \text{ Change in area} = \frac{.558 - .510}{.558}(100) = 8.6\% \text{ lighter}.$$

To summarize our findings: The redesigned strap was 8.6% lighter and yet its allowable column strength was 13.8% stronger than the original flat strap design. Clearly, by using return flanges, the compression allowables, crippling as well as column stresses, improved while the new strap design also saved weight. When one considers the above arguments (the uncertainties and accidentals of column design), failure in such cases can be prevented by assuming some conservatism of their designs; that is, when in doubt, or in the absence of reliable test data, assume the column pinned-ended. And in the future, other premature failures may be prevented.

7.6 Problem for Solution. (a) Using the column test results of Example 7-3 and the cross-sectional area of Fig. 7-25, determine the benefits that would be derived by fixing the column ends of the upper spar cap. (*Hint:* Compare the critical column allowables and the required thicknesses for optimum strap design for each column end-condition.) (b) Make a strength and weight comparison of your results. (c) Repeat parts (a) and (b) for a pinned-ended column.

CHAPTER 8

Shear-Resistant Beams

8.1 Introduction. In this chapter, the methods and principles of structural analysis of "shear-resistant" beams are studied. Their designs are particularly common to riveted structural panels (thin sheet or plate aircraft members) where stability is of prime importance to the reliability and structural integrity of the aircraft. For example, the front, rear, and main spar webs of an aircraft wing, the outer covering of the fuselage and wing surfaces, pressure bulkheads, and various rib type of structures, just to name a few, all represent flat or curved panels that must meet prescribed buckling requirements of the aircraft structure. These structural types are illustrated in Fig. 8-1.

A beam is referred to as being "shear-resistant" if the "web" portion of its structure is stable, i.e., not buckled, at a certain specified loading. For most structures, this loading is designated at limit or at some percentage less than limit load, rarely are these webs designed to be shear-resistant above limit load values. Above limit load, the resulting weight penalty from a shear-resistant web would generally prohibit their use in real aircraft structure. Aerodynamic effects due to surface aberrations caused by a buckled panel on the outer covering of the wing or fuselage skin can to a certain degree reduce the performance characteristics of an aircraft, missile, or, for that matter, any smooth-surface vehicle structure. To avoid this occurrence, and thus presume a less costly, more effective type of structure, the external surfaces of the wing and fuselage are made shear-resistant at normal

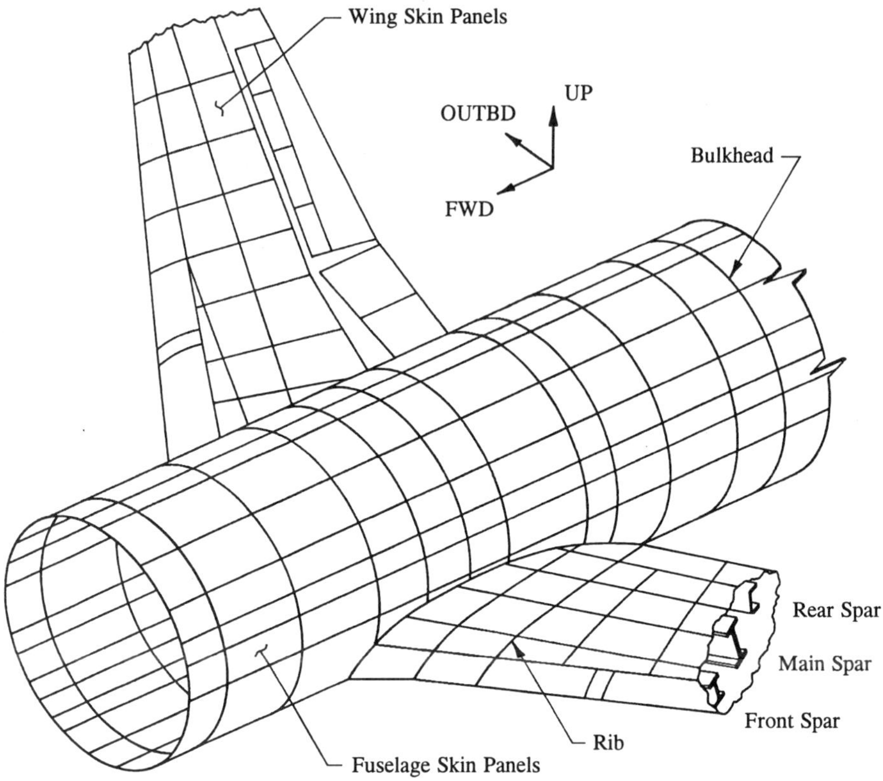

FIGURE 8-1 Aircraft structure showing various structural members.

operating loads (limit loads). Although shear-resistant structures, in general, are not weight-efficient compared to structural members with buckled webs or panels, their usefulness and practical importance to aircraft structures are still indispensable. The degree of resistance to buckling is of course a function of the particular design requirements for each specific design problem.

It is therefore the main intent and purpose of this chapter to examine these and other similar loading configurations as they relate specifically to the structural design behavior of (1) shear-resistant, flat panel designs and (2) shear-resistant, curved panel designs. The standard methods of analysis predominantly used by the aerospace industry in the solution of shear-resistant plate or beam designs will be the preferred method of analysis. The structural approaches and limitations imposed in this chapter on their designs must be clearly understood if shear-resistant beams are to be fully comprehended and their designs incorporated in actual structure. Several example problems will be presented in this chapter to fully illustrate the proper and correct use of these methods of analysis.

For the most part, because shear-resistant beams must have relatively thick webs to actually prevent buckling, these members do not necessarily produce

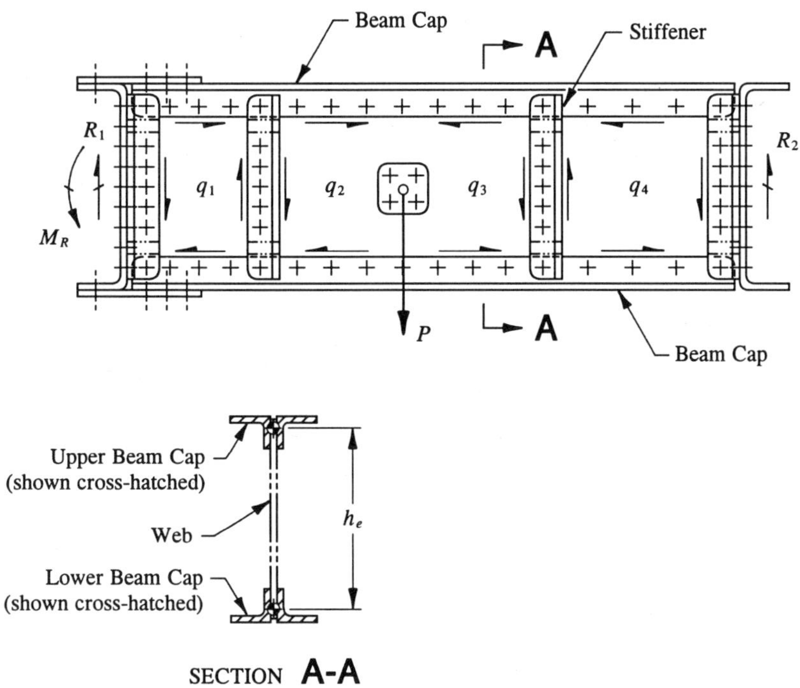

FIGURE 8-2 Panels formed by the boundary support structure of a deep beam.

highly weight-efficient structures. Without going into detail now, let us just say that the strength-to-weight ratio of nonbuckled webs (also commonly referred to as stable webs) makes their designs a poor alternative. Nevertheless, their importance to the safety and reliability of the structure as a whole does warrant special consideration in their proper applications—some of which are particularly significant, for example, to the general aesthetics of the aircraft. Since shear-resistant beams do not actually buckle under load, no outward evidence or appearance of deformity of their surfaces is visible (at least to the naked eye). Although panel buckling is not actually considered a structural failure, its avoidance in normal flight should make passengers somewhat at ease, certainly relieved, to know that such a condition will not presumably occur during actual flight.[1] Stability therefore plays an important role in the design of nonbuckled, shear-resistant beam and panel designs under normal flight and landing conditions. They are recommended in the following design applications: (1) integral fuel tanks where leaking along the boundaries of the structure must be prevented; (2) wing and fuselage skins where under normal flying and landing conditions these members must remain nonbuckled; and (3) wing and fuselage skin panels where visual inspection by passengers and well-

[1] Even while an aircraft is taxiing, landing, or completely stationary, no evidence of buckling of its wing or fuselage skin surfaces should be visible to pilots or boarding passengers.

trained professional pilots would certainly lessen the aesthetics of the aircraft, if not completely weaken the entire faith of these individuals in the structural performance and airworthiness of the aircraft in general, if this condition (premature buckling) were not totally avoided.

Figure 8-2 shows a typical deep beam structure with transverse web stiffeners, beam caps, and riveted web (sheet or plate) used to attach these members and the beam caps together. The panels, formed by these boundary members, are shear-resistant if, under the corresponding design shear flows indicated in this figure by the values q_1, q_2, q_3, and q_4, the panels remain unbuckled. The standard notation for internal panel shear flows is always drawn such that the vector shear flows are indicated head-to-head or tail-to-tail at the corners of the panels. Internal panel shear flows are determined from internal loads analysis using the equations of static equilibrium, or by drawing internal shearing forces opposing the reactions R_1 and R_2 and then completing the force picture by drawing the shear flows as described above: head-to-head and tail-to-tail. Internal panel shear flows are always drawn opposing applied or reactive loads. For this beam, this is shown by the shear flows q_1 and q_4 opposing the reactions R_1 and R_2, respectively, at the ends of the beam structure. From these values, the complete internal shear flows picture is drawn. The shear flows represent the load felt by the boundary structure of the beam from the attached web.

To determine the magnitude of the internal shear flows, let us first describe the average applied shearing stress of the beam.[1] Then, from basic definitions, the shear flow follows directly from Eq. 4-5 ($f_s = q/t$). The applied shearing stress f_s used in the design of shear-resistant webs is normally taken as the average shearing stress measured between cap centroids of the beam structure. For a beam having well-defined beam caps, this corresponds to the following equation:

$$f_s = \frac{V}{h_e t} \tag{8-1}$$

where: f_s = average applied shearing stress
V = applied web vertical shear[2]

---

[1] The buckling strength of a panel is best described by its average shearing stress. The maximum or peak value, as would be determined by Eq. 4-2, would be too conservative for practical engineering design. It should be recalled that in Sec. 4.2 we analyzed the capability of the web structure of a beam in terms of its ultimate strength capacity. Nothing at the time was mentioned regarding the stability of these members at limit load. In fact, it was assumed in that section that most beams were shear-resistant even at ultimate load. In general, if a structure is shear-resistant above limit load, the engineer should consider the structure "overweight" and begin to initiate potential weight reduction and cost-savings to correct the structural inefficiency.

[2] It will be shown in Sec. 8.6 that the beam caps of a tapered beam, e.g., spars of a conventional wing structure, can actually relieve the applied internal web shear that is carried by the web structure. This reduction in web shear should help realize some weight reduction and cost-savings where small negative margins of safety have occurred for panels that are slightly buckled. This relieving action of tapered beam structures should be considered for optimal web design.

t = web or panel thickness

h_e = effective depth of the beam measured between cap centroids (neglect the effective web area as shown in Fig. 8-2 when making this calculation).[1]

In terms of shear flow, if we substitute f_s from Eq. 4-5, $f_s = q/t$, into Eq. 8-1, we obtain:

$$\frac{q}{t} = \frac{V}{h_e t}$$

which then simplifies to the following expression for shear flow:

$$q = \frac{V}{h_e} \tag{8-2}$$

where these terms are the same as those previously defined above for Eq. 8-1.

Bulkhead webs, the webs of deep beams, wing and fuselage skin surfaces are just a few of the possible plate members that are normally investigated for buckling. For those members that are allowed to buckle below limit load, a lower limit cutoff for their designs is usually recommended. To a certain extent, every panel is designed to be shear-resistant at some prescribed value. For example, to prevent fatigue-related problems of a structure, a structural panel may be designed not to buckle, say, below 70% limit load. Some other criterion or special condition may even limit buckling to lower values. The engineer must use his discretion based on past experience or company policy to establish the particular criterion to use for each panel design. To arrive at a safe and reliable aircraft structure, some limiting value is usually prescribed for panel buckling, whether a panel of an aircraft wing or fuselage, whether the web of a deep beam, the possibility of buckling must be fully considered.

There are three standard buckling formulas which are particularly important to the design stability of thin, flat plate members. These formulas, based on theoretical observations, are derived from empirical test data of simple shear, compression, and bending tests. These loading conditions will be the basis for the solution of plates analyzed for shear resistance. Although these equations are formulated in terms of the inelastic stress behavior of the plate material, they can also be extended to the special case of elastic stability of plates. In addition, plate members subjected simultaneously to shear and compression, shear and bending, and compression and bending will also be fully investigated. These particular topics will be covered in Sec. 8.4 (see page 490, "Stability of Thin, Flat Plate Members in Compression, Shear, Bending, and Under Combined Loading Conditions").

Although a riveted structural panel made from sheet or plate material may be shear-resistant at some prescribed stress level, usually a value corresponding to

---

[1] For an integral I-beam, the value of h_e is measured between flange centroids.

limit load, these panel members must be further evaluated in their buckled states at ultimate load. The ultimate strength of thin, buckled flat plates will not however be covered in this book. The engineer is referred to an advanced textbook on this subject, specifically, "Semi-Diagonal Tension-Field Analysis," where thin web structural members are allowed to buckle at ultimate load.[1] The remainder of the chapter will focus on the stability of thin, curved sheets, Sec. 8.5, and the theory of tapered beam structures, discussed briefly in Sec. 8.6.

8.2 Edge-Support Conditions and Standard Loading Types of Flat Plate Members. The buckling strength of a flat plate may depend on several factors contributing to its satisfactory performance and design: (1) the type of loading which causes the plate to buckle, (2) the edge-support conditions at the edges of the plate, (3) the geometric properties of the plate, and (4) the material properties of the plate. These parameters are each a related system of variables which help to define the strength and stiffness characteristics of the plate. Each one contributes to a certain degree to the reliability and performance of the plate and its surrounding structure. To assure the true structural performance of the plate member, these variables must be correctly defined as they would actually be perceived in real structure. In most cases, however, such an appraisal of the structure is not so easily perceived or standardized, even by the most sagacious engineers. In fact, for most aircraft structures, the true physical behavior of an unknown support can only be accurately appraised through structural testing of the plate and its boundary structure under simulated loading conditions. For this reason, it is recommended that some degree of conservatism be achieved for their designs, which, by aircraft standards, would be necessary to satisfy and govern the reliability and structural integrity of the plate structure as a whole. Such conservatism can be resolved, however, if new designs can be correlated from existing plate structure, or perhaps by actually substantiating their designs by structural testing. Such evidence based on structural test data should then be sufficient to assume the true structural behavior of these members in actual structure.

Edge-Support Conditions

Two ideal conditions of support are considered in standard riveted plate construction. The edges of a plate are either assumed to be simply-supported or fixed-supported depending on the physical structure surrounding the plate and the method of attaching these members together. Such construction features are illustrated in Fig. 8-3. Note, particularly, the physical characteristics of each support and their effective panel depths.[2] Such distinctive properties are noted as follows: A fixed-supported edge is restrained from any rotational movement along its

---

[1] Kuhn, Peterson, Levin, "A Summary of Diagonal Tension," Part 1, "Methods of Analysis," *NACA TN 2661*, Part 2, "Experimental Evidence," *NACA TN 2662*.

[2] A welded aircraft structural panel is assumed to have fixed-supported edges along its boundary structure.

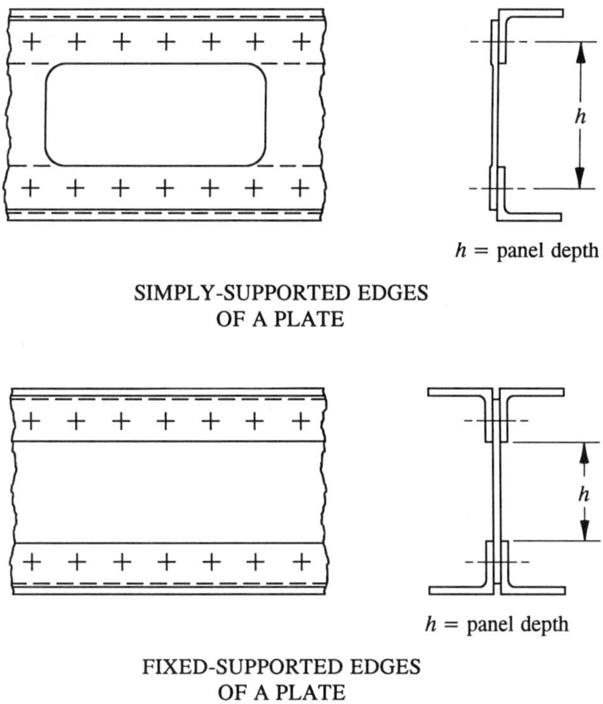

FIGURE 8-3 Edge-support conditions for standard riveted plate construction.

boundaries. For this type of support, bending moments develop along the supported edges of the plate. In contrast to this, simply-supported edges are free to rotate about the centerline of the plate. Hence, no bending moments develop for this support. It can also be assumed that fixed- and simply-supported edges of a plate remain essentially straight throughout all stress levels of the loaded structure.

Most plate members of an aircraft structure, e.g., the panel sections of a wing or fuselage skin, the web of a built-up beam structure, are supported along their boundary edges by riveted structural members. Although a multitude of support types are physically possible, only two standard types are normally considered for the evaluation of plate designs. If the engineer chooses to consider these intermediate edge-support types for his designs, the degree of uncertainty of the edge-restraints must be structurally verified by static testing before their intermediate values are used to accurately define the boundaries of the plate structure for analysis. In most cases, without reliable test data to substantiate the plate edge-conditions, some degree of conservatism should be considered. That conservatism is usually arrived at by assuming the edges of the plate to be either simply-supported or fixed-supported, unless, of course, structural test data proves contrary to their assumed behavior. Then, the intermediate edge-support conditions of the tested structure should be used instead. This basic approach to the design of plate structures should prove satisfactory for most aircraft structural panels where the edge-support conditions are not known with great certainty.

To arrive at the true edge-conditions of the plate, those either correlated from tested structure or those assumed from engineering experience, the supported edges of the plate must be prevented from (1) inter-rivet buckling between rivets,[1] (2) shearing failure of the plate boundary rivets, and (3) bearing failure of the riveted plate and attached boundary structures.[2]

The edge-conditions of a plate can influence strength and stiffness of a plate member considerably. The supported edges of a plate depend on the stiffness of the supporting structure to which the plate member is attached. A simply-supported edge is free to rotate or pivot about the centerline of the supported edges of the plate. The rotational restraint of this support is zero. On the other hand, a fixed-supported edge physically restrains the edges; hence, this support will develop a bending moment (or fixed-end moment) along its supported edges. Although intermediate support types can also physically occur for plate members, these support types are usually verified from structural test data. Independent investigations are usually recommended to establish the true structural behavior for these support types. Some conservatism is usually recommended and necessary if reliability of designed plate members is to be assured. Without reliable test data to substantiate one's assumptions, perceptions, and judgments, the engineer should approach the problem by assuming the edge-support conditions of the supported plate member to be pinned (i.e., simply-supported). In most cases, this assumption should prove conservative, unless, of course, the plate was actually unsupported on one side. In that event, the plate would act more like a flange of a structural shape than a flat plate member, and therefore, if compressed, its structural behavior would instead be analyzed for crippling failure (analysis details are provided in Sec. 6.4). Fortunately, most plate members are generally supported on all edges by a boundary structure. For questionable or unknown supported plate edges, the assumption of simply-supported edges should however prove more than satisfactory, at least, until the supported edges of the plate can be confirmed—structurally proved or verified by test.

Standard Plate-Loading Types

The outer skin covering of a wing and fuselage are examples of thin, buckled members subjected to aerodynamic forces on their surfaces that can produce a multitude of different loading combinations in the plane of their surfaces. Although a complex system of combined loads can occur for shear-resistant plate or beam designs, only three standard types are normally considered: (1) when

[1] It is usually better to be on the conservative side when analyzing a riveted plate member than to risk premature failure of the plate (or surrounding support structure) by unnecessarily weakening the plate due to this undesirable condition.

[2] The proper size and spacing requirements of rivets must be designed in accordance with prescribed methods of analysis to prevent shearing and bearing failures. These failure checks were specifically described in Sec. 3.2.

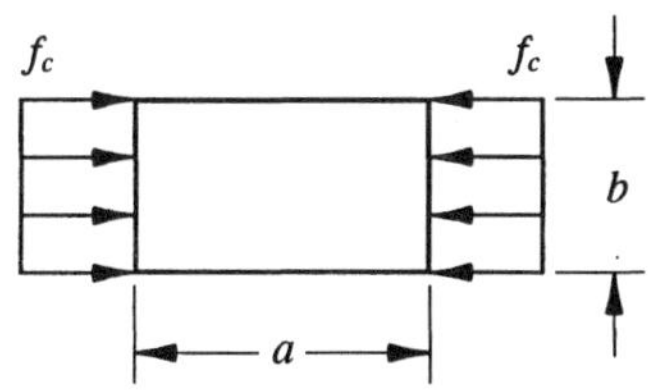

(a) Plate loaded in pure compression.

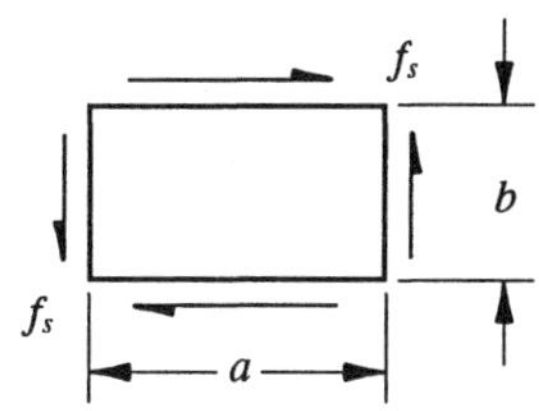

(b) Plate loaded in pure shear.

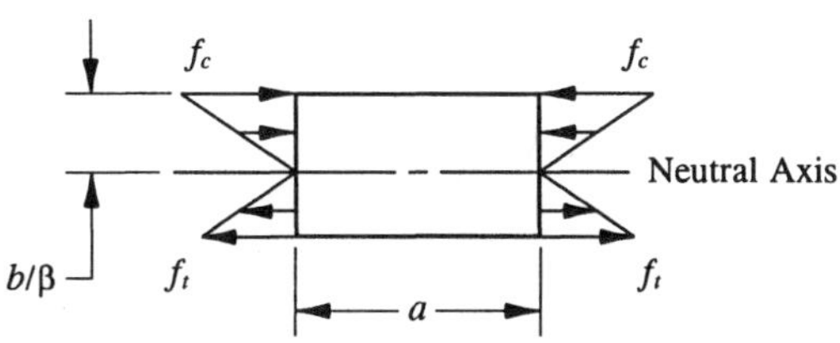

(c) Plate loaded in pure bending.

FIGURE 8-4 Standard loading conditions for plates: (a) in pure compression, (b) in pure shear, and (c) in pure bending.

opposite edges of a plate are stressed in compression, (2) when shear is uniformly distributed along the supported edges of the plate, and (3) when opposite edges of a plate are stressed in bending. Examples of these standard loading types are illustrated as shown in Fig. 8-4. These loading types will be investigated in detail in Sec. 8.4 using general buckling formulas developed from general plate theory of elasticity. From these standard types, other loading combinations are also possible, e.g., plate members simultaneously loaded in shear and compression, shear and bending, and compression and bending. The web of a bulkhead or rib, or web of a deep beam structure and others, are examples of thin plate members which can cause direct buckling of these members at critical loading combinations. Independent studies have evolved some simple, practical methods to use to solve these problems. Combined loading conditions will be solved indirectly using interaction equations for their solutions (see ahead to Table 8-3, page 519, for specific formulas). More about rectangular plate designs is presented in Sec. 8.4.

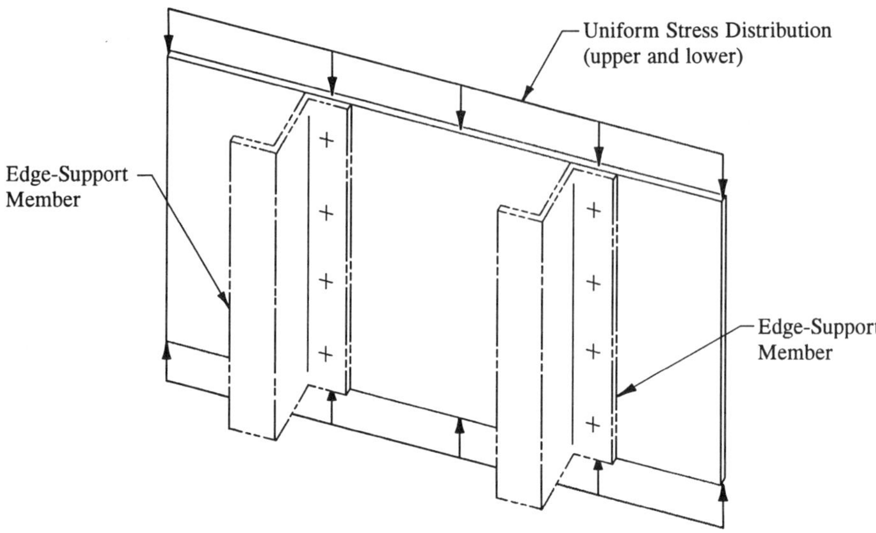

FIGURE 8-5 Compression-loaded flat plate.

8.3 Instability Behavior of Plate Members. Observe the compression-loaded rectangular, flat plate of Fig. 8-5. The plate is uniformly compressed at its ends and simply-supported along its (unloaded) edges by single rows of attachments. Such a member is, however, structurally inefficient as far as its ability to carry compression loads. This can be seen from the low allowable buckling stresses developed for flat plate members in compression compared to the higher buckling allowables of formed and extruded structural shapes (refer to Sec. 6.4, "Crippling of Built-up Sections in Compression"). Similar analogies can be made for buckling of a flat sheet or plate member in shear or bending.

In Sec. 8.4 it will be shown that flat sheets and plates are also weak in their ability to carry not only shear, compression, and bending but simple interaction combinations of shear and compression, shear and bending, and compression and bending. Regardless of which loading types occur, prior to buckling, the plate exhibits a uniform internal stress distribution of the magnitude indicated by the applied loading across the plate edges in Fig. 8-5. Essentially, simple strains occur in the material in the direction of the compression load applied.

Now assume that the plate is laterally unstable and buckles at the compression load indicated. The stress distribution across the width of the buckled plate is now as shown in Fig. 8-6. This distribution arises from the ability of the plate to sustain the compression load which caused the plate to buckle. The plate remains shear-resistant (nonbuckled) until the buckling stress of the plate has been reached. Then the plate undergoes distortion of its surfaces. However, total collapse of the plate structure does not (as yet) actually occur. The deflected shape of the plate is a temporary condition not to be confused with actual structural failure. This structural

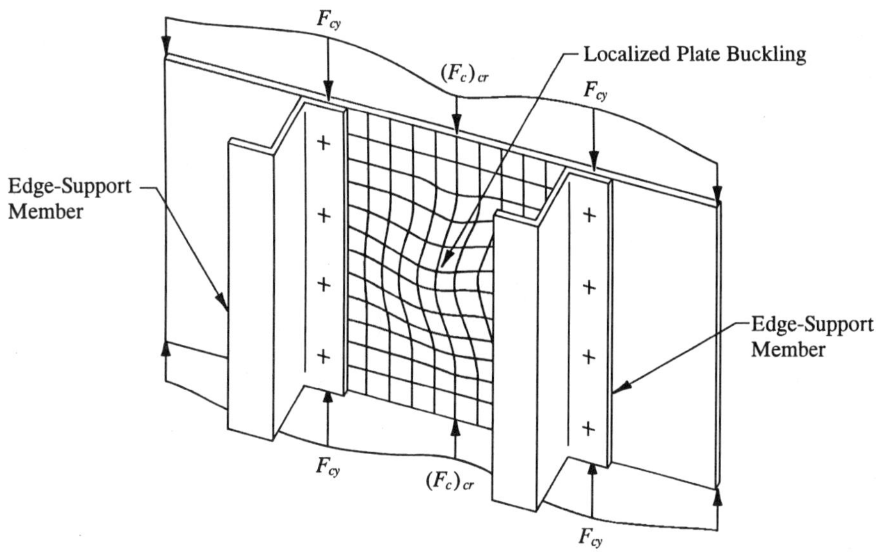

FIGURE 8-6 Compression stress distribution of a buckled plate.

phenomenon occurs because the supported edges of the plate have the additional inherent ability to carry more load than that which precipitated the plate to initially buckle. Structurally, this occurs because the edges of the plate are supported by riveted members, themselves inherently stiffer than the weaker middle portion of the plate structure. From this argument, one can deduce that the deflected shape of the plate may not actually indicate structural failure, but because of its supported edges, the plate has the unique ability to carry additional load: more load than that which caused the plate to initially buckle. One can generalize this behavior further by saying that the additional increase in load is shed (transferred) from the middle (weaker) portion of the plate to the undeflected, stiffer supported edges.[1] When the supported edges of the plate have yielded, the plate will then fail.

Most plate members of this kind are simply-supported by rivets attached along the boundaries of the plate structure. The stiffer supported sides provide additional support that the weaker middle portion of the plate cannot. Below the allowable compression buckling stress, the plate remains essentially undeflected (flat, shear-resistant). But then, as the load is increased, the member initially buckles at a value corresponding to the allowable compression buckling stress of the plate. At this time, the edges of the plate strain rapidly with increasing load, causing the rate of deflection in the direction of the load to be much greater during this

[1] Basically, this condition describes a redistribution of loads to more rigid members supporting the basic plate structure. The stiffness of the supporting structure (for example, a stiffener, a stringer, a bulkhead cap, or a frame cap) around the boundary of the supported plate can help to control the overall stability of the plate structure. Thus, the restraint capability of the plate is assured by providing relatively stiff boundary members for the overall plate design.

moment of deformation than before buckling occurred. And the simple stress-strain relationship which preceded buckling is no longer valid for the plate in this deflected shape. From this behavior, an obvious and logical design criterion for the buckling of plates can be drawn: that is, to determine a maximum compression load which a plate can sustain without initial buckling of its surfaces. This condition is commonly referred to as "shear-resistant beam design."

The boundary conditions of the plate, such as the supporting structure and attachment rivets, also play an exceedingly important role in shear-resistant beam design. This is as important, it can be said, as the plate structure itself to which these boundary members are attached. Unlike columns that fail suddenly, plates initially buckle first. Then, at higher loads, the plate undergoes excessive deflections, even inducing other loads (commonly referred to as secondary bending loads) into localized regions of the supporting structure. However, the member can still provide some ability to carry compression loads in its buckled state. In fact, at ultimate load, the web severely buckles, converting most of the applied shear loading into diagonal tension stresses.[1] Although shear-resistant beams produce no such secondary effects on the supporting structure, the efficiency or stiffness of the plate is also influenced by the rotational restraint of the supported plate edges. The restraint capability of these edges is structurally verifiable by observing the torsional weakness (or strength) of the supporting structure. The assumption of simply-supported edges for most aircraft plate structures should not be made haphazardly or carelessly. Sometimes this assumption is not conservative, which can lead to a low degree of correlation with existing design criteria of shear-resistant beam or plate designs.

In general, riveted supported edges of a plate can safely be assumed to be simply-supported if the plate is supported at the edges by riveted stiffeners. However, the stiffeners should not be torsionally weak under the applied system of loads. If simply-supported edges of a panel are stiffened by hat-section stiffeners, the assumption of simply-supported edges is valid. However, if open-section stiffeners are used to support the edges of the panel, the assumption of simply-supported edges may be too optimistic. This evaluative judgment for support edges of the plate structure is in part based on the torsional stiffness of the supporting structure. In Sec. 8.4, the supporting structure is optimized in terms of a minimum stiffener moment of inertia. To prevent torsional weakness of the supported edges of a simply-supported or fixed-supported panel, the panel is normally stiffened using closed-section stiffeners, as shown in Fig. 8-7. In this way, the assumption of simply-supported edges, not explicitly verified by analysis or test, can with some degree of certainty and confidence be safely assured, even though support conditions of a panel can only be reliably predicted through structural testing. Increasing the torsional stiffness of the plate edges will in theory help to increase the buckling

[1] The NACA carried on a comprehensive study and testing program to develop a method of analysis for engineers to use for their detailed solutions. The engineer is referred to an aerospace industry structures manual or to an advanced textbook on this subject. These beams, commonly referred to as "intermediate" diagonal tension-field beams, are not specifically covered in this book.

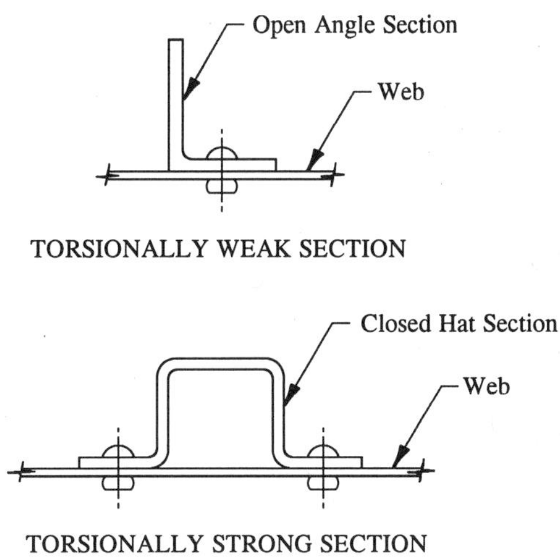

FIGURE 8-7 Torsional stiffness of the supported edges of a plate provided by: (a) an open angle section and (b) a closed hat section.

strength of the plate structure. It will therefore, exhibit a reasonable consistency in results obtained for the allowable buckling stress of the plate structure and safely guarantee all of the assumptions that went into its determination.

Now, let us look at the boundary rivets of a plate structure (wing or fuselage skin). In keeping with our general ideas and assumptions of simply-supported and fixed-supported edges, the plate material between rivets along the supported edges of the plate must preclude inter-rivet buckling at prescribed stress levels corresponding to the shear-resistant capability of the supported plate structure. To do this, a similar criterion as that which was adopted in Sec. 6.2 for riveted compression members is formulated here in this section for compression-loaded plate members. As a brief review of that topic: It was shown in that section that to prevent inter-rivet buckling of a riveted compression member, that member must satisfy the inequality $F_{ir} \geq F_{cc}$, where F_{ir} is the allowable inter-rivet buckling stress of the riveted material between rivets and F_{cc} is the allowable crippling stress of the compression member. In so doing, the damaging effects of premature inter-rivet buckling have been avoided. For plates, a similar expression can also be formulated. Here, to prevent premature inter-rivet buckling along the boundary rivets, and thus avoiding a reduction in plate bending stiffness, boundary members must satisfy the following inequality:

$$F_{ir} \geq (F_c)_{cr}$$

where: F_{ir} = allowable inter-rivet buckling stress of the riveted material between rivets (use Eq. 6-4, page 364, for this calculation)

$(F_c)_{cr}$ = critical compression buckling stress of the plate (its value will be determined by the methods of Sec. 8.4).

If this equation is not satisfied, and premature inter-rivet buckling does occur, such a condition can detrimentally influence plate behavior—causing the plate to buckle at a lower compression buckling stress than that which would presumably have occurred for a plate with standard supported edges along its boundary structure. Since no known method has been devised to date to account for this reduction in plate stiffness, all attempts should be made to avoid its occurrence in actual structure.[1]

8.4 Stability of Thin, Flat Plate Members in Compression, Shear, Bending, and Under Combined Loading Conditions. In this section, the equations of buckling of flat, rectangular plates subjected to compression, shear, and bending are presented. To account for a reduction in bending stiffness of these plates when critical buckling stresses exceed the proportional limit of the material, a plasticity correction factor η is incorporated. These equations are generalized to include the solutions of inelastic plate members by incorporating specific correction factors for their particular loading types. For example, simply by including this factor in Eqs. 8-4, 8-5, and 8-13 which follow in this section, plate buckling is generalized to include the solutions of inelastic plate members. These formulas, derived from empirical test data, provide valuable information for the solution of shear-resistant panel designs. Essentially they form the basis for the evaluation of inelastic or elastic stability of plate members. Specifically, these equations will be used to determine the solution of critical buckling stresses of these (standard loading types) and other critical plate-loading combinations, such as compression and shear, compression and bending, and shear and bending. Their combined solutions are arrived at through interaction equations used to determine the critical buckling stress of plate members. Only the stability requirements of shear-resistant, flat, thin plate members will be considered (analyzed) in this section. They are, for example, any thin structural member that is used as an outer covering, like the wing and fuselage skins of an aircraft; or the web of a deep beam, like the main spar web of an aircraft wing. Typically, these are examples of members that are investigated for sheet or plate buckling.

However, other design requirements (some of which have already been mentioned earlier in this section) will usually determine whether a particular shear panel should be designed to be shear-resistant or not. Shear-resistant design refers to any thin, nonbuckled, riveted structural panel, while intermediate diagonal-tension webs are thin buckled panels. In general, a diagonal-tension web or beam is preferred for its weight-efficient structure. However, several design factors, none of which may consider the lightest-weight structure, may influence or dictate the engineer's decision to use a particular web design criterion for panel design. The

[1] The structural deficiency caused by premature inter-rivet buckling of a riveted plate member in compression can only be verified by structural test.

engineer must carefully evaluate these factors according to their immediate and primary functions to the overall performance and reliability of the aircraft structure. No matter which criterion is chosen, the plate structure must still meet the expected requirements of its corresponding analytical solution in either its buckled or nonbuckled state. Although the outer skin covering of a wing and fuselage skin are not actually flat surfaces, if they are assumed to be flat, the analysis of these members should be conservative. Most curved panels of conventional aircraft structures are analyzed first by flat panel theory, then by curved panel theory if the analysis warrants a more detailed investigation. A curved sheet with a high radius of curvature is only slightly stiffer than a flat panel, and thus its stiffness is reflected by a slightly higher allowable buckling stress. The analysis of curved, thin plate members will be considered in Sec. 8-5, where stiffness of a curved sheet will be shown to be directly proportional to its radius of curvature.

Our solution of plate instability is further complicated by the fact that plate stresses can be inelastic (stresses which occur above the proportional limit of the material) even when a plate is designed to be shear-resistant at limit load. However, this added complication of their designs actually poses no real problem for the analyst. The engineer simply accounts for the inelastic behavior of these members by using published instability buckling curves for specific material types. Thus, the engineer will avoid having to "reinvent the wheel," so to speak, for each new material considered in his proposed plate designs.

A buckled sheet depends upon many factors, such as (1) the type of loading to which the panel is subjected to, (2) the size of the panel dimensions, (3) the design material, (4) the operating temperatures, and (5) the edge-support conditions of the plate edges. For this reason, it is critical to the structural integrity of the buckled member to determine the loads or stresses at which these structural members buckle. A member is shear-resistant if its surfaces are stable (undeflected) at loads up to the allowable buckling stress of the plate. Before presenting the critical buckling stress equations for the design of plates in compression, shear, and bending, let us determine the required stiffener moment of inertia to use with a shear-resistant panel.

Minimum Stiffener Moment of Inertia

The equations of plate buckling that are used to determine web or panel stability are not sufficient alone to adequately design a web or panel to be shear-resistant. Some consideration must be given to the boundary structure of the panel. For example, their primary functions are to prevent panel buckling by maintaining adequate panel size, to provide proper restraint capability of the supported edges, and to maintain overall web stability. A shear-resistant panel therefore assumes that the boundary structure is stiff enough to support the panel in an undeflected, nonbuckled state. For this reason, some regard to the required stiffness of transverse stiffeners in a web or bulkhead design and longitudinal stringers in a wing or fuselage design must be made to preclude premature panel buckling.

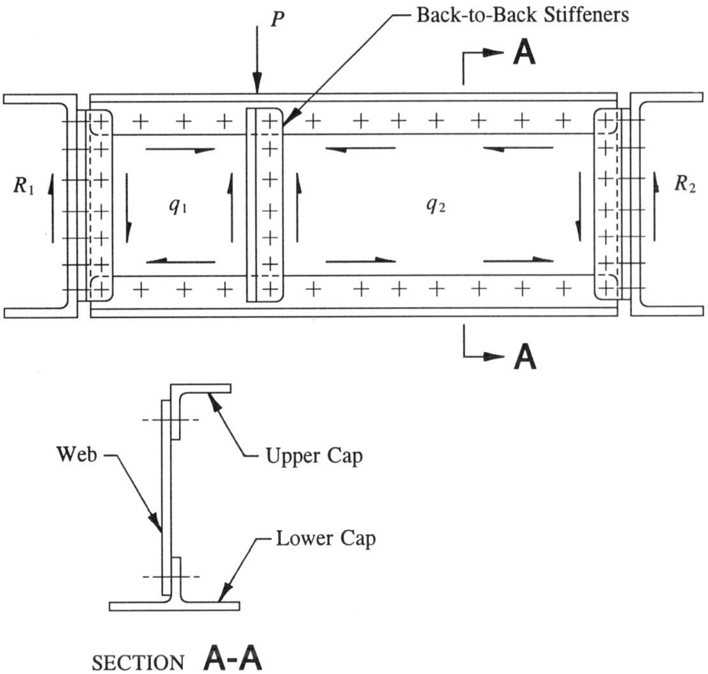

FIGURE 8-8 Stiffener of the beam structure serves as a panel breaker to maintain the web panels shear-resistant.

A stiffener is basically a panel breaker which divides a larger panel into two smaller ones. In so doing, it provides the reinforcement of the smaller panels required to maintain the panels shear-resistant. This can be seen from the beam structure depicted in Fig. 8-2 (refer back to page 479). The back-to-back stiffeners in Fig. 8-8, however, serve a dual purpose: (1) as panel breakers and (2) they distribute the applied load P uniformly into the beam structure, and thus they prevent the collapse of the web structure locally. The required stiffness of a panel breaker is measured by the moment of inertia of its section area around the centroidal axis of the member parallel to its web structure (see ahead to Eq. 8-3). Unless loads are directly applied to the stiffener, this member essentially carries no load. An exception to this rule occurs when the adjacent panels of this structure buckle; here, the wrinkling effect of the panel in its buckled state induces tension stresses into the boundary structure which compresses the stiffener.

Shear-resistant webs are considered fully effective in bending, which means, in effect, that their cross-sectional areas can effectively resist in-plane bending moments. As a natural consequence of this occurrence, the moment of inertia of the web structure can be included with the moment of inertia of the total cross-sectional area. For the most part, it can be said that the general instability of a plate structure is principally governed by an adequate number and size of panel

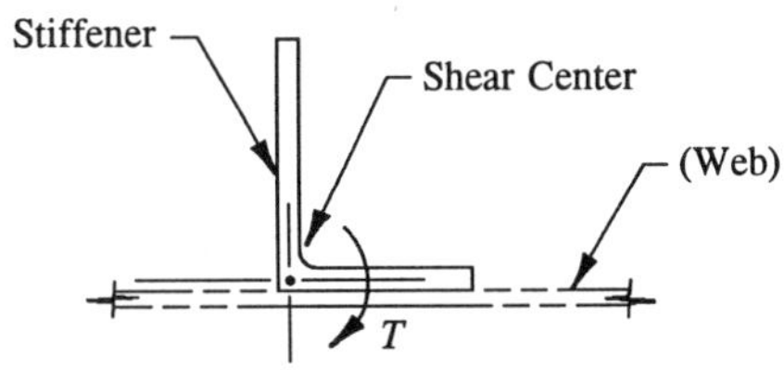

J = polar moment of inertia.

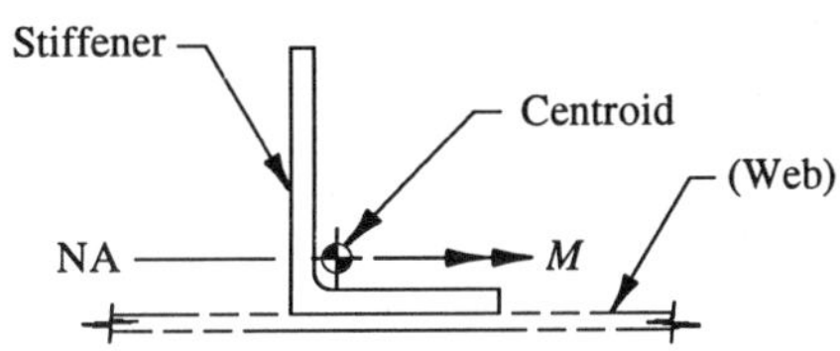

I_{na} = rectangular moment of inertia (see Appendix F).

FIGURE 8-9 (a) Polar moment of inertia for beams in torsion. (b) Rectangular moment of inertia for beams in bending.

breakers[1]. Moreover, without the proper rotational stiffness[2] and bending stiffness required from these members to prevent panel buckling, a panel might not necessarily develop a shear-resistant structure, even if general plate theory would predict otherwise (the equations of plate buckling are presented later in this section, see Eqs. 8-4, 8-5, and 8-13 for reference now). (Also see Appendix F for rectangular moment of inertia I_{na} calculations and to an advanced textbook[3] for polar moment of inertia J calculations.) These terms are described in Fig. 8-9. Even at higher loads, when the panel does buckle, the panel breakers (shown as stiffeners in Fig. 8-8) actually prevent buckling from extending to adjacent panels. Two separate panels are said to be stiffer than one panel of the same surface area (compare the buckling allowables for different size panels). In conjunction with general plate theory, to prevent plate buckling, the following equation is used to determine the minimum required moment of inertia[4] to establish a panel shear-resistant:

$$I_s = \frac{2.29d}{t}\left[\frac{Vh_{\text{web}}}{33E_c}\right]^{4/3} \tag{8-3}$$

[1] Panel breakers are used here in a general sense which could include stiffeners, stringers, and main structural members composed of beam cap members held together by an included web.

[2] Rotational stiffness of edge members of a plate can also be referred to as torsional stiffness. In any case, its determination is beyond the scope and main intent of this text.

[3] See E.F. Popov, *Mechanics of Materials,* Chapter 3, "Torsion," Prentice-Hall, Inc., Englewood Cliffs, N.J., 1952.

[4] H. Wagner, *ASME paper,* 1930.

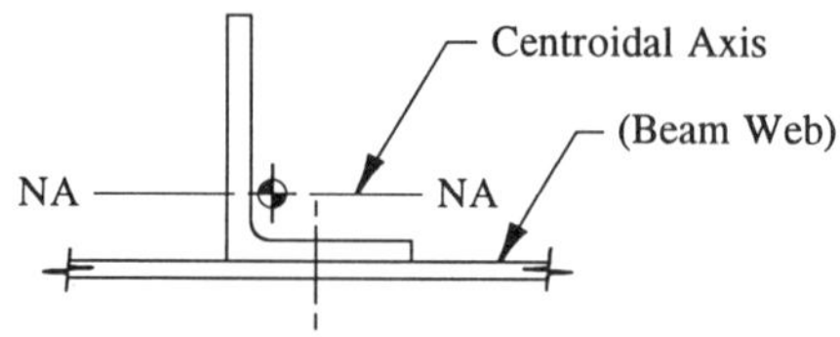

SINGLE ANGLE STIFFENER

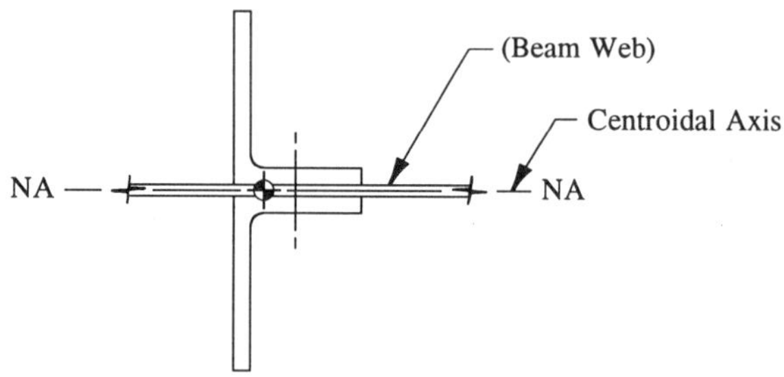

BACK-TO-BACK ANGLE STIFFENERS

FIGURE 8-10 (a) Single angle stiffener. (b) Back-to-back angle stiffeners.

where: I_s = minimum required moment of inertia of the panel breaker acting alone
V = applied web vertical shear force
d = distance measured between panel breakers
h_{web} = height of the web
t = web or panel thickness
E_c = elastic or Young's modulus of elasticity in compression.

Since the solution of this equation for I_s is based on the panel breaker acting alone, do not include any effective web or skin area in the computations for the rectangular moment of inertia I_{na} of the panel breaker (see equation below). Also, remember to calculate this value through the centroidal axis of the cross-sectional area parallel to the plane of the attached web or skin surfaces. For a system of back-to-back panel breakers, consider the moment of inertia of both members about the centroidal axis of their combined sections (also exclude the effective web area in this computation). This structural arrangement of members is viewed in Fig. 8-10. Now, compare the value of I_s obtained from Eq. 8-3 with the moment of inertia I_{na} of the panel breaker(s) acting alone (i.e., excluding the effective sheet areas).

$$\text{Margin of Safety} = \text{M.S.} = \frac{I_{na}}{I_s} - 1$$

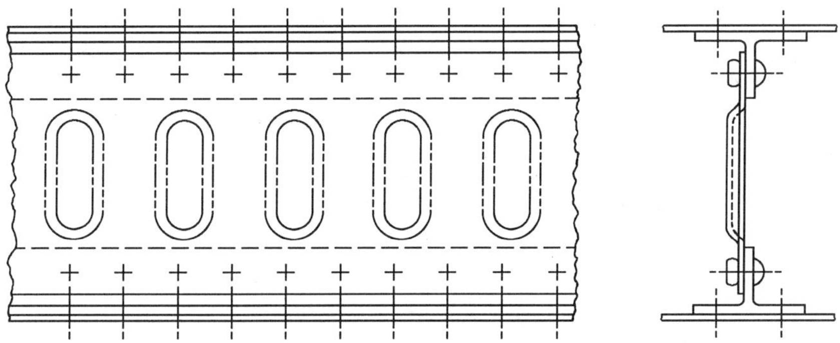

FORMED VERTICAL BEADS

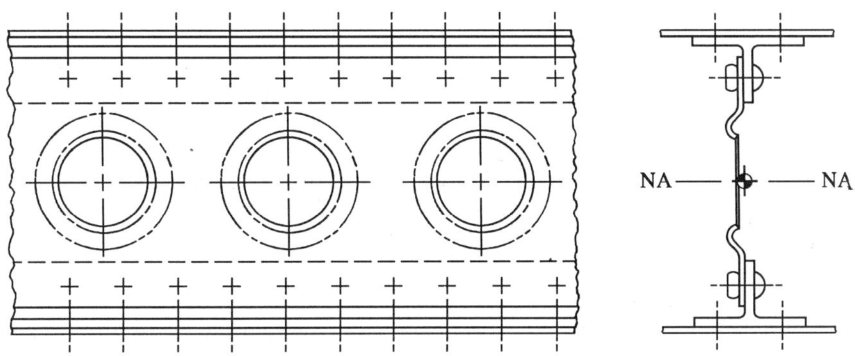

FLANGED LIGHTENING HOLES

FIGURE 8-11 Types of reinforced, shear-resistant webs.

where: I_s = minimum required moment of inertia of the panel breaker(s) acting alone

I_{na} = rectangular moment of inertia of the panel breaker(s) about the centroidal axis parallel to the plane of its attached web or skin surfaces (do not include effective sheet areas).

In general, although panel breakers play an important role in the ability of a riveted aircraft structural panel to maintain its nonbuckled state at limit load and to maintain its adequate strength at ultimate load, their designs are not particularly very efficient from a weight and cost standpoint. A shear-resistant panel is considerably heavier than a panel which is allowed to buckle. The panel breakers only aggravate this problem, since the additional parts required and the increased man-hours required for assembly of these members increase the disadvantage of their use considerably.

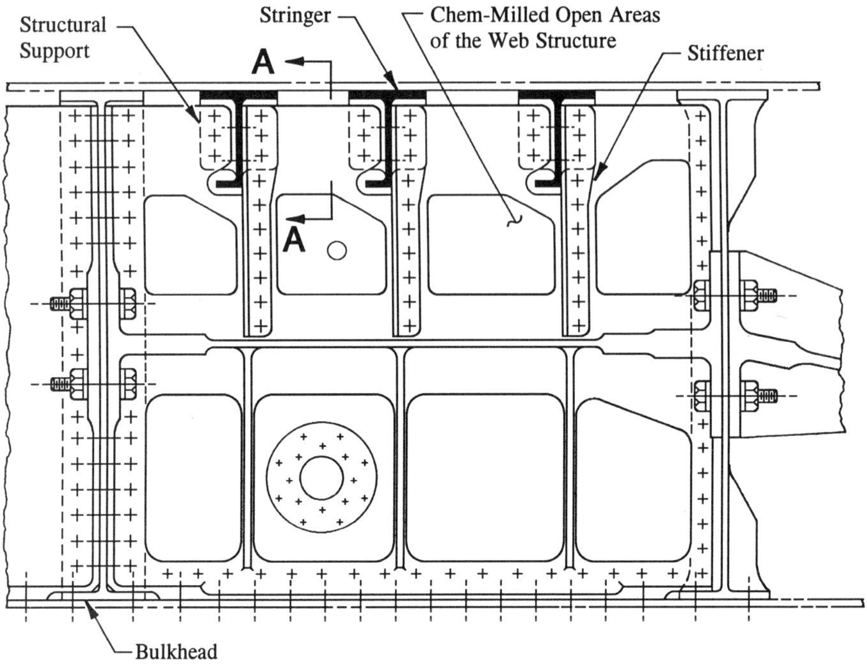

FIGURE 8-12(a) Close-out rib.

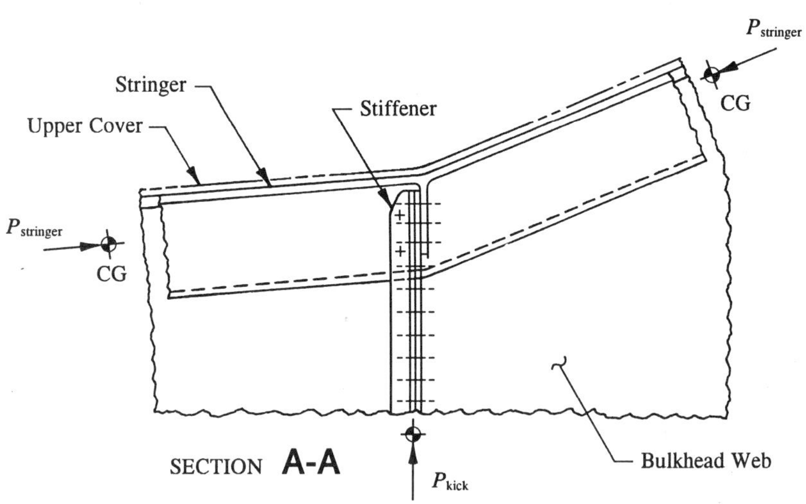

FIGURE 8-12(b) In this view, the structure reveals that an attached stiffener is required to react the stringer kick load. From statics, this load is determined to be compression for the stringer loads given in this figure.

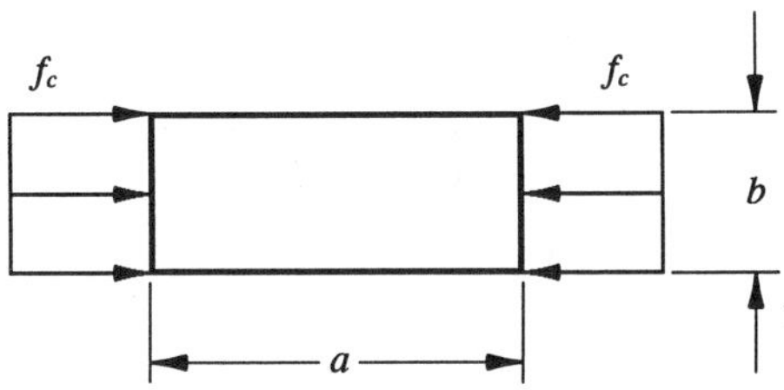

FIGURE 8-13 Thin, flat plate in pure compression.

Types of shear-resistant webs that are considered more cost-effective and practical in actual use than externally attached panel breakers are shown in Fig. 8-11. These designs represent an entirely different class of problems unique to the aerospace industry. Here, the method of stiffening is formed by either vertical beads or flanged lightening holes that are integral with the basic web structure. In some cases, their designs may even be slightly heavier than a web structure with attached stiffeners, but the added weight penalty, if one occurs at all, is usually small compared to the savings in manufacturing costs realized by eliminating the attached stiffeners altogether. Their designs are also used to stiffen a panel or beam web by preventing initial buckling or deflection of their surfaces. For their solutions, the engineer should consult an aerospace company structures manual. Normally, empirical solutions are provided for these and other structural types from published design curves based on structural test data of different material types.

A final note when designing panel breakers: Provide a panel breaker whenever external loads are applied to the structure. For example, the close-out rib shown in Fig. 8-12(a) requires separately attached stiffeners to react stringer kick loads. For the loads given in Fig. 8-12(b), the kick load P_{kick} will compress the attached stiffener. Physically, the load is transferred through the five connection rivets attaching this member to the structural support. From there, the load will shear from the stiffener into the basic web structure. The stiffeners are also utilized to prevent panel buckling. Additionally, the stiffeners must be stiff enough to prevent the influence of loads from one panel to another. And, most importantly, the stiffeners must be analyzed for column instability.

When analyzing the panels for buckling, assume the thicknesses of the panels to be uniform and of the same thickness as those indicated by their chem-milled areas. Although the results are slightly conservative, the panel designs should prove consistent with structural theory (and practice). Increased stiffness of a panel can be achieved by: (l) increasing the thickness of the panel, (2) increasing the stiffness of the supporting structure, (3) tighter or closer spacing of boundary rivets, (4) using a stiffener as a panel breaker, or (5) changing the panel (i.e., rib structure) to a higher strength material.

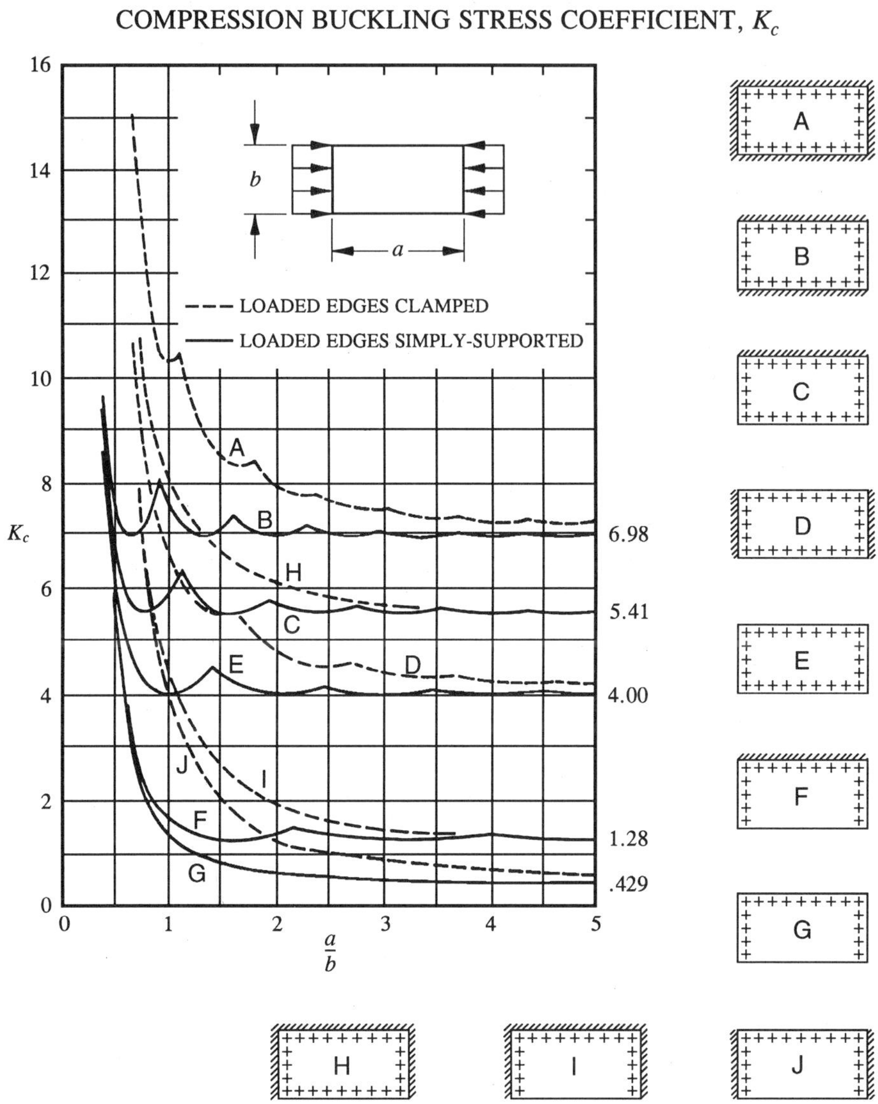

FIGURE 8-14 Compression buckling stress coefficients versus aspect ratios of thin, flat plates.

Stability of Thin, Flat Plate Members in Pure Compression

The critical buckling stress of a thin, flat plate member in pure compression, as shown in Fig. 8-13, is expressed by the following equation:

$$\frac{(F_c)_{cr}}{\eta_c} = \frac{\pi^2 K_c E_c}{12(1-\mu^2)}\left[\frac{t}{b}\right]^2 \tag{8-4}$$

where: K_c = compression buckling stress coefficient from Fig. 8-14 (see page 498)
η_c = plasticity correction factor for plates in pure compression
μ = Poisson's ratio (physical property of the material found in the mechanical-property tables of MIL-HDBK-5)
b = distance measured along the axially loaded edges of the plate
E_c = elastic or Young's modulus of elasticity in compression
t = web or panel thickness.

In this form, this equation represents the "theoretical" buckling stress $(F_c)_{cr}/\eta_c$ of a plate in pure compression. To determine its "true" value, the plasticity correction value η_c must be determined. For stresses within the elastic range of a stress-strain diagram (or low stresses), the plasticity correction factor η_c is a constant, or a value of 1.0. However, if stresses exceed the proportional limit of the material, the material goes plastic and the plate undergoes a reduction in bending stiffness. This reduction is accounted for by the plasticity correction factor η_c. Although its actual numerical value is now less than 1.0, its value need not be calculated directly if the following procedure is used to determine $(F_c)_{cr}$:

(1) Begin by calculating the theoretical compression buckling stress $(F_c)_{cr}/\eta_c$ of the plate using Eq. 8-4. For convenience, this equation is again repeated here below:

$$\frac{(F_c)_{cr}}{\eta_c} = \frac{\pi^2 K_c E_c}{12(1-\mu^2)}\left[\frac{t}{b}\right]^2.$$

(2) With the value of $(F_c)_{cr}/\eta_c$, enter a compression plasticity correction curve, $(F_c)_{cr}/\eta_c$ vs. $(F_c)_{cr}$, for a specific material and determine the true compression buckling stress of the plate or $(F_c)_{cr}$. Use Fig. 8-15 for clad 2024-T3 sheet (QQ-A-250/5) at room-temperature. For curves of other material types, the engineer should consult an aerospace company structures manual. Additionally, these same curves can also be used to determine the true buckling stresses of plates loaded in pure shear and to plates loaded in pure bending. (More about this as we continue our discussions of this subject for other standard loading types.)

Instability of the plate in pure compression is then predicted as follows:

$$\text{Margin of Safety} = \text{M.S.} = \frac{(F_c)_{cr}}{f_c} - 1$$

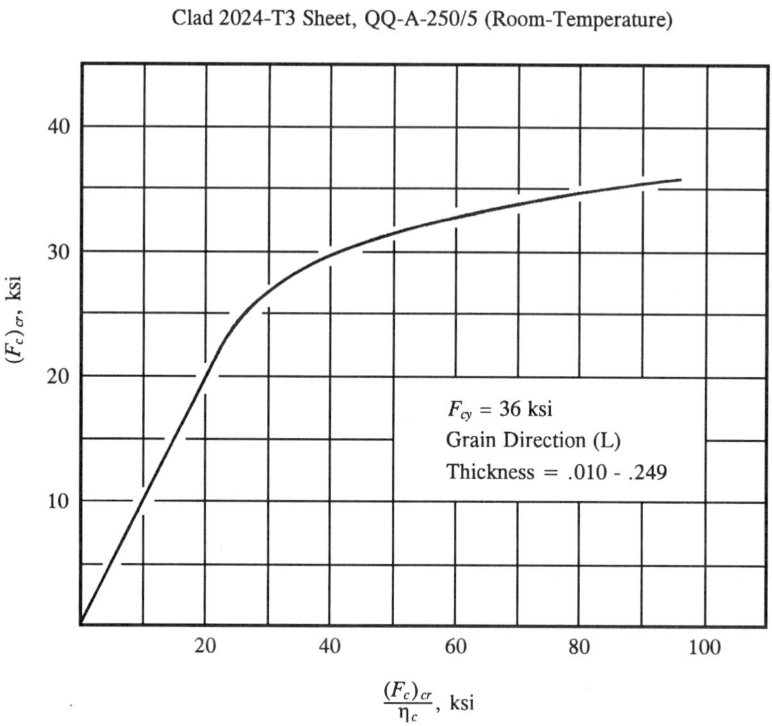

FIGURE 8-15 Plasticity correction curve for compression buckling.

where: $(F_c)_{cr}$ = critical buckling stress of a thin, flat plate member in pure compression

$f_c = P/A$ = applied axial compression stress

P = applied axial compression load

$A = bt$ = cross-sectional area of the plate in the direction of the applied axial load

b = distance measured at the loaded edges of the plate

t = web or panel thickness.

Stability of Thin, Flat Plate Members in Pure Shear

The critical buckling stress of a thin, flat plate member in pure shear, as shown in Fig. 8-16, is expressed by the following equation:

$$\frac{(F_s)_{cr}}{\eta_s} = \frac{\pi^2 K_s E_c}{12(1-\mu^2)}\left[\frac{t}{b}\right]^2 \tag{8-5}$$

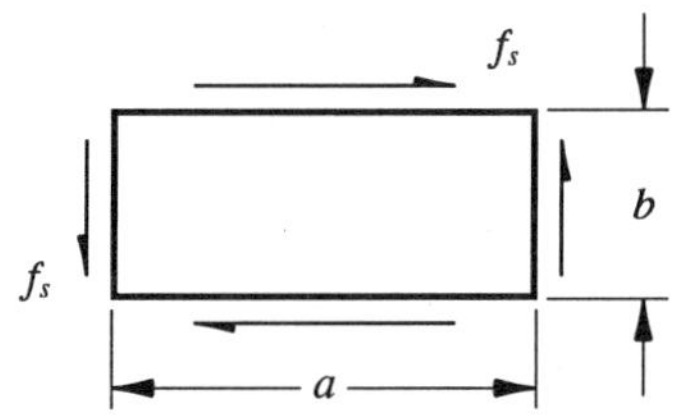

FIGURE 8-16 Thin, flat plate in pure shear.

where: K_s = shear buckling stress coefficient from Fig. 8-18
η_s = plasticity correction factor for plates in pure shear
μ = Poisson's ratio (physical constant of the material found in the mechanical-property tables of MIL-HDBK-5)
b = shorter dimension of the plate[1]
E_c = elastic or Young's modulus of elasticity in compression
t = web or panel thickness.

Notice how similar looking this equation is to the equation of a flat plate acting in pure compression (see Eq. 8-4). Like compression buckling, this equation also represents the "theoretical" buckling stress $(F_s)_{cr}/\eta_s$ of the plate, but, in this case, the plate is loaded in pure shear. To determine its "true" value, or $(F_s)_{cr}$, the plasticity correction factor η_s in pure shear must be found. It should be recalled that when stresses occur within the elastic range of a stress-strain diagram, the plasticity correction factor η_s is 1.0. For stresses above the proportional limit of the material, a value less than 1.0 is usually indicated. To determine this value and thus determine the true shear buckling stress of the plate, the following procedure is devised:

(1) Begin by calculating the theoretical shear buckling stress $(F_s)_{cr}/\eta_s$ of the plate using Eq. 8-5, or

$$\frac{(F_s)_{cr}}{\eta_s} = \frac{\pi^2 K_s E_c}{12(1-\mu^2)}\left[\frac{t}{b}\right]^2.$$

[1] In the case of a beam that has its beam depth h greater than its stiffener spacing d (these terms are defined in Fig. 8-17), the stiffener spacing is taken as the "b dimension" in the solution of Eq. 8-5. Expressed as an inequality:

If $h > d$, use d as the "b dimension" in the solution of Eq. 8-5.

Alternatively, if the depth h of the beam is less than its stiffener spacing d, the shorter dimension or beam depth is taken as the "b dimension." Written as an inequality:

If $h < d$, use h as the "b dimension" in the solution of Eq. 8-5.

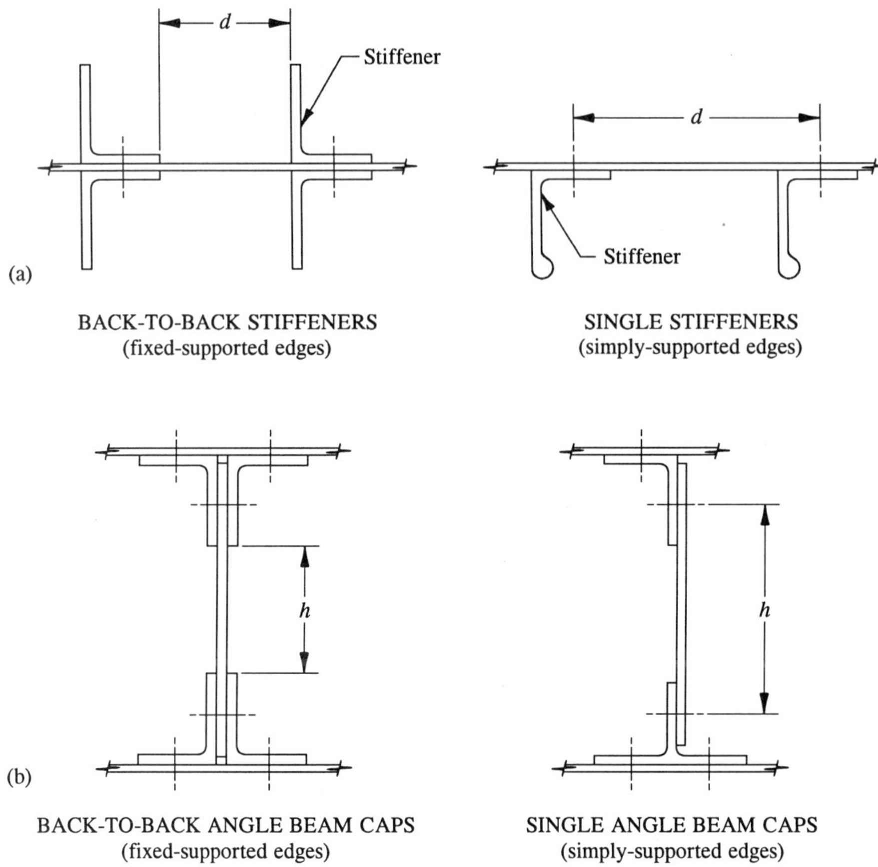

FIGURE 8-17 (a) Stiffener spacing and (b) panel height for different support conditions of a panel.

(2) For most ductile materials, the allowable yield shearing stress F_{sy} can be conveniently expressed in terms of the allowable tensile yield stress F_{ty} of the material as follows: $F_{sy} = F_{ty}/\sqrt{3}$. From this general stress relationship that exists between tension and shear,[1] an analogous relationship for the theoretical compression buckling stress of a plate in terms of its corresponding theoretical shear buckling stress is formulated. Solve for this value:

$$\frac{(F_c)_{cr}}{\eta_c} = \frac{(F_s)_{cr}}{\eta_s}\sqrt{3}\,. \tag{8-6}$$

[1] From this simple relationship that exists between certain ductile materials, derives the solution to Eq. 8-5.

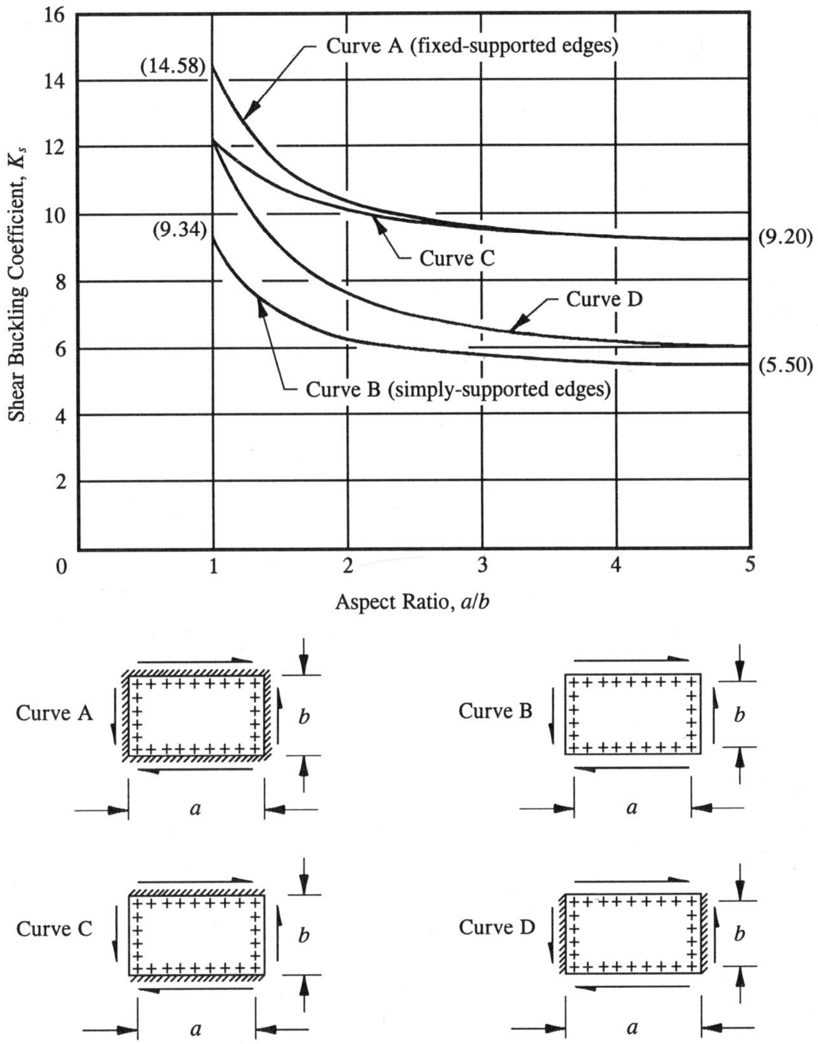

FIGURE 8-18 Shear buckling stress coefficients versus aspect ratios of thin, flat plates.

(3) With the value of $(F_c)_{cr}/\eta_c$, enter a compression plasticity correction curve, $(F_c)_{cr}/\eta_c$ vs. $(F_c)_{cr}$, for a specific material and determine the true compression buckling stress of the plate or $(F_c)_{cr}$. Such a curve is shown in Fig. 8-15 for clad 2024-T3 sheet (QQ-A250/5) at room-temperature. For curves of other material types, the engineer should consult an aerospace company structures manual.

(4) Divide the value of $(F_c)_{cr}$ obtained in step 3 by $\sqrt{3}$.

$$(F_s)_{cr} = \frac{(F_c)_{cr}}{\sqrt{3}}. \tag{8-7}$$

Thus, the true shear buckling stress $(F_s)_{cr}$ of the plate is arrived at without actually having to determine the value of η_s from shear plasticity correction curves for specific material types.

The constant K_s in Eq. 8-5 is a function of the plate dimensions, i.e., the aspect ratio a/b, and the edge-support conditions of the plate. Its value is determined from the following equations for simply-supported edges and fixed-supported edges of a plate:[1]

For simply-supported plate edges (see Curve B, page 503):

$$K_s = 5.34 + 4.00\left[\frac{b}{a}\right]^2. \tag{8-8}$$

For fixed-supported plate edges (see Curve A, page 503):

$$K_s = 8.98 + 5.60\left[\frac{b}{a}\right]^2. \tag{8-9}$$

Equations 8-8 and 8-9 are plotted in Fig. 8-18 in terms of the shear buckling coefficient K_s versus the aspect ratio a/b of the plate. These curves can also be used to compare the stiffnesses of riveted structural panels having different support conditions. For example, if we consider panels of the same aspect ratio, say, $a/b = 1.0$, it can be seen from these curves that a fixed-supported plate (Curve A) is approximately 56% stiffer than a simply-supported plate (Curve B). (Compare values of K_s for each support condition.)

A more important question to answer is as follows: Is a square panel stiffer than a rectangular panel of the same surface area? Use Fig. 8-18 and Eq. 8-5 to help you arrive at your prediction. Are the results in agreement with what you perceived to be true? Instability of the plate in pure shear is then predicted as follows:

$$\text{Margin of Safety} = \text{M.S.} = \frac{(F_s)_{cr}}{f_s} - 1$$

where: $(F_s)_{cr}$ = critical buckling stress of a thin, flat plate member in pure shear

$f_s = \frac{q}{t}$ = average applied shearing stress

q = average applied panel shear flow (for beams, use $q = V/h_e$)

V = applied vertical web shear force

t = web or panel thickness

---

[1] Bleich, *Buckling Strength of Metal Structures*, p. 395.

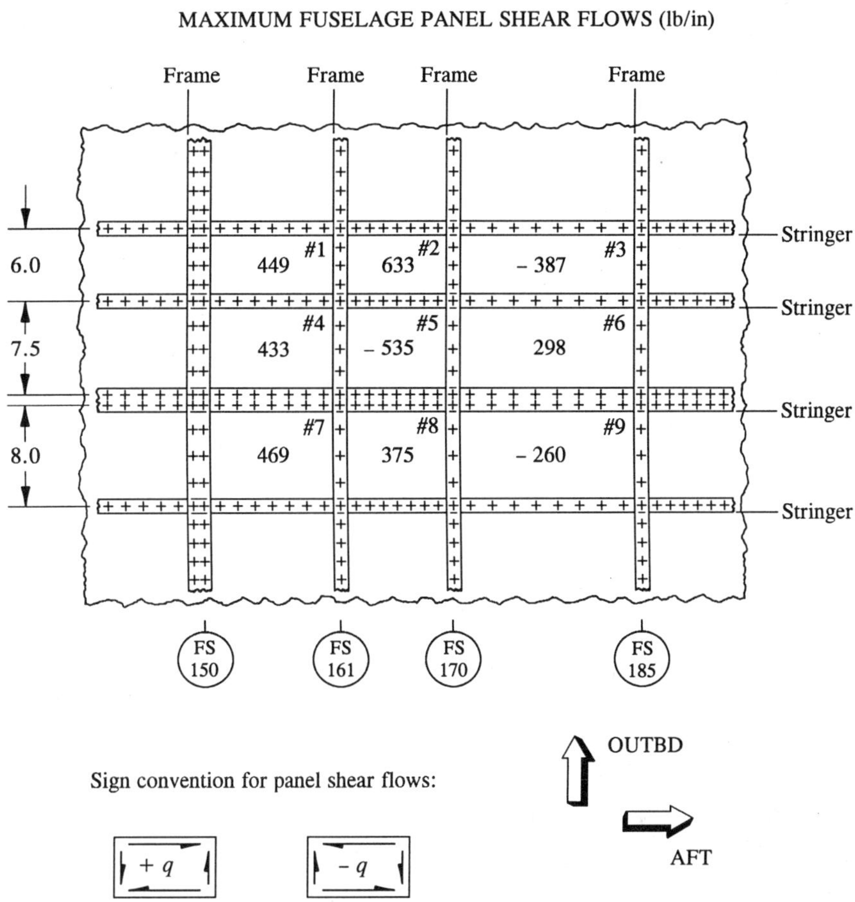

FIGURE 8-19 Skin panel shear flows for the fuselage shell between FS 150 and FS 185.

h_e = effective depth of the beam measured between cap centroids (neglect the effective web area, see Fig. 8-2).

Example 8-1 Using the shear flows given in Fig. 8-19, determine a constant skin thickness for the fuselage shell for the regions indicated in this figure. For fatigue design reasons, the skin panels, formed by the intersection of the frames and stringers of the fuselage shell, are required to be shear-resistant at 70% limit load. Assume the following conditions also apply to these panels: (1) all boundary members are of sufficient stiffness to prevent panel buckling, (2) inter-rivet buckling is prevented along the frames and stringers, and (3) all fuselage panels are essentially flat plates. The panel shears (or shear flows) represent a maximum envelope of all flight and landing conditions that the aircraft experiences during its normal expected service life. The fuselage skin is made of clad 2024-T3 aluminum alloy sheet material (QQ-A-250/5).

SOLUTION: Although under normal flight and landing conditions the fuselage may experience the effects of combined loads, for fatigue design of buckled skin panels, only *shear loading* is normally considered. Hence, from the shear flows given in Fig. 8-19, the fuselage panels are checked for premature shear buckling and their values are tabulated as shown in Table 8-1. Following this summary table, a sample calculation illustrating the detailed solution of panel #7 for shear buckling requirements at 70% limit load will be presented.

TABLE 8-1 CRITICAL SHEAR BUCKLING STRESSES

Panel No.	q	f_s* (limit)	$.70f_s$	a	b	K_s (Eq. 8-8)	$(F_s)_{cr}$ (Eq. 8-5)	Shear Buckling MS
1	449	6,324	4,427	11.0	6.0	6.53	9,030	+ 1.04
2	633	8,915	6,241	9.0	6.0	7.12	9,846	+ 0.58
3	- 387	5,451	3,815	15.0	6.0	5.98	8,270	+ 1.17
4	433	6,099	4,269	11.0	7.5	7.20	6,372	+ 0.49
5	- 535	7,535	5,275	9.0	7.5	8.12	7,187	+ 0.36
6	298	4,197	2,938	15.0	7.5	6.34	5,611	+ 0.91
7	469	6,606	4,624	11.0	8.0	7.46	5,803	+ 0.25
8	375	5,282	3,697	9.0	8.0	8.50	6,612	+ 0.79
9	- 260	3,662	2,563	15.0	8.0	6.48	5,041	+ 0.97

* $f_s = q/t$ (refer back to Eq. 4-5).

Sample calculation for panel #7:

The critical shear buckling stress of panel #7 is found by solving Eq. 8-5 for $(F_s)_{cr}$. A trial-and-error approach is used to solve for the solution of a standard gage thickness for the fuselage skin. Let us try $t = .071$ for which $E_c = 10.7 \times 10^6$ psi and $\mu = .33$ are found for this panel (see the mechanical-property tables given in MIL-HDBK-5F for clad 2024-T3 aluminum alloy sheet material). Based on the panel conditions provided above, the edges of the panel are assumed to be simply-supported. Thus, we can use Curve B of Fig. 8-18 to determine the shear buckling coefficient K_s. This value can also be determined by solving Eq. 8-8 directly. This equation is repeated here below:

$$K_s = 5.34 + 4.00\left[\frac{b}{a}\right]^2.$$

Regardless of panel orientation in the structure, the shorter dimension of the panel is always taken as the "b dimension" in the solution of Eq. 8-5 (refer back to the inequality expressions given on page 501). For panel #7, this corresponds to $b = 8.0$. Hence, substituting, $b = 8.0$, and the other dimension of the plate, $a = 11.0$, into this expression and simplifying gives:

$$K_s = 5.34 + 4.00\left[\frac{8.0}{11.0}\right]^2 = 7.46.$$

Now, substituting this and all known values into Eq. 8-5, we obtain:

$$\frac{(F_s)_{cr}}{\eta_s} = \frac{\pi^2 K_s E_c}{12(1-\mu^2)}\left[\frac{t}{b}\right]^2 = \frac{\pi^2 (7.46)\,10.7 \times 10^6}{12\left[1-(.33)^2\right]}\left[\frac{.071}{8.0}\right]^2 = 5,803 \text{ psi.}$$

Using the general stress relationship between compression and shear buckling for ductile materials, determine the theoretical compression buckling stress $(F_c)_{cr}/\eta_c$ of the plate. From Eq. 8-6, we obtain directly the following value:

$$\frac{(F_c)_{cr}}{\eta_c} = \frac{(F_s)_{cr}}{\eta_s}\sqrt{3} = 5,803\sqrt{3} = 10,051 \text{ psi.}$$

With this value, enter a compression plasticity correction curve, $(F_c)_{cr}/\eta_c$ vs. $(F_c)_{cr}$, for clad 2024-T3 aluminum alloy sheet material and determine a value for $(F_c)_{cr}$. Such a curve is shown in Fig. 8-15. Since this value actually corresponds to the elastic portion of this curve, $\eta_c = 1.0$, and

$$(F_c)_{cr} = 10,051 \text{ psi.}$$

Then, if we divide this value by $\sqrt{3}$, the true critical shear buckling stress of panel #7 is determined:

$$(F_s)_{cr} = \frac{(F_c)_{cr}}{\sqrt{3}} = \frac{10,051}{\sqrt{3}} = 5,803 \text{ psi.}$$

To meet the criterion of shear buckling at 70% limit load, the critical shear buckling stress $(F_s)_{cr}$ is compared to the applied shearing stress f_s of panel #7 at 70% limit load. As a margin of safety, this comparison is written as follows:

$$\text{Margin of Safety} = \text{M.S.} = \frac{(F_s)_{cr}}{.70 f_s} - 1 = \frac{5,803}{4,624} - 1 = +.25$$

where: $(F_s)_{cr} = 5,803$ psi

$f_s = \frac{q}{t} = 6,606$ psi limit; $4,624$ psi @ 70% limit

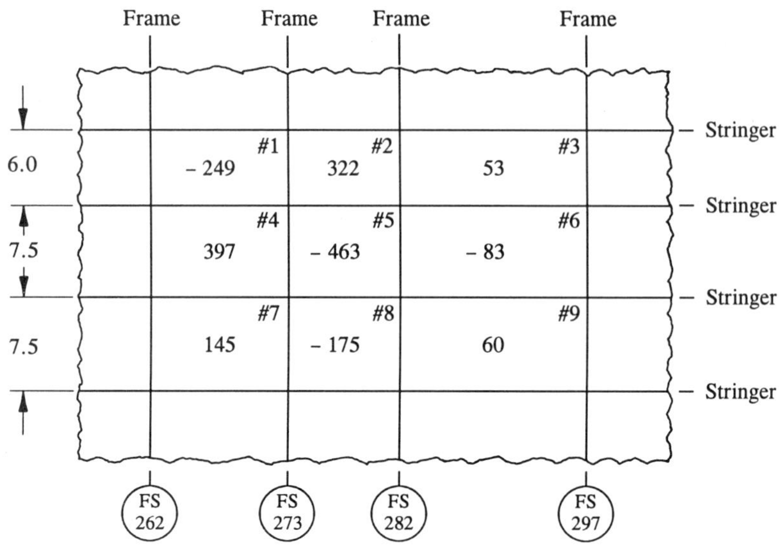

FIGURE 8-20 Fuselage panel limit shear flows.

q = 469 lb/in limit (refer to the maximum limit shear flows given in Fig. 8-19 for panel #7)
t = .071 in (proposed fuselage skin thickness).

Table 8-1 shows the numerical computations of panels #1 through #9 and a summary of the shear buckling margins of safety for these panels at 70% limit load. Observe in this table that panel #7 is critical since it has the least margin of safety of all the panels investigated, or M.S. = + .25. Therefore, this panel will govern the design thickness of the fuselage shell. Normally, a panel that is designed to be shear-resistant at limit load (or 70% limit load), if not overdesigned too much, will buckle at ultimate load. *If this occurs, such panels must be analyzed for the effects of diagonal tension at these higher loads.*

As a second try, if the fuselage skin is made one-gage thinner, or t = .063, panel #7 would then buckle at 70% limit load (or M.S. = − .12) and be unsubstantiated for the fatigue design buckling requirements of this problem. (Verification of this margin of safety is left as an exercise for the engineer to complete.) Hence, the .071 in thick material (M.S. = + .25) proves adequate for the fuselage shell.

Example 8-2 After a careful review of all flight and landing conditions, the fuselage skin between Frame Station 262 and Frame Station 297 was found to be critical for wing down-bending loads.[1] Panel shear flows given for the fuselage

[1] When the wing undergoes down-bending, the fuselage, which simultaneously balances the

skin in lb/in limit are indicated in Fig. 8-20. Much like the panel analysis that was performed and tabulated for the fuselage skin of Example 8-1, the fuselage panels here are similarly analyzed and tabulated for review. The results of that analysis are summarized in Table 8-2. It should be observed from this table that panels #1, #2, #4, and #5 are not shear-resistant at limit load (this is indicated by the negative margins of safety in this table for these panels). (a) What thickness of panel reinforcement would be required to maintain these panels shear-resistant at limit load? (b) If an aluminum reinforcement is used in part (a) to stiffen the critical panels, what pattern of field rivets would be required to prevent premature buckling of these panels at limit load? The fuselage shell is constructed of .050 in clad 2024-T3 aluminum alloy sheet material (QQ-A-250/5).

TABLE 8-2 CRITICAL SHEAR BUCKLING STRESSES

Panel No.	q	f_s (limit)	a	b	K_s (Eq. 8-8)	$(F_s)_{cr}$* (Eq. 8-5)	Shear Buckling MS
1	− 249	4,980	11.0	6.0	6.53	4,478	− 0.10
2	322	6,440	9.0	6.0	7.12	4,883	− 0.24
3	53	1,060	15.0	6.0	5.98	4,101	+ 2.87
4	397	7,940	11.0	7.5	7.20	3,160	− 0.60
5	− 463	9,260	9.0	7.5	8.12	3,564	− 0.62
6	− 83	1,660	15.0	7.5	6.34	2,783	+ 0.68
7	145	2,900	11.0	7.5	7.20	3,160	+ 0.09
8	− 175	3,500	9.0	7.5	8.12	3,564	+ 0.02
9	60	1,200	15.0	7.5	6.34	2,783	+ 1.32

* Use values of $E_c = 10.7 \times 10^6$ psi and $\mu = .33$ for the panels in this column (see the mechanical-property tables given in MIL-HDBK-5F for clad 2024-T3 aluminum alloy sheet material). Based on the low critical shear buckling stresses for these panels (second to last column in Table 8-2), theoretical buckling stresses (those calculated from Eq. 8-5) should correspond to true elastic shear values. And, therefore, the shear plasticity correction factor η_s for elastic shear buckling of these panels is 1.0.

SOLUTION: To maintain the fuselage skin shear-resistant at limit load, the critical panels, indicated by the negative margins of safety in Table 8-2, must be reinforced. The reinforced area of the fuselage shell shall overlay or cover panels #1, #2, #4, and #5, as shown in Fig. 8-21. Also note how the reinforcement is attached to the boundary structure in Fig. 8-22. The required thickness of the reinforcement is found by solving the shear buckling equation, Eq. 8-5, for the panel thickness t. As is customarily assumed for the design of panels subjected to shear, boundary members provide simply-supported edges for the reinforced panels. Other assump-

aerodynamic forces of the wing, will experience up-bending loads. Therefore, it can be said that wing down-bending is analogous to fuselage up-bending and, conversely, wing up-bending is analogous to fuselage down-bending.

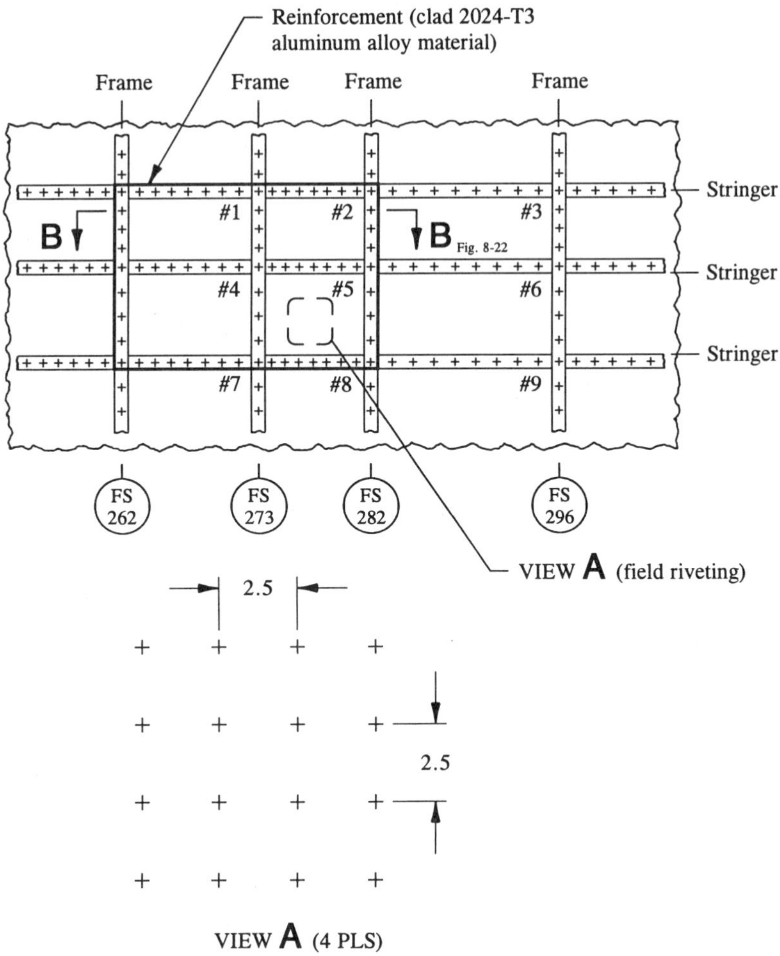

FIGURE 8-21 Reinforcement is field riveted to the fuselage shell.

tions follow from basic definitions and general theory of flat plate analysis, such as (1) boundary members are of sufficient stiffness to prevent panel buckling, (2) inter-rivet buckling of the supported edges of the plate and boundary structure are prevented, and (3) curved fuselage panels are considered essentially flat plate members. These requirements help to establish the support conditions favorable to the analysis of fuselage panels.

The reinforcement shall be constructed of the same material as the fuselage skin (clad 2024-T3 aluminum alloy material) and be of a constant thickness. To pinpoint the required thickness of the most critical panel, and thus avoid a trial-and-error approach to the analysis, let us take a slightly different plan of attack to our solution. Instead of assuming several different values of panel thickness t and

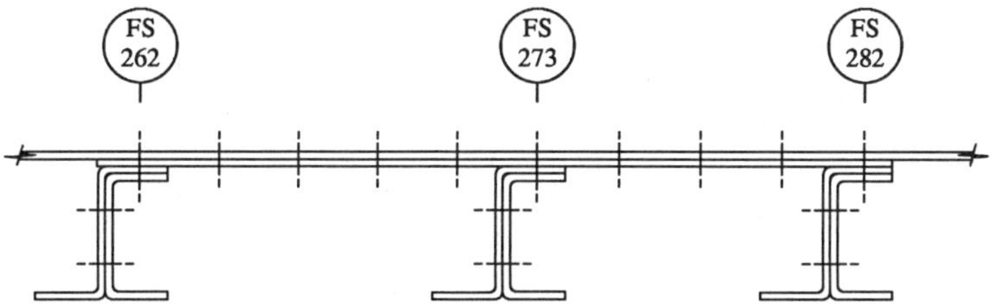

FIGURE 8-22 Installation of the reinforcement to the boundary structure.

then solving for the corresponding values of $(F_s)_{cr}$ to converge upon a zero (0) margin of safety for the most critical panel, the thickness dimension t in Eq. 8-5 will be directly solved for. To do this correctly, all terms in this equation containing the variable t must be included. From this expression, the required panel thickness can then be determined for the most critical panel—that of course occurs for panel #5 which indicates a negative margin of safety of 62% for this panel. To rapidly converge to a zero (0) margin of safety, the applied shearing stress for panel #5 is designed for. This means substituting or replacing the critical shear buckling stress $(F_s)_{cr}$ in Eq. 8-5 with the applied shearing stress f_s. Since the value of f_s is sensitive to the thickness of the panel, this value must also be expressed in terms of the variable t. Hence, from definitions, we have $f_s = q/t = 463/t$, where $q = 463$ lb/in limit. Now, substituting this and all known values into Eq. 8-5 (most values are found listed in Table 8-2) and solving for the required thickness, we obtain:

$$\frac{(F_s)_{cr}}{\eta_s} = \frac{\pi^2 K_s E_c}{12(1-\mu^2)}\left[\frac{t}{b}\right]^2$$

$$\frac{463/t}{1.0} = \frac{\pi^2 (8.12)\, 10.7 \text{ x } 10^6}{12\left[1-(.33)^2\right]}\left[\frac{t}{7.5}\right]^2$$

$$t^3 = .000325$$

$$t = .069 \text{ in.}$$

Since the skin is already .050 in thick, the difference, or .019 in, would be necessary to prevent premature buckling of panel #5 at limit load. Since most aircraft designs utilize standard gage material, let us consider an .025 in thick aluminum sheet of the same basic fuselage skin material for the proposed reinforcement.

Note that the panel analysis above assumes that the reinforcement physically acts together with the fuselage skin. To realize this physical action of the structure, the reinforcement must be properly field riveted to the fuselage skin. If inadequate rivet spacing is provided for the reinforcement, much like inadequate spacing of rivets in built-up beam construction reduces the stiffness (or moment of inertia) of the overall beam structure, the combined stiffness of the fuselage skin and reinforcement likewise would be reduced. Consequently, their combined thickness could not be used in the solution of Eq. 8-5. More about the effectivity of these members acting together when our solution to the second part of this problem—What pattern of field rivets would be required to prevent premature buckling of the reinforced panels at limit load?—is continued. Reinforcements of dissimilar materials, for example, steel and aluminum, are discussed later in this chapter along with an example problem to illustrate the theoretical and practical applications of their designs.[1]

Design of Field Rivets for the Aluminum Reinforcement:

Up to this point in our analysis of this problem, we have determined that a .025 in thick aluminum reinforcement will prevent buckling of the critical panels of the fuselage at limit load. However, if the above panel analysis is to be valid, the reinforcement plate must also be properly attached to the fuselage skin so that the combined structure, reinforcement plus fuselage skin, can physically act together as a structural unit and carry the loads (shear flows) intended. Whenever a structure is beefed up like our proposed aluminum reinforcement plate, invariably, some redistribution of loads will occur to the reinforcement and to the local surrounding structure because of the stiffer reinforced panels in the immediate area. However, this structural tendency for the most part should be overlooked, since its occurrence is somewhat small compared to the largeness of the overall fuselage structure. In theory, a sufficient number of field fasteners are required to make the reinforcement act in composite (integrally) with the fuselage skin. Real structure, however, does not behave so simply. Nevertheless, the reinforced structure is considered fully effective if properly and adequately field riveted to the fuselage skin. In other words, if we provide a sufficient number of fasteners, then the combined thickness of the reinforcement and the fuselage skin can be used in the solution of Eq. 8-5. It should be recalled from simple beam theory that if a built-up beam section is not properly attached with a sufficient number and size of fasteners, the moment of inertia of the total beam section could not be used in the solution of bending stresses. This was shown quite dramatically in Appendix H, where it was shown in that section how important the requirements of size and spacing of fasteners are to the basic design requirements of an efficient structure. The same line of reasoning holds true here for the field rivets of our aluminum reinforcement.

To establish a structurally weight-efficient reinforced panel, some criterion must be established for the reinforcement to effectively simulate an integral (composite) panel structure. Since panel buckling at limit load is our buckling criterion

[1] Since galvanic action can occur between dissimilar materials, such designs are not usually recommended for aircraft production use. Nontheless, their designs are important in aircraft structural situations where modifications of the existing structure, perhaps a test structure, is required for temporary repair.

for the fuselage skin, it seems logical to assume a criterion for the attached reinforcement which can at least duplicate or exceed this general requirement. If we consider the latter course of action—to exceed the limit shear buckling requirements of the fuselage skin—then let us assume that the panels bounded by the spacing of field rivets of the reinforcement plate are shear-resistant at ultimate load. Hence, from Fig. 8-20, the shear flow in the most critical panel will determine the appropriate field riveting for the combined structure. This occurs for panel #5, where the shear flow exceeds that of the other critical panels. As a first try, let us assume 2.5 in spacing for the field rivets. For two separately attached members, the panel shear flow is assumed to divide proportionally between: (1) the shear flow that is carried by the fuselage skin and (2) the shear flow that is carried by the reinforcement. Mathematically, this assumption is expressed as follows:

$$q = q_{\text{skin}} + q_{\text{plate}} \tag{8-10}$$

where: q = total shear flow that is carried by the composite panel
q_{skin} = shear flow that is carried by the skin
q_{plate} = shear flow that is carried by the reinforcement plate.

For the reinforcement plate and fuselage skin to physically act together, the reinforcement plate must be adequately field riveted to the fuselage skin. In this way, the combined panel thickness of these members can be fully utilized in Eq. 8-5 to determine the critical shear buckling stress of the combined structure.

$$t = t_{\text{skin}} + t_{\text{plate}} \tag{8-11}$$

where: t = total thickness of the composite panel
t_{skin} = thickness of the skin
t_{plate} = thickness of the reinforcement plate.

To design the reinforcement plate for field riveting, the design shear flow carried by the reinforcement must be determined. A simple ratio of thicknesses should determine the distribution of shear flow to this member. The magnitude of which is determined by the following expression:

$$q_{\text{plate}} = q\left[\frac{t_{\text{plate}}}{t_{\text{skin}} + t_{\text{plate}}}\right] \tag{8-12}$$

where: q_{plate} = shear flow carried by the reinforcement plate
q = total shear flow carried by the panel
t_{plate} = thickness of the reinforcement plate
t_{skin} = thickness of the skin.

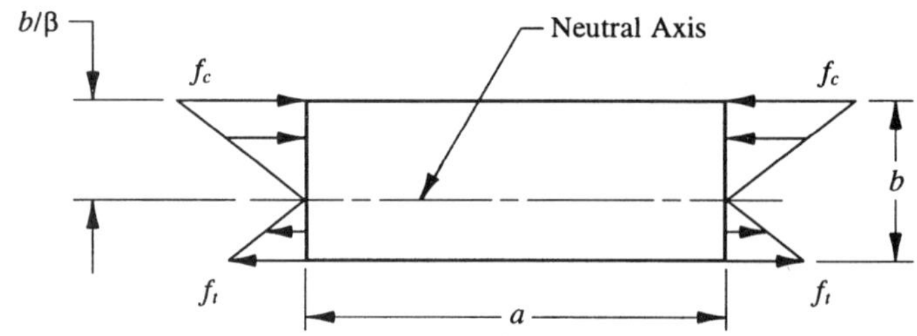

FIGURE 8-23 Thin, flat plate in pure bending.

Substituting values into Eq. 8-12, we obtain:

$$q_{\text{plate}} = 463\left[\frac{.025}{.050 + .025}\right] = 154 \text{ lb/in limit}$$

where: $q = 463$ lb/in limit (from Table 8-2 for panel #5)
$t_{\text{plate}} = .025$ in (proposed thickness of the reinforcement plate)
$t_{\text{skin}} = .050$ in.

Since the field fasteners are spaced 2.5 in apart, $b/a = 1.0$, and from Eq. 8-8 the shear buckling coefficient is obtained:

$$K_s = 5.34 + 4.0\left[\frac{b}{a}\right]^2 = 5.34 + 4.0(1.0)^2 = 9.34$$

where $b = 2.5$ in and $a = 2.5$ in.

Now, if we idealize a 2.5 x 2.5 square panel reinforcement (refer to View A in Fig. 8-21), the solution of Eq. 8-5 becomes:

$$\frac{(F_s)_{cr}}{\eta_s} = \frac{\pi^2 K_s E_c}{12(1-\mu^2)}\left[\frac{t}{b}\right]^2 = \frac{\pi^2 (9.34)\, 10.7 \times 10^6}{12\left[1-(.33)^2\right]}\left[\frac{.025}{2.5}\right]^2 = 9,224 \text{ psi}.$$

Using Fig. 8-15 and the stress relationship that exists between shear buckling and compression buckling (Eqs. 8-6 and 8-7), the shear plasticity correction factor η_s is found. From this, the true shear buckling stress of the reinforcement plate is determined:

$$(F_s)_{cr} = 9,224 \text{ psi}.$$

Buckling of this member at ultimate load is then predicted as follows:

$$\text{Margin of Safety} = \text{M.S.} = \frac{(F_s)_{cr}}{f_s} - 1 = \frac{9,224}{9,240} - 1 = -.00$$

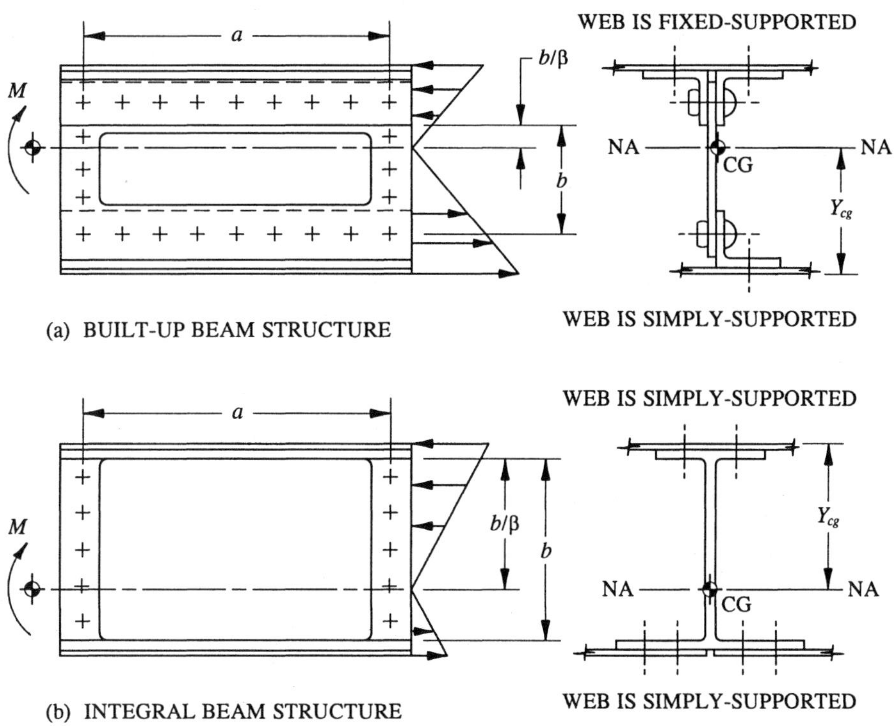

FIGURE 8-24 Supported edges of a web: (a) for a built-up beam and (b) for an integral beam.

where:
$$
\begin{aligned}
(F_s)_{cr} &= 9{,}224 \text{ psi} \\
f_s &= \frac{q_{\text{plate}}}{t_{\text{plate}}} = \frac{154}{.025} = 6{,}160 \text{ psi limit; } 9{,}240 \text{ psi ultimate} \\
q_{\text{plate}} &= 154 \text{ lb/in limit} \\
t_{\text{plate}} &= .025 \text{ in.}
\end{aligned}
$$

Based on the arbitrariness of our buckling criterion at ultimate load for the spacing of field rivets of the reinforcement plate, a slightly negative margin of safety should pose no real problem for most engineers accepting this solution. However, if the design engineer feels somewhat reluctant about accepting the results without conclusive proof, then some reduction in field riveting should be made. Or, perhaps, the design engineer may find that fastener spacing may actually have to be tightened anyway once rivets are actually equally spaced on the real structure. This solution therefore represents the minimum acceptable spacing to prevent buckling of the reinforcement plate at ultimate load, and at the same time maintains the fuselage skin and reinforcement plate shear-resistant at limit load.

BENDING BUCKLING STRESS COEFFICIENT, K_b

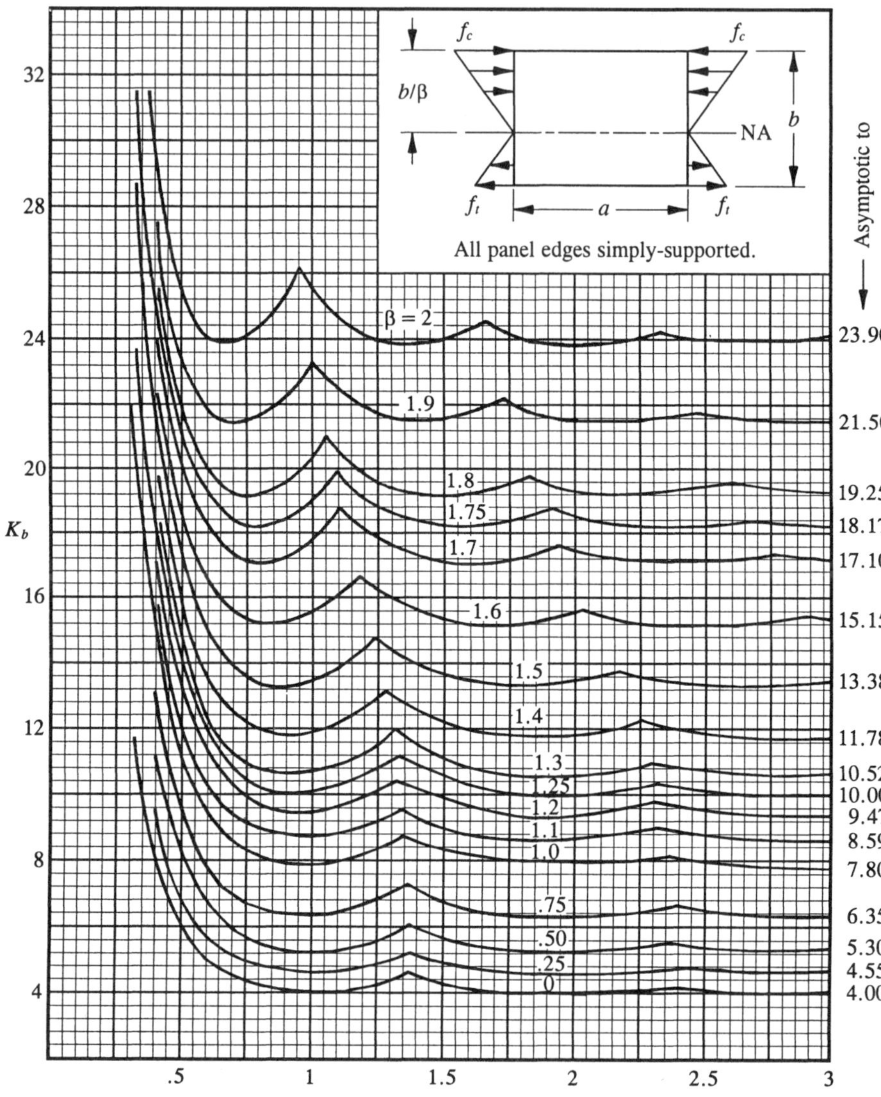

FIGURE 8-25 Bending buckling stress coefficients vs. aspect ratios of thin, flat plates.

Stability of Thin, Flat Plate Members in Pure Bending

The critical buckling stress of a thin, flat plate member in pure bending, as shown in Fig. 8-23, is expressed by the following equation:

$$\frac{(F_b)_{cr}}{\eta_b} = \frac{\pi^2 K_b E_c}{12(1 - \mu^2)} \left[\frac{t}{b}\right]^2 \tag{8-13}$$

where: K_b = bending buckling stress coefficient from Fig. 8-25
η_b = plasticity correction factor for plates in pure bending
μ = Poisson's ratio (physical constant of the material found in the mechanical-property tables of MIL-HDBK-5)
b = distance measured along the loaded edges of the plate
E_c = elastic or Young's modulus of elasticity in compression
t = web or panel thickness.

Notice how similar looking this equation is to Eqs. 8-4 and 8-5 for thin, flat plate members acting in pure compression and pure shear, respectively. The idealized plate structure of Fig. 8-23 could have been taken from a built-up beam structure loaded in pure bending, as shown in Fig. 8-24(a), or from an integral beam structure, Fig. 8-24(b). In each case, note particularly how the edges of the included webs are supported: in one case, by the beam flanges, and in the other, by the flange-to-web rivets. In accordance with recommended design practices for the buckling analysis of thin, flat plate members, the webs of these beams can safely be assumed to be supported by the particular structural arrangement of members indicated (in this figure) for their designs. Like compression and shear buckling, this equation represents the "theoretical" buckling stress $(F_b)_{cr}/\eta_b$ of the plate in pure bending. To determine its "true" value, or $(F_b)_{cr}$, the plasticity correction factor η_b in pure bending must be found. It should be recalled that when stresses occur within the elastic range of a stress-strain diagram, the plasticity correction factor η_b is 1.0. For stresses above the proportional limit of the material, a value less than 1.0 is indicated. Without available test data to determine the effects of plasticity on the bending of plates, the following (conservative) procedure is recommended to determine the true bending buckling stress $(F_b)_{cr}$:

(1) Calculate the theoretical bending buckling stress $(F_b)_{cr}/\eta_b$ of the plate using Eq. 8-13.

(2) Assume that $(F_c)_{cr}/\eta_c = (F_b)_{cr}/\eta_b$.

(3) With this value, enter a compression plasticity correction curve, $(F_c)_{cr}/\eta_c$ vs. $(F_c)_{cr}$, for a specific material and determine the true compression buckling stress of the plate $(F_c)_{cr}$. Such a curve is shown in Fig. 8-15 for clad 2024-T3 aluminum alloy sheet material (QQ-A-250/5) at room-temperature. For curves of other material types, the engineer should consult an aerospace company structures manual.

(4) This value then corresponds to the true bending buckling stress $(F_b)_{cr}$ of the plate.

Buckling coefficients K_b for simply-supported, flat, rectangular plates loaded in pure bending are given in Fig. 8-25. The curves can also be used for the included webs of unsymmetrically loaded beams. For example, from geometry and the loading structure of the beam, the value of beta (β) is found. From this and the aspect ratio a/b of the included web, the bending buckling coefficient K_b is also found. With this and all other known values substituted into Eq. 8-13, the critical bending buckling stress of this member is determined.

Instability of the included web in pure bending is predicted as follows:

$$\text{Margin of Safety} = \text{M.S.} = \frac{(F_b)_{cr}}{f_b} - 1$$

where: $(F_b)_{cr}$ = critical buckling stress of a thin, flat plate member in pure bending

$f_b = \dfrac{Mc}{I_{na}}$ = applied compression bending stress

M = internal bending moment

I_{na} = moment of inertia of the total beam cross-sectional area (include the entire web structure in this computation)[1]

c = distance measured from the neutral axis of the section area to the compression edge of the plate.

Stability of Thin, Flat Plates Under Combined Loading Conditions

In general, the skin or outer covering of the fuselage and wing surfaces are subjected to loads producing shear, compression, and bending stresses in the plane of their surfaces. At critical loads, the skin surfaces wrinkle (or buckle) causing aerodynamic disturbances due to surface roughness. From this occurrence, a redistribution of loads to more rigid members of the surrounding structure and increased deflections due to the buckled surfaces of these members are likely. To avoid the occurrence of such abnormalities, riveted aircraft structural panels are designed to be shear-resistant or nonbuckled at certain prescribed loading. This usually corresponds to limit or some percentage of limit load.

Interaction equations provide the means by which combined stress systems are analyzed. They enable the design engineer to substantiate a structure for a complex system of loads. Only the most common types of interaction equations are presented: those particular loading combinations most frequently occurring in actual aircraft structure. Figure 8-26 illustrates those common types for bending and shear, bending and axial compression, and shear and axial compression.

---

[1] Since the web is presumed to be shear-resistant at limit load, the web cross-sectional area is fully effective in bending. Of course, at higher loads, the web will buckle and therefore be less effective in bending. To account for this reduction in bending stiffness due to web buckling, the effective area of the web is normally considered. Effective area calculations of thin compression members that buckle under light loading are treated in Sec. 6-3.

TABLE 8-3 INTERACTION EQUATIONS FOR THE STABILITY OF PLATES UNDER COMBINED LOADING CONDITIONS

Type of Loading	Interaction Equation	Margin of Safety Equation	Ref.
Bending and Shear	$R_b^2 + R_s^2 = 1.0$	$\dfrac{1}{\sqrt{R_b^2 + R_s^2}} - 1$	Fig. 8-27
Bending and Axial Compression	$R_b^{1.75} + R_c = 1.0$	(Use the interaction curve on page 522.)	Fig. 8-28
Shear and Axial Compression	$R_c + R_s^2 = 1.0$	$\dfrac{2}{R_c + \sqrt{R_c^2 + 4R_s^2}} - 1$	Fig. 8-29

All terms in Table 8-3 are defined as stress ratios as follows:

$$R_c = \frac{f_c}{(F_c)_{cr}}, \quad R_s = \frac{f_s}{(F_s)_{cr}}, \text{ and } R_b = \frac{f_b}{(F_b)_{cr}}$$

where: $(F_c)_{cr}$ = critical buckling stress of a thin, flat plate member in pure compression (use Eq. 8-4, page 499, for this evaluation)

$(F_s)_{cr}$ = critical buckling stress of a thin, flat plate member in pure shear (use Eq. 8-5, page 500, for this evaluation)

$(F_b)_{cr}$ = critical buckling stress of a thin, flat plate member in pure bending (use Eq. 8-13, page 517, for this evaluation).

Note how each term above is expressed as a separate nondimensional ratio of the applied stresses f_c, f_s, and f_b to their corresponding allowable plate buckling stresses $(F_c)_{cr}$, $(F_s)_{cr}$, and $(F_b)_{cr}$, respectively. The applied stresses are defined as follows:

(1) $f_c = -\dfrac{P}{A}$ (axial compression stress, Eq. 2-2, page 57).

(2) $f_s = \dfrac{V}{h_e t}$ (average applied shearing stress, Eq. 8-1, page 480).

(3) $f_b = -\dfrac{Mc}{I_{na}}$ (compression bending stress at the supported edge of the included web of a beam, Eq. 2-5, page 63).

THIN, FLAT PLATES UNDER COMBINED LOADING CONDITIONS

TYPE OF LOADING	LOADING CONFIGURATION	REF.
Bending and Shear	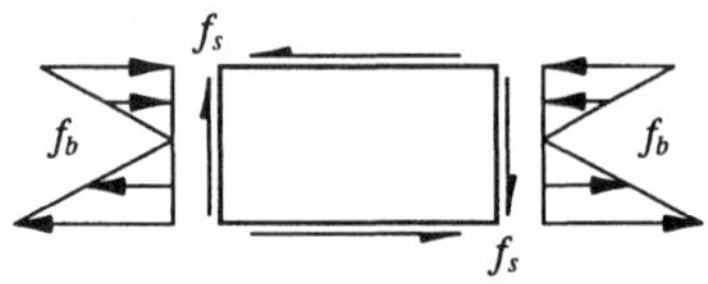	Fig. 8-27
Bending and Axial Compression	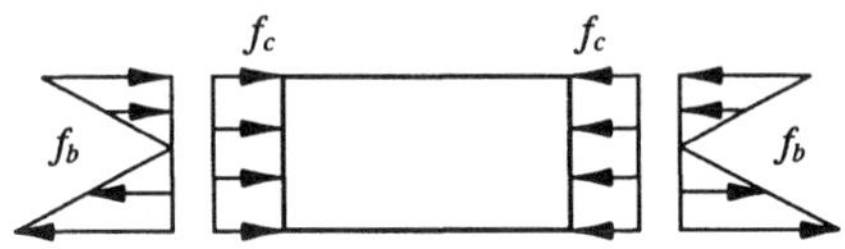	Fig. 8-28
Shear and Axial Compression	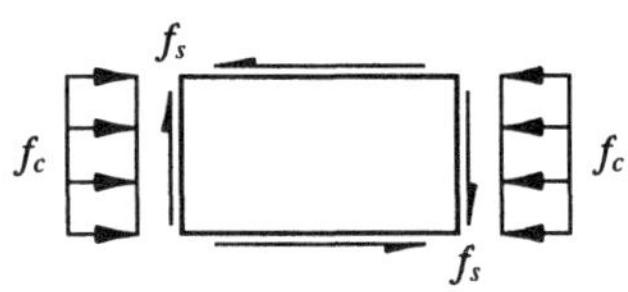	Fig. 8-29

FIGURE 8-26 Thin, flat plates under combined loading conditions.

Earlier treatment of panel buckling in this section emphasized the separate solutions of web instability of panels subjected to compression, shear, and bending. Rarely do such loading conditions occur in these purest of forms. For the most part, in real structure, combinations of standard loading types commonly occur. For this reason, interaction equations have been developed to determine solutions for their complex loading behavior (see Table 8-3). These equations will serve as a rapid design method for their solutions. This will provide a convenient way of determining the buckling stiffness of plates without the complexities of a rigorous analysis solution involved. Note that for each loading combination given in this table, a corresponding interaction curve can be drawn. These curves are used to design plate and panel structures for stability (and strength requirements) under combined loading conditions.

Interaction curves are determined by actual testing of plate members under combined loading conditions. Interaction formulas are derived from these tests by curve fitting of the test data from the tested structure. A simple plot of their stress ratios will reveal whether or not the plate members are shear-resistant for the prescribed loads intended. For example, if the stress ratios R_b and R_s, R_b and R_c, and R_c and R_s are plotted as interior points of their respective interaction design curves, their loading combinations will produce positive margins of safety; whereas, if the stress ratios are plotted as exterior points, their loading combinations will produce

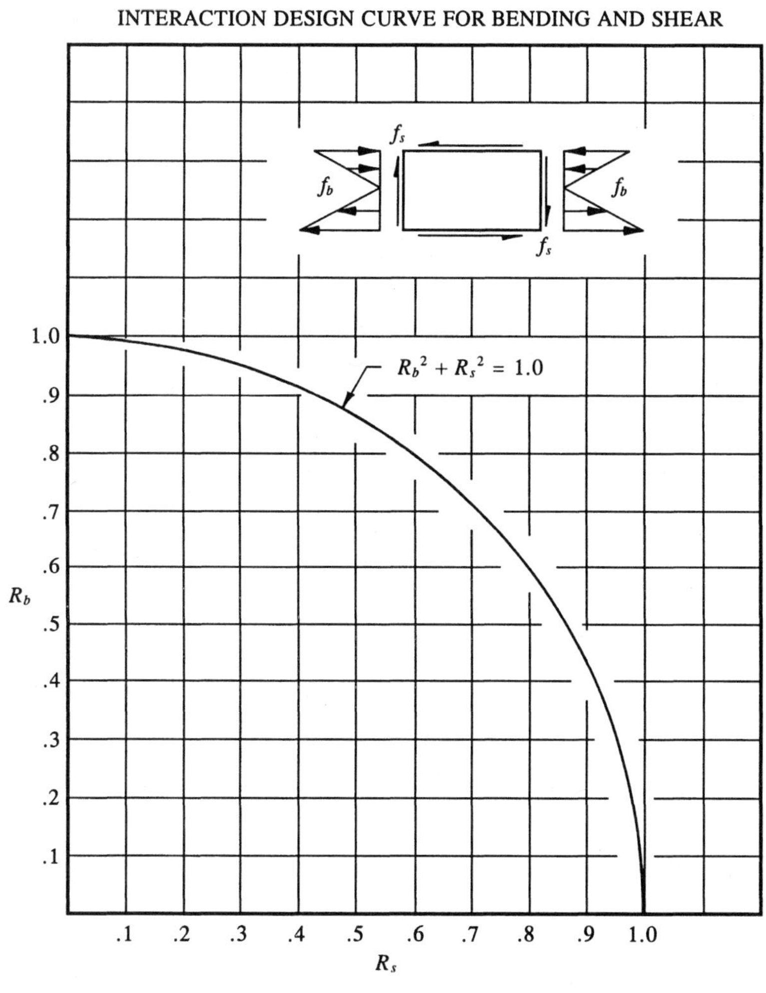

FIGURE 8-27 Stability of thin, flat plates in combined bending and shear.

negative margins of safety; on the other hand, if the stress ratios fall directly on the curve, the margins of safety are zero (0). The magnitude of these margins are determined mathematically from margin of safety expressions used to determine their specific values (refer to the second to last column of Table 8-3). If an expression is not given (for example, refer to the case for bending and axial compression in this table), a solution can always be arrived at graphically.[1] Moreover, an important point to keep in mind when designing for shear-resistant members—if limit shear is the criterion for panel buckling, then at ultimate load the panel must

[1] If this procedure is not familiar to the engineer, review the material presented in Chapter 5, Sec. 5.4 (see pages 347 and 348), for details and methodology of its graphical solution.

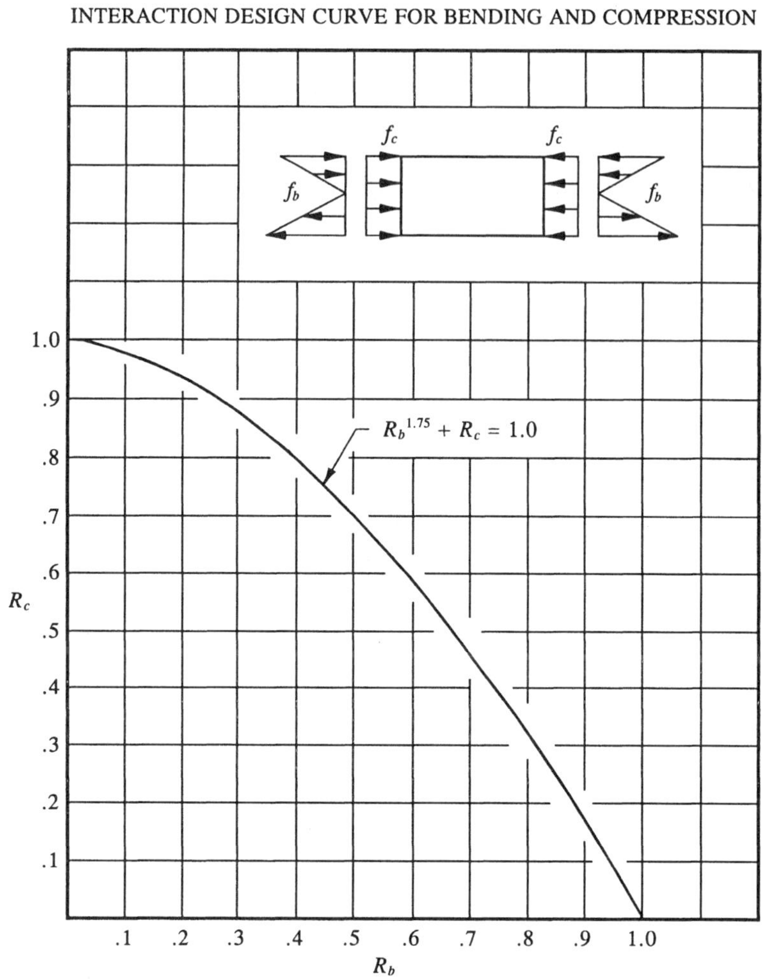

FIGURE 8-28 Stability of thin, flat plates in combined bending and compression.

be designed for combined loading effects (whether or not the panel actually buckles at these higher loads).

Designing for Ultimate Strength of Shear-Resistant Beams

Knowing whether the web of a beam is shear-resistant or not is not enough to determine the structural integrity of the web structure. Of equal importance in the design of these members is the determination of ultimate strength. A thorough knowledge and examination of this subject is essential to the design of shear-resistant panels. Unlike the buckled web of a beam that must be analyzed by

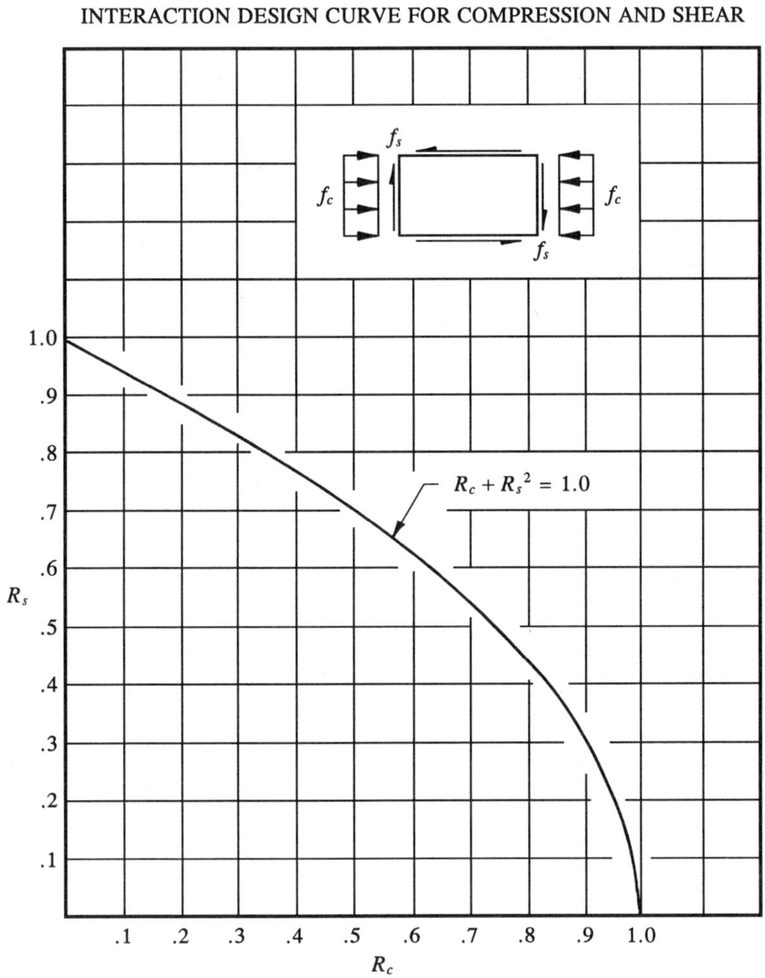

FIGURE 8-29 Stability of thin, flat plates in combined compression and shear.

diagonal tension-field analysis methods, a shear-resistant beam design is analyzed by conventional methods of stress analysis. Where they apply, these requirements will be referenced to particular sections or equations in this book. Actual numerical computations are performed for many example problems throughout the previous chapters of this book. The engineer is encouraged to again review specific examples in these chapters if certain topics presented which follow seem somewhat unfamiliar at first glance. The steps outlined in the following paragraphs will serve as a review or summary of the strength requirements needed to substantiate a shear-resistant web structure.

The actual stress analysis will not be performed. Instead, it is recommended that the engineer formulate in his mind a mental picture of the problem as it specifically correlates to the particular design phases of substantiation of the structure. Let these findings then be used to analyze other similar designs. This approach will provide the engineer with greater flexibility in solving most complex beam design problems. It will also provide the engineer with more efficient and productive use of his engineering time. After a clear and precise understanding of the entire problem has been formulated mentally, then the actual stress analysis solution can be performed with a greater sense of confidence and self-determination. Let us begin this review.

(1) Calculate the maximum shearing stress $(f_s)_{max}$ at the neutral axis of the beam using the shear stress equation.

$$(f_s)_{max} = \frac{VQ}{I_{na}\, t} \quad \text{(for definition of terms, refer back to Eq. 4-2, page 227).}$$

(2) Determine the net shearing stress along the web rivets of the upper and lower beam cap members. Then compare these values with the ultimate allowable shearing stress F_{su} of each material.

$$(f_s)_{net} = \frac{q}{t}\left[\frac{s}{s - D}\right]$$

where: $q = VQ/I_{na}$ (from Eq. 4-3, page 227)
s = fastener spacing
D = fastener diameter (for rivets, use the nominal hole diameter)
t = web or flange thickness.

(3) Check the beam compression caps for crippling as well as column failures. (Refer to the analysis methods in Chapters 6 and 7, respectively.)

a. For shallow beams, use an Mc/I_{na} stress distribution for their designs.
b. For deep beams, use an $(M/H)/A$ stress distribution for their designs.

(4) Check for shearing failure of the flange-to-web rivets and bearing failure of the web and beam cap members:

a. Shearing failure of the flange-to-web rivets:

$$\text{Margin of Safety} = \text{M.S.} = \frac{P_{su}}{p_s\, k} - 1$$

where the terms in this expression are defined in Chapter 3 (refer specifically to Eq. 3-1, page 145).

b. Bearing failure of the web and beam cap members:

$$\text{Margin of Safety} = \text{M.S.} = \frac{P_{bru}}{p_s k} - 1$$

where the terms in this expression are defined in Chapter 3 (refer specifically to Eqs. 3-2 and 3-3 on pages 151 and 152, respectively).

(5) Determine the ultimate bending stresses across the beam cross-sectional area. Tension stresses are compared to the ultimate allowable tension stress F_{tu} of the material, while compression stresses are compared to the appropriate compression allowables for strength and instability failures (see 3 above).

$$f_b = \pm \frac{Mc}{I_{na}} \quad \text{(for definition of terms, refer to Eq. 2-5, page 63).}$$

8.5 Stability of Thin, Curved Sheets or Plates in Compression, Shear, and in Combined Compression and Shear. Compression buckling and shear buckling acting separately or in combination will be the main loading types considered for curved panel designs in this section. The surfaces of the fuselage and wing represent curved panels subjected to aerodynamic forces during flight and landing conditions. The fuselage is stiffened by longitudinal stringers and transverse frames to support the thin shell of the fuselage under load. The wing surface is likewise supported by longitudinal stringers and transverse ribs. Without these stiffening members to help reinforce the thin panels formed by the intersection of these members, the skin surfaces would buckle dramatically at extremely low stresses. With the structural panel securely attached around its boundaries, the panel becomes considerably stiffer and less likely to exhibit permanent set from oil-canning caused by excessive deformations of the buckled structure. As load is gradually applied to the stiffened panel, the middle portion of the panel will buckle but the panel will not fail (refer back to Fig. 8-6). Some redistribution of load occurs at this time—causing the surrounding structure to increase in load while the panel sustains the portion of load which caused it to initially buckle. Panel buckling essentially converts the internal shearing stresses of the panel into diagonal tension stresses. These stresses then induce compression into the stiffeners and bending, if a beam structure, into the main cap members. Failure occurs when the composite structure (including the panel) fails simultaneously at ultimate load from diagonal-tension effects.

Stability of Thin, Curved Plate Members in Pure Shear

A flat panel can be stiffened merely by bending its width or length to a prescribed curvature. The greater the curvature, the more resistant the curved sheet will be to initial buckling, and therefore the higher resistance to shear buckling it

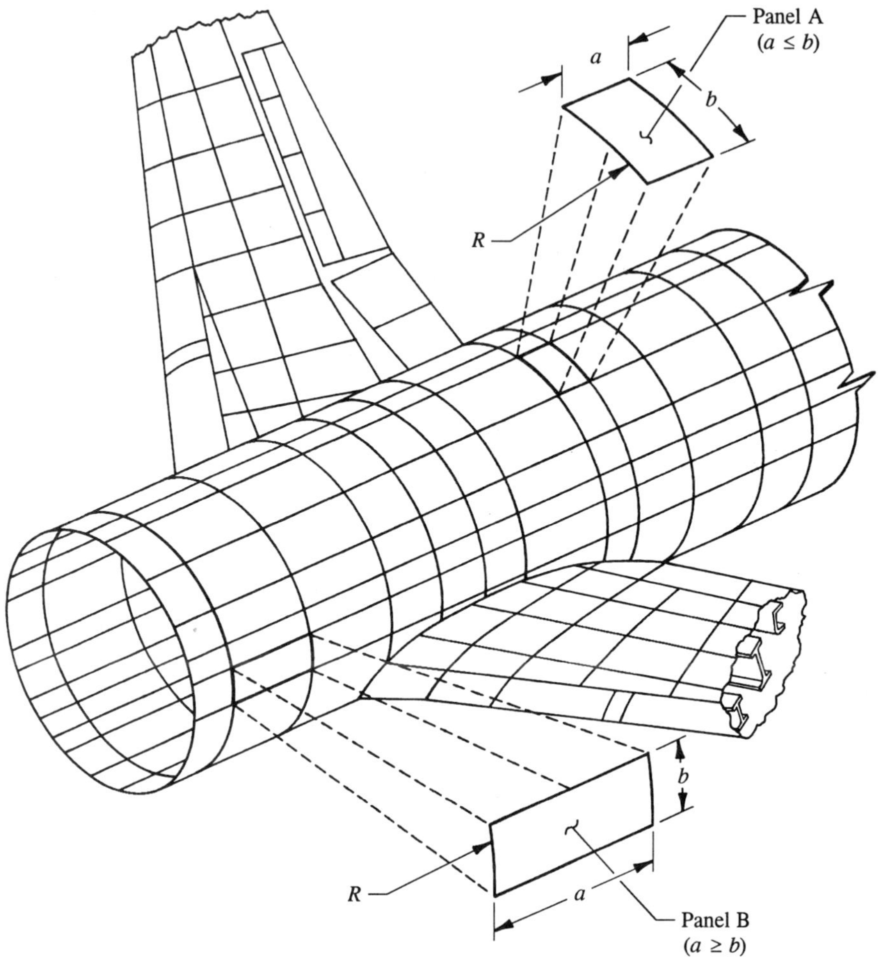

FIGURE 8-30 Curved fuselage panels.

will become. The main emphasis of this section is to determine the stresses which cause curved panels to initially buckle (the point at which the panel loses its ability to remain shear-resistant). A shear-resistant structure, the web of a deep beam, the skin panels of a wing or fuselage, simply prevents the original shape of the structure from visible signs of deformation. Internal strains do occur however, but their effects are minimal as far as instability of the structure is concerned.

Consider the curved fuselage panels in the exploded views of Fig. 8-30. By definition, a = the linear distance of the straight side of the plate and b = the circumferential distance of the curved edge of the plate. The critical buckling stresses for panels A and B in pure shear are expressed by the following equations depending on whether $a \le b$ or $a \ge b$:

For panel A ($a \leq b$):

$$\frac{(F_s)_{cr}}{\eta_s} = \frac{\pi^2 K_s E_c}{12(1-\mu^2)}\left[\frac{t}{a}\right]^2 \tag{8-14}$$

where: K_s = shear buckling stress coefficient from Fig. 8-31
η_s = plasticity correction factor for plates in pure shear
μ = Poisson's ratio (physical constant of the material found in the mechanical-property tables of MIL-HDBK-5)
a = linear distance of the straight side of the plate
E_c = elastic or Young's modulus of elasticity in compression
t = web or panel thickness.

The shear buckling coefficient K_s is a function of the plate dimensions (i.e., aspect ratio a/b), edge-support conditions, and curvature of the plate. Before its value can be determined for panel A, the following equation for the curvature parameter Z must be solved for:

$$Z = \frac{a^2}{Rt}\sqrt{1-\mu^2} \tag{8-15}$$

where: a = linear distance of the straight side of the plate
μ = Poisson's ratio (as defined in Eq. 8-14)
R = radius of curvature
t = web or panel thickness.

Now, with the curvature parameter Z and the aspect ratio a/b known for panel A, the shear buckling coefficient K_s may be read directly from Fig. 8-31. Similarly, we obtain:

For panel B ($a \geq b$):

$$\frac{(F_s)_{cr}}{\eta_s} = \frac{\pi^2 K_s E_c}{12(1-\mu^2)}\left[\frac{t}{b}\right]^2 \tag{8-16}$$

where: K_s = shear buckling stress coefficient from Fig. 8-32
η_s = plasticity correction factor for plates in pure shear
μ = Poisson's ratio (physical constant of the material found in the mechanical-property tables of MIL-HDBK-5)
b = circumferential distance of the curved edge of the plate
E_c = elastic or Young's modulus of elasticity in compression
t = web or panel thickness.

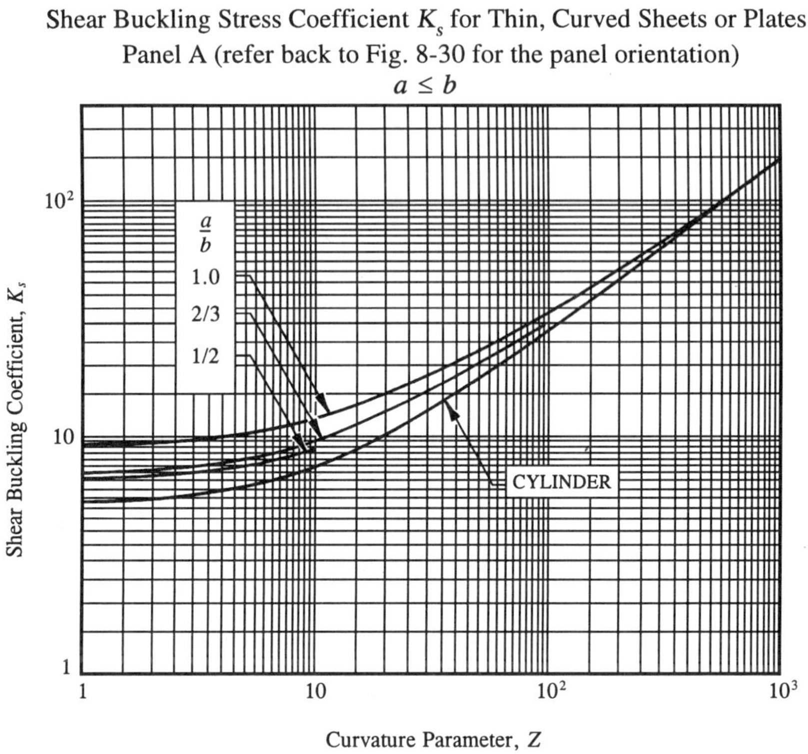

FIGURE 8-31 Shear buckling stress coefficient K_s for thin, curved, simply-supported sheets or plates.

Before the shear buckling coefficient K_s for panel B can be determined, the following equation for the curvature parameter Z must be solved for:

$$Z = \frac{b^2}{Rt}\sqrt{1 - \mu^2} \tag{8-17}$$

where: b = circumferential distance of the curved edge of the plate
μ = Poisson's ratio (as defined in Eq. 8-16)
R = radius of curvature
t = web or panel thickness.

The shear buckling equations (Eqs. 8-14 and 8-16) represent the "theoretical" buckling stress $(F_s)_{cr}/\eta_s$ of curved panels in pure shear. To determine their "true" values, or $(F_s)_{cr}$, the plasticity correction factor η_s must be evaluated for each design solution. For stresses within the elastic range of a stress-strain diagram, η_s is 1.0. However, if stresses exceed the proportional limit of the material, the material goes plastic and the plate undergoes a reduction in bending stiffness. This reduction is accounted for by the plasticity correction factor η_s. Although its actual numerical value is now less than 1.0, its value need not be calculated directly if the following procedure is used to determine its true value:

(1) Begin the analysis by calculating the theoretical shear buckling stress $(F_s)_{cr}/\eta_s$ of the plate using either Eq. 8-14 or 8-16 depending on whether $a \leq b$ or $a \geq b$, respectively.

(2) From the general stress relationship that exists between tension and shear,[1] an analogous relationship for the theoretical compression buckling stress of a plate in terms of its corresponding theoretical shear buckling stress is formulated. Solve for this value.

$$\frac{(F_c)_{cr}}{\eta_c} = \frac{(F_s)_{cr}}{\eta_s}\sqrt{3}\,.$$

(3) With the value of $(F_c)_{cr}/\eta_c$, enter a compression plasticity correction curve, $(F_c)_{cr}/\eta_c$ vs. $(F_c)_{cr}$, for a specific material and determine the true compression buckling stress of the plate or $(F_c)_{cr}$. Such a curve is shown in Fig. 8-15 for clad 2024-T3 sheet (QQ-A-250/5) at room-temperature. For curves of other material types, the engineer should consult an aerospace company structures manual.

(4) Divide the value of $(F_c)_{cr}$ obtained in step 3 by $\sqrt{3}$.

$$(F_s)_{cr} = \frac{(F_c)_{cr}}{\sqrt{3}}\,.$$

Hence, the true shear buckling stress $(F_s)_{cr}$ of the plate is arrived at without having to determine the value of η_s from established shear plasticity correction curves for specific material types.

Instability of the plate in pure shear is predicted as follows:

$$\text{Margin of Safety} = \text{M.S.} = \frac{(F_s)_{cr}}{f_s} - 1$$

where: $(F_s)_{cr}$ = critical buckling stress of a thin, flat plate member in pure shear

$f_s = \dfrac{q}{t}$ = average applied shearing stress

q = average applied panel shear flow (for beams, use $q = V/h_e$)

V = applied web vertical shear force

---

[1] For most ductile materials, the allowable yield shearing stress F_{sy} can be conveniently expressed in terms of the allowable tensile yield stress F_{ty} of the material (refer back to page 502).

Shear Buckling Stress Coefficient K_s for Thin, Curved Sheets or Plates
Panel B (refer back to Fig. 8-30 for the panel orientation)
$a \geq b$

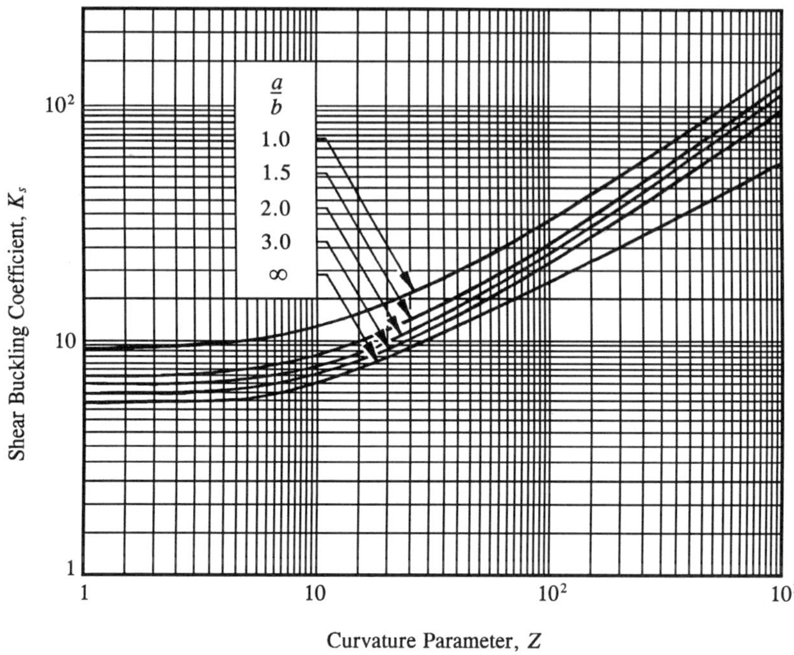

FIGURE 8-32 Shear buckling stress coefficient K_s for thin, curved, simply-supported sheets or plates.

t = web or panel thickness
h_e = effective depth of the beam measured between cap centroids (neglect the effective web area, see Fig. 8-2).

As a first approximation to the analysis of a curved panel: consider idealizing such a member as a flat panel. This assumption would of course depend on the degree of curvature of the panel and on its intended application for design. Since a curved panel is somewhat stiffer than a flat panel, a flat panel analysis of a curved panel will always be conservative. The degree of conservatism will depend upon the amount of curvature neglected for the curved panel. In most cases, a flat panel analysis is perfectly justified in those cases where the degree of curvature is large. Here, the panel (with the large curvature) becomes less stiff, and ultimately approaches that of a flat panel design. Conversely, though, as the curvature of the panel is increased, for example, the leading-edge (L.E.) surfaces of a wing, a flat panel analysis there would be too conservative for practical design, and therefore would produce an undesirable weight penalty for the leading-edge (L.E.) curved

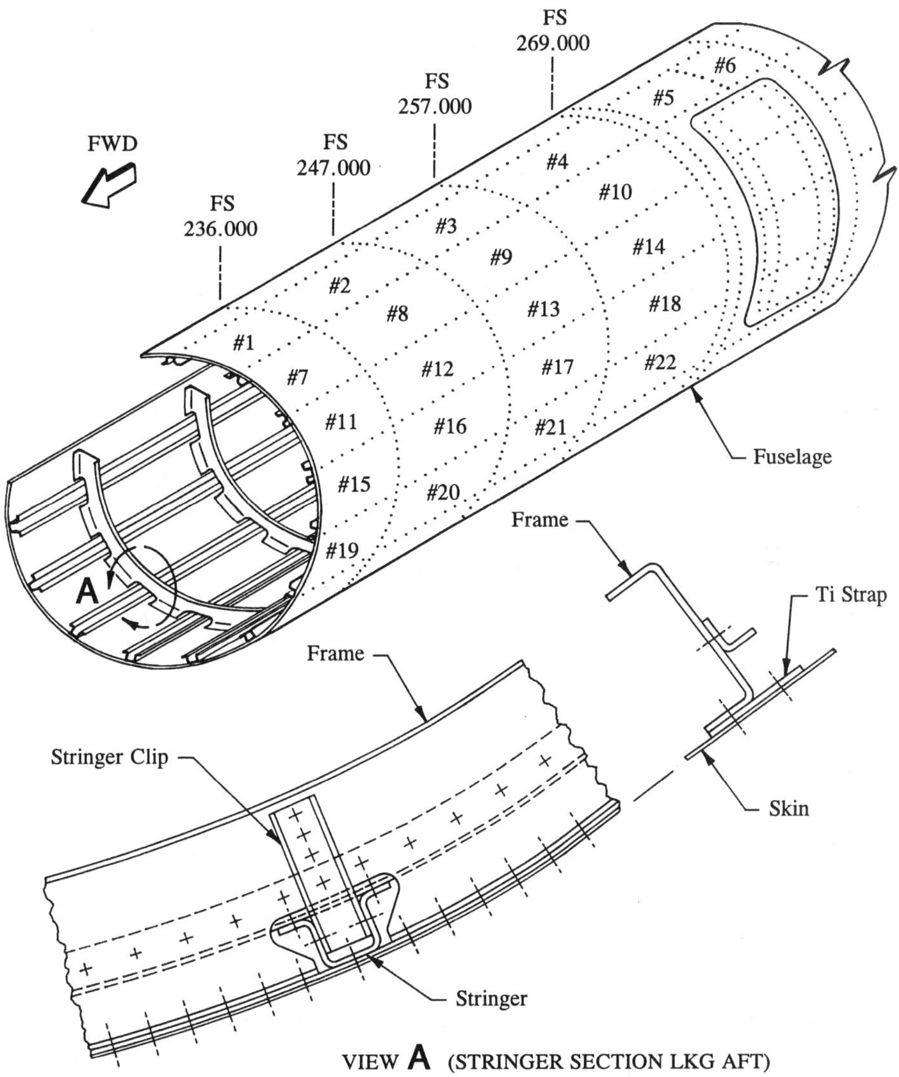

FIGURE 8-33 Structural arrangement of main members of a stiffened fuselage shell.

panels of the wing. And for this reason, a curved panel analysis would be required for these panels.

Example 8-3 The fuselage structure of Fig. 8-33 is critical for fuselage up-bending. A partial summary of skin shear flows for this structure is shown in Fig. 8-34. Panel shear flows are indicated for this structure in lb/in limit. (a) Provide an .016 in steel reinforcement (301 stainless steel, 1/2 hard) for panel #12 to prevent the fuselage skin from buckling at limit load. Perform a flat panel analysis for this structure first and then compare the results obtained from this solution with that of a curved panel analysis. (Use a fuselage diameter of 145 in.) The fuselage shell is constructed of .071 in clad 2024-T3 aluminum alloy sheet material (QQ-A250/5). Assume simply-supported edges for the reinforced panel. Along with the above panel analysis, what other structural checks must be made to substantiate the panel shear-resistant at limit load?

SOLUTION: The analysis of the fuselage shell is normally based on the assumption that skin curvature of the fuselage is essentially flat. In keeping with this assumption, let us now perform a flat panel analysis of panel #12 for dissimilar materials. After this analysis is completed, a curved panel analysis of the same panel structure with dissimilar materials will be performed and the results compared.

Flat Plate Analysis of a Reinforced Panel of Dissimilar Materials (Panel #12):

When a flat panel is reinforced by another flat panel of dissimilar material,[1] the plate combination must be designed somewhat differently. Its solution is arrived at by modifying the shear buckling equation (Eq. 8-5) in a slightly different format. The physical constants E_c and μ in this equation are replaced in terms of equivalent values, denoted by the quantities $(E_c)_{eq}$ and μ_{eq}, respectively. Hence, the buckling strength of a flat plate combination of dissimilar materials can be mathematically expressed by the following equation:

$$\frac{(F_s)_{cr}}{\eta_s} = \frac{\pi^2 K_s (E_c)_{eq}}{12(1 - \mu_{eq}^2)} \left[\frac{t}{b}\right]^2 \qquad \textbf{(8-18)}$$

where: K_s = shear buckling stress coefficient from Fig. 8-18
η_s = plasticity correction factor for plates in pure shear
μ_{eq} = equivalent Poisson's ratio
b = shorter dimension of the plate (see footnote on page 501)
$(E_c)_{eq}$ = equivalent elastic or Young's modulus of elasticity in compression
t = total thickness of the composite panel (this includes the thickness of the panel reinforcement).

For this solution, b = 7.7 in, a = 11.0 in, and t = .087 in. Therefore a/b = 1.43, and, from Fig. 8-18 (page 503), Curve B, K_s = 7.3. Or, this constant can be determined from Eq. 8-8 for simply-supported edges of the panel:

[1] Flat reinforced plates of similar materials in pure shear with simply-supported edges are designed by the method of analysis presented in Sec. 8.4 using conventional flat plate analysis. Such a solution is illustrated in Example 8-2 (see page 508).

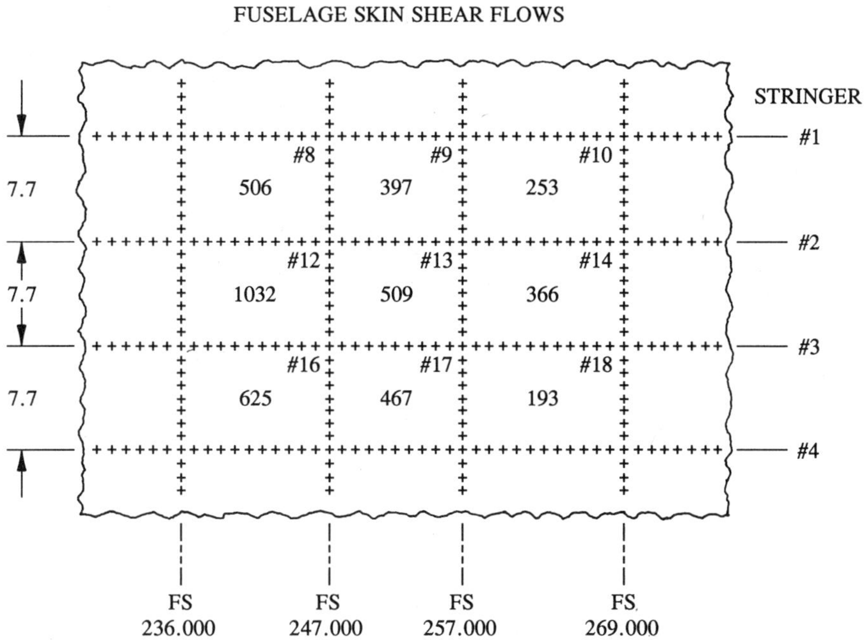

FIGURE 8-34 Summary of skin shear flows for the fuselage shell.

$$K_s = 5.34 + 4.00\left[\frac{b}{a}\right]^2 = 5.34 + 4.00\left[\frac{7.7}{11.0}\right]^2 = 7.30.$$

Equivalent Plate Physical Properties $(E_c)_{eq}$ and μ_{eq}:

To determine the equivalent physical properties of the composite plates (fuselage skin plus reinforcement), a weighted-average stiffness of the separate members is taken. It should be recalled from the critical shear buckling equation, Eq. 8-5, that instability (or buckling) of a plate is independent of the strength properties of the plate material. This can be seen from the fact that no strength terms appear in this expression. Hence, buckling, it can be said, is dependent on the stiffness properties of the plate members. And from this reasoning, the following equations have been formulated to determine the combined stiffness of these members:

$$(E_c)_{eq} = \frac{E_{\text{steel}}\, t_{\text{steel}} + E_{\text{alum}}\, t_{\text{alum}}}{t} \tag{8-19}$$

where: $(E_c)_{eq}$ = equivalent elastic compression modulus of elasticity
E_{steel} = elastic or Young's modulus of elasticity in compression for steel
E_{alum} = elastic or Young's modulus of elasticity in compression for aluminum

t_{steel} = thickness of the steel reinforcement
t_{alum} = thickness of the aluminum skin
t = combined thickness of the aluminum skin and stainless steel reinforcement.

$$G_{eq} = \frac{G_{\text{steel}}\, t_{\text{steel}} + G_{\text{alum}}\, t_{\text{alum}}}{t} \tag{8-20}$$

where: G_{eq} = equivalent elastic shear modulus of elasticity
G_{steel} = elastic shear modulus of elasticity for steel
G_{alum} = elastic shear modulus of elasticity for aluminum
t_{steel} = thickness of the steel reinforcement
t_{alum} = thickness of the aluminum skin
t = combined thickness of the aluminum skin and stainless steel reinforcement.

From MIL-HDBK-5F, we find $E_{\text{steel}} = 26.0 \times 10^6$ psi and $G_{\text{steel}} = 10.5 \times 10^6$ psi for the stainless steel material. For the aluminum material, $E_{\text{alum}} = 10.7 \times 10^6$ psi, but G_{alum} is not given. To obtain its value, we can use the following relationship for elastic stress design:

$$G = \frac{E}{2(1 + \mu)} \tag{8-21}$$

where: G = elastic shear modulus of elasticity
E = elastic or Young's modulus of elasticity in compression or tension
μ = Poisson's ratio.

Substituting $E_c = 10.7 \times 10^6$ psi and $\mu = .33$ in this equation, we obtain the shear modulus of elasticity for the fuselage skin, or

$$G_{\text{alum}} = \frac{10.7 \times 10^6}{2(1 + .33)} = 4.02 \times 10^6 \text{ psi.}$$

In terms of equivalent physical properties of the composite plate members, Eq. 8-21 becomes:

$$\mu_{eq} = \frac{E_{eq}}{2\, G_{eq}} - 1. \tag{8-22}$$

The application of Eqs. 8-19 and 8-20 determines the values of E_{eq} and G_{eq}, respectively, which are then substituted in Eq. 8-22 to find μ_{eq}.

$$(E_c)_{eq} = \frac{E_{steel}\,t_{steel} + E_{alum}\,t_{alum}}{t}$$

$$(E_c)_{eq} = \frac{\left[26.0 \text{ x } 10^6(.016) + 10.7 \text{ x } 10^6(.071)\right]}{.016 + .071} = 13.514 \text{ x } 10^6 \text{ psi.}$$

$$G_{eq} = \frac{G_{steel}\,t_{steel} + G_{alum}\,t_{alum}}{t}$$

$$G_{eq} = \frac{\left[10.5 \text{ x } 10^6(.016) + 4.02 \text{ x } 10^6(.071)\right]}{.016 + .071} = 5.212 \text{ x } 10^6 \text{ psi.}$$

Substituting these values in Eq. 8-22 gives:

$$\mu_{eq} = \frac{E_{eq}}{2\,G_{eq}} - 1 = \frac{13.514 \text{ x } 10^6}{2(5.212 \text{ x } 10^6)} - 1 = .30$$

where: $E_{eq} = (E_c)_{eq} = 13.514 \text{ x } 10^6$ psi
$G_{eq} = 5.212 \text{ x } 10^6$ psi.

The theoretical shear buckling stress of the composite plates are then found by substituting all values into the shear buckling equation, Eq. 8-18, or

$$\frac{(F_s)_{cr}}{\eta_s} = \frac{\pi^2 K_s (E_c)_{eq}}{12(1 - \mu_{eq}^2)}\left[\frac{t}{b}\right]^2$$

$$\frac{(F_s)_{cr}}{\eta_s} = \frac{\pi^2(7.30)(13.514 \text{ x } 10^6)}{12\left[1 - (.30)^2\right]}\left[\frac{.016 + .071}{7.7}\right]^2 = 11,383 \text{ psi.}$$

Using the general stress relationship between compression buckling and shear buckling,[1] we obtain:

$$\frac{(F_c)_{cr}}{\eta_c} = \frac{(F_s)_{cr}}{\eta_s}\sqrt{3} = 11,383\sqrt{3} = 19,716 \text{ psi.}$$

With this value, enter a compression plasticity correction curve, $(F_c)_{cr}/\eta_c$ vs. $(F_c)_{cr}$, for clad 2024-T3 aluminum alloy sheet and determine the value of $(F_c)_{cr}$ (use Fig. 8-15). It can be seen from this curve that η_c is 1.0. And so, since this corresponds to the elastic range of stresses, the value of $(F_c)_{cr}$ is also 19,716 psi. The true shear buckling stress is then obtained by dividing this value by $\sqrt{3}$. Hence

$$(F_s)_{cr} = \frac{(F_c)_{cr}}{\sqrt{3}} = \frac{19,716}{\sqrt{3}} = 11,383 \text{ psi.}$$

---

[1] Refer to Eq. 8-6 on page 502.

Stability of the plate combination is then predicted by comparing this value with the applied limit shearing stress f_s of panel #12:

$$\text{Margin of Safety} = \text{M.S.} = \frac{(F_s)_{cr}}{f_s} - 1 = \frac{11,383}{11,862} - 1$$

$\text{M.S.} = -.04$ (flat panel analysis of the fuselage shell)

where: $(F_s)_{cr} = 11,383$ psi
$f_s = q/t = 1,032/.087 = 11,862$ psi limit
$q = 1{,}032$ lb/in limit (skin shear flow for panel #12, see Fig. 8-34)
$t = .016 + .071 = .087$ in (combined thickness of both plate members).

A negative margin of safety results. Instead of increasing the thickness of the steel reinforcement and bumping the contour of the fuselage skin further, the plates will be analyzed as composite curved panels. Hopefully, this additional refinement of the analysis will help to increase the allowable (or shear buckling stress) of these members to an acceptable value sufficient to prevent the redesign (increase in thickness) of the reinforcement.

Curved Plate Analysis of a Reinforced Panel of Dissimilar Materials (Panel #12):

When a curved panel is reinforced by another curved panel of dissimilar material, the plate combination of their design must be investigated somewhat differently than a flat panel design of dissimilar materials (previously). Their solutions for buckling strength may be written in equivalent form by modifying Eqs. 8-16 and 8-17 to account for their composite behavior. The physical constants E_c and μ in these equations are replaced in terms of equivalent values. These are denoted by the quantities $(E_c)_{eq}$ and μ_{eq}, respectively. This provides the general theory for the buckling strength of curved plate combinations of dissimilar materials. And thus, from this, the structural tendency of these members to buckle as a unit can be mathematically formulated:

For panel #12 ($a \geq b$):

$$\frac{(F_s)_{cr}}{\eta_s} = \frac{\pi^2 K_s (E_c)_{eq}}{12(1 - \mu_{eq}^2)}\left[\frac{t}{b}\right]^2 \qquad \textbf{(8-23)}$$

where: K_s = shear buckling stress coefficient from Fig. 8-32
η_s = plasticity correction factor for plates in pure shear
μ_{eq} = equivalent Poisson's ratio (see Eq. 8-22)
b = circumferential distance of the curved edge of the plate

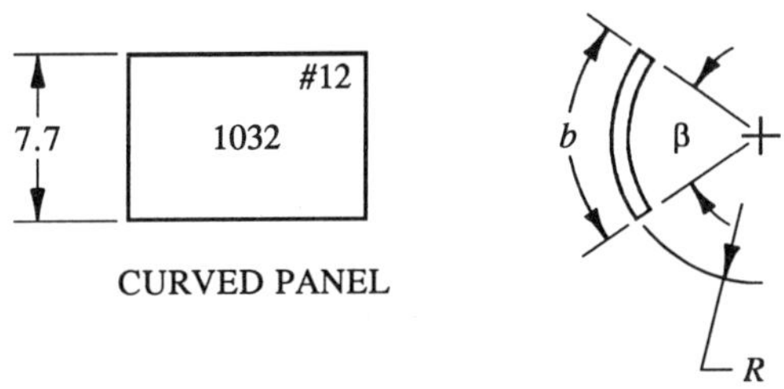

From trigonometry:

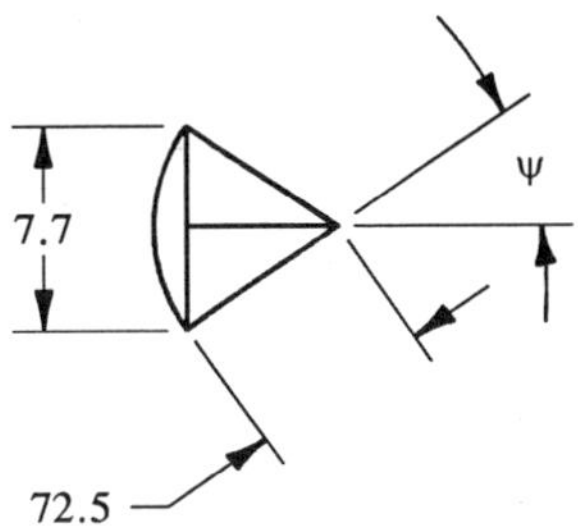

$$\sin \psi = \frac{7.7/2}{72.5} = .0531$$

$$\psi = 3.044°$$

$$2\psi = \beta = 6.088°$$

FIGURE 8-35 Circumferential distance of a curved panel.

$(E_c)_{eq}$ = equivalent elastic or Young's modulus of elasticity in compression
t = total thickness of the composite panel (this also includes the thickness of the panel reinforcement).

$$Z = \frac{b^2}{Rt}\sqrt{1 - \mu_{eq}^2} \tag{8-24}$$

where: b = circumferential distance of the curved edge of the plate
μ_{eq} = equivalent Poisson's ratio (see Eq. 8-22)
R = radius of curvature
t = total thickness of the composite panel (this also includes the thickness of the panel reinforcement).

Before solving Eqs. 8-23 and 8-24, let us determine the circumferential distance b of the panel. This value, as shown in Fig. 8-35, is determined from the following equation (see mensuration formula in a mathematics textbook for the length of an arc of a circle for an included angle β):

$$b = R\beta$$

where: b = circumferential distance of the panel (in)
R = radius of the panel (in)
β = included angle of the panel (rad).

Hence

$$b = R\beta = 72.5(.106) = 7.685 \text{ in}$$

where: $R = D/2 = 145/2 = 72.5$ in
$D = 145$ in (fuselage diameter, see page 532)
$\beta = 6.088^\circ \left(\frac{\pi}{180^\circ}\right) = .10626$ rad.

Next, the critical shear buckling stress $(F_s)_{cr}$ is found by first determining the curvature parameter Z from Eq. 8-24. Hence

$$Z = \frac{b^2}{Rt}\sqrt{1 - \mu_{eq}^2} = \frac{(7.685)^2}{72.5(.087)}\sqrt{1 - (.30)^2} = 8.93$$

where: $b = 7.685$ in
$\mu_{eq} = .30$ (calculated value from page 535)
$R = 72.5$ in (from $D/2 = 72.5$ in, where D is the fuselage diameter)
$t = .016 + .071 = .087$ in (combined thickness of both plate members).

With this value and $a/b = 11.0/7.685 = 1.43$, enter Fig. 8-32 and find the shear buckling coefficient for the plate combination, $K_s = 8.9$. Now, the solution of Eq. 8-23 is applied as follows:

$$\frac{(F_s)_{cr}}{\eta_s} = \frac{\pi^2 K_s (E_c)_{eq}}{12(1 - \mu_{eq}^2)}\left[\frac{t}{b}\right]^2$$

$$\frac{(F_s)_{cr}}{\eta_s} = \frac{\pi^2 (8.9)\, 13.514 \text{ x } 10^6}{12\left[1 - (.30)^2\right]}\left[\frac{.087}{7.685}\right]^2 = 13,932 \text{ psi}.$$

From Eqs. 8-5 and 8-6 and Fig. 8-15, it can be logically reasoned that theoretical shear buckling stresses $(F_s)_{cr}/\eta_s$ are elastic and therefore the plasticity correction factor η_s is 1.0. Which then also follows that

$$(F_s)_{cr} = 13,932 \text{ psi}.$$

Stability of the plate combination is then predicted by comparing this value with the applied limit shearing stress f_s of panel #12 (see page 536):

$$\text{Margin of Safety} = \text{M.S.} = \frac{(F_s)_{cr}}{f_s} - 1 = \frac{13,932}{11,862} - 1$$

M.S. = + .17 (curved panel analysis of the fuselage shell).

This result proves conclusively that a curved panel has a greater stiffness than a flat panel configuration for the same size and thickness of panel, type of loading, and material selection. Remarkably, the curved panel analysis has a positive margin of safety of 17% for the same reinforced panel, which presumes that the .016 in steel reinforcement is adequately field riveted to panel #12 to be satisfactory for its actual design use as a reinforcement (this is left as an exercise for the engineer to complete). And thus, we have avoided an increase in the thickness of the reinforcement that would have been required if the results obtained from the flat panel analysis (M.S. = − .04) would have instead been used to needlessly improve (beef up) this design. Comparing shear buckling allowables from the flat panel analysis and that of the curved panel analysis, we find that the curved panel is, as would be expected, stiffer. This would of course be anticipated for a curved panel by the very nature of its more efficient structural shape. The increase in stiffness is measured as follows:

$$\% \text{ Increase} = \frac{13,932 - 11,383}{11,383}(100) = 22.4\ \%$$

where: $(F_s)_{cr}$ = 11,383 psi (critical buckling stress for panel #12, analyzed as if it were a flat reinforced panel)

$(F_s)_{cr}$ = 13,932 psi (critical buckling stress for panel #12, analyzed as a curved reinforced panel).

For the curvature of the fuselage shell given, the critical shear buckling stress of the reinforced panel is actually 22.4% greater for a curved panel analysis than for a similar flat panel analysis of that same structure. Or, quite simply, one could say that the curved panel is 22.4% stiffer. In any case, the results are good. In general, the greater the radius of curvature for a panel, the less stiff the panel becomes, approaching that of a flat panel when the radius of that member becomes infinite.

Design of Field Rivets for Curved Reinforced Panels of Dissimilar Materials

Proper field riveting of a reinforcement is essential to the correct analysis of a curved reinforced panel of dissimilar materials. It was shown in Sec. 8.4 that to consider the reinforcement as an effective member of the reinforced panel, a sufficient number and size of field rivets must be provided.[1] The criterion of no buckling at ultimate load forms the basis for the determination of the proper field riveting for the reinforcement. This criterion was established in Sec. 8.4 for flat panels; likewise, it should also prove quite reliable and satisfactory to use for curved panels.

There is essentially no difference between the method of attack of a flat reinforced panel and that of a curved reinforced panel. The required stiffness of the

[1] The engineer is referred to Example 8-2 for specific details of how to analyze and design for field rivets of a flat reinforced panel (specifically, see page 512).

boundary members of the plate structure must also be verified for the panel to be shear-resistant as predicted by the foregoing analysis. Additionally, like most problems of this type, in actual structure, the above analysis assumes that (1) the boundary members are of sufficient stiffness to prevent panel buckling of the reinforced panel and (2) inter-rivet buckling along compression riveted members is prevented. Hence, if these additional requirements to the above analysis are substantiated, the reinforced panel of dissimilar materials can be considered shear-resistant at limit load.

Stability of Thin, Curved Plate Members in Pure Compression

The critical buckling stress of a thin, curved plate member in pure compression is expressed by the following equation:

$$\frac{(F_c)_{cr}}{\eta_c} = \frac{\pi^2 K_c E_c}{12(1-\mu^2)}\left[\frac{t}{b}\right]^2 \qquad \textbf{(8-25)}$$

where: K_c = compression buckling stress coefficient from Fig. 8-36
η_c = plasticity correction factor for plates in pure compression
μ = Poisson's ratio (physical constant of the material found in the mechanical-property tables of MIL-HDBK-5)
b = circumferential distance of the curved edge of the plate (this also corresponds to the loaded edges of the plate)
E_c = elastic or Young's modulus of elasticity in compression
t = web or panel thickness.

In this form, this equation represents the "theoretical" buckling stress $(F_c)_{cr}/\eta_c$ of a curved panel in pure compression. To determine its "true" value, the plasticity correction factor η_c must be determined. Plasticity correction factors for curved panels are the same as those used for flat panels. In general, a curved panel is much stiffer than a flat panel and therefore its behavior is more likely to experience inelastic than elastic buckling in its full range of loading. When critical buckling stresses occur in the elastic range of a stress-strain diagram, the plasticity correction factor is 1.0. However, if stresses exceed the proportional limit of the material, the material goes plastic and the plate undergoes a reduction in bending stiffness. This reduction is accounted for by the plasticity correction factor η_c. Although its actual numerical value is now less than 1.0, its value need not be calculated directly if the following procedure is used to determine its true value:

(1) Begin by calculating the theoretical compression buckling stress $(F_c)_{cr}/\eta_c$ of the plate using Eq. 8-25.

(2) With the value of $(F_c)_{cr}/\eta_c$, enter a compression plasticity correction curve, $(F_c)_{cr}/\eta_c$ vs. $(F_c)_{cr}$, for a specific material and determine the true

Compression Buckling Stress Coefficient K_c for Thin, Curved Sheets or Plates

$a/b > .5$

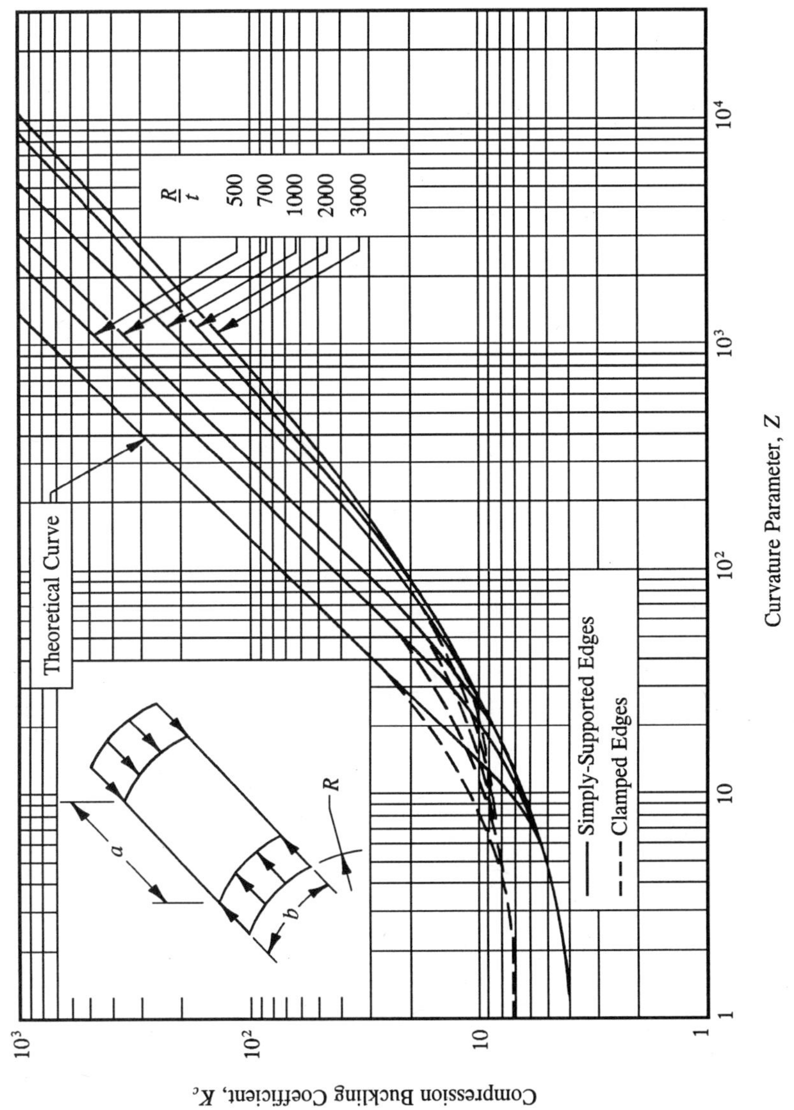

FIGURE 8-36 Compression buckling stress coefficient K_c for thin, curved sheets or plates.

compression buckling stress of the plate or $(F_c)_{cr}$. Use Fig. 8-15 for clad 2024-T3 sheet (QQ-A-250/5) at room-temperature. For curves of other material types, the engineer should consult an aerospace company structures manual.

Instability of the plate in pure compression is then predicted as follows:

$$\text{Margin of Safety} = \text{M.S.} = \frac{(F_c)_{cr}}{f_c} - 1$$

where: $(F_c)_{cr}$ = critical buckling stress of a thin, curved plate member in pure compression

$f_c = P/A$ = applied axial compression stress

P = applied axial compression load

$A = bt$ = cross-sectional area of the plate in the direction of the applied axial load

b = circumferential distance of the curved edge of the plate (this distance must also correspond to the loaded edges of the plate)

t = web or panel thickness.

Stability of Thin, Curved Plates in Combined Compression and Shear

Interaction equations again provide the means by which combined loading conditions are analyzed. For the combined loading effects of compression and shear, the engineer is referred to Table 8-3, page 519. The same procedure and equations are used in the solution of curved panels as are used in the solution of combined loading conditions for flat panels. Also refer to Fig. 8-29, page 523, for a graphical solution for plates (flat or curved) subjected to combined compression and shear using an interaction curve.

For the same surface area, compare shear buckling coefficients K_s for a thin, curved, simply-supported panel in pure shear (Fig. 8-31, page 528) with that of a thin, flat panel for the same loading and support conditions (Fig. 8-18, Curve B, page 503). Buckling coefficients of curved panels are noticeably higher than those of flat panel designs. In general, a curved sheet or panel such as the upper and lower surfaces of a wing are examples of curved surfaces which are analyzed as flat panels. However, the leading-edge (L.E.) panels of a wing are somewhat stiffer by virtue of their small curvature and for their design a curved panel analysis would be justified. For large values of curvature R or small values of the parameter Z, a curved panel is considered essentially flat.

8.6 Concepts and Theory of Tapered, Deep Beam Structures. Up to this point in our study of stability of flat plates, we have primarily concerned ourselves with the solution of rectangular plate sections, completely ignoring the entire problem of tapered, deep beam designs. When they occur, this latter group is as important to a weight-efficient, cost-effective structure as any main structural member of an aircraft. In this section, we will focus our attention on where the wing structure reduces in size as it tapers outboard. The wing, horizontal and vertical stabilizers of an aircraft are a few examples of tapered, deep beam structures. These major components of the aircraft structure are supported internally by tapered beams called "spars." The web design of these tapered spars are studied in this section. The

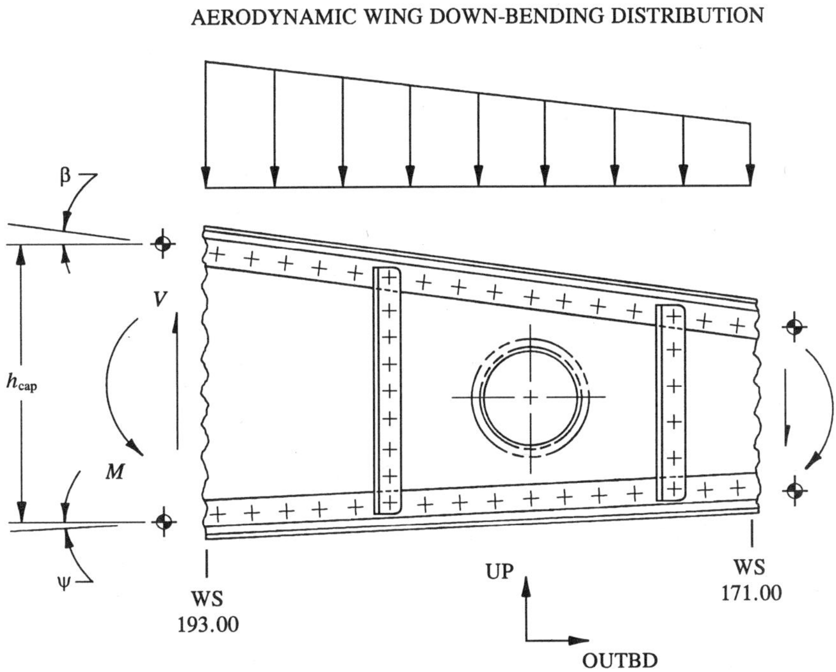

FIGURE 8-37 Tapered beam structure.

essential problem confronting us in the solution of these members is to find the true web shear carried by these structural members. Most internal loads are derived from a computer solution which presents the loaded structure in terms of internal loads (shears and bending moments) at specified locations along the loaded structure. These loads, whether they were generated from a computer solution, or whether they were hand-calculated by the design engineer, were all basically derived from the same equations of static equilibrium.

Most conventional beam structures are constructed with parallel beam caps. For such a member, the vertical shear is primarily carried by the web, little or no shear is actually carried by the horizontal beam caps. This concept was illustrated in Sec. 4.2 of Chapter 4 (see Fig. 4-14). The main point of discussion of this section will be the following: If a beam is designed with sloping flanges, no longer is the web the only appreciable member to carry the vertical shear; the beam caps can also share in their ability to carry part of this load. The greater the degree of slope, the greater are the vertical shears carried by the beam caps, and the greater is the vertical shear relieved to the web. This is unique to tapered beam construction. Rectangular beams for the most part, do not normally behave in this way; for example, when a beam is constructed with parallel beam caps, except for certain structural shapes,[1] the vertical shear is principally carried by the web. Although most tapered beam structures are (conservatively) designed with the full internal shear carried by the web, sometimes a slightly negative margin of safety in shear for the web can be corrected by reducing the web portion of the vertical shear slightly. Thus, the reduction in web shear can reduce the overall weight of the main structure by reducing the weight of the web. In simple terms, it can be said that if a beam structure is tapered, its beam caps carry part of the vertical shear. In fact, the vertical shear carried by these members actually relieves the shear carried by the web.

In the next few paragraphs, a method of analyzing a tapered beam structure will be presented. A tapered beam is a unique structure which by its geometric shape can either increase or decrease the internal vertical shear that is carried by the web. A reduction in web shear is what normally occurs for most conventional aircraft designs. Clearly, the wing spars and spars of the tail section are a couple of examples of cantilevered tapered beam construction where this occurs. For practical design, these beams are conservatively designed by conventional methods of stress analysis which ignore their tapering effects.

For the tapered beam structure shown in Fig. 8-37, the total web vertical shear V at any point along the structure is made up of the shear carried by the web V_{web} and the shear that is carried by the vertical shear components $(V_c)_{\text{upper}}$ and $(V_c)_{\text{lower}}$ of the upper and lower beam caps, respectively (see ahead to Fig. 8-38). The tapering direction of a wing will tend to relieve the vertical shear carried by the web. Let us take a specific example, wing down-bending loads, and develop some very important equations used to determine web vertical shear loads.[2]

Before proceeding ahead with the theoretical aspects of tapered beam construction, the general theory and observations of internal loads analysis at an exposed section of beam need to be more clearly defined. From our earlier study, regardless of whether a beam is tapered or not, the fundamental principles of shears and bending moments at a section of beam are theoretically the same. Expanding these principles now to tapered beams, it can be said that vertical shears and bending moments at different sections of these tapered members are composed of one part that is carried by the web and the other part that is carried by the beam caps. Mathematically, this is formulated by the following two equations below:

$$V = V_{\text{caps}} + V_{\text{web}} \tag{8-26}$$

---

[1] For some structural shapes, even though the beam caps are parallel, the configuration of these shapes can also increase or decrease the web vertical shear. However, since these particular shapes are somewhat rare in common aircraft use, they will not be investigated in this section. Instead, the engineer is encouraged to review the theory of shearing stresses for these structural shapes from an advanced college textbook on this subject.

[2] Whether the wing loading is up-bending or down-bending, the same equations will hold true. However, the equations are not applicable to a beam tapered in the reverse direction. Similar to the derivation that follows, it can be shown that a beam with a reverse taper will actually increase the web vertical shear. Other than for its purely academic considerations, this type of beam is purely hypothetical and serves no particular importance or practical consideration to real aircraft structure. Most aircraft structures are not tapered like this.

where: V = total vertical shear carried by the beam section (from a statics solution of internal loads)
V_{web} = web vertical shear
V_{caps} = upper and lower beam cap vertical shears

and

$$M = M_{caps} + M_{web} \tag{8-27}$$

where: M = total bending moment carried by the beam section (from a statics solution of internal loads)
M_{web} = bending moment carried by the web
M_{caps} = bending moment carried by the upper and lower beam caps.

The vertical shears carried by the upper and lower beam caps are shown in Fig. 8-38, where their values are determined from the shear components of the beam couple-force or P_{couple}. Notice the direction of these shears, essentially confirming the very nature of tapered beam designs: that the slope of a tapered wing relieves the vertical shear carried by the web. For wing up-bending, the vertical shear is also relieved by the conventional taper direction of a cantilevered wing.[1] (See Fig. 8-39 for the internal loads depiction for this exposed section of beam.) If both the upper and lower beam caps of Figs. 8-38 and 8-39 are sloped, each cap will contribute to the total vertical shear at the section. Mathematically, this says that

$$V_{caps} = (V_c)_{upper} + (V_c)_{lower}.$$

And from trigonometry, the vertical components of shear for these cap members (at the exposed section) are formulated as follows:

$$(V_c)_{upper} = P_{couple} \tan\beta$$

$$(V_c)_{lower} = P_{couple} \tan\psi.$$

Now, substituting these values into the equation above for V_{caps} and factoring gives:

$$V_{caps} = P_{couple}(\tan\beta + \tan\psi).$$

---

[1] On the other hand, if the same loading condition was applied to a beam with a reverse taper, either for wing up-bending or down-bending, the opposite effect would result, the web vertical shear would be increased. This is shown in Fig. 8-40. Notice that the vertical shears carried by the beam caps are in the same direction as the aerodynamic wing down-bending load distribution of the wing. Fortunately, such a structure is highly uncommon to aircraft designs.

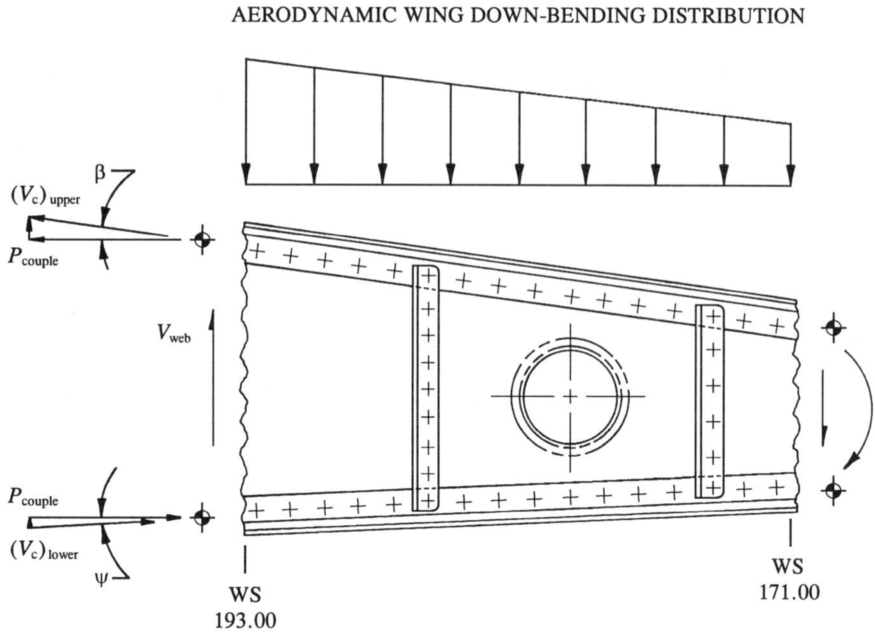

FIGURE 8-38 Web vertical shear in a tapered beam for wing down-bending.

And substituting this expression into Eq. 8-26 and solving for V_{web} gives:

$$V_{\text{web}} = V - P_{\text{couple}}(\tan\beta + \tan\psi). \qquad \textbf{(8-28)}$$

In terms of the bending moment at the beam section, we obtain from the couple-force relationship of a moment:

$$P_{\text{couple}} = \frac{M_{\text{caps}}}{h_{\text{cap}}} \qquad (1)$$

where: P_{couple} = horizontal component forces of the beam caps
M_{caps} = bending moment carried by the beam caps
h_{cap} = distance measured between beam cap centroids.

From Eq. 8-27, solving for M_{caps}, we obtain:

$$M_{\text{caps}} = M - M_{\text{web}}.$$

A buckled web offers very little bending resistance to its beam structure. Therefore, assuming the web is ineffective in bending, $I_{\text{web}} = 0$, and this equation

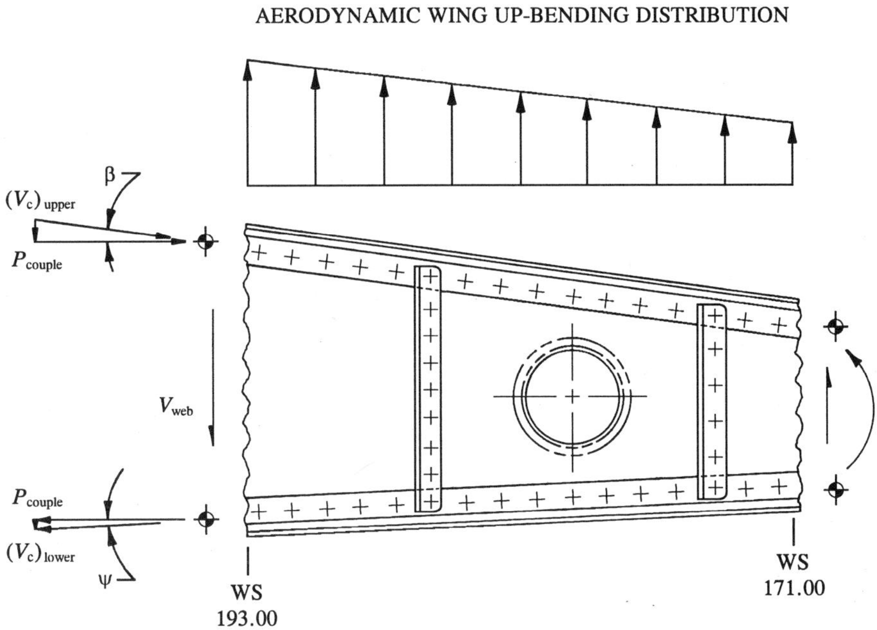

FIGURE 8-39 Web vertical shear in a tapered beam for wing up-bending.

reduces further to:

$$M_{\text{caps}} = M.$$

In terms of this moment, Eq. (1) becomes:

$$P_{\text{couple}} = \frac{M}{h_{\text{cap}}}.$$

Substituting this value in Eq. 8-28, we obtain:

$$V_{\text{web}} = V - \frac{M}{h_{\text{cap}}}(\tan\beta + \tan\psi) \tag{8-29}$$

where: V_{web} = web vertical shear
V = total vertical shear carried by the beam section (from a statics solution of internal loads)
M = total bending moment carried by the beam section (from a statics solution of internal loads)
h_{cap} = distance measured between beam cap centroids
β = slope of the upper beam cap (as defined in Figs. 8-38 and 8-39)

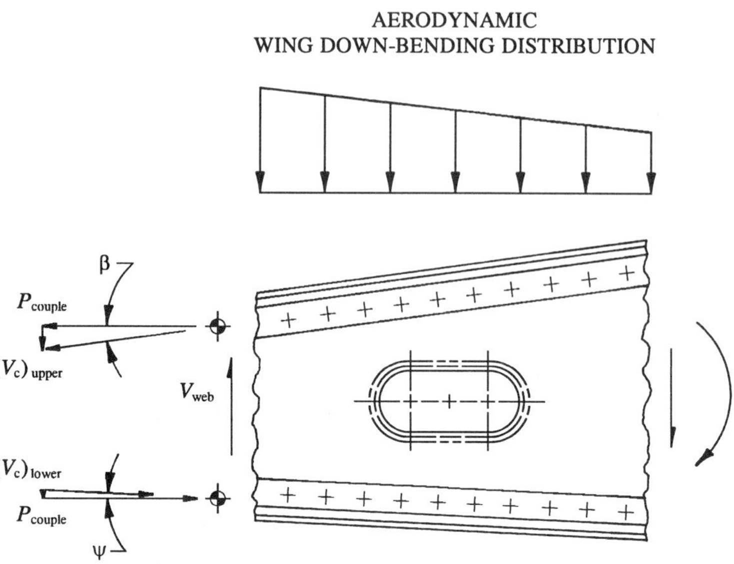

FIGURE 8-40 Web vertical shear in a beam with a reverse taper for wing down-bending.

ψ = slope of the lower beam cap (as defined in Figs. 8-38 and 8-39).

Designing for Web Stability:

$$f_s = \frac{V_{\text{web}}}{h_e t} \quad \text{(see Eq. 8-1)}$$

where: V_{web} = web vertical shear (from Eq. 8-29)
h_e = effective depth of the beam measured between cap centroids (neglect the effective web area, see Fig. 8-2)
t = web or panel thickness.

Instability of the web in pure shear is then predicted as follows:

$$\text{Margin of Safety} = \text{M.S.} = \frac{(F_s)_{cr}}{f_s} - 1$$

where: $(F_s)_{cr}$ = critical buckling stress of a thin, flat plate member in pure shear
f_s = average applied shearing stress (see equation above).

In summary, Eq. 8-29 is applicable to a beam structure with both upper and lower sloping beam caps and whose web structure has buckled. However, the nature of buckling of beam webs (tapered or not) precludes their structure from being analyzed by conventional methods of stress analysis. Instead, these beams (with buckled webs) are analyzed by diagonal tension-field analysis methods. Now, commensurate with the subject of shear-resistant beam design in this section, let us derive an alternative expression to Eq. 8-29 for tapered beam structures with stable webs. If the web is stable, this member will proportionately carry some of the bending moment that exists at an exposed section of beam, the magnitude of which is usually taken as a simple ratio of moments of inertia.

$$M_{web} = M\left[\frac{I_{web}}{I_{total}}\right] \tag{8-30}$$

where: M_{web} = bending moment carried by the web

M = bending moment carried by the beam section (from a statics solution of internal loads)

I_{web} = moment of inertia of the web

I_{total} = moment of inertia of the total beam section.

Let us now look at a special case of a shear-resistant web of a tapered beam design. A shear-resistant web is effective in carrying bending in the plane of its web. Using Fig. 8-37 once again, the bending moment at the exposed section of beam is described in two parts: the bending moment that is carried by the web and the bending moment that is carried by the beam caps.

$$M = M_{caps} + M_{web} \quad \text{(from Eq. 8-27).}$$

Substituting Eq. 8-30 into this expression.

$$M = M_{caps} + M\left[\frac{I_{web}}{I_{total}}\right].$$

Solving for M_{caps} and factoring, we obtain:

$$M_{caps} = M\left[1 - \frac{I_{web}}{I_{total}}\right].$$

Substituting this expression in the equation for P_{couple} gives:

$$P_{couple} = \frac{M_{caps}}{h_{cap}} = \frac{M}{h_{cap}}\left[1 - \frac{I_{web}}{I_{total}}\right].$$

Now substituting P_{couple} into Eq. 8-28 gives:

$$V_{\text{web}} = V - \frac{M}{h_{\text{cap}}}\left[1 - \frac{I_{\text{web}}}{I_{\text{total}}}\right](\tan\beta + \tan\psi) \qquad \textbf{(8-31)}$$

where: V_{web} = web vertical shear
V = total vertical shear carried by the beam section (from a statics solution of internal loads)
M = total bending moment carried by the beam section (from a statics solution of internal loads)
h_{cap} = distance measured between beam cap centroids
I_{web} = moment of inertia of the web
I_{total} = moment of inertia of the total beam section
β = slope of the upper beam cap (as defined in Figs. 8-38 and 8-39)
ψ = slope of the lower beam cap (as defined in Figs. 8-38 and 8-39).

This equation is applicable to a tapered beam structure whose web structure is shear-resistant.

Designing for Web Stability:

$$f_s = \frac{V_{\text{web}}}{h_e t} \quad \text{(see Eq. 8-1)}$$

where: V_{web} = web vertical shear (from Eq. 8-31)
h_e = effective depth of the beam measured between cap centroids (neglect the effective web area, see Fig. 8-2)
t = web or panel thickness.

Instability of the web in pure shear is then predicted as follows:

$$\text{Margin of Safety} = \text{M.S.} = \frac{(F_s)_{cr}}{f_s} - 1$$

where: $(F_s)_{cr}$ = critical buckling stress of a thin, flat plate member in pure shear
f_s = average applied shearing stress (see equation above).

8.7 Problem for Solution. The rib structure in Fig. 8-41 is part of a fuel-cell compartment. To prevent leakage, upper and lower end-panels are designed to be shear-resistant at limit load. To save weight, the rib structure was chem-milled in open areas of the web. Find: (a) The buckling margin of safety at limit load for the upper panel loaded as shown in this figure. Assume that a pad thickness of at least twice the thickness of the chem-milled web (a purely subjective judgment) is sufficient to provide a simply-supported edge along the edge of the pad. Consider a design load factor of 1.5. (b) The required thickness of this panel to prevent

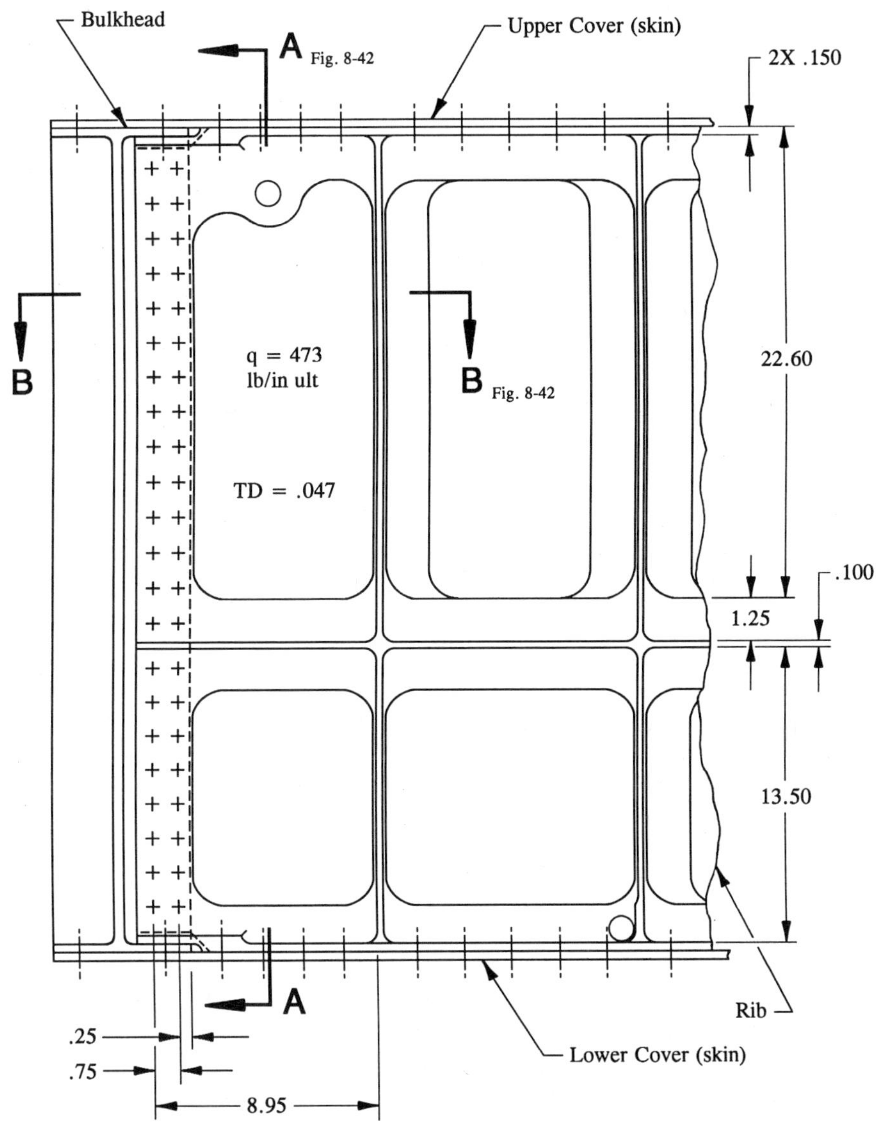

FIGURE 8-41 Machined forged rib structure with integral supports.

buckling at limit load. (c) Should the design requirement of this panel change to prevent buckling at ultimate load, what panel thickness would then be needed?

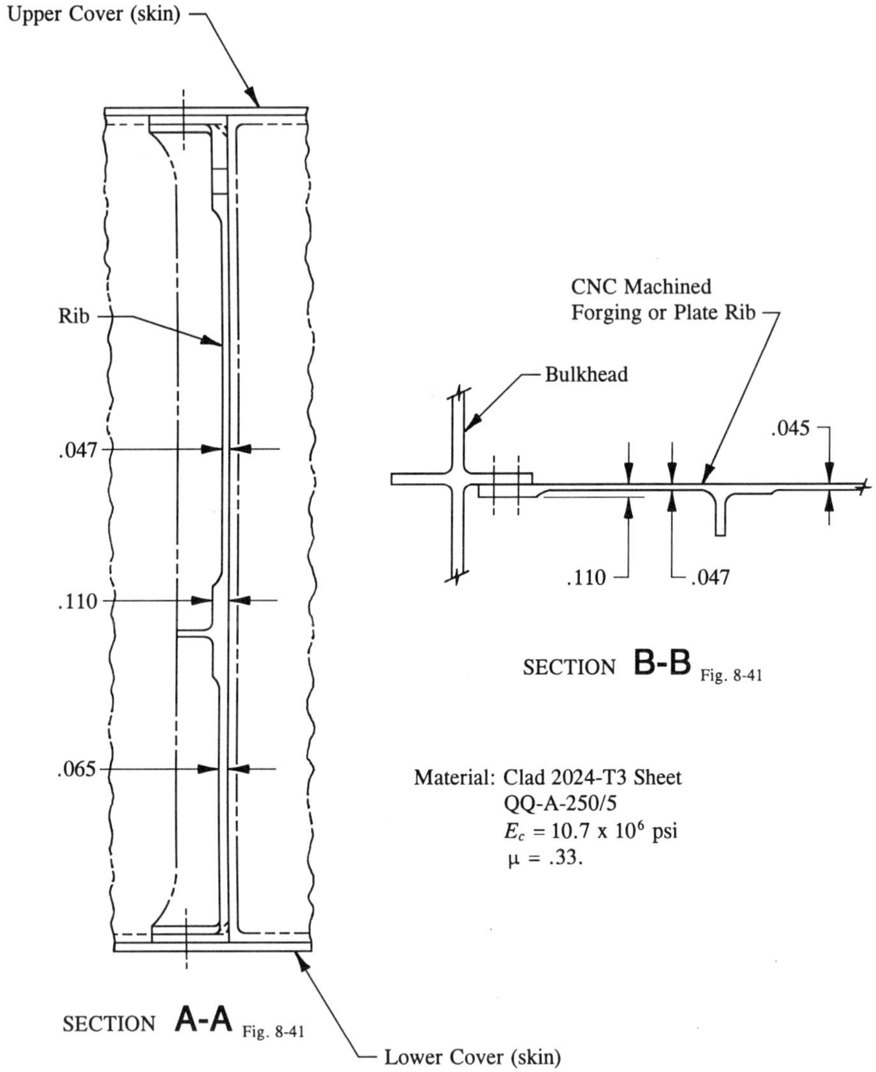

FIGURE 8-42 Cross-sectional areas of the CNC machined forged rib.

CHAPTER

9

Cutouts and Hole Reinforcements

9.1 Introduction. In the last chapter, besides giving the general theory of shear-resistant beams and panels, we investigated in detail the behavior of tapered beam structures. Expressions were given to obtain the critical buckling stresses for flat and curved panels in compression, shear, and bending. From these, other combinations were studied and their solutions determined using interaction equations. In this chapter, these same expressions are again used, but this time, to analyze flat and curved panels with circular cutouts, i.e., panels with holes, with or without a riveted ring reinforcement in (1) a diagonal tension-field and (2) in a shear-resistant web or panel. Also included in this chapter, Sec. 9-4, is a practical study of nonstructural door cutouts, i.e., the design and analysis of pressure doors and the edge-support members around the door, which are normally composed of vertical frames and horizontal sill beams for these structural openings.

The structural methods and approaches of small- and medium-size circular cutouts and hole reinforcements are studied in this chapter. Their practical applications to aircraft designs are many, such as (1) small cutouts—used for hydraulic and electrical lines, control cable lines, fuel slosh, drain, etc., (2) medium cutouts—used for fuel access openings, windows, engine servicing doors, etc., (3) large cutouts—used for cargo doors, passenger doors, baggage doors, etc. It is the subject of this chapter, therefore, to examine these and other similar types of configurations as they relate specifically to the structural design behavior of

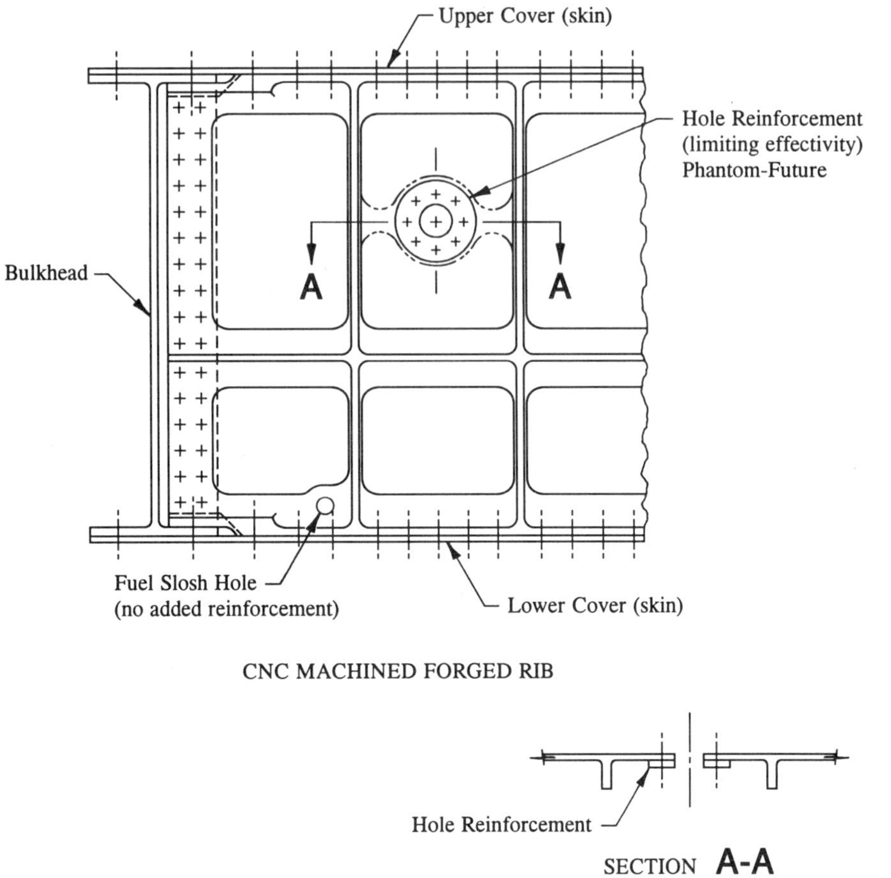

FIGURE 9-1 Riveted ring doubler in the web of a CNC machined forged rib.

commonly used aircraft hole reinforcements. To fully understand the principles and theories of this chapter, the design engineer must have a thorough and broad understanding of the basic assumptions and approaches of shear-resistant beams that were discussed in the previous chapter. The standard methods of analysis that are predominantly used by the aerospace industry in the solution of hole reinforcements will be presented in this chapter. The applications of these methods to industry-related aircraft designs are fully discussed and illustrated in the many example problems contained within this chapter. These problems should provide the engineer with a step-by-step procedure to the solution of cutouts and doors normally encountered in actual engineering aircraft designs.

Consider the hole reinforcement in Fig. 9-1. Without the stabilizing effect of the hole reinforcement around the hole, the panel will buckle prematurely, i.e., the panel will buckle at a critical buckling stress lower than that which would normally be expected for a panel without a hole. However, if the reinforcement sufficiently reinforces the hole, then the weakening effect of the hole or loss in structural stiffness of the panel, as far as the buckling strength of the panel goes, can thus be minimized and therefore neglected in the buckling analysis of the panel. This means that structurally, the panel can be assumed to be sufficiently reinforced to be analyzed by the buckling equations of Chapter 8 as if the panel had no hole. The FAA requires a fitting factor of 1.15 to comply with the structural integrity of the reinforcement, its fasteners, and bearing upon the joined members when no structural test data have been proved.

The design philosophy of most categories of cutouts will require at least one of the following loading conditions to be considered for their design: (1) loads due to burst pressure at ultimate load, (2) loads due to body shears[1] from ultimate flight and landing conditions, or (3) loads due to combined limit pressure and body shears from ultimate flight and landing conditions. Many aerospace companies have adopted a universal criterion in which most doors are designed to carry only burst pressure; or limit pressure when combined with flight and landing conditions. This type of door is usually referred to as being "nonstructural." Additionally, for this type of door, the longitudinal and hoop tension loads due to limit pressure when combined with ultimate flight loads and due to burst pressure alone are carried around the door by frame and sill members. For large nonstructural doors, however, this criterion can make the design of these members rather impractical to manufacture—causing the framework of the door to be unusually heavy and oversize. So, to minimize the loss of structural stiffness and reduce the weight penalty created by large nonstructural access doors, the loads due to limit pressure and ultimate flight conditions are combined together and carried by the door itself, thereby achieving a more optimum design of the door and boundary structures. This type of load-carrying member is termed "structural." More about this in Sec. 9.3 (see page 582).

9.2 Small, Circular Holes or Cutouts and Their Applications to Shear-Resistant Webs or Panels. It is the purpose of this section to investigate the structural behavior of small cutouts with or without hole reinforcements in shear-resistant webs or panels. A small, circular hole or cutout may either be (1) unreinforced, (2) reinforced with an integral flange, or (3) reinforced with a riveted ring doubler. The following requirements are suggested to achieve the best structural design possible for most cutouts:

(1) Provide generous radii for the reinforcement and attaching structure.
(2) Minimize the loss of structural stiffness.
(3) Minimize the size and weight of the reinforcement.
(4) Locate the cutout in an area of low stress intensity.
(5) Minimize stress concentrations.

---

[1] Body shears refer to shear loads resulting from aerodynamic forces on the surfaces of the fuselage, which are ultimately counterbalanced by the wings of the aircraft.

The methodologies and procedures for their solutions will be discussed throughout this section and several example problems will be included illustrating their detailed solutions. The methods and approaches to their stress analysis are outlined below in accordance with acceptable design solutions recognized by industry practicing engineers.

Unreinforced Cutout in a Shear-Resistant Web

Requirements for unreinforced cutouts[1] should be obtained from the structural analysis group in charge of issuing such policy directives governing their design. Several design philosophies or factors are usually applied to an unreinforced cutout. If no such policy directives are detailed for their solutions, the following suggested guidelines (purely subjective) will help to insure their structural reliability:

(1) Provide a shear stress margin of safety greater than 25% using the net area of the panel.

$$\text{Margin of Safety} = \text{M.S.} = \frac{F_{su}}{(f_s)_{max}} - 1 > 25\%$$

where: F_{su} = ultimate allowable shear stress of the material (see published values in MIL-HDBK-5 for commonly used material types)

$(f_s)_{max}$ = q/t (for a beam, use Eq. 4-2, $(f_s)_{max} = VQ/I_{na}t$)

q = maximum panel shear flow

t = web or panel thickness.

(2) The area of the hole should represent approximately less than 5% of the gross surface area of the web or panel.

$$\frac{A_{hole}}{A_{gross}}(100) < 5\%$$

where: $A_{hole} = \pi D^2/4$ = area of the hole

$A_{gross} = hw$ = surface area of the web or panel

D = hole diameter

h = web or panel height

w = web or panel width.

(3) The hole should be located at or near the center of the panel (for a beam,

[1] Unreinforced cutouts or access holes are quite common in web designs where hydraulic, electrical, and control lines must pass through the structure. Or sometimes they are merely provided for as hand clearance or working space for routine aircraft servicing.

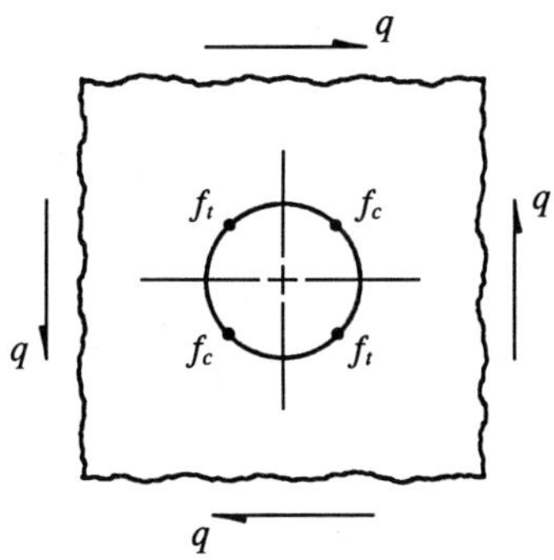

FIGURE 9-2 Circular hole in an infinitely wide, shear-resistant, thick plate in pure shear.

locate the hole close to the neutral axis of the cross-sectional area).

Since most aircraft structures are usually idealized from simplifying assumptions, exact stress-concentration factors resulting from open holes or cutouts are seldom accurately realized for their designs. In such cases, a conservative approach to the analysis of hole reinforcements is advised. Reliable results can frequently be obtained from fatigue testing or sometimes their solutions can be determined from a mathematical model using a computer model analysis solution. Much experimental work has been done to describe the state of stress of a circular hole in a shear-resistant plate subjected to pure shear. Such a plate is shown in Fig. 9-2, where the maximum stresses f_c and f_t that occur at the diagonal edges of the hole are denoted.[1] These stresses are written in equation form as follows:

$$f_t = 4\frac{q}{t} = 4f_s \tag{9-1}$$

$$f_c = -4\frac{q}{t} = -4f_s \tag{9-2}$$

$$(f_s)_{\max} = 2\frac{q}{t} = 2f_s . \tag{9-3}$$

From these stresses, predicted structural failures are formulated for tension, compression, and shear:

Tension Failure:

$$\text{Margin of Safety} = \text{M.S.} = \frac{F_{tu}}{f_t} - 1.$$

[1] The maximum stresses were obtained from Peterson, R.E., *Stress-Concentration Factors,* Fig. 165, page 236, New York: John Wiley and Sons, 1974.

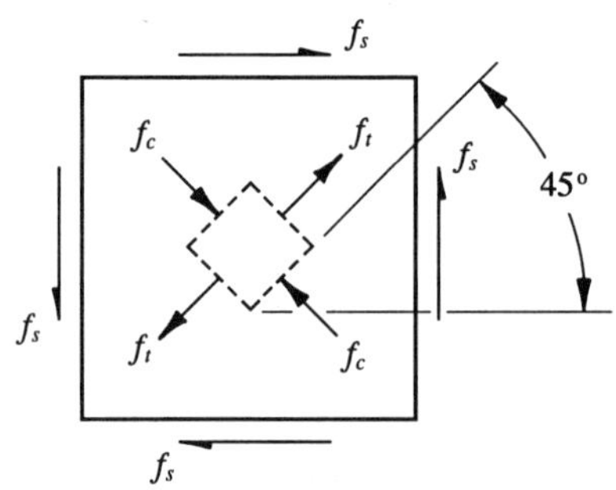

FIGURE 9-3 Maximum normal stresses or "principal stresses."

Compression Failure:

$$\text{Margin of Safety} = \text{M.S.} = \frac{F_{cy}}{f_c} - 1.$$

Shear Stress Failure:

$$\text{Margin of Safety} = \text{M.S.} = \frac{F_{su}}{(f_s)_{\max}} - 1.$$

Important Transformation of Stress

Shear is the most common type of loading considered for small cutout design. For this reason, an important transformation of pure shearing stresses is conveniently described into an alternative state of stress where "principal stresses" occur. The principal stresses are maximum normal stresses, as shown in Fig. 9-3 by the values f_t and f_c, and numerically are equal to the shearing stresses f_s, but act on planes 45 degrees to the shearing planes. Note that the planes on which the principal stresses act are completely free of shearing stresses, i.e., $(f_s)_{\max} = 0$.

$$f_t = f_s \tag{9-4}$$

$$f_c = -f_s \tag{9-5}$$

$$(f_s)_{\max} = 0. \tag{9-6}$$

Redistribution of Shear Around an Unreinforced Cutout

Sometimes engineering requirements demand that rather large openings be provided in various main structural members of an aircraft. For instance, the web of a deep beam, such as a bulkhead, or skin panels of the fuselage or wing surfaces are very often considered for large access openings. Although the openings are plugged by windows and doors, these members are designed to carry only cabin pressurization loads. These structural types are termed nonstructural since they carry no body shears[1] in their planes. Structurally, this means that body shears (from flight and landing conditions) are carried around the opening or cutout by the adjacent boundary structure, usually composed of frame, sill, and panel members. Often these members are modeled from loads generated from computer solutions of an entire wing or fuselage section. Computer runs of large sections of fuselage or wing structure are, however, extremely costly and therefore additional computer runs are normally avoided or minimized, if possible. In most cases, if a large cutout is made to an existing structure which has been computer modeled, the cost of an additional computer run of that new structure (with the large cutout) would be too cost prohibitive.

For such cases, a necessary compromise would be to initiate a "hand-calculated solution" to distribute panel shears to the localized cutout area. This approach would be far less costly and more desirable in the long run than to initiate a full-blown computer run of the new structure with the large cutout. In other words, instead of using costly computer runs to distribute skin panel shear flows, this section (the paragraphs which follow) will present a method of analysis to rapidly distribute skin shears around a large unreinforced cutout. The design engineer should become familiar with this method of analysis so that, if someday he should be called upon to perform or discuss the effect of incorporating a large cutout in a web or panel, he will be able to do so with a high degree of confidence. This method, if followed closely, should provide the design engineer with one additional method by which he can gain a better understanding of the behavior of structure from a redistribution of loads standpoint.

For example, let us assume that a large unreinforced cutout was made in panel #10 of the fuselage structure of Fig. 9-4. Instead of providing a computer run to redistribute the shear this panel carried before the cutout was made, a hand redistribution of shear flows is made to the adjacent panels. Panel shear flows indicate the load felt by the boundary structure from the web. To accomplish this, the load carried by panel #10 (center panel) is distributed to the adjacent panels: (1) above and below the center panel, (2) to the left and right of the center panel, and (3) to the corner panels. The following procedure is illustrated using a system of self-balancing shear flows for the center and adjacent panels, as shown in Fig. 9-5.

Since a large, unreinforced cutout in panel #10 essentially prevents this member from carrying any load, the load this panel carried before the cutout was made or 400 lb/in must now be distributed to the adjacent panels. To do this, an equal and opposite shear flow of 400 lb/in is assumed in this panel and this value distributed to the adjacent panels. The self-balancing system of shear flows obtained from this procedure (those values indicated in Fig. 9-5) is then combined (algebraically) with the original system of design shear flows from Fig. 9-4. The resulting

[1] The aerodynamic forces on the external surfaces of a flight vehicle structure are ultimately transferred into the internal structure of the aircraft as "body shears."

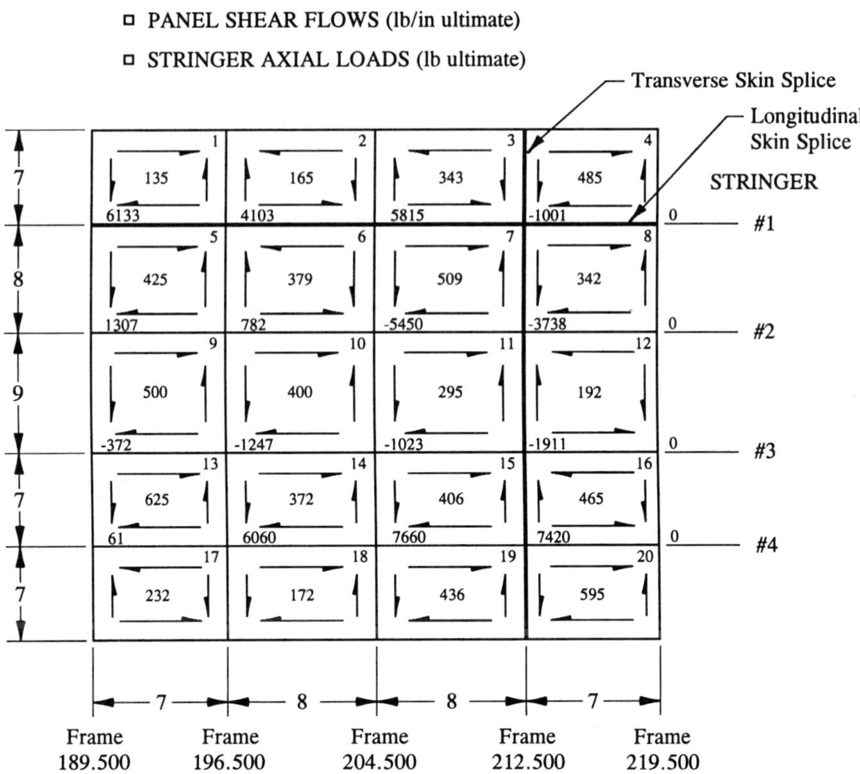

FIGURE 9-4 Panel shear flows and stringer axial loads.

system of shear flows will then correspond to zero (0) shear flow in panel #10 (see ahead to Fig. 9-6).

Procedure Used to Redistribute Shear Around an Unreinforced Cutout

(1) Determine which adjacent structural panels will carry the shear load that was carried by the panel with the unreinforced cutout before the cutout was made in that member.

(2) Using the shear load from step 1 that was carried by the panel with the unreinforced cutout, applied in the opposite direction, determine a system of self-balancing shear flows to the adjacent structural panels.

(3) Combine the self-balancing shear flows (step 2) with the original panel shear flows, thereby obtaining a final set of shear flows with "zero" shear flow in the panel with the unreinforced cutout.

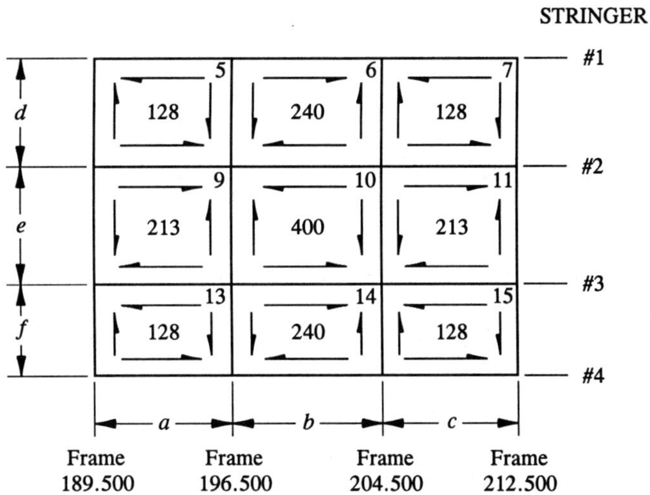

FIGURE 9-5 System of self-balancing internal shear flows.

The standard notation for internal panel shear flows is always head-to-head or tail-to-tail at the corners of a panel. Internal panel shear flows are always drawn opposing applied or reactive loads. To avoid inconsistencies in our solution, assume that the panels above and below the center panel, and left and right of the center panel, have the same magnitude of shear flow. Distribution is achieved by forcing the shear flow in the center panel to balance (1) the panels above and below the center panel, (2) the panels left and right of the center panel, and (3) the corner panels. Specifically, equilibrium is achieved from a horizontal and vertical balance of shear flow in the center panel. In simpler terms, the shear flow in the center panel is proportionally distributed by length to the adjacent panels.

Left and right of the center panel:

$$q_9 = q_{11} = \frac{q_{10}\, b}{a + c} = \frac{400(8)}{7 + 8} = 213 \text{ lb/in ultimate}.$$

Above and below the center panel:

$$q_6 = q_{14} = \frac{q_{10}\, e}{d + f} = \frac{400(9)}{7 + 8} = 240 \text{ lb/in ultimate}.$$

Distribution is completed by taking these shear flows and determining a vertical balance of shear flows in the corner panels as follows:

$$q_7 = q_{15} = \frac{q_{11}\, e}{d + f} = \frac{213(9)}{7 + 8} = 128 \text{ lb/in ultimate}$$

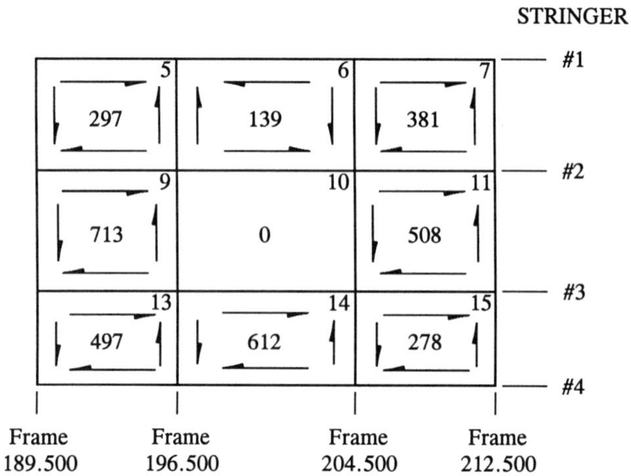

FIGURE 9-6 Final system of panel shear flows.

$$q_5 = q_{13} = \frac{q_9 e}{d + f} = \frac{213(9)}{7 + 8} = 128 \text{ lb/in ultimate.}$$

Or, these values can be verified by a horizontal balance of shear flows:

$$q_5 = q_7 = \frac{q_6 b}{a + c} = \frac{240(8)}{7 + 8} = 128 \text{ lb/in ultimate}$$

$$q_{13} = q_{15} = \frac{q_{14} b}{a + c} = \frac{240(8)}{7 + 8} = 128 \text{ lb/in ultimate.}$$

Now, combining the system of self-balancing shear flows, Fig. 9-5, with the panel shear flows in Fig. 9-4, we obtain the final system of panel shear flows as indicated in Fig. 9-6.

The redistribution of shear flow from panel #10 to the adjacent panels clearly shows that the final system of shear flows in panels #9, #11, and #14 are now greater than the shear flows which occurred for these panels before the cutout was made. Hence, these panels must be investigated (analyzed once again) for panel buckling for the higher shear loads. Additionally, the following stability requirement for panel stability and possible structural failures must be checked: (1) panel buckling at ultimate load (refer to a company structures manual for the analysis of diagonal tension-field beams), (2) frame and stringer axial tension and compression loads, (3) shearing of the skin rivets, and (4) bearing of the fuselage skin and attaching structures.

A structure substantiated from theory (like our example here) can usually be modified later from empirical data (static test results obtained from structural testing). Test data can also be obtained from strain-gauge studies of a flight test

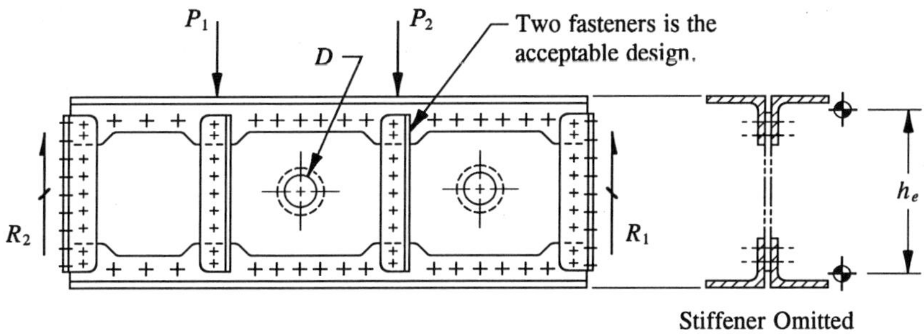

FIGURE 9-7 Flanged lightening holes in the shear web of a beam.

aircraft during various maneuvers and flight conditions. In fact, most analyses of critical structures are eventually substantiated by static testing. In the final analysis, to be certified by the FAA, an aircraft structure must be shown to return to its original configuration once limit loads have been removed from the structure. Deflection indicators are used to monitor permanent set or deformation of the tested structure at crucial or sensitive locations of the aircraft. From limit load tests, results can then be extrapolated to predict ultimate failure. If the structure is in good agreement with analytical predictions, then the structure can be safely tested to ultimate. Of course, the tested structure should be monitored along the way to insure these higher loads—making certain that all monitored strain gauges are still in good agreement with expected (calculated) values. The structure is then substantiated at ultimate load if the structure can be shown to carry these loads for three (3) seconds without catastrophic failure. Failure of minor structure, such as skin rivets, is not considered catastrophic. Hence, if nothing more serious than this happens during structural testing, certification of the aircraft structure is most likely assured. After structural loads have been verified of all test regimes of the aircraft, the structure is then tested to destruction.

Reinforced Cutout with an Integral Flange

The strength of reinforced holes or cutouts with integral flanges is obtained from empirical expressions or sometimes from graphical solutions formulated from test results.[1] Such structures are shown in Fig. 9-7 and are called flanged lightening holes. Specifically, these expressions are used to determine the allowable collapsing shearing stress of the web. The collapsing strength of the web $(F_s)_{cr}$ is then compared to the net shear stress through the hole.

$$\text{Margin of Safety} = \text{M.S.} = \frac{(F_s)_{cr}}{(f_s)_{\text{net}}} - 1$$

[1] Paul Kuhn, "The Strength and Stiffness of Shear Webs with Round Lightening Holes Having 45° Flanges," *NACA*, December 1942.

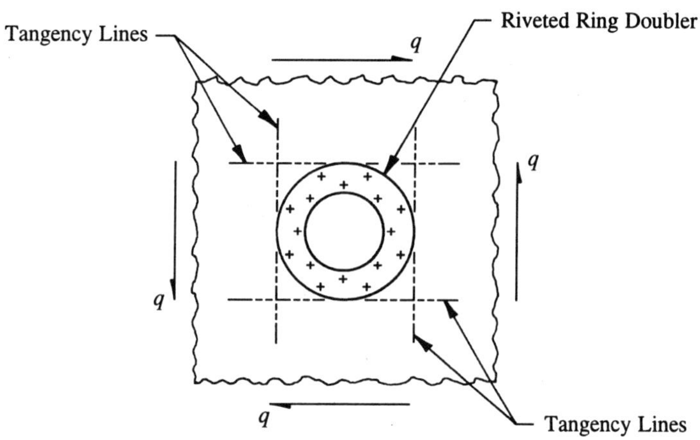

FIGURE 9-8 Reinforced cutout with a riveted ring doubler in a shear-resistant web.

where: $(F_s)_{cr}$ = allowable collapsing shear stress of the web (refer to an aerospace company structures manual for the empirical expression used to determine this value; *do not use the shear buckling equation given in Chapter 8)*

$$(f_s)_{\text{net}} = \frac{V}{(h_e - D)t}$$

D = hole diameter

V = applied vertical design shear through the hole

h_e = effective height measured between cap centroids (neglect the effective web area, see Fig. 9-7)

t = web or panel thickness.

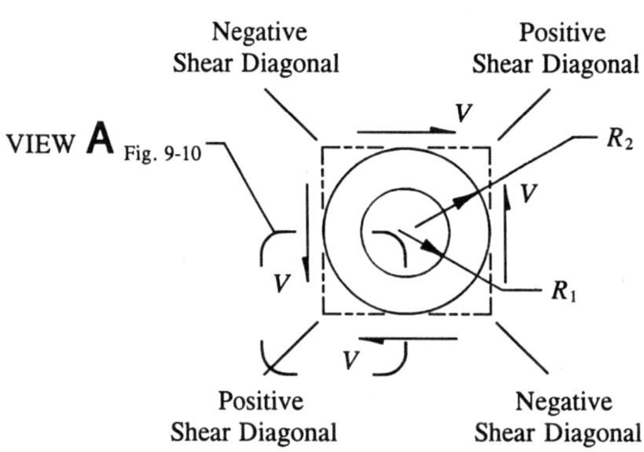

FIGURE 9-9 Free-body diagram of a riveted ring doubler with effective web area.

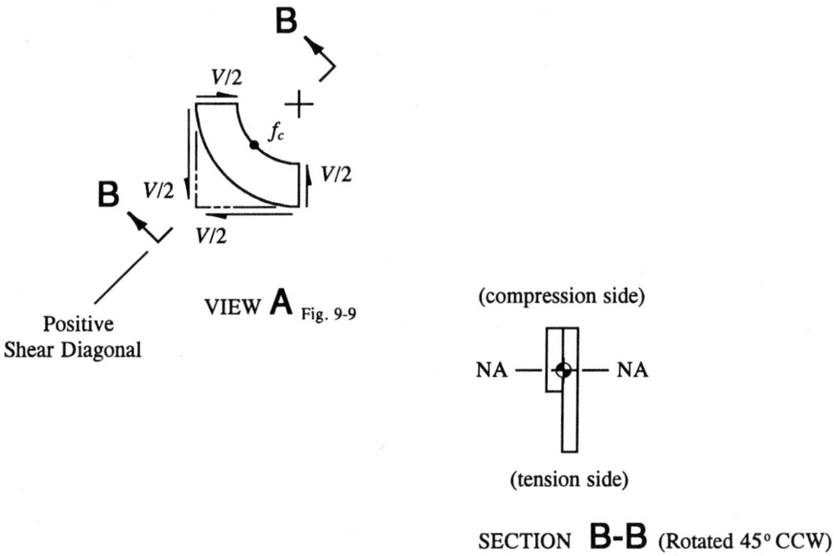

FIGURE 9-10 Quarter segment of web and ring doubler.

Reinforced Cutout with a Riveted Ring Doubler in a Shear-Resistant Web

When empirical data is not available for the analysis of a reinforced cutout with a riveted ring doubler, the following step-by-step method is recommended for its solution. The web is cut along vertical and horizontal tangency lines to the ring doubler, as shown in Fig. 9-8. The encased portion of web and attached ring doubler are then removed and free-bodied, as shown in Fig. 9-9. To the free-body, horizontal and vertical section cuts are taken through the centerline of the hole, isolating a quarter segment of web and ring doubler, as illustrated in Fig. 9-10. From this segment, the section can now be analyzed using standard stress analysis methods. The compression stress at the edge of the hole is located along the positive shear diagonal, as shown in this figure. The internal loads *V*, *P*, and *M* are determined by passing an imaginary line through the segment along the positive shear diagonal, and then applying the equations of static equilibrium at the centroid of Section B-B. Failure is predicted as follows:

$$\text{Margin of Safety} = \text{M.S.} = \frac{F_{cy}}{f_c} - 1$$

where: F_{cy} = allowable yield compression stress

$f_c = -\dfrac{P}{A} - \dfrac{Mc}{I_{na}}$ (combined axial and bending stresses on the compression side at the edge of the hole, as shown in View A, Fig. 9-10).

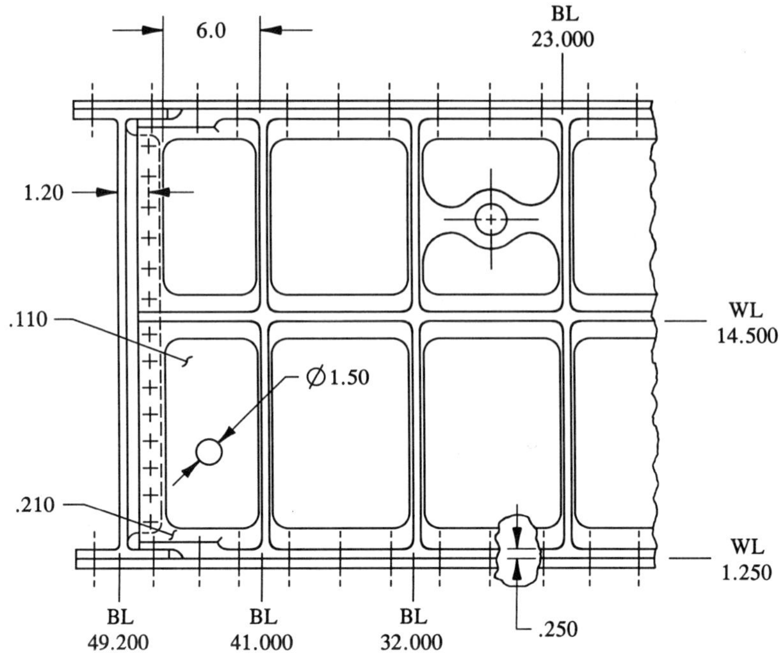

FIGURE 9-11 Machined forged rib structure with integral supports.

The following example problem will help to illustrate the practical application of this method of analysis.

Example 9-1 A 1.5 in diameter hole was located in the chem-milled panel of the rib structure shown in Fig. 9-11. Using a computer model solution of the rib, a maximum shearing stress of 10,000 psi ultimate was determined for this panel (program thickness = .080 in). What type of hole reinforcement, if any, would this panel require for an actual panel thickness of .110 in? Assume that the edge members provide simply-supported edges for the panel. The web material is bare 2024-T351 plate, QQ-A-250/4, F_{cy} = 39 ksi, F_{su} = 38 ksi, and F_{tu} = 64 ksi.

SOLUTION: Without reliable test data to substantiate the loss of structural stiffness of the rib panel with a hole, a rational and conservative approach to the buckling analysis of the panel is advised. Since the solution of the theoretical shear buckling stress, Eq. 8-5, does not account for a reduction in the buckling strength of a flat panel with a circular hole, the following criteria (modified from page 556) are proposed to help justify its use and proper application to this problem and thereby account for the loss of structural stiffness of this panel:

(1) The critical shear buckling stress $(F_s)_{cr}$ of the web should be approx-

imately 25% greater than the net shear stress of the web $(f_s)_{net}$. Written as a margin of safety, this gives:

$$\text{Margin of Safety} = \text{M.S.} = \frac{(F_s)_{cr}}{(f_s)_{net}} - 1 > 25\%$$

where: $(F_s)_{cr}$ = allowable shear buckling stress of the panel (from Eq. 8-5)

$(f_s)_{net} = (f_s)_{gross}\left[\dfrac{w}{w - D}\right]$

$(f_s)_{gross} = \dfrac{V}{ht}$ (this value need not be calculated since the maximum shearing stress of the panel is given)

w = width of the panel

D = diameter of the hole

V = applied vertical design shear

h = height of the panel (for a beam, use the distance measured between cap centroids)

t = web or panel thickness.

(2) The area of the hole should represent less than 5% of the gross surface area of the web. Hence

$$\frac{A_{hole}}{A_{gross}}(100) < 5\%$$

where: $A_{hole} = \pi D^2/4$ = area of the hole

$A_{gross} = hw$ = area of the panel

D = hole diameter

t = web or panel thickness

h = panel height

w = panel width.

By satisfying the above criteria, the panel can then be assumed to be shear-resistant (nonbuckled), and the method of analysis proposed on page 565 for a reinforced cutout with a riveted ring doubler in a shear-resistant web can then be applied. The theoretical shear buckling stress of the web is computed as follows:

Critical Shear Buckling Stress

From Eqs. 8-5 and 8-8 (pages 500 and 504, respectively),

$$\frac{(F_s)_{cr}}{\eta_s} = \frac{\pi^2 K_s E_c}{12(1 - \mu^2)}\left[\frac{t}{b}\right]^2$$

where: $K_s = 5.34 + 4.00\left[\frac{b}{a}\right]^2$ (this corresponds to a panel with simply-supported edges, refer to page 503, Curve B)

$E_c = 10.9 \times 10^6$ psi (from MIL-HDBK-5F)

$\mu = .33$ (see MIL-HDBK-5F)

$a = 13.0$ in (height of panel, see Fig. 9-11)

$b = 7.0$ in (width of panel, see Fig. 9-11)

$t = .110$ in (given).

Solving for K_s first, we obtain:

$$K_s = 5.34 + 4.00\left[\frac{7.0}{13.0}\right]^2 = 6.50$$ (this value can also be verified from Curve B of Fig. 8-18).

Next, substituting this value and all known values into Eq. 8-5 gives:

$$\frac{(F_s)_{cr}}{\eta_s} = \frac{\pi^2 (6.50)(10.9 \times 10^6)}{12\left[1 - (.33)^2\right]}\left[\frac{.110}{7.0}\right]^2 = 16,148 \text{ psi.}$$

The true shear buckling stress $(F_s)_{cr}$ is determined from the following relationship:

$$\frac{(F_c)_{cr}}{\eta_c} = \frac{(F_s)_{cr}}{\eta_s}\sqrt{3} = 16,148\sqrt{3} = 27,969 \text{ psi.}$$

Using a compression plasticity correction curve for bare 2024-T351 plate, we obtain $(F_c)_{cr} = 26,000$ psi.[1] The true shear buckling stress is then obtained by dividing this value by $\sqrt{3}$. Thus

$$(F_s)_{cr} = \frac{(F_c)_{cr}}{\sqrt{3}} = \frac{26,000}{\sqrt{3}} = 15,011 \text{ psi.}$$

First Criterion (from page 566)

To satisfy the first criterion for panel buckling (or shear-resistant design) of a flat panel with a circular hole, let us determine the following values:

$$(f_s)_{\text{net}} = (f_s)_{\text{gross}}\left[\frac{w}{w - D}\right] = 7,273\left[\frac{7.0}{7.0 - 1.5}\right] = 9,257 \text{ psi ultimate}$$

where: $(f_s)_{\text{gross}} = (f_s)_{\text{program}}\left[\frac{t_{\text{program}}}{t}\right] = 10,000\left[\frac{.080}{.110}\right]$

[1] The engineer is referred to an aerospace company structures manual for this material.

$(f_s)_{gross}$ = 7,273 psi ultimate, refer to Eq. 4-7 and to a discussion of program shearing stresses in Chapter 4.

Comparing this stress to the true shear buckling stress of the web:

$$\text{Margin of Safety} = \text{M.S.} = \frac{(F_s)_{cr}}{(f_s)_{net}} - 1 = \frac{15{,}011}{9{,}257} - 1 = +.62.$$

Since the margin of safety of the panel is greater than 25%, the first criterion is substantiated.

Second Criterion (from page 567)

The percent of surface area removed by the 1.5 in diameter hole is determined as follows:

$$\text{Area of Hole, } A_h = \pi R^2 = \pi\left[\frac{1.5}{2}\right]^2 = 1.767 \text{ in}^2$$

$$\text{Gross Area of Web, } A_w = 7.0\,(13.0) = 91.0 \text{ in}^2$$

$$\%\text{ Surface Area Removed} = \frac{1.767}{91.0}(100) = 1.9\%.$$

Since the percent of area removed is less than 5%, the second criterion established for this problem is also satisfied. Now, having satisfied both criteria, it can be safely reasoned that the loss of structural stiffness of the panel due to a 1.5 in diameter hole is minimal. Hence, the web can be assumed to be nonbuckled, and therefore a detailed analysis of the hole can be performed with the web considered as the reinforcement around the hole. If the effective web material around the hole can be shown to structurally support the hole, no additional reinforcement would then be needed. A most desirable consequence to a weight-efficient, cost-effective structure.

Isolating the Hole and Effective Material Around the Hole

Now, if we isolate the hole with effective web material around the hole, as shown in Fig. 9-12, we obtain a balanced system of panel shears for the isolated plate segment.

$$V = qL_e$$

where L_e is bounded by $2D$ effective web material around the hole. (More about this in the paragraph which follows.) Thus, since by definition $q = f_s t$, for our solution this corresponds to $q = (f_s)_{gross}\, t$. Substituting this expression into the previous equation gives:

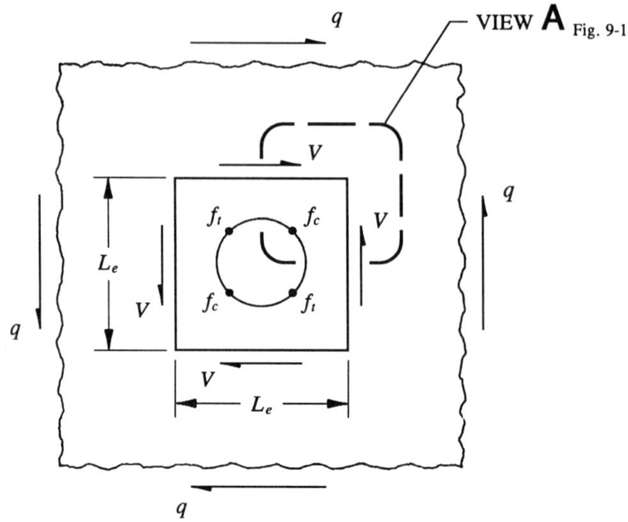

FIGURE 9-12 Isolated hole with effective web material around the hole.

$$V = (f_s)_{\text{gross}}\, tL_e = 7,273(.110)(3.0) = 2,400 \text{ lb}$$

where: $(f_s)_{\text{gross}} = 7,273$ psi ultimate (see page 569)

$t = .110$ in (given)

$L_e = 2D = 2(1.5) = 3.0$ in (this value corresponds to the effective web material around a hole in an infinite plate).

In no case shall more than 2*D* web material be taken as effective around the hole. The reason is that no matter how much web material exists or is assumed effective around the hole, calculated stresses (by our proposed method here) can never be less than the stresses that would theoretically occur or develop for a circular hole in an infinite plate case (refer back to Eqs. 9-1, 9-2, and 9-3). Written as an inequality, this says that if $L_e \geq 2D$, then use these equations, representing stresses at the edges of the hole, for ultimate strength computations. For easy reference, these equations are again conveniently written below:

$f_t = 4f_s$ (tension stress)

$f_c = -4f_s$ (compression stress)

$(f_s)_{\max} = 2f_s$ (shearing stress).

On the other hand, if $L_e < 2D$, the method of analysis described on page 565 for a reinforced cutout with a riveted ring doubler in a shear-resistant web is used. Consistent with our discussions here so far is the notion that, since 2*D* effective

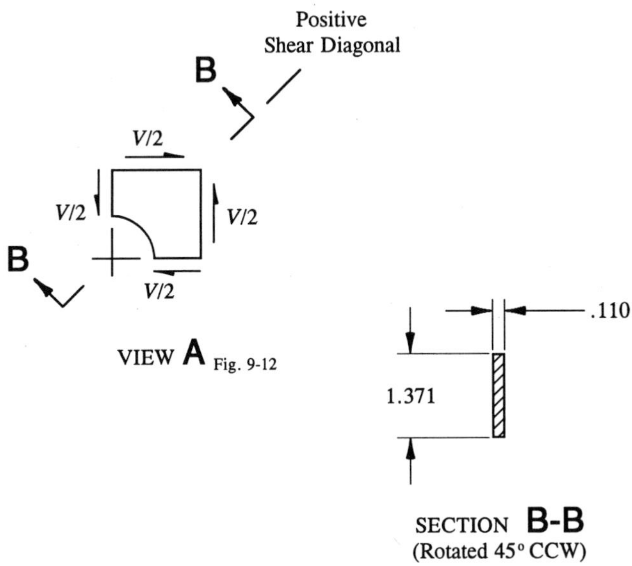

FIGURE 9-13 Isolated quarter segment of hole and the section area along the positive shear diagonal.

web material is taken around the hole, calculated stresses should be in good agreement with stresses for a circular hole in an infinite plate case. This will be shown to be true in subsequent paragraphs.

Notice that the compression and tension stresses are the same. These stresses can be verified along the positive shear diagonal of the section for compression, along the negative shear diagonal of the section for tension, and through a vertical or horizontal section across the hole for (calculated) shearing stresses. When one compares the compression stress f_c at the edge of the hole and the tension stress f_t at the corner of the effective web material around the hole, clearly the former (or compression case) should produce a failure combination at the edge of the hole that is far more critical. Ultimately the hole is designed by this condition (compare the mechanical properties of different materials in compression and tension). Essentially, this means that since the compression and tension stresses are the same, but the compression allowable is lower, the hole only needs to be designed for compression. This critical combination then designs the hole.

Free-Body of a Quarter Segment of Hole and the Internal Loads Acting Along the Positive Shear Diagonal

Isolating a quarter segment of the hole, Fig. 9-12, and taking the cross-sectional properties along the positive shear diagonal of this quarter segment (Section B-B), as shown in Fig. 9-13, we obtain:

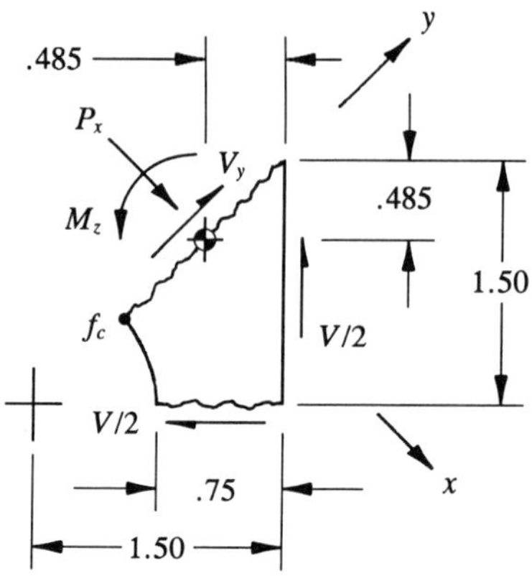

FIGURE 9-14 Equilibrium forces along the positive shear diagonal (segment of hole taken from View A, Fig. 9-13).

Cross-Sectional Properties of Section B-B:

$$A = 1.371(.110) = .151 \text{ in}^2$$

$$I_o = \frac{.110(1.371)^3}{12} = .024 \text{ in}^4.$$

An additional section cut is taken along the positive shear diagonal, isolating the segment of hole as shown in Fig. 9-14. The exposed system of internal forces occurring there are now used to describe the equilibrium of this segment of the open hole. The system of internal forces to maintain the segment in equilibrium consists of an axial force P_x, a shearing force V_y, and a bending moment M_z. The stresses these internal loads produce were discussed in previous chapters of this text. For example, the stresses caused by an axial force were investigated in Chapter 2, the shearing stresses caused by a vertical shear were described in Chapter 4, and also in Chapter 2, the nature of the stresses caused by a bending moment in a beam was discussed. The internal forces may be obtained by the equations of statics (see equations below). From earlier discussions, use $V = 2{,}400$ lb, and then make the appropriate substitution of this quantity into these equations:

$$\Sigma F_x = 0, \qquad P_x - 2\left[\frac{V}{2}\right]\cos 45^\circ = 0, \quad P_x = 1697 \text{ lb}$$

$$\Sigma F_y = 0, \qquad \frac{V}{2}\cos 45^\circ - \frac{V}{2}\cos 45^\circ + V_y = 0, \quad V_y = 0 \text{ lb}$$

$$\Sigma M_{cg} = 0, \qquad \circlearrowleft\!+ \quad -M_z + \frac{V}{2}(1.5 - .485) - \frac{V}{2}(.485) = 0$$

$$M_z = 636 \text{ in-lb}.$$

Axial and Bending Stresses at the Compression Edge of the Hole:

Axial and bending stresses (at Section B-B) are calculated from Eq. 2-9.

$$f = \pm \frac{P}{A} \pm \frac{Mc}{I_{na}}$$

$$= -\frac{1697}{.151} - \frac{636\left[\dfrac{1.371}{2}\right]}{.024} = -11,238 - 18,166$$

$$f_c = -29,404 \text{ psi ultimate.}$$

Compression failure is predicted as follows:

$$\text{Margin of Safety} = \text{M.S.} = \frac{F_{cy}}{f_c} - 1 = \frac{39,000}{29,404} - 1 = +.33.$$

Shearing Stresses Across the Horizontal Shear Plane of the Hole:

The average shearing stress distribution across the horizontal (or vertical) shear plane of the hole is approximated from basic stress principles. Simplification of shearing stresses is permissible and is consistent with the design theory of plate structures. Hence

$$f_s = \frac{V}{A_{\text{shr}}} = \frac{1,200}{.0825} = 14,545 \text{ psi}$$

where: $V = 2,400/2 = 1,200$ lb (the shear divides equally across the hole)
$A_{\text{shr}} = ht = .75(.110) = .0825 \text{ in}^2$
$h = .75$ in
$t = .110$ in.

Shearing failure is predicted as follows:

$$\text{Margin of Safety} = \text{M.S.} = \frac{F_{su}}{f_s} - 1 = \frac{38,000}{14,545} - 1 = +1.61.$$

Since a positive compression margin of safety (M.S. = + .33) and a positive shear margin of safety (M.S. = + 1.61) result, no reinforcement is therefore required for the hole.

It is interesting to note the shear and compression stresses that would have resulted for a hole in an infinite plate. The results of that comparison should be in very good agreement, as they should be, with the detailed solution obtained here. The compression stress f_c at the edge of the hole for an infinite plate is given by:

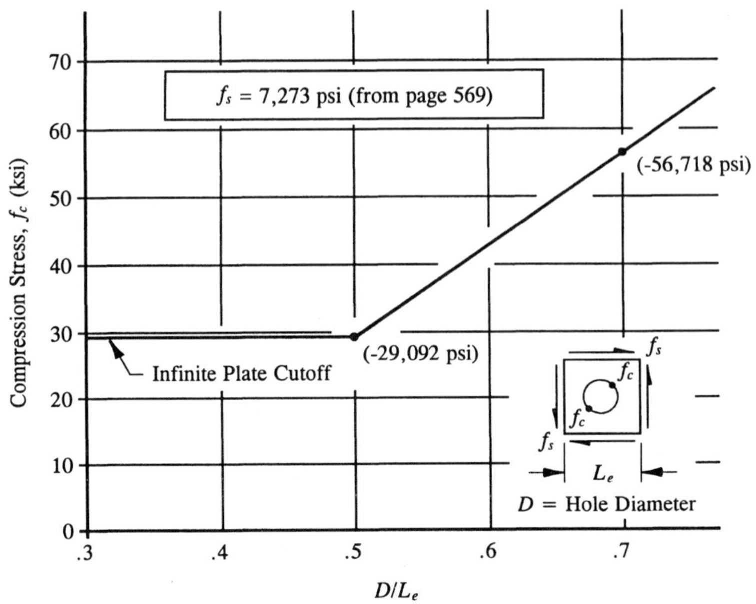

Maximum Compression Stress for an Unreinforced Hole Loaded in Pure Shear in a Shear-Resistant Web. (Do not linearly extrapolate for compression stresses below values of $D/L_e < .5$.)

FIGURE 9-15 Design curve to determine the maximum compression stress at the edge of an open hole.

$$f_c = -4f_s = -4(7,273) = -29,092 \text{ psi} \quad \text{(from Eq. 9-2)}$$

where $f_s = 7,273$ psi (see page 569). This stress is in good agreement with the calculated compression stress (from page 573). Hence, this verifies the notion that an infinite plate has 2*D* effective material around the hole. Comparing compression stresses,

$$\% \text{ Error} = \frac{29,404 - 29,092}{29,092}(100) = 1.1\,\% \quad \text{(slightly conservative)}.$$

Likewise, the maximum shearing stress f_s for an infinite plate is

$$(f_s)_{\max} = 2f_s = 2(7,273) = 14,546 \text{ psi} \quad \text{(from Eq. 9-3)}.$$

Similarly, comparing shearing stresses,

$$\% \text{ Error} = \frac{14,546 - 14,545}{14,546}(100) = 0\,\%.$$

Graphical Method to Determine the Compression Stresses for an Open Hole in a Shear-Resistant Web or Panel

To determine whether a reinforcement is required for an open hole in a shear-resistant web, the foregoing procedure may be applied graphically using a parametric design curve. This is essentially equivalent to applying the basic equations except that a graphical method is considerably quicker in its application. Such a curve is shown in Fig. 9-15 where the results of Example 9-1 are plotted in terms of D/L_e versus f_c. The construction of this curve is left as an exercise for the engineer to complete. Basically, the procedure goes as follows: For a shearing stress of 7,273 psi and panel thickness of .110 in, determine the compression stresses f_c for different values of D/L_e. Starting with Example 9-1, we have for a value of $D/L_e = .7$ a compression stress of $-56,718$ psi, established by following through Example 9-1 again using the same shear stress and panel thickness (as before) but this time with different values of D/L_e. Note that the lower limit of this curve is cut off for that stress corresponding to an unreinforced hole in an infinite plate. How do we use Fig. 9-15 for different values of shearing stress? Using the linear relationship of shearing stress in the solution of Example 9-1, we can formulate an expression for the compression stress at the edge of an unreinforced hole for different values of shearing stress. For instance, by noting that shearing stress is directly proportional to the calculated compression stress at the edge of the hole, the following expression is formulated:

$$(f_c)_{\text{design}} = f_c\left[\frac{(f_s)_{\text{design}}}{7,273}\right] \tag{9-7}$$

where: $(f_c)_{\text{design}}$ = compression stress at the edge of the hole

f_c = compression stress given from Fig. 9-15

$(f_s)_{\text{design}}$ = applied shearing stress.

If the applied shearing stress in Eq. 9-7 is given from a computer model program solution, the value of $(f_s)_{\text{design}}$ is determined as follows:

From Eq. 4-6 (see page 231),

$$q = (f_s)_{\text{program}}\, t_{\text{program}}\,. \tag{1}$$

Since $f_s = q/t$, in terms of a design shearing stress, this gives:

$$(f_s)_{\text{design}} = q/t\,.$$

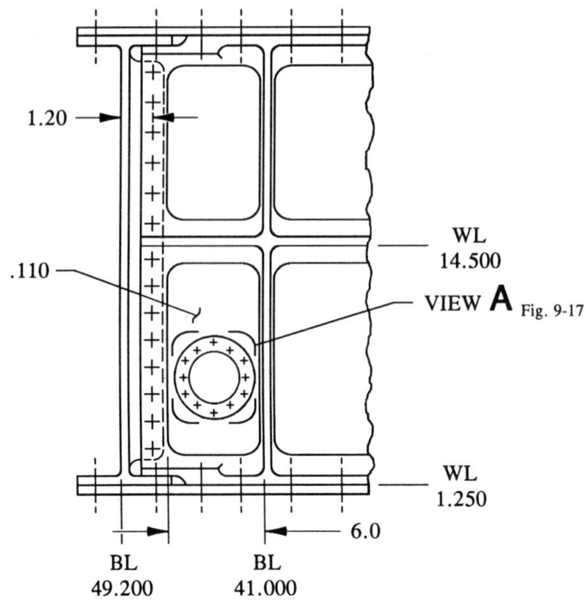

FIGURE 9-16 Reinforced hole with a riveted ring doubler in a machined forged rib.

Substituting for q, we obtain:

$$(f_s)_{\text{design}} = \frac{(f_s)_{\text{program}}\, t_{\text{program}}}{t}$$

where: $(f_s)_{\text{program}}$ = output shearing stress given from a computer program solution
t_{program} = program input panel thickness
t = design panel thickness.

If, instead, the applied shear flow q (also generated from a computer program solution) was given, $(f_s)_{\text{design}}$ would be determined directly from the following relationship derived in Chapter 4 (see Eq. 4-5, page 230):

$$(f_s)_{\text{design}} = q/t.$$

The main purpose in developing a design curve for an unreinforced hole in a shear-resistant web is to have a quick and reliable procedure for determining whether a hole in a shear-resistant web requires reinforcing. A graphical solution should provide a simple and direct way of determining the design requirements. The following example problem will help to illustrate this procedure for a riveted ring doubler.

Example 9-2 Using the analysis method of this section for a reinforced cutout with a riveted ring doubler in a shear-resistant web, determine (a) the stability state of the chem-milled panel of Example 9-1 for an increased hole diameter of 3.0 in (consult the design curve of Fig. 9-15 for this determination), (b) the proper size ring doubler required if the hole in part (a) in fact does need reinforcing, and (c) the particular size and pattern of rivets required if a ring doubler in part (b) was used. Analyze the ring doubler for an average panel ultimate shearing stress of 20,000 psi. Assume this value was given from a computer solution of the rib structure using a program thickness of .080 in. The rib structure with the proposed reinforcement around the hole is shown in Fig. 9-16.

SOLUTION: Using Equation (1) on page 575, the applied shear flow is

$$q = (f_s)_{\text{program}}\, t_{\text{program}} = 20,000(.080) = 1,600 \text{ lb/in.}$$

From this, the actual gross shearing stress is

$$(f_s)_{\text{design}} = \frac{q}{t} = \frac{1,600}{.110} = 14,545 \text{ psi.}$$

The critical shear buckling stress $(F_s)_{cr}$ is 15,011 psi, as determined for the chem-milled panel of Example 9-1 without the hole (see page 568). Before a particular size reinforcement is determined, let us determine the stability of the web. That is, whether the web is buckled or whether it is shear-resistant at the ultimate design shearing stress indicated. Comparing this stress to the critical shear buckling stress of the web,

$$\text{Margin of Safety} = \text{M.S.} = \frac{(F_s)_{cr}}{(f_s)_{\text{design}}} - 1 = \frac{15,011}{14,545} - 1 = +.03.$$

Although a positive margin of safety results, based on the loss of structural stiffness as a result of a 3.0 in diameter hole in the web, the panel will probably buckle. However, providing a reinforcement around the hole should help to stabilize the web. Hence, the reinforced hole can be analyzed as if it were in a shear-resistant web. This hypothesis should prove sufficient from the known fact of the problem to determine whether or not a hole reinforcement is in fact necessary. This assertion is used as a basis for further investigation. The procedure outlined previously using Fig. 9-15 is employed now for this determination. If we enter Fig. 9-15 with a value of $D/L_e = 3.0/5.0 = .6$, we obtain $f_c \approx 43,000$ psi. The compression stress at the edge of the hole is determined from Eq. 9-7. Hence

$$(f_c)_{\text{design}} = f_c\left[\frac{(f_s)_{\text{design}}}{7,273}\right] = 43,000\left[\frac{14,545}{7,273}\right] = 85,994 \text{ psi}$$

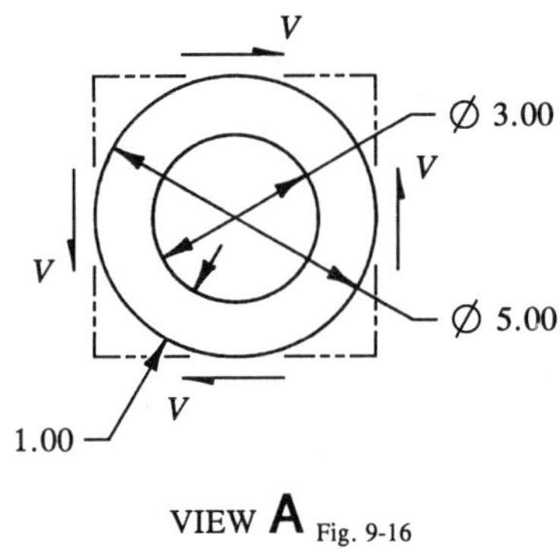

FIGURE 9-17 Free-body diagram of the riveted ring doubler with effective web area.

where: $(f_s)_{\text{design}} = 14,545$ psi (from the previous page)
$f_c = 43,000$ psi (value determined from Fig. 9-15).

If we compare this value to the compression yield stress of the material or $F_{cy} = 39,000$ psi, clearly, a reinforcement is required! The next step in our solution is to design a reinforcement to stabilize the 3.0 in diameter hole so that the web can be considered shear-resistant. The web and ring doubler are free-bodied along the vertical and horizontal tangency lines to the ring doubler, as shown in Fig. 9-17. The shear V is

$$V = qL_e = (f_s)_{\text{design}}\,tL_e = 14,545(.110)(5.0) = 8,000 \text{ lb}$$
$$\frac{1}{2}V = \frac{1}{2}(8,000) = 4,000 \text{ lb}$$

where: $q = (f_s)_{\text{design}}\,t$
$(f_s)_{\text{design}} = 14,545$ psi (see previous page)
$t = .110$ in (given, see Example 9-1)
$L_e = 5.0$ in (see figure above).

Let us now isolate the upper right-hand quarter segment of web and ring doubler, as shown in Fig. 9-18. The internal loads *V, P,* and *M* are determined by passing an imaginary line through the segment along the positive shear diagonal of the reinforced hole, and then applying the equations of static equilibrium at the centroid of the exposed section area (this corresponds to Section A-A in this figure). First, let us calculate the moment of inertia of this section.

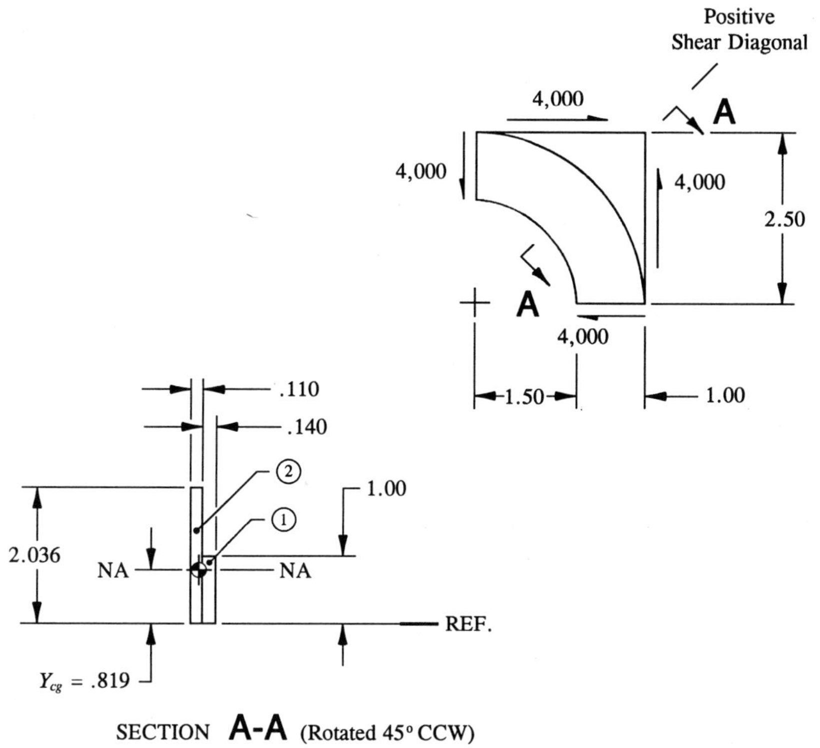

FIGURE 9-18 Quarter segment of web and ring doubler is isolated from the web structure (from Fig. 9-17).

TABLE 9-1 MOMENT OF INERTIA I_{na} AROUND THE NEUTRAL AXIS OF SECTION A-A

Element	b	h	y	A	Ay	Ay^2	I_o
1	0.140	1.000	0.500	0.140	0.070	0.035	0.012
2	0.110	2.036	1.018	0.224	0.228	0.232	0.077
			Total	0.364	0.298	0.267	0.089

$$Y_{cg} = \frac{\Sigma\, Ay}{\Sigma\, A} = \frac{.298}{.364} = .819 \text{ in}$$

$$I_{cg} = \Sigma\, I_o + \Sigma\, Ay^2 - Y_{cg}\,(\Sigma\, Ay) = .089 + .267 - .819(.298) = .112 \text{ in}^4.$$

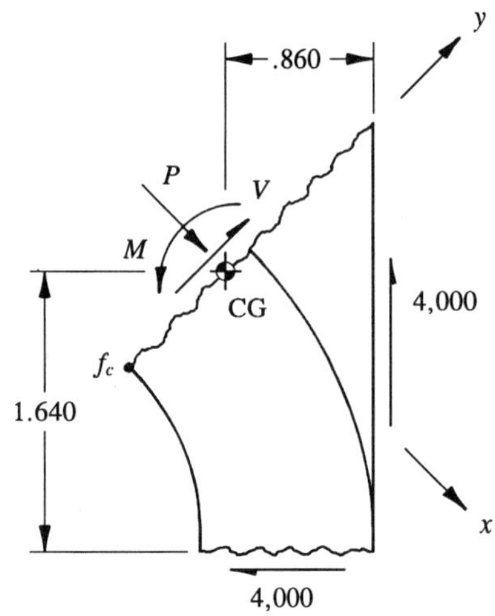

FIGURE 9-19 Internal loads for the riveted ring doubler are indicated along the positive shear diagonal at Section A-A (from Fig. 9-18).

For elastic stress design,

$$I_{na} = I_{cg} = .112 \text{ in}^4.$$

Internal loads *V*, *P*, and *M* at Section A-A:

The internal loads *V*, *P*, and *M* are found by applying the equations of static equilibrium at Section A-A. These calculations are made from Fig. 9-19.

$$\Sigma F_x = 0, \quad P - 4,000 \cos 45^\circ - 4,000 \cos 45^\circ = 0, \quad P = 5,657 \text{ lb}$$

$$\Sigma F_y = 0, \quad V + 4,000 \cos 45^\circ - 4,000 \cos 45^\circ = 0, \quad V = 0 \text{ lb}$$

$$\Sigma M_{cg} = 0, \quad (+) \quad -M - 4,000(.860) + 4,000(1.640) = 0$$

$$M = 3,120 \text{ in-lb}.$$

Axial and Bending Stresses at the Compression Edge of the Hole:

From Eq. 2-9, combined axial and bending stresses at the compression edge of the hole at Section A-A are computed.

$$f = \pm \frac{P}{A} \pm \frac{Mc}{I_{na}}$$

$$= -\frac{5,657}{.364} - \frac{3,120(.819)}{.112} = -15,541 - 22,815$$

$$f_c = -38,356 \text{ psi ultimate}.$$

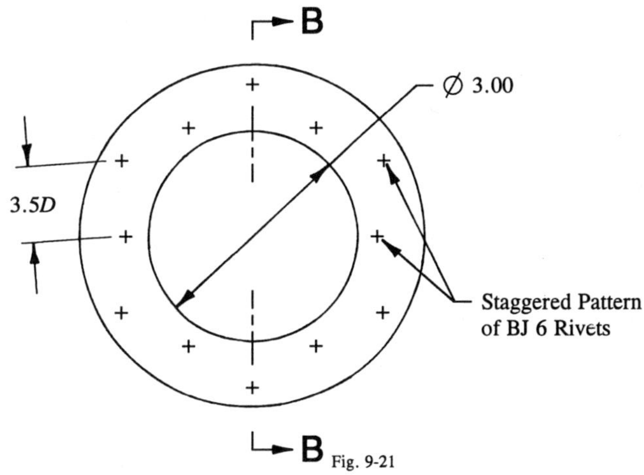

FIGURE 9-20 Staggered pattern of rivets around the riveted ring doubler.

Compression failure is then predicted as follows:

$$\text{Margin of Safety} = \text{M.S.} = \frac{F_{cy}}{f_c} - 1 = \frac{39,000}{38,356} - 1 = +.02.$$

Rivet Design:

Using a staggered pattern of BJ 6 rivets around the doubler, as shown in Fig. 9-20, let us find the shear flow q along this rivet pattern. Failure is then predicted

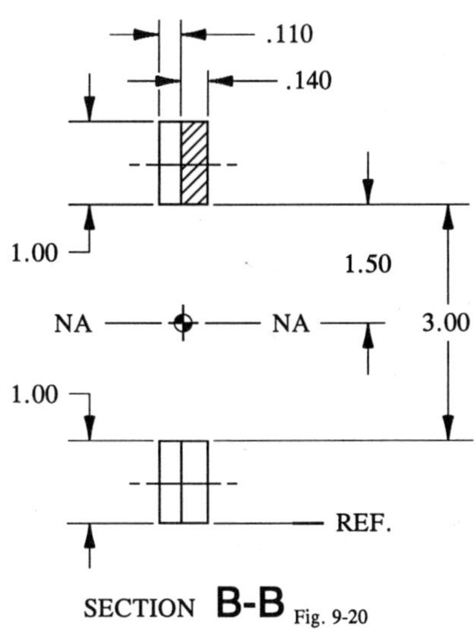

FIGURE 9-21 Section area of web and ring doubler across the hole.

from the ultimate capacity of the joint: Essentially, this means determining the bearing and shearing margins of safety for the most critical rivet. To do this, the shear flow equation, Eq. 4-3 ($q = VQ/I_{na}$) is solved. The values of Q and I_{na} are determined from Section B-B, Fig. 9-21. First, the moment of inertia I_{na} is calculated for the entire section (including the 3.0 in diameter hole) and deducting the moment of inertia for the hole. If this shortcut procedure is unfamiliar, instead, the engineer may wish to determine this value in tabular form as is usually done for most cross-sectional areas or the engineer may wish to review Example A-4 of Appendix F to learn this shortcut approach. Continuing along, from the symmetry of the geometrically shaped section,

$$I_{na} = I_{cg} = \frac{(.110 + .140)(5.0)^3}{12} - \frac{(.110 + .140)(3.0)^3}{12}$$

$$I_{na} = I_{cg} = 2.604 - .562 = 2.042 \text{ in}^4.$$

The partial area shown cross-hatched in Fig. 9-21 is used to determine the value of Q. Consider this member shearing from the basic web structure. It should be recalled (from Chapter 4, Sec. 4.4) that the static moment of area Q is defined as the area of the reinforcement acting around the neutral axis of the total beam section. For our solution, this gives:

$$Q = \Sigma A\bar{y} = 1.0(.140)(1.50 + .500) = .280 \text{ in}^3.$$

From Eq. 4-3, with the total shear $V = 8,000$ lb (refer back to page 578) and to the values computed from above,

$$q = \frac{VQ}{I_{na}} = \frac{8,000(.280)}{2.042} = 1,097 \text{ lb/in ult}.$$

The interconnection shearing forces of these rivets are computed from Eq. 4-10 (see Chapter 4, page 254),

$$p_s = qs = 1,097(.656) = 720 \text{ lb ult}$$

where s = rivet spacing at $3.5D$ or 3.5(6/32) = .656 in.

The rest of this problem involves formulating margins of safety for (1) shearing failure of the reinforcement rivets, (2) bearing failure of the reinforcement, and (3) bearing failure of the web. Refer to Chapter 3 or to specific example problems in this book where these particular failures are investigated.

9.3 Small, Circular Holes or Cutouts Reinforced with Riveted Ring Doublers in Diagonal Tension-Field Webs. The methods and principles of structural

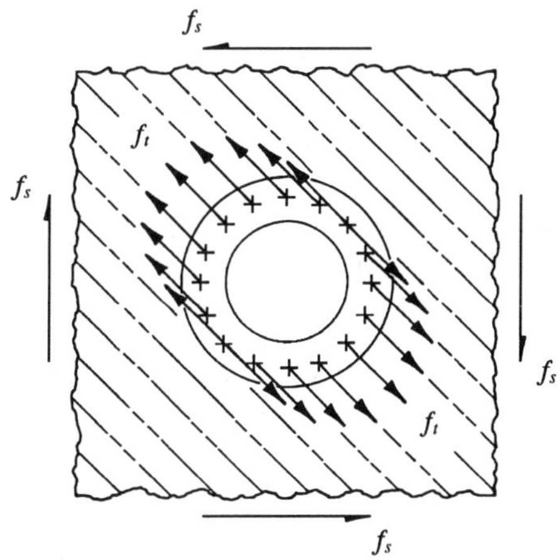

FIGURE 9-22 Shear-loaded flat, rectangular plate in a pure diagonal tension-field web.

analysis of reinforced cutouts with riveted ring doublers in "diagonal tension-field webs or panels" are studied in this section. Reinforced cutouts in a tension field are particularly common to aircraft designs where tension loads predominately govern their design (more about this later). Prescribed buckling requirements are usually established for the outer covering of the fuselage and wing surfaces, pressure bulkheads, ribs, and generally most plate or thin sheet members. If designed efficiently, that is, with due regard to weight reductions and cost-savings, these members will buckle above limit load.

Unlike the previous section where a beam, panel or web was considered shear-resistant at some prescribed stress level, usually corresponding to limit load or some percentage of limit, in this section, a panel becomes buckled at higher loads (investigation of these loads is usually made at ultimate). Such a panel, if loaded in pure shear, has converted part of its applied strain energy in shear into diagonal tension stresses (see representation of these loads in Fig. 9-22). This is only true in its buckled state or configuration. Rarely are webs or panels of this nature exclusively designed to be shear-resistant above limit load. At these higher load levels, shear-resistant webs are not generally weight-efficient and thus their designs are not normally considered for practical design use. The reason buckled webs or panels are more weight-efficient compared to structural members that do not buckle is due to higher allowables being more prevalent in tension (for buckled webs) than in shear-only applications (for shear-resistant webs). When they occur, buckled webs must warrant special attention and consideration. In general, diagonal-tension webs or panels do buckle, hence some deformity of their surfaces is visible to the naked eye (hopefully, not to the close scrutiny of the public). When

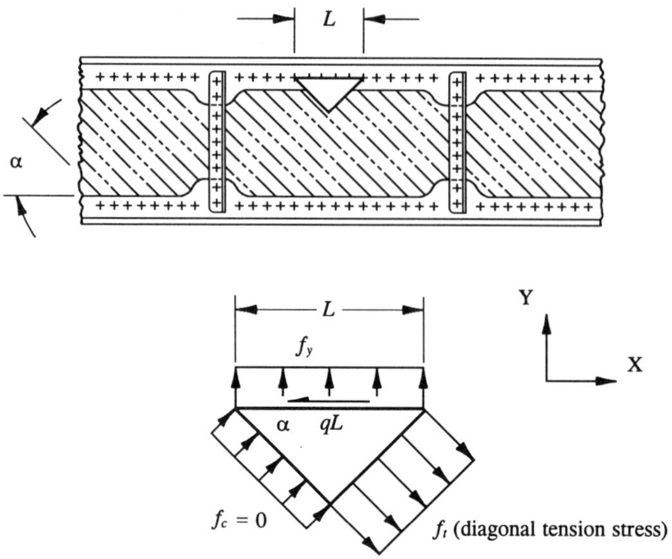

FIGURE 9-23 Triangular element of buckled web is used to develop a mathematical relationship between shearing stresses and diagonal tension stresses.

a panel buckles, it does not fail, it merely sustains the load which precipitated deformity of its surfaces.

Observe the shear-loaded flat, rectangular plate of Fig. 9-22 in a pure diagonal tension-field web. The applied shearing stress f_s is shown carried by (internal) diagonal tension stresses f_t in the web. In pure shear, the plate exhibits a uniform internal shearing stress distribution of the magnitude indicated by the applied loading across the plate edges in that figure. Now assume that the plate is laterally unstable and buckles at the shear loading indicated. The internal stress distribution across the width of the buckled plate is now in tension as shown in this figure by the tension forces across the reinforcement. This distribution arises from the ability of the plate to convert shear load into tension load. The plate remains shear-resistant, nonbuckled until the buckling stress of the plate has been reached. Then the plate undergoes distortion of its surfaces. However, total collapse or failure of the plate structure does not actually occur at this point, some but not all of the applied shear is converted to tension. The deflected shape of the plate is not to be confused with actual structural failure. In fact, even at ultimate load, the web will not necessarily excessively buckle—thus, converting only some of the applied shear loading into diagonal tension stresses. Furthermore, if most of the applied shear loading is converted to diagonal tension stresses, this occurrence is referred to as "complete diagonal tension."

To determine a mathematical relationship between the shearing stresses and the diagonal tension stresses carried by the web, a small triangular element of buckled web in a partial, as opposed to a complete, diagonal tension-field will be isolated and free-bodied, as shown in Fig. 9-23.

The compression stress f_c that caused the web to buckle will be neglected. This assumption is valid since a thin web has relatively little compression stress ability up to the shear buckling stress $(F_s)_{cr}$ of the web.

From statics,

$$\Sigma F_x = 0, \qquad -qL + f_t \cos\alpha (L \sin\alpha) t = 0$$

$$f_t = \frac{q}{t \cos\alpha \sin\alpha}.$$

Using the standard trigonometric function for multiple angles, $\sin 2\alpha = 2 \sin\alpha \cos\alpha$, this equation further simplifies to:

$$f_t = \frac{2q}{t \sin 2\alpha}. \tag{9-8}$$

Next, it is convenient to express the total applied shear flow q as two separate terms: (1) the shear flow that is carried by the web in pure diagonal tension, or q_{tension}; and (2) the shear flow that is carried by the web in pure shear, or q_{shear}. Thus

$$q = q_{\text{tension}} + q_{\text{shear}}. \tag{9-9}$$

Now, if we let k represent a percentage of the total applied shear flow that is carried by the web in diagonal tension, then a factor $1 - k$ would represent the percentage of the shear flow that remains or that portion of the total shear flow that is carried by the web in shear.[1] From these simple definitions, the following general expression can be formulated:

$$q_{\text{tension}} = kq. \tag{9-10}$$

Substituting Eq. 9-10 into Eq. 9-9, and solving for q_{shear}, we also obtain:

$$q_{\text{shear}} = (1 - k)q. \tag{9-11}$$

Note, as the diagonal tension-field factor k increases in this equation, the shear flow carried by the web in pure shear, or q_{shear}, decreases. In terms of the diagonal tension stress f_t (solving for q in Eq. 9-8), Eqs. 9-10 and 9-11 can be rewritten as follows:

---

[1] When a web or panel is analyzed for diagonal tension-field effects, the value of k is commonly referred to as the diagonal-tension factor.

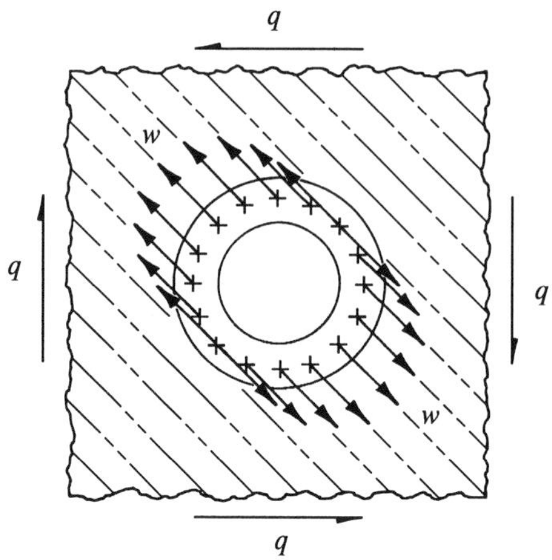

STRESS DISTRIBUTION

FIGURE 9-24 A ring doubler in a pure diagonal tension-field web.

$$q_{\text{tension}} = \frac{k f_t t \sin 2\alpha}{2} \tag{9-12}$$

$$q_{\text{shear}} = \frac{(1 - k) f_t t \sin 2\alpha}{2}. \tag{9-13}$$

In a pure diagonal tension-field, $k = 1$, $\alpha = 45°$, and these equations reduce to:

$$q_{\text{tension}} = \frac{f_t t}{2} \tag{9-14}$$

$$q_{\text{shear}} = 0. \tag{9-15}$$

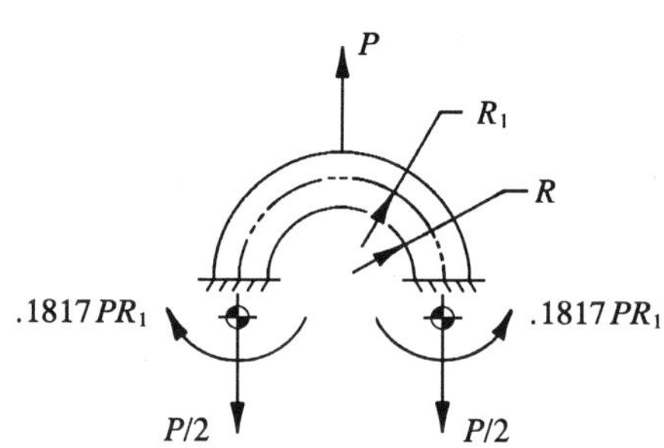

FIGURE 9-25 Equilibrium forces of a thick ring loaded by a concentrated load.

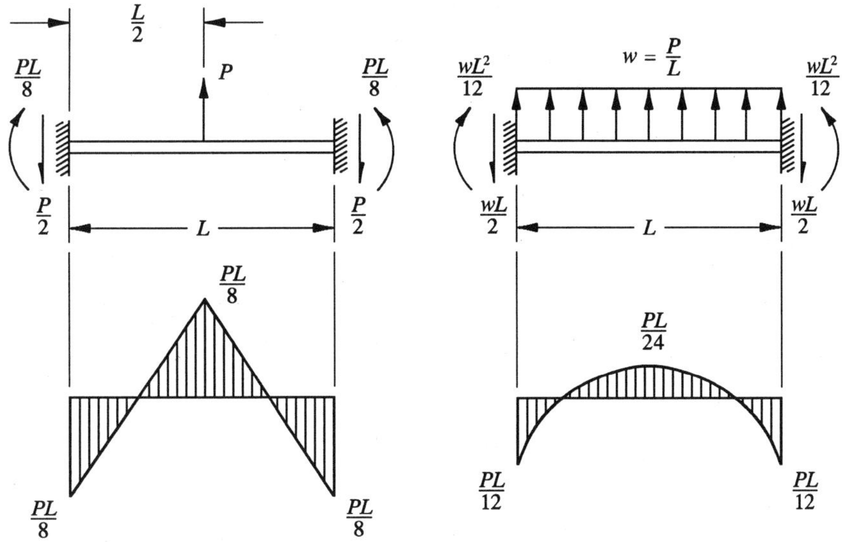

FIGURE 9-26 Comparison of bending moments for a fixed-fixed beam loaded by a concentrated load at center span versus the same beam loaded by an equivalent uniform load.

Substituting Eqs. 9-14 and 9-15 into Eq. 9-9, and solving for f_t, we obtain:

$$f_t = \frac{2q}{t} = 2f_s. \tag{9-16}$$

This equation states that in a pure diagonal tension-field, the diagonal tension stresses are equal to twice the applied shearing stresses of the web. Using this result and the results obtained from the solution of a ring loaded by a concentrated load, Fig. 9-25, similar analogies can be drawn which would lead to the solution of a riveted ring doubler in a pure diagonal tension-field web.

In summary, thin buckled webs are acceptable because of their effectiveness in carrying tension loads. In other words, even though thin webs can maintain the compression stress that induced the web to buckle in the first place, the diagonal tension stress can continue to accept an increasing applied shear load. The higher allowable tension stresses for most materials also make diagonal-tension webs very desirable from a weight reduction standpoint. A ring doubler in a pure diagonal tension-field web is shown in Fig. 9-24. Multiplying both sides of Eq. 9-16 by the web or panel thickness t gives:

$$f_t t = 2f_s t$$

$$w = 2q \tag{9-17}$$

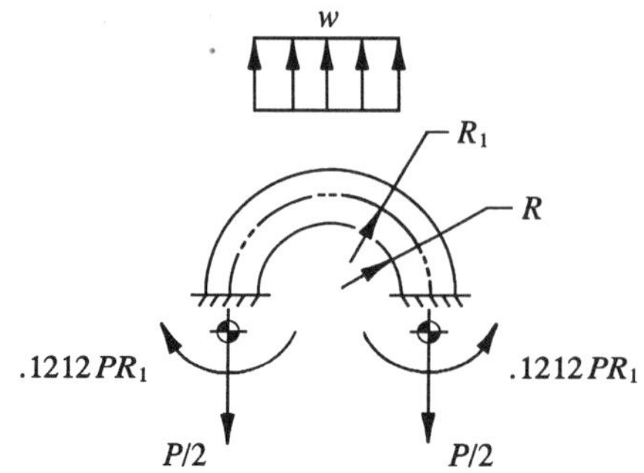

FIGURE 9-27 Free-body diagram of a ring doubler in a pure diagonal tension-field.

where: $w = f_t t$
$q = f_s t$.

A ring loaded by a concentrated load P at the center of the ring has a moment equal to $.1817PR_1$, as shown in Fig. 9-25.[1] Since a ring doubler in a diagonal tension-field is actually loaded by a uniform load w or $2q$, and not by a concentrated load P, the moment in the ring due to diagonal tension-field effects must be reevaluated. This is done by modifying the moment in accordance with straight beam theory. Here, the moments for the ring doubler will be assumed to vary in the same proportion as that of a straight beam. To further simplify our solution, let us compare the end moments of a beam fixed at both ends loaded by a concentrated load at center span versus the same beam loaded by an equivalent uniform load. These beams and their corresponding moment diagrams are compared in Fig. 9-26, and the results of that comparison mathematically formulated as follows:

$$\% \text{ Reduction in End Moments} = \frac{\frac{PL}{8} - \frac{PL}{12}}{\frac{PL}{8}} = 33.3\,\%.$$

Now, using the same reduction in end moments for a ring doubler in a diagonal tension-field, we obtain:

$$M = .1817PR_1 - (33.3\,\% \text{ of } .1817PR_1) = .1212PR_1 \qquad \textbf{(9-18)}$$

where: $P = wL = 2q(2R) = 4qR$
R_1 = radius measured to the centroidal axis of the ring

[1] See Raymond J. Roark, *Formulas for Stress and Strain*, Table VIII, "Formulas for Circular Rings and Arches," Case 1, p. 172, McGraw-Hill Book Company, New York, 1965, Fourth Edition.

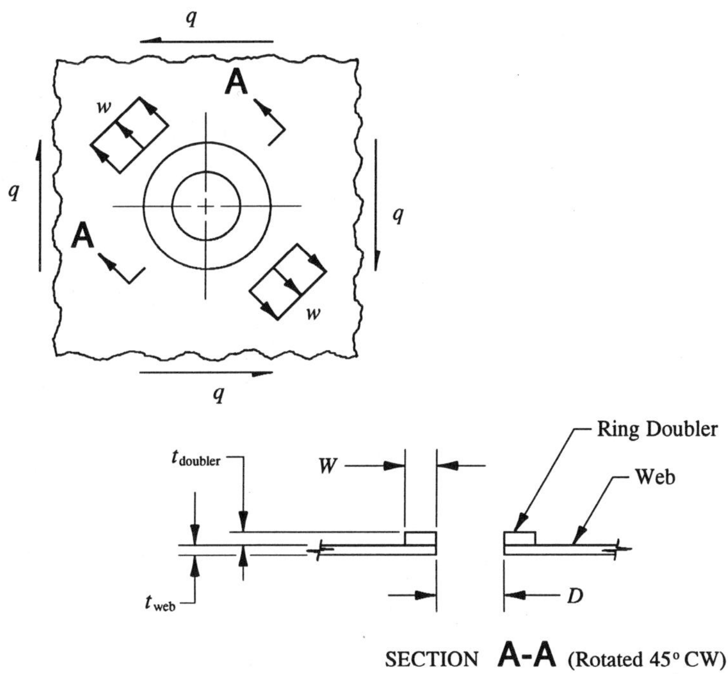

FIGURE 9-28 Cross-sectional properties of the hole and doubler.

q = applied shear flow
R = inside radius of the ring.

The foregoing results are drawn on a free-body diagram of the ring in a diagonal tension-field through the center section of the ring. This is viewed in Fig. 9-27. From the internal loads designated there, an analysis of the ring doubler can be done by conventional stress analysis methods, i.e., by combining axial tension and bending stresses at the inner edges of the hole and reinforcement. The cross-sectional area of the ring doubler including some effective web material should be used to carry the load that the web would have carried if the cutout had not been made in this member. The engineer is referred to Example 9-3 where the detailed solution of a ring doubler in a diagonal tension-field is illustrated. Before this example problem is presented, however, a brief discussion of the principles and methods of approximate analysis to the solution of a reinforced cutout in a diagonal tension-field web or panel is reviewed.

Ring Doubler Approximation Method

To approximate the solution of a riveted ring doubler in a pure diagonal tension-field web or panel, the cross-sectional area removed by the hole across its

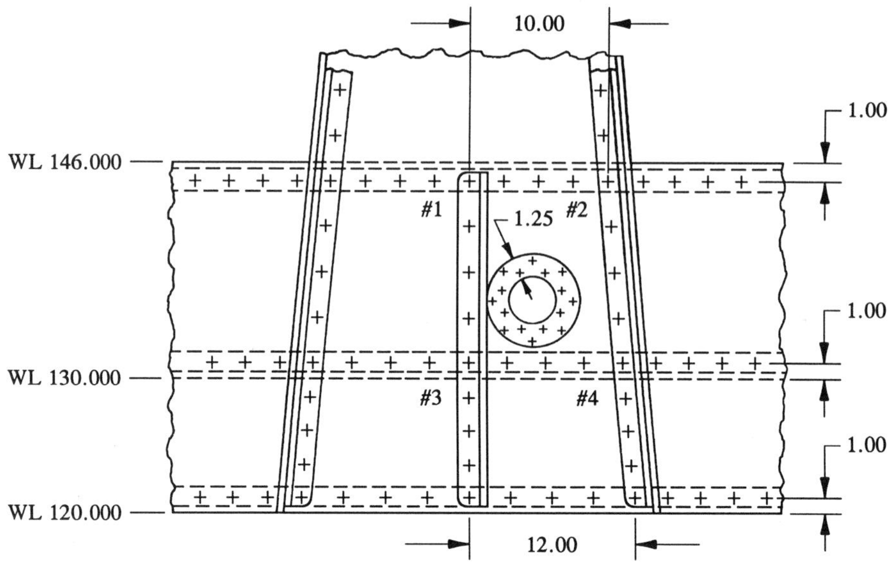

FIGURE 9-29 Riveted ring doubler in the web of a vertical tail spar.

diameter is replaced by a ring doubler of equivalent cross-sectional area. In equation form, this equality says that

$$A_{\text{hole}} = A_{\text{doubler}}.$$

From Fig. 9-28, the geometric properties of the hole and doubler are substituted into this expression. This gives:

$$D\,t_{\text{web}} = 2\,W t_{\text{doubler}}.$$

Next, solving for t_{doubler},

$$t_{\text{doubler}} = \frac{D\,t_{\text{web}}}{2\,W} \tag{9-19}$$

where: D = diameter of the hole

W = width of the ring doubler

t_{web} = web or panel thickness

t_{doubler} = thickness of the ring doubler.

This equation should be used during the initial structural analysis effort of the preliminary design concept. It is extremely important to an efficiently designed structure to make preliminary stress analysis computations. The simplification of

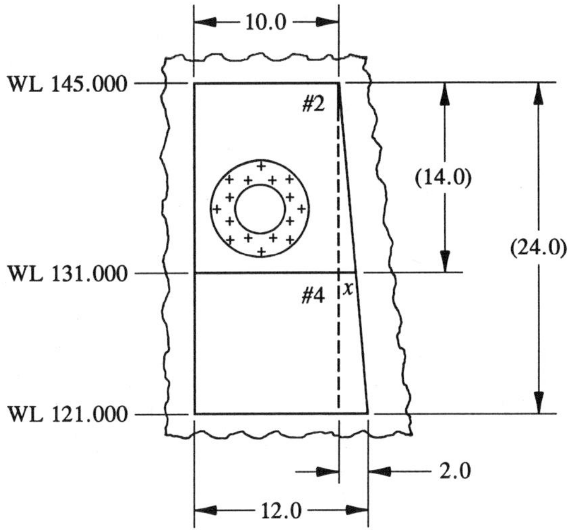

FIGURE 9-30 Dimensions of the panel are determined from the simple geometry of the trapezoidal shape.

stress analysis of a complex solution can serve to assist and support the design engineer in his selection of the final design concept. Of course, it is also important that the engineer differentiate between these approximations and those of more exact methods of detailed stress analysis. An approximate solution is therefore only the "first step" used in the creative and intelligent thought process of truly successful aircraft designs.

Example 9-3 A 4.0 in diameter hole is located in the web of the vertical tail spar shown in Fig. 9-29. For a maximum shear flow of 490 lb/in limit and a web thickness of .063 in, what size ring reinforcement would be required for the hole at ultimate load? Use Eq. 9-19 for rough sizing and then verify the results by a detailed analysis of the reinforcement for combined axial tension and bending stresses at the inner edges of the hole. Assuming that buckling requirements at limit load have been previously met by analysis, determine a staggered pattern of rivets for the ring doubler at ultimate load to securely attach this member around the hole. The vertical tail spar web is constructed of clad 2024-T3 aluminum alloy sheet material (QQ-A-250/5). Use the following mechanical properties given from MIL-HDBK-5F for this material: $F_{tu} = 62,000$ psi, $F_{cy} = 37,000$ psi, $F_{su} = 38,000$ psi, $F_{bru} = 125,000$ psi ($e/D = 2.0$), $F_{bry} = 84,000$ psi ($e/D = 2.0$), $E_c = 10.7 \times 10^6$ psi, and $\mu = .33$. To meet strain compatibility requirements, it is recommended that the ring doubler be made from the same material as the web. Assume a factor of safety of 1.5 for ultimate design and a fitting factor of 1.15 as recommended by the FAA for riveted joint designs.

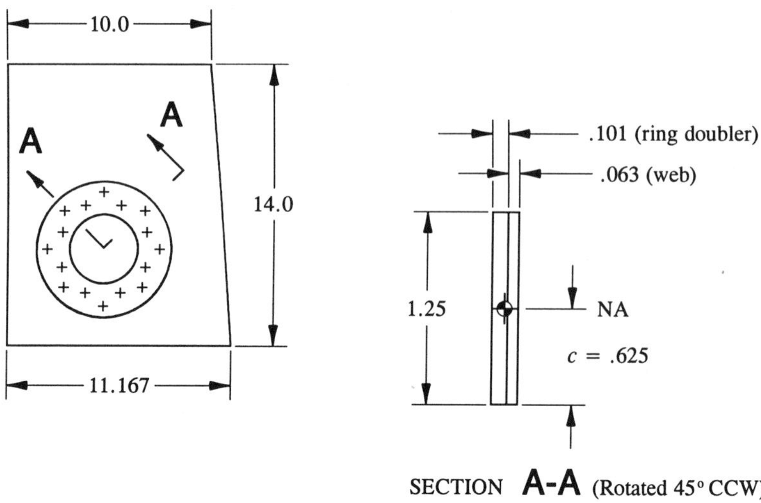

FIGURE 9-31 Panel dimensions and sectional area detail of the web and riveted doubler.

SOLUTION: Before analyzing a ring doubler in a diagonal tension-field web, let us find out if panel #2 is, in fact, buckled at ultimate load. To do this, the theoretical shear buckling stress of the web is computed and compared to the applied ultimate shearing stress of the panel. The panel is buckled if the applied ultimate shearing stress is shown to be greater than the theoretical shear buckling stress. The solution follows by applying Eqs. 8-5 and 8-8 and comparing the result with the applied ultimate shearing stress of the panel. Although the panel may be only slightly buckled at ultimate load, it is customary to assume a pure diagonal tension-field condition for the web. The analysis of the ring doubler is then performed by the procedure outlined previously for a pure diagonal tension-field web. To assume a ring doubler in a shear-resistant web would be unconservative.[1]

Critical Shear Buckling Stress for Panel #2:

$$\frac{(F_s)_{cr}}{\eta_s} = \frac{\pi^2 K_s E_c}{12(1 - \mu^2)} \left[\frac{t}{b}\right]^2$$

where: $K_s = 5.34 + 4.00\left[\frac{b}{a}\right]^2$ (this corresponds to a panel with simply-supported edges, refer to page 503, Curve B)

[1] This observation was made by comparing the compression margin of safety for a ring doubler in a shear-resistant web with the tension margin of safety for that same ring doubler in a diagonal tension-field web. The latter analysis was found to be more critical in all cases where this comparison was made. The engineer is encouraged to verify this by making his own margin of safety comparisons of different size reinforced cutouts. Use the methods outlined in this section for this purpose.

E_c = 10.7 x 10^6 psi
μ = .33
a = 14.0 in (height of panel)
b = 10.583 in[1] (average width of panel, see calculations below)
t = .063 in (web thickness).

From similar triangles, the following ratio is formulated and the value of x determined:

$$\frac{14}{24} = \frac{x}{2}$$

$$x = 1.167 \text{ in.}$$

From this, the end dimension of the panel (at WL 131) is calculated to be 11.167 in. The rest of the panel dimensions are shown in Fig. 9-31.

To determine the critical shear buckling stress for a trapezoidal-shaped panel, let us assume an average value for the shorter b dimension of the panel. This gives:

$$b = \frac{10.0 + 11.167}{2} = 10.583 \text{ in.}$$

Solving for K_s first, we obtain:

$$K_s = 5.34 + 4.00\left[\frac{10.583}{14.0}\right]^2 = 7.626.$$

Now, substituting this value and all other known values into the theoretical shear buckling stress gives:

$$\frac{(F_s)_{cr}}{\eta_s} = \frac{\pi^2 (7.626)(10.7 \text{ x } 10^6)}{12\left[1 - (.33)^2\right]}\left[\frac{.063}{10.583}\right]^2 = 2,669 \text{ psi.}$$

Using Fig. 8-15 and the stress relationship that exists between compression and shear for ductile materials, Eq. 8-6, the value of $(F_s)_{cr}/\eta_s$ can be verified to correspond to the elastic portion of the compression plasticity correction curve for clad 2024-T3 aluminum alloy sheet material, hence, η_s = 1.0.[2] Thus, the true shear buckling stress is

$$(F_s)_{cr} = 2,669 \text{ psi.}$$

[1] From Fig. 9-30, the average value for the shorter dimension of panel #2 is figured from simple geometry of a trapezoidal shape. Also, consider the panel dimensions as measured from the boundary rivets of the panel.

[2] This essentially confirms that the theoretical shear buckling stress corresponds to the true elastic shear buckling stress of the panel for low values of shearing stress.

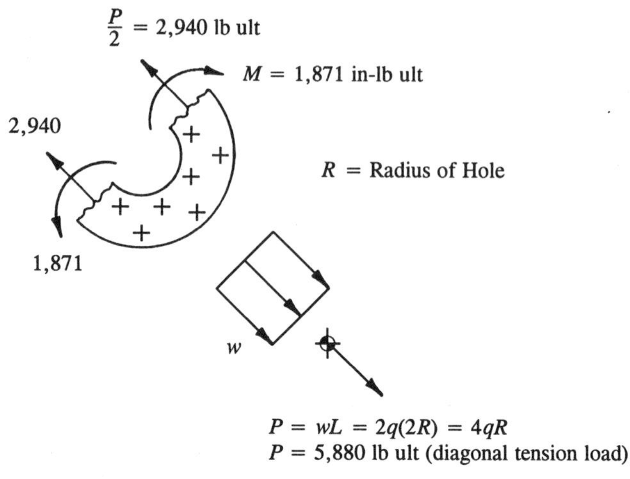

FIGURE 9-32 Using Eq. 9-18, a statics solution of the doubler and effective web material is determined.

From the definition of shearing stress, Eq. 4-5, the applied shearing stress is

$$f_s = \frac{q}{t} = \frac{490}{.063} = 7,778 \text{ psi limit; } 11,667 \text{ psi ultimate}.$$

The magnitude of this value clearly indicates that the web is buckled at ultimate load and that the analysis of a reinforced cutout with a riveted ring doubler in a pure diagonal tension-field web is therefore applicable to our further solution of this problem. The actual degree of buckling is verified by comparing the ultimate shearing stress f_s to the critical shear buckling stress $(F_s)_{cr}$ calculated from the previous page. Substitution of these values into the margin of safety expression gives:

$$\text{Margin of Safety} = \text{M.S.} = \frac{(F_s)_{cr}}{f_s} - 1 = \frac{2,669}{11,667} - 1$$

$$\text{M.S.} = -.77 \quad \text{(this verifies that buckling does occur)}.$$

Now, to get some general sense of direction as to the thickness of ring doubler required around the hole, let us begin our analysis of this problem by solving Eq. 9-19 (see page 590).

$$t_{\text{doubler}} = \frac{D\,t_{\text{web}}}{2\,W} = \frac{4.0(.063)}{2(1.25)} = .101 \text{ in.}$$

From this solution, the section properties of the ring doubler and effective web material acting together are determined. Section property calculations are referred to in subsequent paragraphs of this example solution.

Internal loads:

The diagonal tension loads across the hole are found from the general theory of internal loads analysis, i.e., from a statics solution of the doubler and effective web material, or from Eq. 9-18, where the calculated values of the internal axial load and bending moment are determined. These loads are shown in Fig. 9-32, where the doubler and effective web material are isolated and free-bodied.

$$P = wL = 2q(2R) = 4qR = 4(490)(2) = 3,920 \text{ lb limit; } 5,880 \text{ lb ultimate}.$$

From this, the internal axial load is $P/2$ or 1,960 lb limit; 2,940 lb ultimate (see Fig. 9-32), and the bending moment is

$$\begin{aligned} M &= .1212 PR_1 \quad \text{(see Eq. 9-18 on page 588)} \\ &= .1212(5,880)(2.625) \\ M &= 1,871 \text{ in-lb ultimate (this value is also shown in Fig. 9-32).} \end{aligned}$$

Combined axial and bending stresses:

From Section A-A, Fig. 9-31, the distance from the neutral axis to the tension edge of the hole is .625 in, hence the value, $c = .625$. The area and moment of inertia of this section are computed for a combined rectangular section (i.e., doubler plus effective web). In addition, for elastic stresses, $I_{na} = I_{cg}$, and therefore by using the moment of inertia for a rectangular-shaped section (see Appendix F, Table A-5, $I_o = bh^3/12$), we obtain:

$$I_{na} = I_{cg} = \frac{bh^3}{12} = \frac{(.101 + .063)(1.25)^3}{12} = .027 \text{ in}^4$$

$$A = bh = (.101 + .063)1.25 = .205 \text{ in}^2.$$

The combined axial tension and bending stresses are calculated from Eq. 2-9.

$$f = \pm\frac{P}{A} \pm \frac{Mc}{I_{na}}$$

$$f_t = +\frac{2,940}{.205} + \frac{1,871(.625)}{.027} = 14,341 + 43,310 = 57,651 \text{ psi}.$$

At the opposite extreme fibers of this cross-sectional area, compression stresses, usually much lower, are not investigated. Consequently, only tension

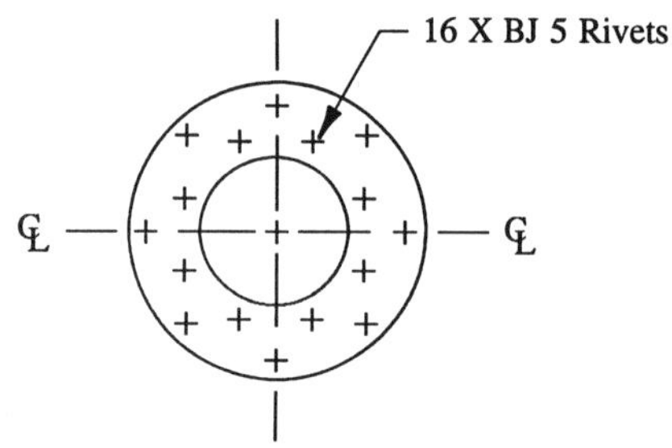

FIGURE 9-33 Staggered pattern of rivets around a riveted ring doubler.

failure of the section along the tension edges of the hole needs to be substantiated. That is,

Tension failure:

$$\text{Margin of Safety} = \text{M.S.} = \frac{F_{tu}}{f_t} - 1 = \frac{62{,}000}{57{,}651} - 1 = +.08.$$

Clearly, with a margin of safety of 8%, the .101 in ring doubler is of adequate size and strength to effectively reinforce the hole, and therefore no further refinement of the analysis is necessary.

Rivet pattern:

If the buckled web is fully effective in a diagonal tension-field web, the load transferred to the ring by the web, or P_{ring}, can be determined by taking a percentage of the load that the web carried before the hole was made. To determine this value, the following ratio of thicknesses[1] is taken:

$$P_{\text{ring}} = P\left[\frac{t_{\text{ring}}}{t_{\text{ring}} + t_{\text{web}}}\right] \tag{9-20}$$

$$P_{\text{ring}} = 5{,}880\left[\frac{.101}{.101 + .063}\right] = 3{,}621 \text{ lb ultimate}$$

where: $t_{\text{ring}} = .101$ in (ring doubler thickness)
$t_{\text{web}} = .063$ in (web thickness)
$P = 5{,}880$ lb ultimate (calculated from page 595).

[1] Equation 9-20 is actually developed from a ratio of area terms, not thicknesses. However, since the widths of the ring and effective web are the same, the width terms in this equation cancel, which will then lead to the reduced expression indicated.

From the centerline bisector of the ring and the total number of rivets given, Fig. 9-33, it can be reasoned that eight (8) rivets transfer load from the web to the doubler, and another eight (8) transfer load from the doubler across the hole back to the web. Hence, from this simple reasoning, it can be deduced that eight (8) reinforcement rivets will share the ring load P_{ring}, or in terms of the shearing force per rivet,

$$p_s = \frac{P_{\text{ring}}}{8} = \frac{3,621}{8} = 453 \text{ lb ultimate.}$$

The prevailing attitude of experienced engineers assumes that a buckled web is structurally less effective in a diagonal tension-field, and for this reason, it is common to see assumptions made of reduced web structural effectivity (or partial loss in structural stiffness) for this member. For example, if we assume the web is 80% effective, which is probably based on the design engineer's own personal judgment and experience for that particular design case, Eq. 9-20 would be modified slightly as follows:

$$P_{\text{ring}} = P\left[\frac{t_{\text{ring}}}{t_{\text{ring}} + .80\,t_{\text{web}}}\right] \qquad \textbf{(9-21)}$$

where: P = diagonal tension load (see Fig. 9-32)
t_{ring} = ring doubler thickness
t_{web} = web thickness.

For extremely buckled webs, where the critical shear buckling stress $(F_s)_{cr}$ is much less than the ultimate applied shearing stress f_s of the web, assumptions of 50% web effectivity are quite common. The engineer must use his own discretion as to how conservative he may wish his designs to be. In the final analysis, each design will ultimately be verified by some form of structural testing. Which is of course a necessary prerequisite to general aircraft certification.

Ultimate Allowable Shearing Strength of the Reinforcement Rivets:

$$P_{su} = F_{su} A_{shr} C_r = 596(1.0) = 596 \text{ lb}$$

where: $F_{su} A_{shr}$ = 596 lb (from Table 3-1)
C_r = 1.0 (from Table 3-2 in .063 in sheet thickness).

Shearing failure is then predicted by:

$$\text{Margin of Safety} = \text{M.S.} = \frac{P_{su}}{p_s k} - 1 = \frac{596}{(453)1.15} - 1 = +.14.$$

Ultimate Allowable Bearing Strength of the Vertical Tail Spar Web:

Since $F_{bru} < 1.5F_{bry}$, Eq. 3-2 is correctly chosen for the computation of ultimate allowable bearing strength of the vertical tail spar web.

$$P_{bru} = F_{bru}tD = 125,000(.063)(.159) = 1,252 \text{ lb}$$

where: $F_{bru} = 125,000$ psi (QQ-A-250/5, $e/D = 2.0$)
$F_{bry} = 84,000$ psi (QQ-A-250/5, $e/D = 2.0$)
$t = .063$ in
$D = .159$ in (nominal hole diameter).

Bearing failure is then predicted by:

$$\text{Margin of Safety} = \text{M.S.} = \frac{P_{bru}}{p_s k} - 1 = \frac{1,252}{(453)1.15} - 1 = +1.40.$$

Ultimate Allowable Bearing Strength of the Ring Doubler:

Although the ultimate allowable bearing strength of the ring doubler should prove to be less bearing critical than the web itself, and therefore should require no analytical substantiation (note that this member is slightly thicker), for the sake of completeness, its detailed analysis will nevertheless be performed. For the same material, $F_{bru} < 1.5F_{bry}$, and once again Eq. 3-2 is applied, this time, for the computation of ultimate allowable bearing strength of the ring doubler.

$$P_{bru} = F_{bru}tD = 125,000(.101)(.159) = 2,007 \text{ lb}$$

where: $F_{bru} = 125,000$ psi (QQ-A-250/5, $e/D = 2.0$)
$F_{bry} = 84,000$ psi (QQ-A-250/5, $e/D = 2.0$)
$t = .101$ in
$D = .159$ in (nominal hole diameter).

Bearing failure is then predicted by:

$$\text{Margin of Safety} = \text{M.S.} = \frac{P_{bru}}{p_s k} - 1 = \frac{2,007}{(453)1.15} - 1 = +2.85.$$

9.4 Medium, Circular Holes or Cutouts in Shear-Resistant and Diagonal Tension-Field Webs or Panels. This section will present an elementary discussion of the design theories and philosophies of windows, windshields, access doors, passenger doors, baggage doors, etc., all of which are common to that group of members referred to as "nonstructural." Essentially, a nonstructural door is

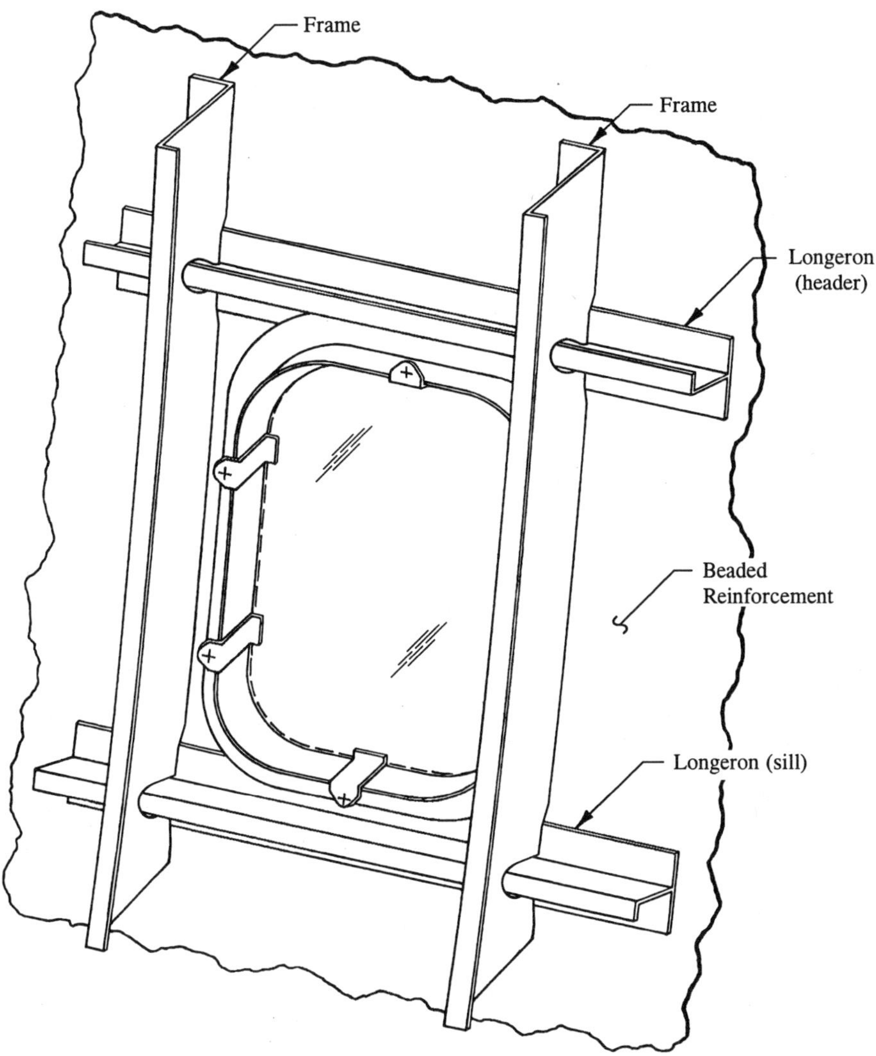

FIGURE 9-34 Simplified fuselage window framing.

designed to carry only pressure loads. Body shears due to normal flight condition loads are carried around the door opening for this type of member. The advanced nature of "structural door cutouts" is left for those engineers who desire a further study of their own on this particular subject. Through aircraft flight service and general aircraft maintenance experience, it has been found that a nonstructural door is easier to operate and service than a structural door. For this reason, most aircraft door designs are nonstructural. However, for large cutouts, such as equipment-handling doors or cargo doors, the structural door is more economical

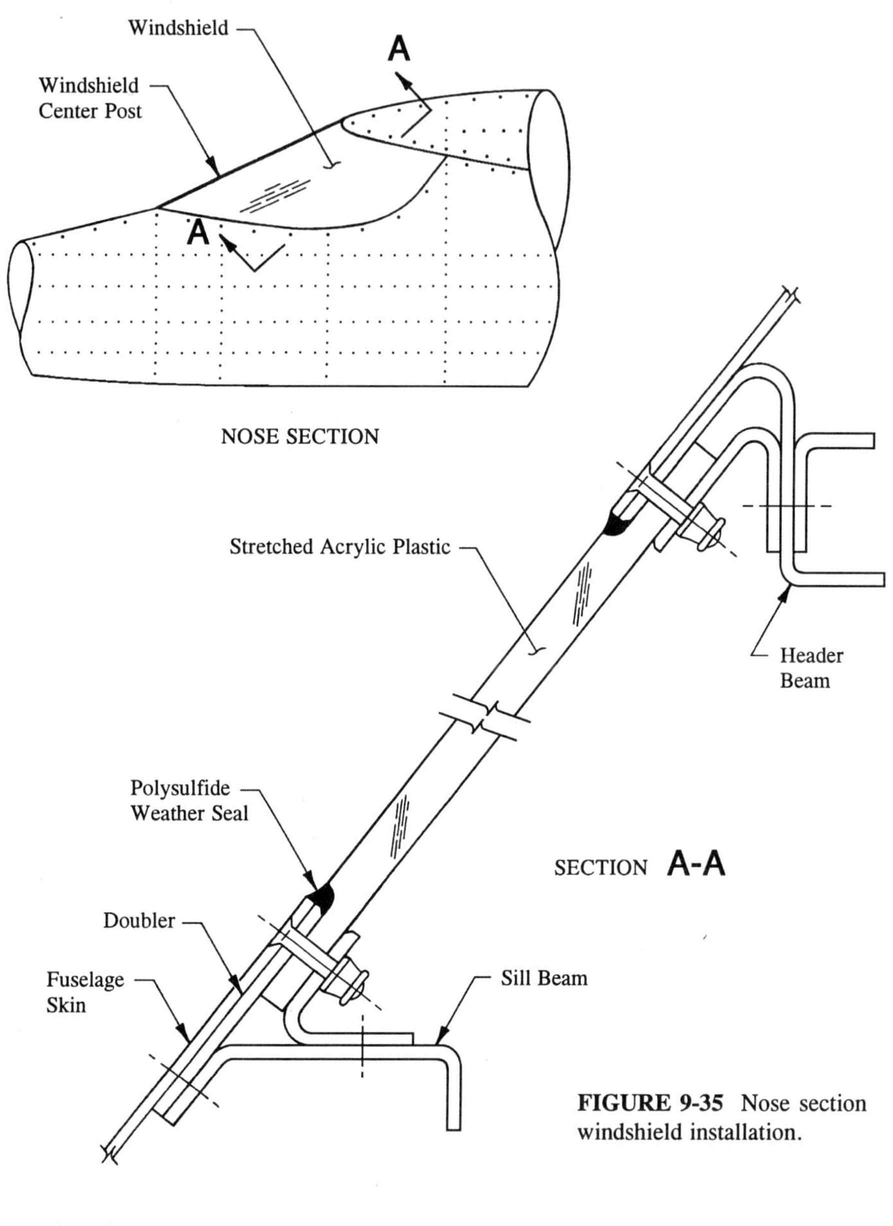

FIGURE 9-35 Nose section windshield installation.

and therefore more desirable (more about this later). If the fuselage is pressurized to permit high-altitude flight, the nonstructural door is designed to carry "only" burst pressure, while the structural door, considered a load-carrying member, must carry ultimate flight loads with limit pressure loads superimposed. Essentially, this means that body shears due to normal flight condition loads as well as longitudinal and hoop tension loads from limit pressure loads are carried through the door for this structural member.

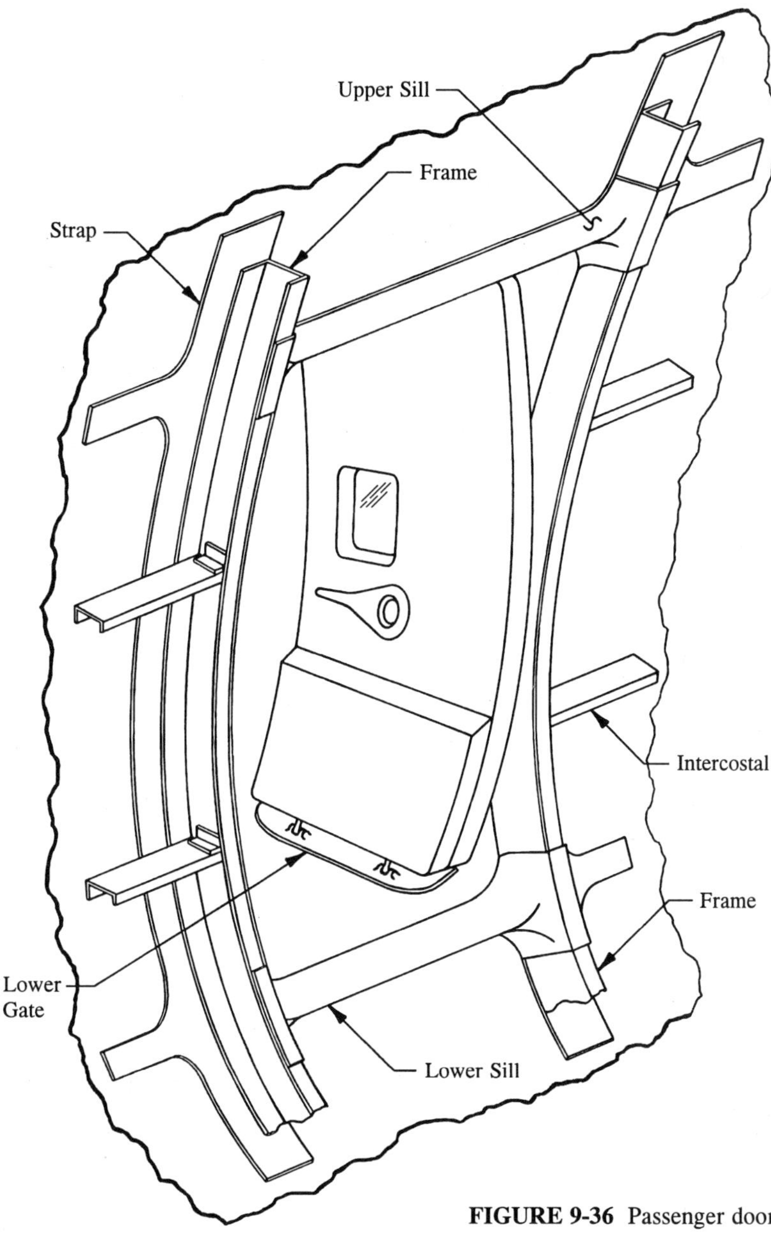

FIGURE 9-36 Passenger door.

A typical framework for a passenger window (nonstructural in this case) for a pressurized aircraft is shown in Fig. 9-34. The opening of the window is reinforced by fuselage frames or rings and by upper and lower extruded longeron members. The longeron members are needed to box in the window opening and thus laterally stabilize the frames from out-of-plane bending. The longerons by themselves are

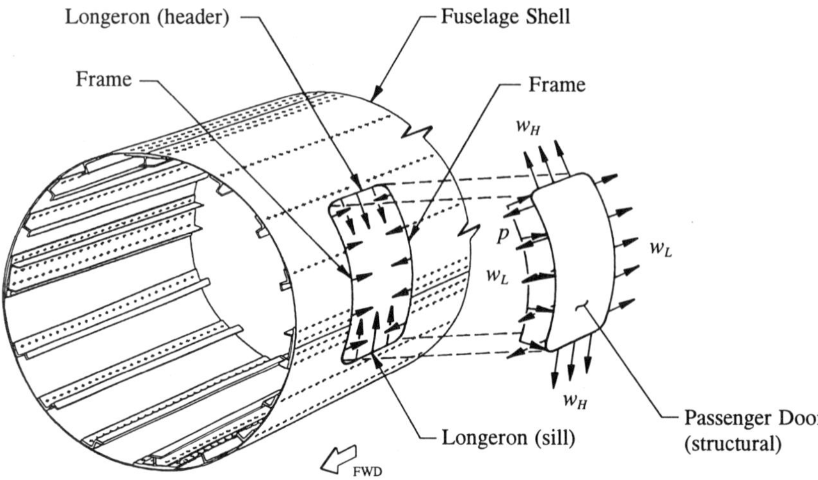

w_L = longitudinal loading, lb/in
w_H = circumferential or hoop loading, lb/in

FIGURE 9-37 Longitudinal and hoop tension loads due to cabin pressurization.

not deep enough to accomplish the additional stiffness required to adequately design the cutout region of the window. Also notice that the paneling around the door is double reinforced with a beaded doubler. This insures that these panels will have sufficient stiffness to prevent panel buckling at prescribed loads. Otherwise, if the panels buckle, the diagonal tension-field effects resulting from this condition will induce out-of-plane loads directly into the frames, causing these members lateral instability. Without longeron members, the frame would have to be beefed up more than the additional weight that longitudinal members would provide if their designs were instead incorporated into the framing structure. Also, the corners of the window should be provided with sufficient radii to prevent high limit stresses, and thus minimize the fatigue damage of the cutout for the normal expected service life of the aircraft.

In cases where a fairly large cutout is made in a skin panel or beam web, a hand redistribution of existing shear flows for the cutout should be contemplated instead of having to make a costly computer rerun of the new design configuration. The method used is quite simple, the existing loads are modified by combining the shear flow of the panel with the relatively large cutout (as far as the panel size goes) with the shear flows of the adjacent panels around the cutout. In effect, for such cutouts, the panel is assumed to have failed. Although some material may actually remain around the cutout, the load the panel carried before it was cut out is basically redistributed to the adjacent structural panels. Sometimes even if a small crack in a panel is stop-drilled, the panel is analyzed as if it had failed. The method of analysis used in Sec. 9-2 (page 558) can be utilized for this determination until a

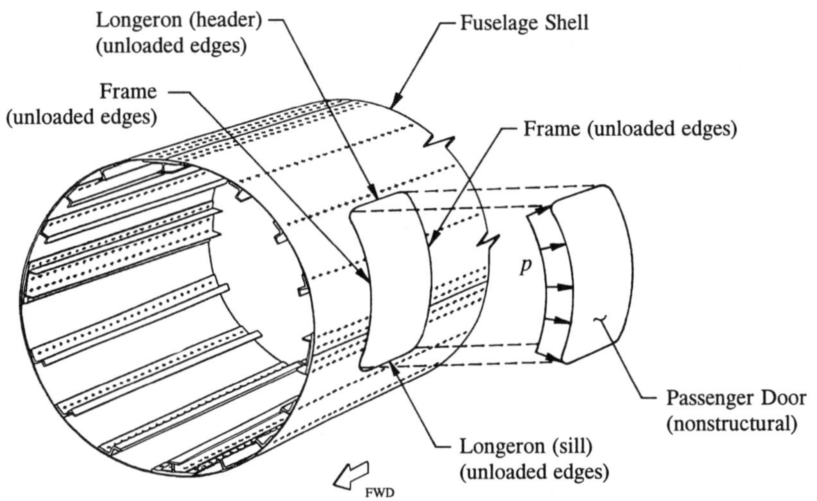

FIGURE 9-38 Pressurized nonstructural door.

computer run can more aptly be justified when more changes have been made and accumulated to the basic aircraft structure. For the most part, a hand-calculated redistribution of loads (i.e., shear flows) should suffice where minor changes to the basic structure have been made.

The windshield installation of a lightweight aircraft is shown in Fig. 9-35. The windshield opening is reinforced by a sill beam, header beam, and center post. The windshield, made of stretched acrylic plastic, is protected with a waterproof adhesive tape around its boundary structure. The sill and header beams are designed without considering any effective windshield material acting in bending with these members. The low allowable strength values of the windshield make the stiffness of this member structurally inefficient. Hence, it is conservatively neglected, omitted from the basic analysis of the framing members. Formed to fit the contour of the aircraft, these members are flanged for increased stiffness and joggled to accommodate the thickness of the window. The window is fitted into the reinforced structure around the opening of the window. These retaining structural members essentially sandwich the window in its properly installed position.

The passenger door of a pressurized executive jet is illustrated in Fig. 9-36. For safety reasons, the door is designed to act as a plug for the door opening. Cabin pressurization actually seats the door against the door framing members. The operation of the door is such that upper and lower hinged gates fold inward causing the door to become smaller than the door opening. This allows the door to move inside the aircraft and the locking mechanism to track the door into its proper closed position. Cabin pressure then seats the door by pushing it outward against the door framing members. The framework around the door opening is constructed of stiff bending members, usually of aluminum alloy material.

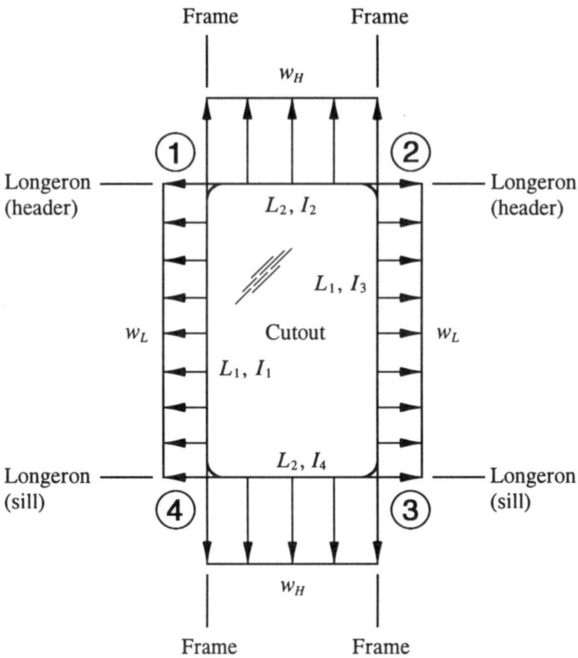

FIGURE 9-39 Longitudinal and hoop tension self-balancing loads carried by the framing structure around the door cutout.

The passenger door of a pressurized executive jet is removed from the fuselage cabin as shown in Fig. 9-37. The longitudinal and hoop tension loads resulting from cabin pressurization are determined from thin-walled, cylindrical pressure vessel theory and applied to the door, longerons, and frame members of the fuselage structure. This illustration shows how the door is maintained in equilibrium against the internal cabin pressure p (psi). If the door is structural, the longitudinal and hoop tension loads are carried through the door.

However, if the door is nonstructural, the longitudinal and hoop tension loads must be carried around the door opening, not through the door. To achieve this loading configuration (see Fig. 9-38), a system of equal and opposite set of self-balancing loads, Fig. 9-39, must be combined with the longitudinal and hoop tension loads of the fuselage edge members. In this way, the edge members are then unloaded so that the door can be removed from the fuselage structure with only the pressure loads acting upon it. The door is then designed for the ultimate cabin pressure p (in psi).

The longitudinal and hoop tension loads are derived from the internal stresses resulting from a cylindrical pressure vessel. Hence, since the fuselage is also a cylindrical-shaped structure, when pressurized, it also acts according to pressure vessel theory. Therefore, from this analogy, the following equations also apply to the fuselage shell:

LONGITUDINAL TENSION LOAD:

$$w_L = \frac{pR}{2} \tag{9-22}$$

where: w_L = longitudinal tension load, lb/in
p = internal cabin pressure, psi
R = radius of the fuselage or pressure vessel (for aircraft or missile design), in.

HOOP TENSION LOAD:

$$w_H = pR \tag{9-23}$$

where: w_H = hoop tension load, lb/in
p = internal cabin pressure, psi
R = radius of the fuselage or pressure vessel (for aircraft or missile design), in.

Structurally, the frame and longeron members must be shown to carry the self-balancing ultimate longitudinal and hoop tension loads around the cutout.[1] The method of moment distribution (or Hardy Cross) for the framing structure of the door will be used to determine the modified corner end-fixity moments. The corner end-fixity moments are then combined with the axial loads due to longitudinal and hoop tension loads from burst pressure using standard strength analysis methods (from simple beam theory, stresses can be predicted by the application of Eq. 2-9 or $f = \pm P/A \pm Mc/I_{na}$). The engineer is also referred to the "elastic center method" in the solution of closed-ring types of rigid structure.[2]

System of Self-Balancing Longitudinal and Hoop Tension Loads Around a Cutout Due to Burst (or Ultimate) Pressure

Based on the Hardy Cross Method of Analysis of redundant structures, the general expression for the modified end-fixity moments (or joint moments) of a framing structure is formulated:

$$M_n = (\text{FEM})_n - \Sigma\, (\text{FEM})_{\text{joint}}\, (\text{DF})_n \tag{9-24}$$

---

[1] Of course, these edge members must also be designed for ultimate flight loads superimposed with longitudinal and hoop tension loads due to limit pressure.

[2] W.M. Fife and J.B. Wilbur, *Theory of Statically Indeterminate Structures*, pp. 114-120, McGraw-Hill Book Company Inc., New York, 1937.

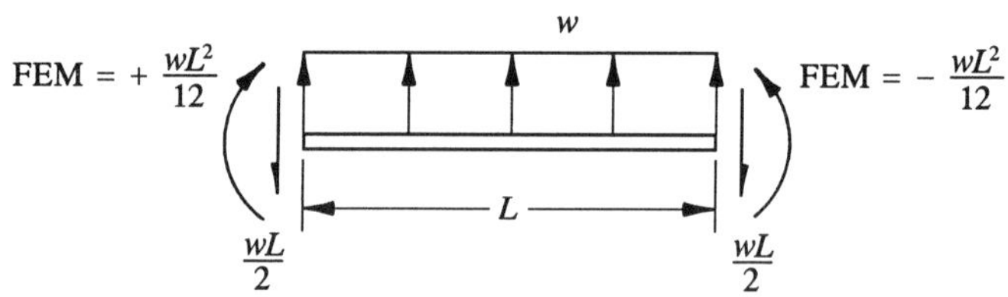

FIGURE 9-40 Sign convention for fixed-end moments (FEM) for a uniformly distributed load.

where: $(\text{FEM})_n$ = fixed-end moment for the framing member meeting at joint n

$\Sigma\ (\text{FEM})_{\text{joint}}$ = summation of fixed-end moments for all members common to joint n

$(\text{DF})_n$ = distribution factor = $\dfrac{I_n/L_n}{\Sigma\ (I_n/L_n)_{\text{joint}}}$

$\Sigma\ (I_n/L_n)_{\text{joint}} = I_1/L_1 + I_2/L_2 + I_3/L_3 + \ldots + I_n/L_n$

M_n = modified end-fixity moment or joint moment at joint n

I_n = moment of inertia of the framing member in the plane of the fuselage skin

L_n = length of the framing member.

The summation symbol Σ in the definitions above for Eq. 9-24 is meant to include all members common to a particular joint. The proper sign convention for fixed-end moments FEM is defined in Fig. 9-40 for a uniformly distributed load w (lb/in).

Longitudinal and Hoop Tension Loads Due to Burst Pressure Carried Around a Medium or Large Cutout

Consider the framing structure of the door cutout of Fig. 9-39. The internal loads carried by the framing members around the cutout due to burst pressure are described using the loading structure of Fig. 9-40. This will help determine the proper signs for the internal loads around the cutout in relation to the standard beam loads given for a beam fixed at both ends. For example, compare the distributed loading indicated in this figure with the longitudinal and hoop tension loading given for burst pressure and draw the corresponding internal loads around the cutout region. This is done in Fig. 9-41. The joint moments are determined from the application of Eq. 9-24 (see Example 9-4 on the next page).

The application of Eq. 9-24 can best be illustrated by a specific example problem. The technique of obtaining the fixed-end moments at the corners of a window or door frame is approached very systematically. Their solutions in the example problem which follows are intended to provide the engineer with a consistent format by which solutions of this kind are solved, and thus avoid having to "reinvent

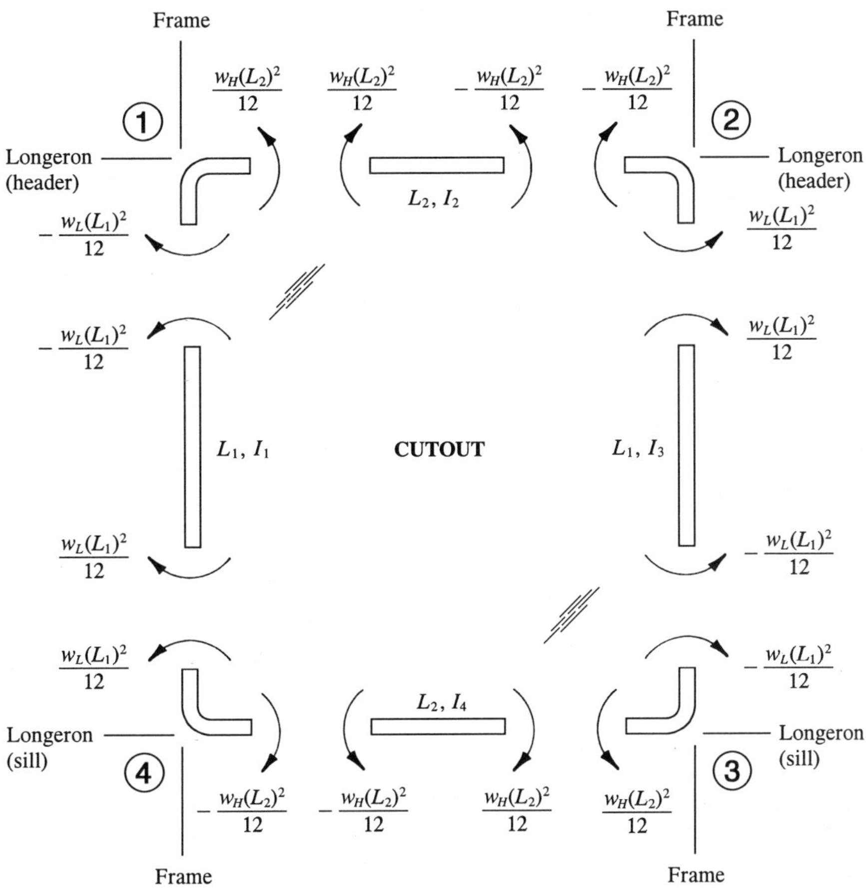

FIGURE 9-41 Fixed-end moments for longitudinal and hoop tension loads.

the wheel," so to speak, for each new problem encountered with burst pressure effects occurring around a cutout. Let these equations provide a standard from which other similar problem solutions can then be solved.

Example 9-4 Using the same size and construction of boundary members for the framing structure around a large cutout due to burst pressure, Fig. 9-39, develop standard moment expressions from Eq. 9-24 at the corners of joints #1, #2, #3, and #4. Also determine the shears and axial loads to properly balance the framing structure for conditions of static equilibrium.

SOLUTION: Fixed-end moments around the frame are established as shown in Fig. 9-41 by comparing the fixed-end moments for the uniformly loaded fixed beam structure of Fig. 9-40 with the loading structure of Fig. 9-39 for burst pressure. The engineer is encouraged to verify these quantities before proceeding ahead with the rest of this solution. From these moments, and Eq. 9-24, the joint moments at the corners of the framing structure are written:

JOINT #1:

Using the upper longeron (horizontal framing member) from node #1 to node #2 of Fig. 9-41:

$$M_1 = \frac{w_H L_2^2}{12} - \left[\frac{w_H L_2^2}{12} - \frac{w_L L_1^2}{12} \right] \frac{I_2/L_2}{I_1/L_1 + I_2/L_2}. \tag{9-25}$$

An alternative expression which gives a numerically similar solution can also be arrived at by using the fuselage frame (vertical framing member) from node #1 to node #4:

$$M_1 = -\frac{w_L L_1^2}{12} - \left[\frac{w_H L_2^2}{12} - \frac{w_L L_1^2}{12} \right] \frac{I_1/L_1}{I_1/L_1 + I_2/L_2}. \tag{9-26}$$

JOINT #2:

Using the upper longeron (horizontal framing member) from node #1 to node #2 of Fig. 9-41:

$$M_2 = -\frac{w_H L_2^2}{12} - \left[\frac{w_L L_1^2}{12} - \frac{w_H L_2^2}{12} \right] \frac{I_2/L_2}{I_3/L_1 + I_2/L_2}. \tag{9-27}$$

An alternative expression which gives a numerically similar solution can also be arrived at by using the fuselage frame (vertical framing member) from node #2 to node #3:

$$M_2 = \frac{w_L L_1^2}{12} - \left[\frac{w_L L_1^2}{12} - \frac{w_H L_2^2}{12} \right] \frac{I_3/L_1}{I_3/L_1 + I_2/L_2}. \tag{9-28}$$

JOINT #3:

Using the fuselage frame (vertical framing member) from node #2 to node #3 of Fig. 9-41:

$$M_3 = -\frac{w_L L_1^2}{12} - \left[\frac{w_H L_2^2}{12} - \frac{w_L L_1^2}{12} \right] \frac{I_3/L_1}{I_3/L_1 + I_4/L_2}. \tag{9-29}$$

An alternative expression which gives a numerically similar solution can also be arrived at by using the lower longeron (horizontal framing member) from node #3 to node #4:

$$M_3 = \frac{w_H L_2^2}{12} - \left[\frac{w_H L_2^2}{12} - \frac{w_L L_1^2}{12}\right] \frac{I_4/L_2}{I_4/L_2 + I_3/L_1}. \tag{9-30}$$

JOINT #4:

Using the lower longeron (horizontal framing member) from node #3 to node #4 of Fig. 9-41:

$$M_4 = -\frac{w_H L_2^2}{12} - \left[\frac{w_L L_1^2}{12} - \frac{w_H L_2^2}{12}\right] \frac{I_4/L_2}{I_4/L_2 + I_1/L_1}. \tag{9-31}$$

An alternative expression which gives a numerically similar solution can also be arrived at by using the fuselage frame (vertical framing member) from node #4 to node #1:

$$M_4 = \frac{w_L L_1^2}{12} - \left[\frac{w_L L_1^2}{12} - \frac{w_H L_2^2}{12}\right] \frac{I_1/L_1}{I_1/L_1 + I_4/L_2}. \tag{9-32}$$

The joint moments from Eqs. 9-25 through 9-32 are shown properly drawn in Fig. 9-42. A numerical evaluation of these quantities for a specific design case will reveal that positive moments occur in a counterclockwise direction, whereas, negative moments occur in a clockwise direction. The actual computations are left as an exercise for the engineer to complete. After these quantities have been verified, the joint moments are then combined with axial loads. For specific details of this evaluation, the engineer is referred to Eq. 2-9 ($f = \pm P/A \pm Mc/I_{na}$) in Chapter 2. From $\Sigma F_y = 0$ and $\Sigma F_x = 0$, the shears and axial loads are determined for the framing members around the cutout as follows:

$$P_1 = V_1 = \frac{w_L L_1}{2} \tag{9-33}$$

$$P_2 = V_2 = \frac{w_H L_2}{2}. \tag{9-34}$$

From conventional stress analysis methods, the framing members are also analyzed for required shear strength. Use Eq. 4-2 ($f_s = VQ/I_{na}t$) in Chapter 4 in making this evaluation.

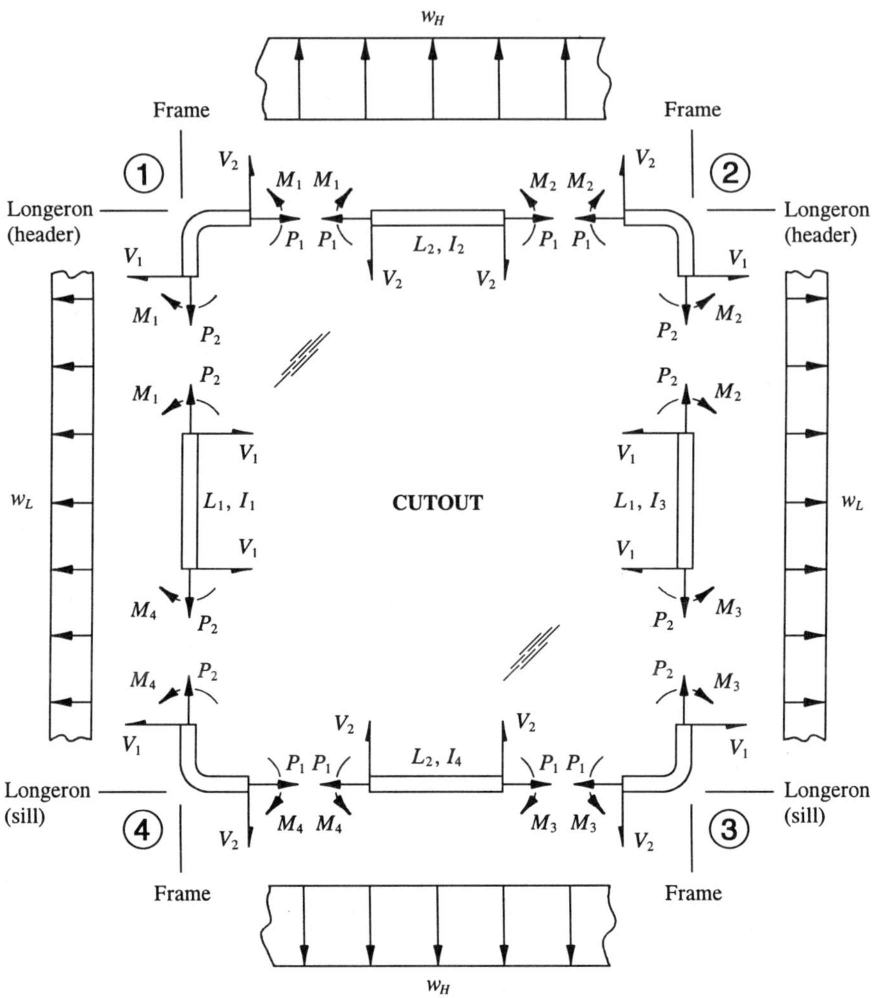

FIGURE 9-42 Longitudinal and hoop tension loads due to burst pressure carried around a large cutout.

Alternative Procedure to Analyzing the Framing Structure Around Large Cutouts:

To achieve a more satisfactory structural design solution, the fuselage skin surrounding most large cutouts is taken as effective in carrying the hoop and longitudinal tension loads around the cutout. See the structural arrangement of members around the large cutout shown in Fig. 9-43. Here, the vertical frames on each side of the cutout, the longeron (header) and longeron, and the longeron (sill) and longeron, in effect, form beams of substantial bending stiffness in the plane of the fuselage skin. The fuselage skin is used to connect these structural members

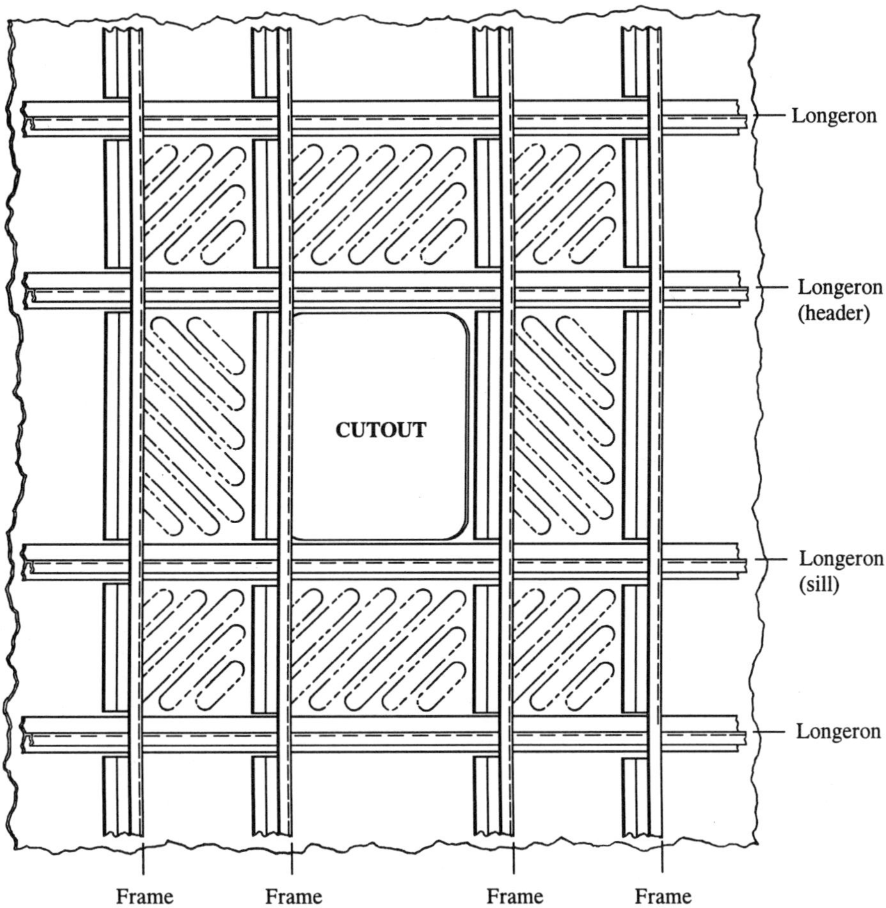

FIGURE 9-43 Structural arrangement around a large cutout.

together. Their analyses result in a more efficiently designed structure around the cutout than supporting the hoop and longitudinal tension loads entirely by a single structural edge member, such as a frame or a longeron (sill) or a longeron (header). And therefore, the end result, if this analysis approach was taken, would be to reduce weight for nonstructural cutouts—windows, windshields, or access doors.

The actual analysis is performed by considering the moment of inertia of the framing members, together with the reinforced fuselage skin, when analyzing the cutout for required bending stiffness. The internal loads arrangement around such a cutout using the fuselage shell as effective in carrying the hoop and longitudinal tension loads around the cutout is depicted in Fig. 9-44. For deep beams, which these are, the upper and lower caps of these beams are taken as axially loaded members, from which the joint moments (Eqs. 9-25 through 9-32) are distributed

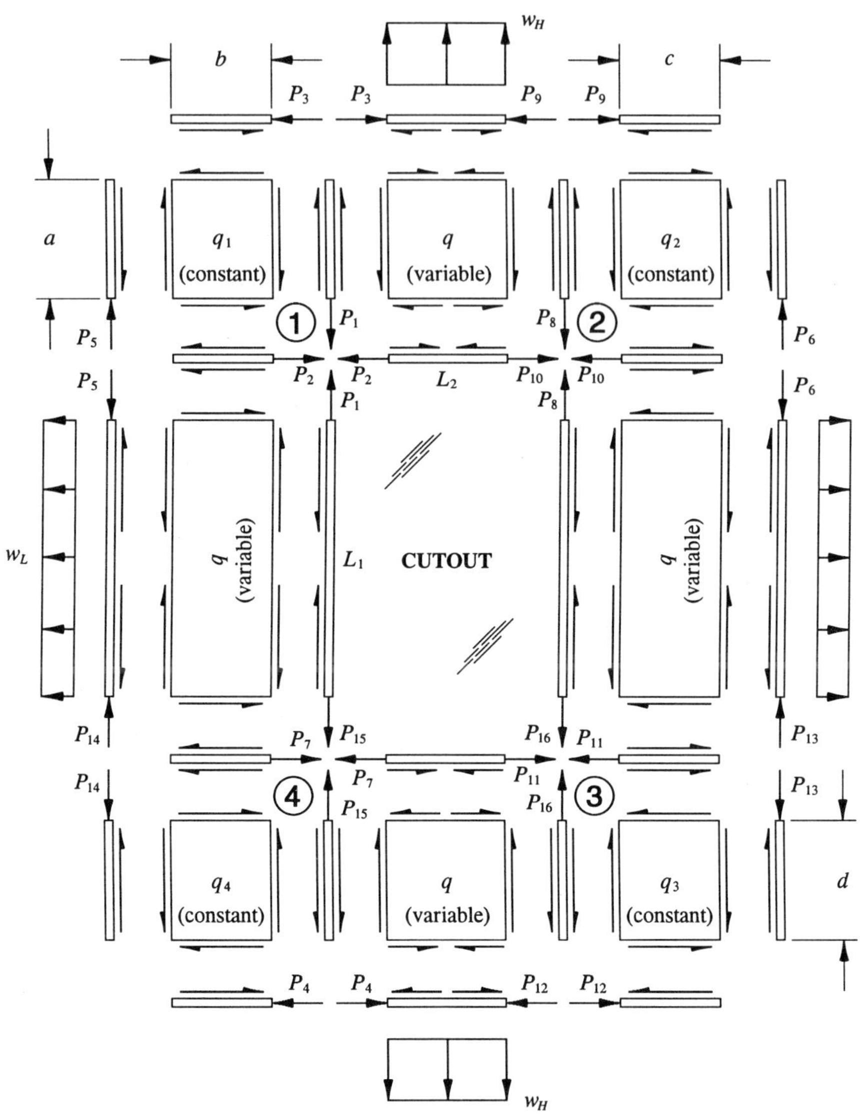

FIGURE 9-44 Longitudinal and hoop tension loads carried around a large cutout using the fuselage shell (as web material) to form beams of substantial bending stiffness.

between the beam caps according to the couple-force relationship of moments or $P_{couple} = M/H$ (from Appendix B, Eq. A-7). That is, the hoop and longitudinal tension loads are exclusively carried as axial loads by the frame, longeron (sill) and longeron (header) edge-support members, while the modified corner end-fixity moments (or joint moments) are coupled between the edge members and the adjacent frames or longerons. The following equations have been formulated from these simple relationships. The engineer is encouraged to verify these equations as they relate specifically to the panel and stick diagram shown in Fig. 9-44.

Frame, Longeron (header), Longeron (sill), and Longeron Axial Loads

$$P_1 = \frac{w_H L_2}{2} + \frac{M_1}{b} \qquad P_5 = -\frac{M_1}{b}$$

$$P_8 = \frac{w_H L_2}{2} + \frac{M_2}{c} \qquad P_6 = -\frac{M_2}{c}$$

$$P_{15} = \frac{w_H L_2}{2} + \frac{M_4}{b} \qquad P_{14} = -\frac{M_4}{b}$$

$$P_{16} = \frac{w_H L_2}{2} + \frac{M_3}{c} \qquad P_{13} = -\frac{M_3}{c}$$

$$P_2 = \frac{w_L L_1}{2} + \frac{M_1}{a} \qquad P_3 = -\frac{M_1}{a}$$

$$P_{10} = \frac{w_L L_1}{2} + \frac{M_2}{a} \qquad P_9 = -\frac{M_2}{a}$$

$$P_7 = \frac{w_L L_1}{2} + \frac{M_4}{d} \qquad P_4 = -\frac{M_4}{d}$$

$$P_{11} = \frac{w_L L_1}{2} + \frac{M_4}{d} \qquad P_{12} = -\frac{M_3}{d}.$$

The panel shear flows q_1, q_2, q_3, and q_4 at the corners of the cutout, Fig. 9-44, are constant values and are determined by beaming out the joint moments M_1, M_2, M_3, and M_4 between the cap centroids of the framing structure (use either the vertical or horizontal deep beam members along the cutout in making these computations). The center panels develop variable shear flows q which can be found using the fundamental equations of static equilibrium at different points along the framing structure (specifically, i.e., consider a beam fixed at both ends loaded by a uniformly distributed load over its entire span, see Appendix D, Table A-1, Case 23 for the standard solution).

Corner Panel Shear Flows

$$(1)\ q_1 = \frac{M_1}{ba} \qquad (2)\ q_2 = \frac{M_2}{ac} \qquad (3)\ q_3 = \frac{M_3}{cd} \qquad (4)\ q_4 = \frac{M_4}{bd}.$$

In the next section, two examples, both in a pressurized aircraft, a nonstructural passenger door and a nonstructural engine access door, will be discussed. Although the doors themselves are designed for ultimate burst pressure loads, the engineer should also include in the substantiation of these types the framework for the following loading conditions: (1) ultimate flight loads and (2) ultimate flight loads plus limit pressure loads.

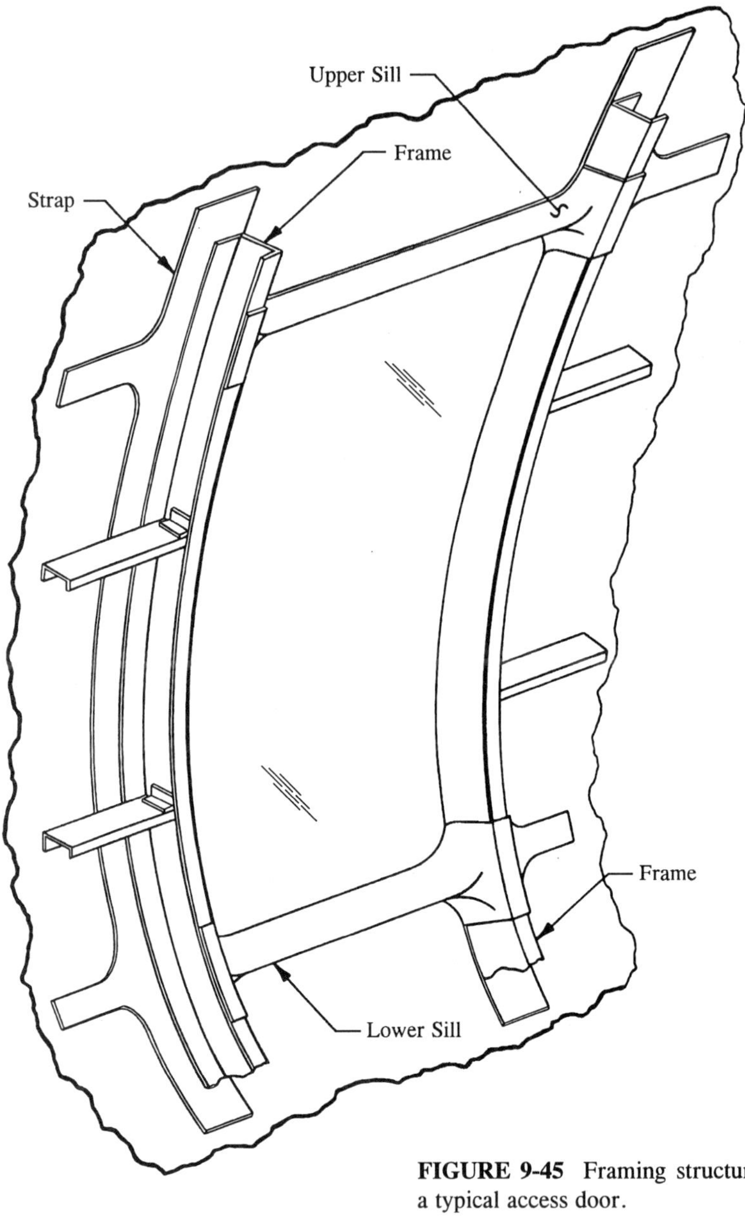

FIGURE 9-45 Framing structure around a typical access door.

9.5 Design and Analysis of Doors in Pressurized Aircraft. A typical access door of an aircraft fuselage is made up of longitudinal members called stringers and transverse members called frames, as shown in Fig. 9-45. In addition to these members, edge beams, themselves part of the door structure, formed to the contour of the fuselage, form the basic support system or framing structure of the door. To

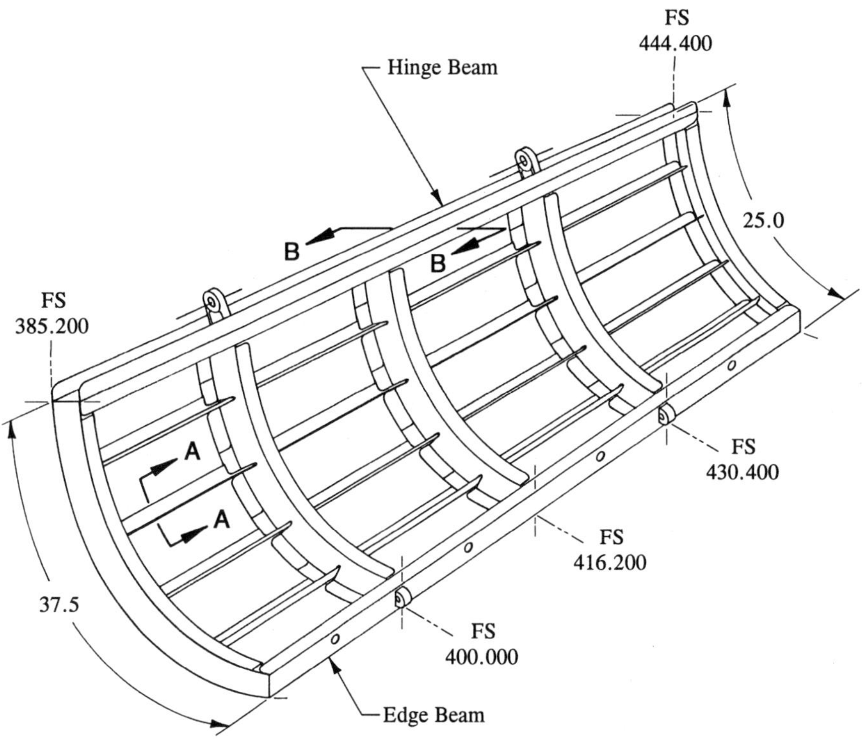

FIGURE 9-46 Structural arrangement of members of an engine access door.

fully develop the required stiffness of the door, these structural members are riveted to the fuselage outer skin along their beam lengths. Generally, the doors of a pressurized aircraft are designed for ultimate burst pressure. Of course, at limit load, the door must also develop sufficient rigidity and stiffness to prevent permanent set which, if not prevented, could eventually cause less than a smooth operation of the door in actual service. Such a condition becomes uneconomical, and therefore, its occurrence should be avoided in practical designs.

Except for Examples 2-1 and 5-5, all the previous examples in this book have had loads applied directly to a beam or panel structure. Just like the floor framing structure of a building, or for that matter the basic floor structure of an aircraft, the framing structure of an aircraft door is similar. Although the pressure loading acts over the entire surface area of the door, it will be assumed that the pressure loading is divided proportionately over each of its longitudinal stringers. Since the stringers are simply-supported by the frames, stringer reactions (or concentrated loads) develop at the intersection of each stringer-frame. These reactions then become applied concentrated loads acting on the frames. The frames then carry the loads to the edge beams, where the loads are finally reacted by the hinges and latching and locking mechanisms of the door.

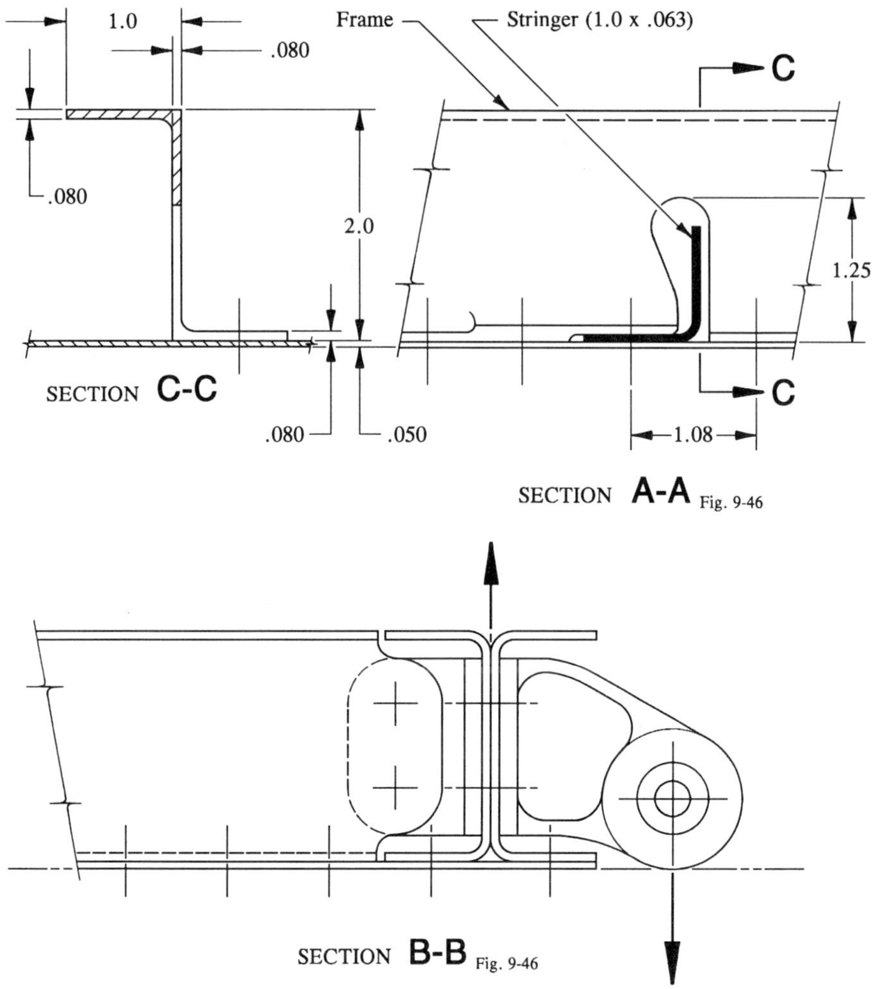

FIGURE 9-47 Cross-sectional areas of the engine access door.

To illustrate the construction of this kind, consider the engine access door shown in Fig. 9-46. Although the fuselage is a curved surface, conservatively, it will be assumed that the door is essentially flat, in which case the loads are applied perpendicular to its surface. The door is designed to carry a reversible pressure of 2.0 psi ultimate. The stringers, frames, and edge beams are analyzed as would any typical beam structure acted upon by direct loads to the beam structure itself. The cross-sectional areas of these members are shown in Fig. 9-47. The engineer is encouraged to investigate on his own the critical combination of loads that result on these structural members. Also indicate any other possible checks that may be required for complete substantiation of this structure. Although the detailed analysis of the door will not be specifically investigated, it is recommended that the engineer should at least mentally prepare the sequence of steps required to perform a complete stress analysis solution.

9.6 Problem for Solution. The engine access door shown in Fig. 9-46 is designed to carry a reversible pressure of 2.0 psi ultimate. Using a simplified[1] distribution of loads as a basis for the solution, investigate the critical loads for the following structural members: (1) frames, (2) stringers, (3) hinge beam, and (4) hinge fitting (*Hint:* isolate and compare members for the critical combinations of maximum load and minimum cross-sectional area.) All stringers are equally spaced.

[1] A more accurate distribution of load is realized by including some distribution of pressure loading carried by the frames. This will produce a more realistic distribution throughout the structure and to supporting members.

APPENDICES

APPENDIX A

Resolution of Forces

A force P may conveniently be represented by two components of force, one acting horizontally p_x and the other acting vertically p_y, as shown in Fig. A-1. To find the magnitude of the component forces, the following trigonometric functions, developed from the right triangle of Fig. A-2, are used:

$$\sin\beta = \frac{\text{opposite side}}{\text{hypotenuse}} = \frac{p_y}{P} \tag{A-1}$$

$$\cos\beta = \frac{\text{adjacent side}}{\text{hypotenuse}} = \frac{p_x}{P} \tag{A-2}$$

$$\tan\beta = \frac{\text{opposite side}}{\text{adjacent side}} = \frac{p_y}{p_x}. \tag{A-3}$$

In plain terms, the way to understand the mathematics of these expressions is to specifically treat each as a simple algebraic equation. That is, if the vertical component of force P is desired, Eq. A-1 is solved for p_y, this gives:

$$p_y = P\sin\beta. \tag{A-4}$$

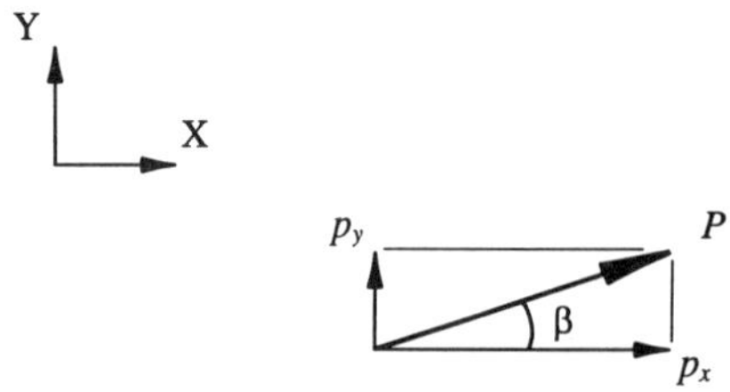

FIGURE A-1 Equivalent components of a force *P*.

If the horizontal component is sought, then Eq. A-2 is solved for p_x, and this gives:

$$p_x = P\cos\beta. \tag{A-5}$$

These equations are also used by the design engineer to find the length of sides of a right triangle. And if their application to these right triangle solutions is clearly understood, their extension to the solution of force vectors should present no additional difficulty.

In the solution of multi-riveted or multi-bolted connections, it will be necessary to combine a system of mutually perpendicular shearing forces p_x and p_y into a single resultant shearing force. This is accomplished by using the Pythagorean theorem of right triangles as it applies to a vector force solution. The theorem in terms of forces states that the sum of the squares of two mutually perpendicular component forces is equal to the square of the resultant force, or mathematically

$$P^2 = p_x^2 + p_y^2$$

where: P = resultant force
p_x = horizontal component force of P (see Fig. A-1)
p_y = vertical component force of P (see also Fig. A-1)

or

$$P = (p_x^2 + p_y^2)^{1/2}. \tag{A-6}$$

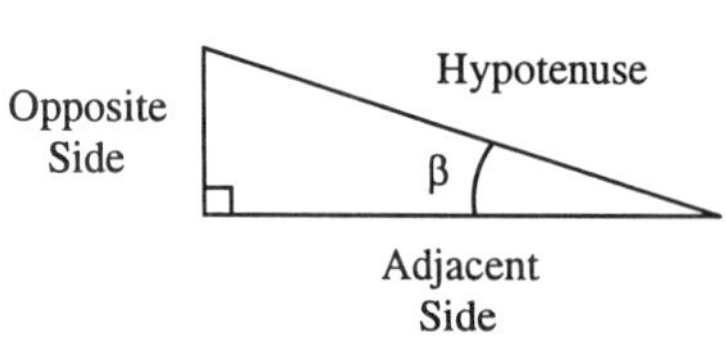

FIGURE A-2 Trigonometric functions of a right triangle.

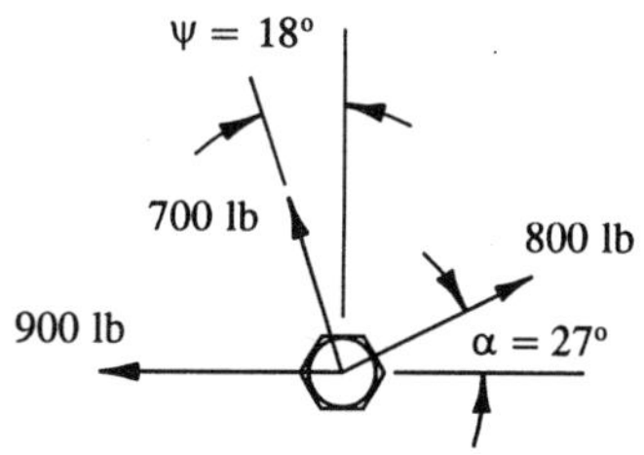

FIGURE A-3 Concurrent applied shearing forces on a Hex bolt.

To help illustrate the method of resolving forces, the following example is presented:

Example A-1 A system of three concurrent applied shearing forces are acting on the bolt shown in Fig. A-3. If these forces are all applied in the same plane, what is the resultant shearing force on the Hex bolt?

SOLUTION: Since the shear strength of a bolt is measured by its shear allowable, it would therefore seem logical to formulate a single applied resultant shearing force from the system of applied shearing forces given in this problem that could directly be compared to this allowable value. Then, from this comparison, the proper selection of bolt could be made. This is exactly how we will proceed here with this solution. The following steps are described to fully illustrate the analysis procedure involved to arrive at a bolt solution. First, each of the shearing forces is resolved into equivalent component shearing forces acting in the direction of the x-

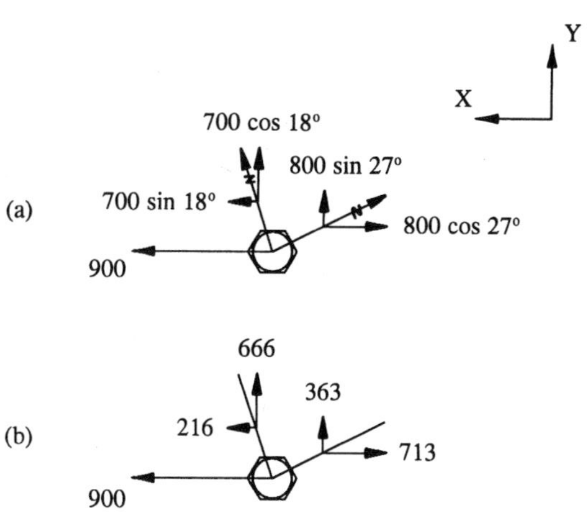

FIGURE A-4 Shearing forces resolved into equivalent component shearing forces.

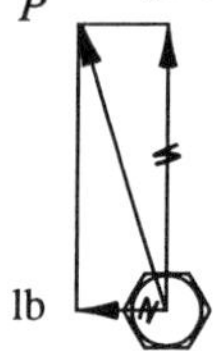

FIGURE A-5 Horizontal and vertical shearing forces represented by a resultant force.

and y-coordinate axes adopted in Fig. A-4. As is customarily the case, the selection of the x- and y-coordinate axes have been chosen completely arbitrarily. Next, to further simplify our solution, the algebraic sum of the horizontal and vertical shearing forces acting in the x- and y-directions, respectively, are taken and their sums denoted in Fig. A-5. Thus

$$\Sigma p_x = 900 + 216 - 713 = 403 \text{ lb}$$

$$\Sigma p_y = 666 + 363 = 1{,}029 \text{ lb}.$$

Now, the Pythagorean theorem is applied to this system of mutually perpendicular component forces to determine the resultant bolt force P. Hence, using Eq. A-6, with $p_x = 403$ lb and $p_y = 1{,}029$ lb, we obtain:

$$P = (p_x^2 + p_y^2)^{1/2} = \left[(403)^2 + (1{,}029)^2\right]^{1/2} = 1{,}105 \text{ lb}.$$

Then, with this resultant force, the proper selection of a bolt of sufficient strength is made by comparing this calculated value to published shear allowables of different size bolts. (The engineer is referred to Chapter 3 where a detailed study of mechanically fastened connections is more appropriately treated.)

APPENDIX B

Couple-Force Relationship of Moments

The couple-force relationship of moments is a mathematical expression used to help the engineer describe the physical effects that internal bending moments produce on a structure. In this appendix, it will be shown that a moment is equivalent to two applied forces of magnitude *M/H* (a couple-force) acting in opposite directions and separated by a distance *H* between them, or

$$P_{\text{couple}} = \frac{M}{H}. \tag{A-7}$$

In Fig. A-6, to demonstrate the usefulness of this relationship, a section of beam is acted upon by an internal moment *M* and is replaced by an equivalent couple-force, P_{couple}, at the upper and lower beam cap centroids. The wavy line through the moment vector means that the moment has been replaced by an equivalent couple-force. Idealized in this way, the engineer is now able to quickly identify a particular moment by its physical action on the structure. In this example, the moment produces tension (or pulling) in the lower cap and compression

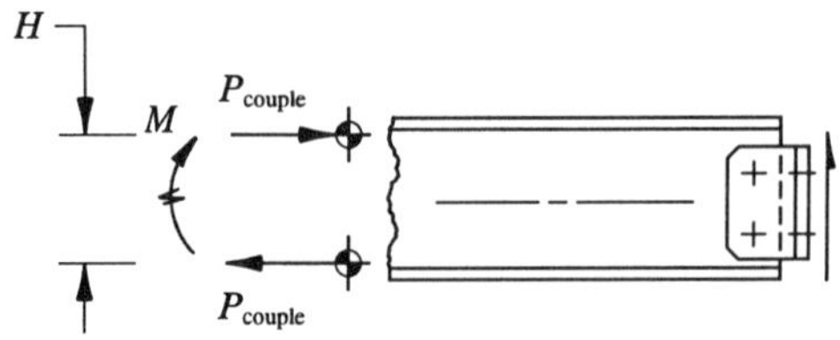

FIGURE A-6 Internal moment replaced by an equivalent couple-force.

(or pushing) in the upper cap. Or, one could simply memorize that the tail end of a moment vector produces tension in the lower cap and the arrowhead end produces compression in the upper cap. Whichever depiction is visualized, the engineer should always remember that bending moments produce bending stresses across the sectional area of a beam, not an equivalent couple-force concentrated at beam cap centroids. Still, as a visual aid, the couple-force does help describe and give the engineer a better understanding as to the physical action of a beam in bending.

To substantiate Eq. A-7, the beam supported as shown in Fig. A-7 will be acted upon by a moment and the reactions necessary to establish equilibrium determined and compared to Fig. A-6. Applying the equations of equilibrium to this structure, we obtain:

$$\Sigma F_x = 0, \qquad R_3 = 0$$

$$\Sigma F_y = 0, \qquad R_1 + R_2 = 0$$

$$\Sigma M_B = 0, \qquad (+ \quad M + R_1(H) = 0$$

and therefore $R_1 = -M/H$. The negative sign of R_1 indicates that the assumed direction of this reaction is incorrect, and is so indicated by circling its arrowhead in Fig. A-7. Now, substituting R_1 into the second equation of equilibrium gives:

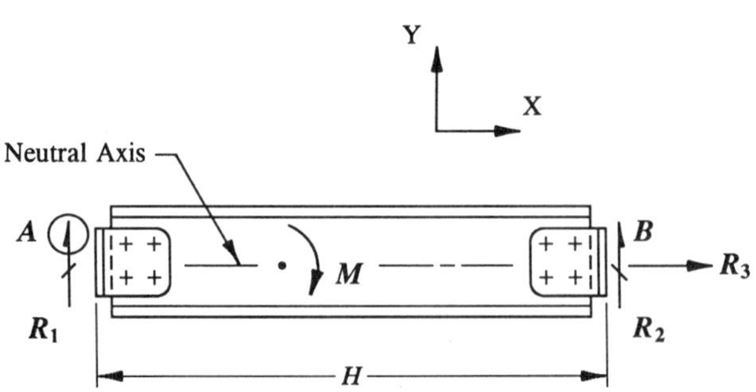

FIGURE A-7 Free-body diagram of unknown reaction forces.

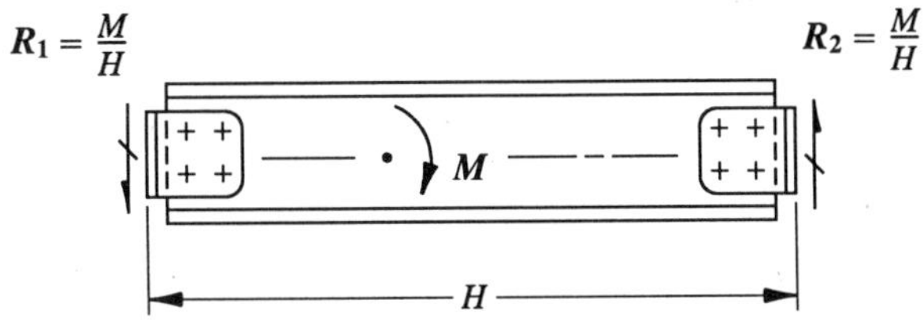

FIGURE A-8 Beam reactions indicated on a properly drawn diagram of the beam.

$$-M/H + R_2 = 0$$
$$R_2 = M/H.$$

In Fig. A-8, the correct free-body diagram is drawn with all loads properly indicated. Our solution is consistent with the basic precepts and theory of Eq. A-7. That is, our solution reveals that the reactions necessary to establish equilibrium is a couple-force of magnitude *M/H* acting in opposite directions and separated by a distance *H* between them. Note that the equivalent couple-force in Fig. A-6 was represented as applied forces, not as reaction forces. This is not at all inconsistent with our results here, since the orientation of a couple-force is normally specified in terms of how the engineer wishes to describe the equivalent forces on the structure; the magnitude of the couple-force is always the same, it is their intended directions that are sometimes used differently.

The meaning is particularly clear, depending upon its particular applications, Eq. A-7 may be represented either as an equivalent (reaction) couple-force or as an equivalent (applied) couple-force. For the most part, this equation is used to generalize and formulate quick, simple solutions to rather complex structural engineering problems. For this reason, its importance to a successful analysis solution should not be underestimated; it serves a very desirable, special purpose and therefore should warrant the design engineer's special consideration and thorough understanding.

APPENDIX C

Construction of Axial, Shear, and Bending Moment Diagrams

The material of Appendix C is presented here to show how the internal loading diagrams for the beam structure of Fig. 1-32 are easily and systematically constructed. The procedure is simple. However, some intuitive reasoning must be used to establish general loading trends for each particular type of loading if their construction is to be accomplished without much difficulty. Before the axial, shear, and bending moment diagrams for the auxiliary wing spar are drawn, however, the spar must be completely balanced by reaction forces. To accomplish this, a free-body diagram of the entire structure under loading is used, as shown in Fig. A-9.

Then, the equations of equilibrium are applied in the usual manner as follows:

$$\Sigma F_x = 0, \qquad R_3 - 800 + 300 = 0, \quad R_3 = 500 \text{ lb}$$

$$\Sigma F_y = 0, \qquad -R_1 + 700 - 500 - 600 + R_2 = 0$$

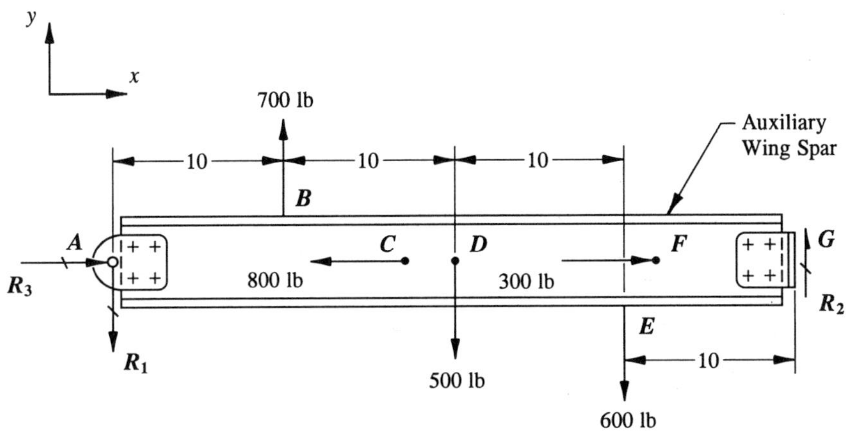

FIGURE A-9 Free-body diagram of unknown reaction forces.

$$\Sigma M_A = 0, \quad \circlearrowleft + \quad -40R_2 + 600(30) + 500(20) - 700(10) = 0$$
$$R_2 = 525 \text{ lb}.$$

Substituting R_2 into the second equation of equilibrium and solving for R_1 gives $R_1 = 125$ lb. The completely balanced structure with all applied and reaction loads properly indicated is shown in Fig. A-10.

Now, to construct the axial, shear, and bending moment diagrams, the method of sections approach to internal loads analysis (see Sec. 1.5) is conveniently and most effectively utilized for this purpose. For convenience sake, the left-hand segment of the beam is chosen for the investigation of internal forces *V*, *P*, and *M* at several exposed sections along the beam. The equations of statics are required to maintain equilibrium of these isolated segments. The computations are performed as shown in Figs. A-11(a), (b), (c), (d), (e), and (f).

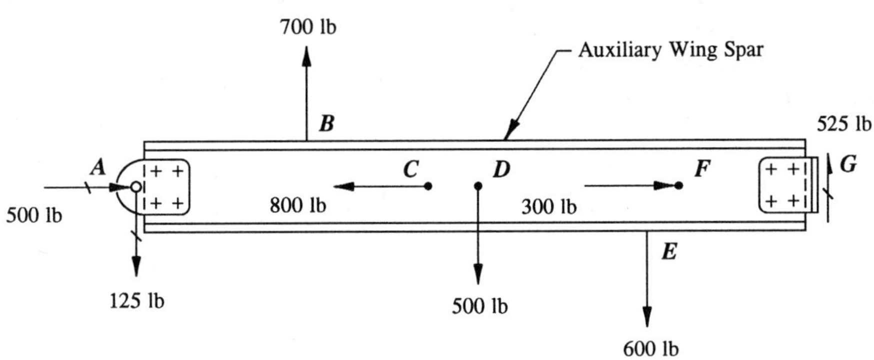

FIGURE A-10 Beam reactions indicated on the auxiliary wing spar.

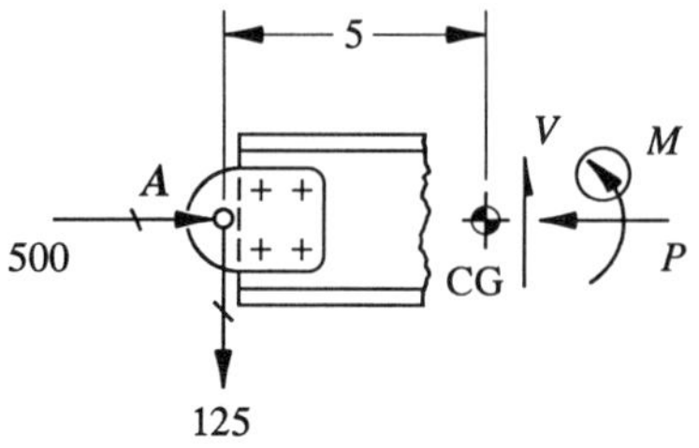

FIGURE A-11(a) Internal forces at an exposed section of the auxiliary wing spar.

$$\Sigma F_x = 0, \quad 500 - P = 0, \quad P = 500 \text{ lb} \quad \text{(compression)}$$

$$\Sigma F_y = 0, \quad -125 + V = 0, \quad V = 125 \text{ lb} \quad \text{(up)}$$

$$\Sigma M_{cg} = 0, \quad \circlearrowleft + \quad -125(5) - M = 0, \quad M = -625 \text{ in-lb.}$$

This moment produces compression stresses on the lower cap of the exposed section area.

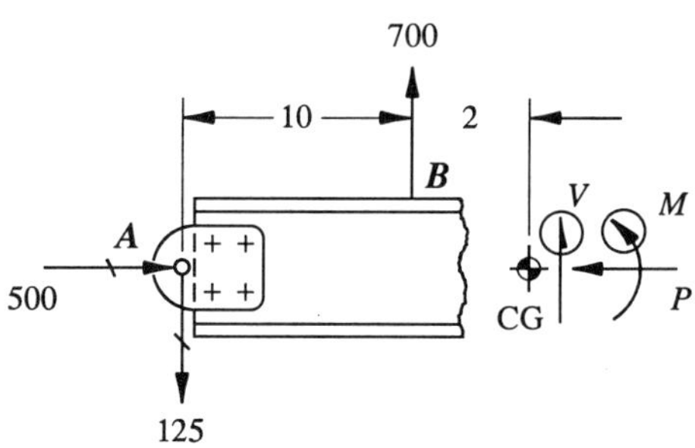

FIGURE A-11(b) Internal forces at an exposed section of the auxiliary wing spar.

$$\Sigma F_x = 0, \quad 500 - P = 0, \quad P = 500 \text{ lb} \quad \text{(compression)}$$

$$\Sigma F_y = 0, \quad -125 + 700 + V = 0, \quad V = -575 \text{ lb} \quad \text{(down)}$$

$$\Sigma M_{cg} = 0, \quad \circlearrowleft + \quad -125(12) + 700(2) - M = 0, \quad M = -100 \text{ in-lb.}$$

This moment produces compression stresses on the lower cap of the exposed section area.

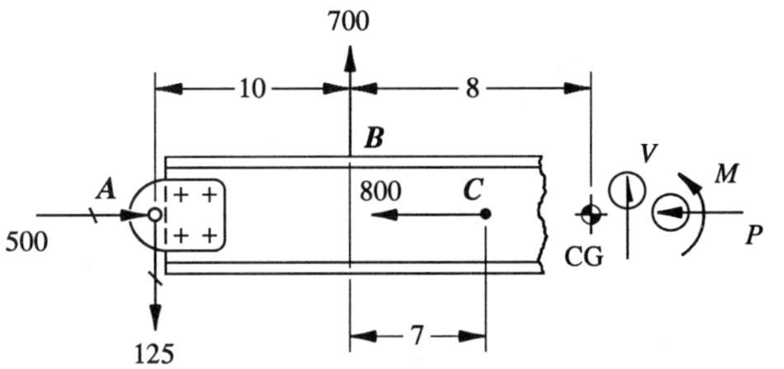

FIGURE A-11(c) Internal forces at an exposed section of the auxiliary wing spar.

$$\Sigma F_x = 0, \quad 500 - 800 - P = 0, \quad P = -300 \text{ lb} \quad \text{(tension)}$$
$$\Sigma F_y = 0, \quad -125 + 700 + V = 0, \quad V = -575 \text{ lb} \quad \text{(down)}$$
$$\Sigma M_{cg} = 0, \quad (+ \quad -125(18) + 700(8) - M = 0, \quad M = 3,350 \text{ in-lb.}$$

This moment produces compression stresses on the upper cap of the exposed section area.

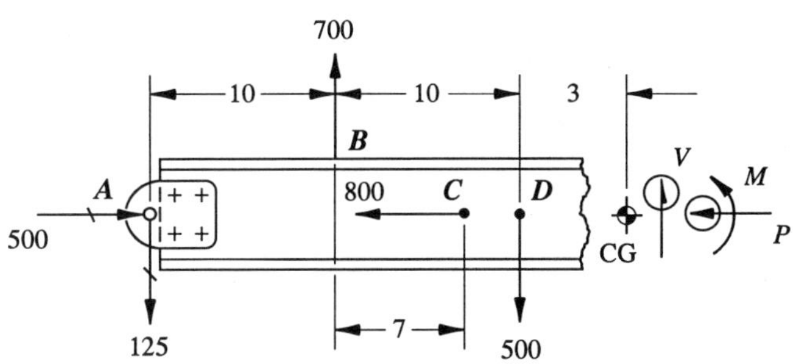

FIGURE A-11(d) Internal forces at an exposed section of the auxiliary wing spar.

$$\Sigma F_x = 0, \quad 500 - 800 - P = 0, \quad P = -300 \text{ lb} \quad \text{(tension)}$$
$$\Sigma F_y = 0, \quad -125 + 700 - 500 + V = 0, \quad V = -75 \text{ lb} \quad \text{(down)}$$
$$\Sigma M_{cg} = 0, \quad (+ \quad -125(23) + 700(13) - 500(3) - M = 0$$
$$M = 4,725 \text{ in-lb.}$$

This moment produces compression stresses on the upper cap of the exposed section area.

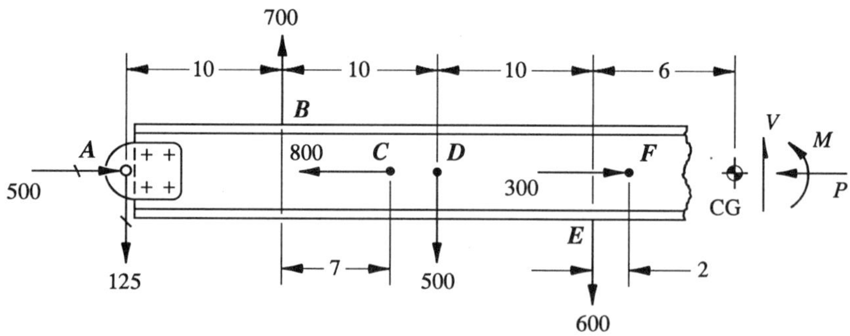

FIGURE A-11(e) Internal forces at an exposed section of the auxiliary wing spar.

$$\Sigma F_x = 0, \quad 500 - 800 + 300 - P = 0, \quad P = 0 \text{ lb}$$
$$\Sigma F_y = 0, \quad -125 + 700 - 500 - 600 + V = 0, \quad V = 525 \text{ lb (up)}$$
$$\Sigma M_{cg} = 0, \quad (+ \quad -125(36) + 700(26) - 500(16) - 600(6) - M = 0$$
$$M = 2,100 \text{ in-lb (compression upper cap).}$$

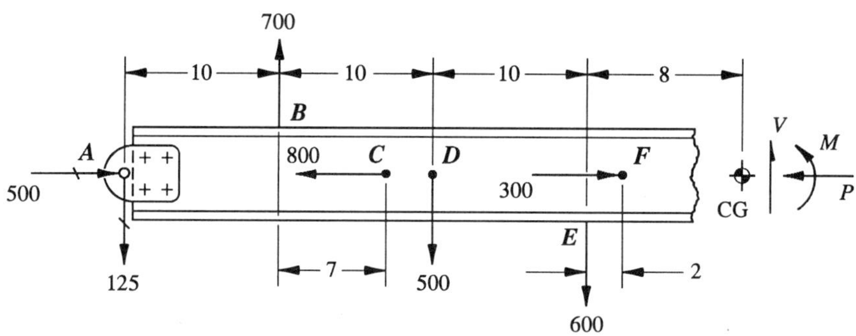

FIGURE A-11(f) Internal forces at an exposed section of the auxiliary wing spar.

$$\Sigma F_x = 0, \quad 500 - 800 + 300 - P = 0, \quad P = 0 \text{ lb}$$
$$\Sigma F_y = 0, \quad -125 + 700 - 500 - 600 + V = 0, \quad V = 525 \text{ lb (up)}$$
$$\Sigma M_{cg} = 0, \quad (+ \quad -125(38) + 700(28) - 500(18) - 600(8) - M = 0$$
$$M = 1,050 \text{ in-lb (compression upper cap).}$$

The values of *V*, *P*, and *M* are now plotted in Fig. A-12. If required, many more intermediate section cuts can be made across the length of the beam to completely reason out the behavior or trend of each particular loading type. It is left as an exercise for the engineer to verify the precise manner in which these loading diagrams have been established. For those engineers who require additional

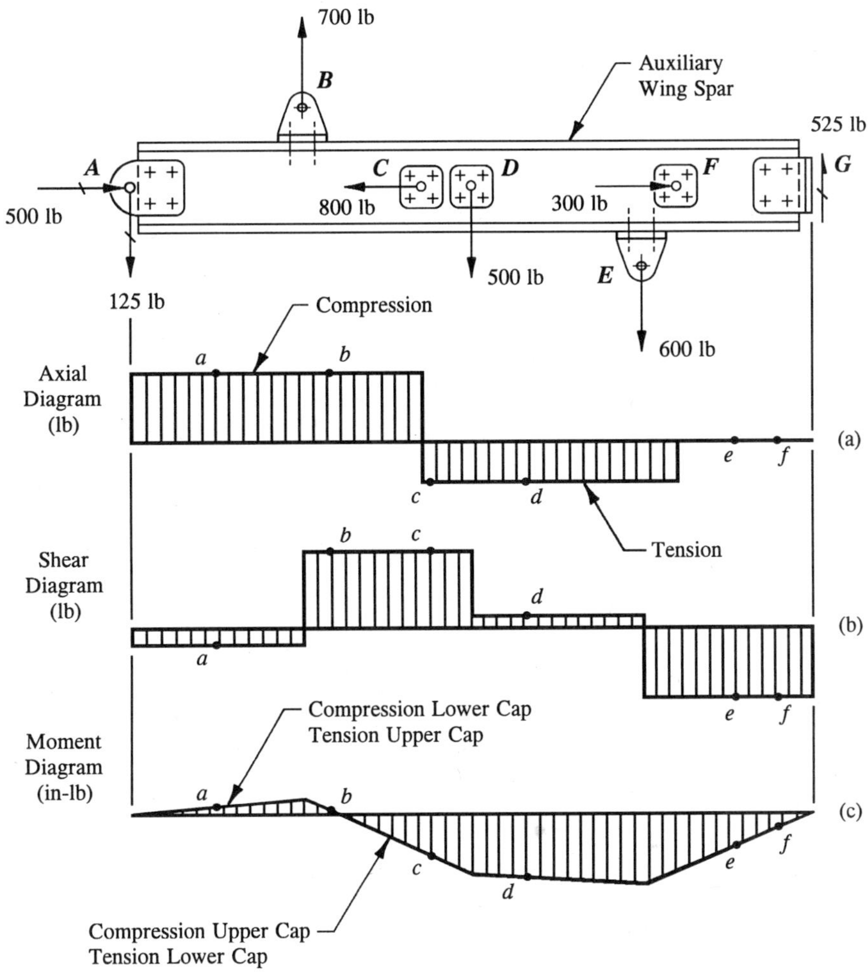

FIGURE A-12 Auxiliary wing spar with accompanying axial, shear, and bending moment diagrams constructed.

practice in constructing these diagrams, refer to Appendix D. Where many more shear and bending moment diagrams of determinate and indeterminate beam structures have been constructed. Start with the simpler loading cases and try to mentally verify their construction. Utilizing the experience gained in their solutions, the fundamental definitions and methods of calculation should follow without much difficulty. Axial, shear, and bending moment diagrams provide a wealth of information to the design engineer regarding the actual structural behavior of his designs. As such, their careful construction plays an important role in the overall design process leading to most successful designs.

APPENDIX D

Reference Beam Formula Solutions

The reference beam formula solutions provided in Table A-1 of this appendix are extremely useful in the design of commonly used aircraft structures. Each solution will attempt to simulate an actual beam structure under idealized loading and various support end-conditions. The equations given for each design solution are also plotted and drawn as shear and bending moment diagrams. From these diagrams, the actual beam structure can be designed for static strength. Other more complex combinations of these solutions can be readily formulated by applying the Principle of Superposition (see Chapter 1, Sec. 1.7). However, to be able to do this, it must be shown that the structure behaves elastically under load; that is, where the structure deforms by stresses below the proportional limit of the material. Moreover, it can be said that if the structure is evaluated in the elastic range of stresses, superposition of these different beam solutions is valid whether the beam structure is determinate or not. Inelastic stress design, a slightly more advanced topic here for discussion, is specifically treated in Appendix J for the design of rectangular beam sections in bending (for more complex shapes, the engineer is referred to an aerospace company structures manual for their solutions).

TABLE A-1 REFERENCE BEAM FORMULA SOLUTIONS

A positive moment $(+M)$ produces tension in the upper cap and compression in the lower cap. A negative moment $(-M)$ produces compression in the upper cap and tension in the lower cap. A positive shear $(+V)$ acts upward on the left side of an exposed section of beam. A negative shear $(-V)$ acts downward on the left side of an exposed section of beam.

Case 1 CANTILEVER BEAM—Concentrated load at the beam end.

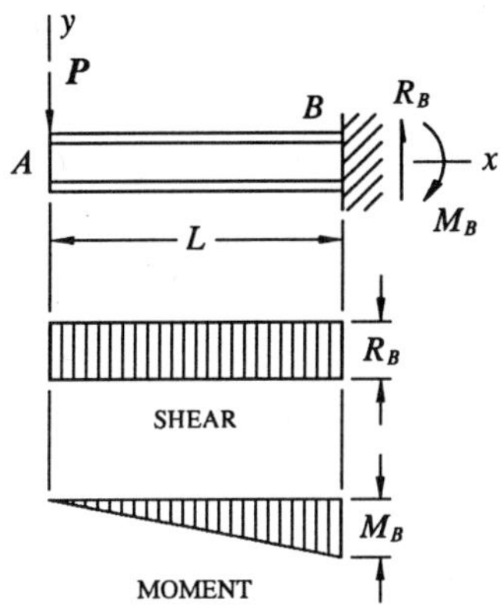

REACTIONS

$R_B = P \qquad M_B = PL$

SHEARS

$V = P$

BENDING MOMENTS

$M = Px$

DEFLECTIONS

$$y = -\frac{P}{6EI}(2L^3 - 3L^2x + x^3)$$

$$y_{max} = -\frac{PL^3}{3EI} \quad \text{at } A$$

Case 2 CANTILEVER BEAM—Concentrated load at any point.

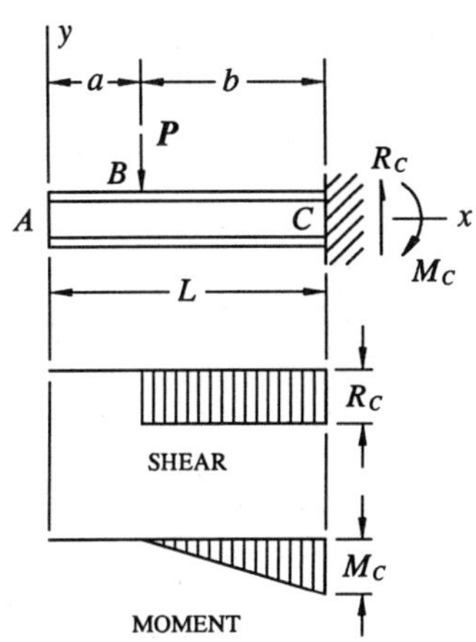

REACTIONS

$R_c = P \qquad M_c = Pb$

SHEARS

$V = 0 \quad (A \text{ to } B)$

$V = P \quad (B \text{ to } C)$

BENDING MOMENTS

$M = 0 \quad (A \text{ to } B)$

$M = P(x-a) \quad (B \text{ to } C)$

DEFLECTIONS

$$y = -\frac{1}{6}\frac{Pb^2}{EI}(3L - b - 3x) \qquad (A \text{ to } B)$$

$$y = -\frac{1}{6}\frac{P}{EI}[(x-a)^3 - 3b^2(x-a) + 2b^3] \qquad (B \text{ to } C)$$

$$y_{max} = -\frac{1}{6}\frac{Pb^2}{EI}(3L - b) \quad \text{at } A$$

TABLE A-1 REFERENCE BEAM FORMULA SOLUTIONS (continued)

Case 3 CANTILEVER BEAM—Uniform load over entire span.

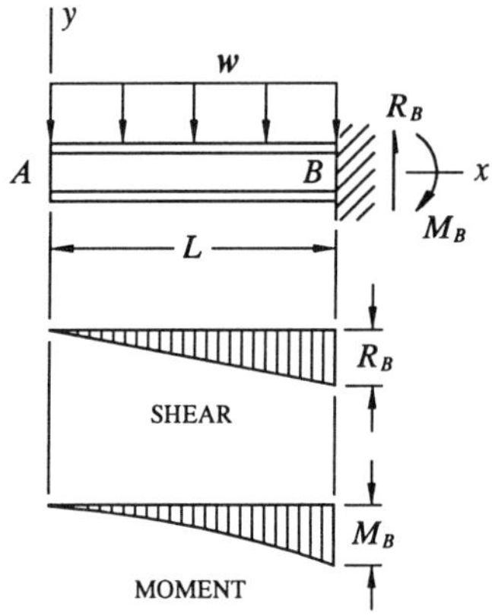

REACTIONS

$$R_B = wL \qquad M_B = \frac{wL^2}{2}$$

SHEARS

$$V = wx$$

BENDING MOMENTS

$$M = \frac{wx^2}{2}$$

DEFLECTIONS

$$y = -\frac{1}{24}\frac{w}{EI}(x^4 - 4L^3x + 3L^4)$$

$$y_{\max} = -\frac{1}{8}\frac{wL^4}{EI} \quad \text{at } A$$

Case 4 CANTILEVER BEAM—Uniform load partially distributed over span.

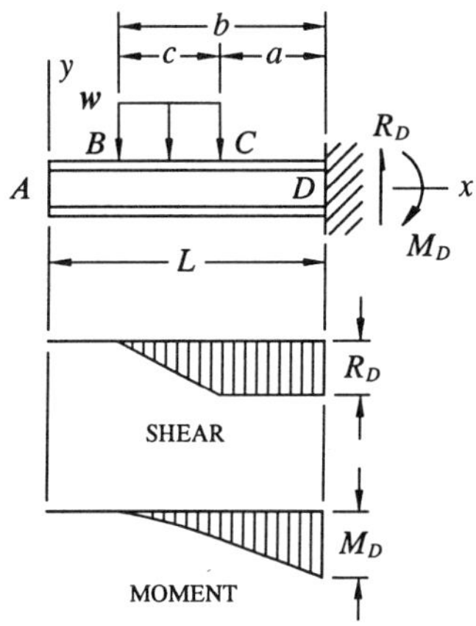

REACTIONS

$$R_D = wc \qquad M_D = \frac{wc}{2}(a+b)$$

SHEARS

$$V = 0 \qquad (A \text{ to } B)$$
$$V = w(x - L + b) \qquad (B \text{ to } C)$$
$$V = wc \qquad (C \text{ to } D)$$

BENDING MOMENTS

$$M = 0 \qquad (A \text{ to } B)$$
$$M = \frac{w}{2}(x - L + b)^2 \qquad (B \text{ to } C)$$
$$M = \frac{wc}{2}(2x - 2L + a + b) \qquad (C \text{ to } D)$$

DEFLECTIONS

$$y = -\frac{1}{24}\frac{wc}{EI}[4(a^2 + ab + b^2)(L - x) - a^3 - ab^2 - a^2b - b^3] \qquad (A \text{ to } B)$$

$$y = -\frac{1}{24}\frac{wc}{EI}\left[6(a+b)(L-x)^2 - 4(L-x)^3 + \frac{(L-x-a)^4}{c}\right] \qquad (B \text{ to } C)$$

$$y = -\frac{1}{12}\frac{wc}{EI}[3(a+b)(L-x)^2 - 2(L-x)^3] \qquad (C \text{ to } D)$$

$$y_{\max} = -\frac{1}{24}\frac{wc}{EI}[4(a^2 + ab + b^2)L - a^3 - ab^2 - a^2b - b^3] \quad \text{at } A$$

TABLE A-1 REFERENCE BEAM FORMULA SOLUTIONS (continued)

Case 5 CANTILEVER BEAM—Uniformly varying distributed load.

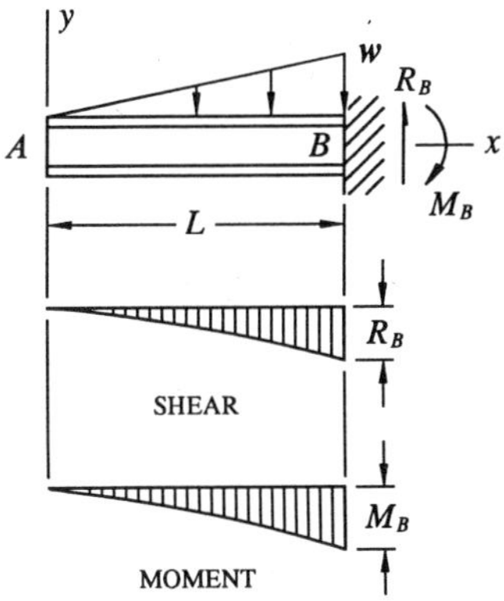

REACTIONS

$$R_B = \frac{1}{2}wL \qquad M_B = \frac{1}{6}wL^2$$

SHEARS

$$V = \frac{1}{2}\frac{wx^2}{L}$$

BENDING MOMENTS

$$M = \frac{1}{6}\frac{wx^3}{L}$$

DEFLECTIONS

$$y = -\frac{1}{120}\frac{w}{EIL}(x^5 - 5L^4x + 4L^5)$$

$$y_{max} = -\frac{1}{30}\frac{wL^4}{EI} \quad \text{at } A$$

Case 6 CANTILEVER BEAM—Uniformly varying partially distributed load.

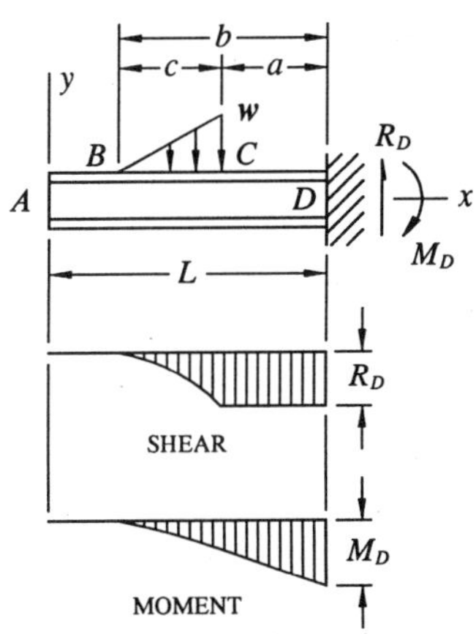

REACTIONS

$$R_D = \frac{1}{2}wc \qquad M_D = \frac{1}{6}wc(2a+b)$$

SHEARS

$$V = 0 \qquad (A \text{ to } B)$$

$$V = \frac{w(x-L+b)^2}{2c} \qquad (B \text{ to } C)$$

$$V = \frac{1}{2}wc \qquad (C \text{ to } D)$$

BENDING MOMENTS

$$M = 0 \qquad (A \text{ to } B)$$

$$M = \frac{w(x-L+b)^3}{6c} \qquad (B \text{ to } C)$$

$$M = \frac{1}{6}wc(3x-3L+b+2a) \qquad (C \text{ to } D)$$

DEFLECTIONS

$$y = -\frac{1}{120}\frac{wc}{EI}[(5b^2+10ba+15a^2)(L-x)-4a^3-2ab^2-3a^2b-b^3] \qquad (A \text{ to } B)$$

$$y = -\frac{1}{120}\frac{wc}{EI}\left[(20a+10b)(L-x)^2-10(L-x)^3+\frac{5(L-x-a)^4}{c}-\frac{(L-x-a)^5}{c^2}\right] \qquad (B \text{ to } C)$$

$$y = -\frac{1}{12}\frac{wc}{EI}(2a+b-L+x)(L-x)^2 \qquad (C \text{ to } D)$$

$$y_{max} = -\frac{1}{120}\frac{wc}{EI}[(5b^2+10ba+15a^2)L-4a^3-2ab^2-3a^2b-b^3] \quad \text{at } A$$

TABLE A-1 REFERENCE BEAM FORMULA SOLUTIONS (continued)

Case 7 CANTILEVER BEAM—Uniformly varying distributed load.

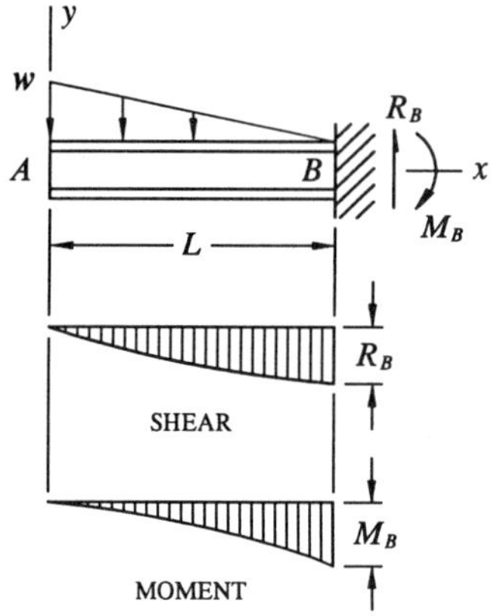

REACTIONS

$$R_B = \frac{1}{2}wL \qquad M_B = \frac{1}{3}wL^2$$

SHEARS

$$V = \frac{1}{2}\frac{wx}{L}(2L-x)$$

BENDING MOMENTS

$$M = \frac{1}{6}\frac{wx^2}{L}(3L-x)$$

DEFLECTIONS

$$y = -\frac{1}{120}\frac{w}{EIL}(11L^5 - 15L^4x + 5Lx^4 - x^5)$$

$$y_{\max} = -\frac{11}{120}\frac{wL^4}{EI} \quad \text{at } A$$

Case 8 CANTILEVER BEAM—Uniformly varying partially distributed load.

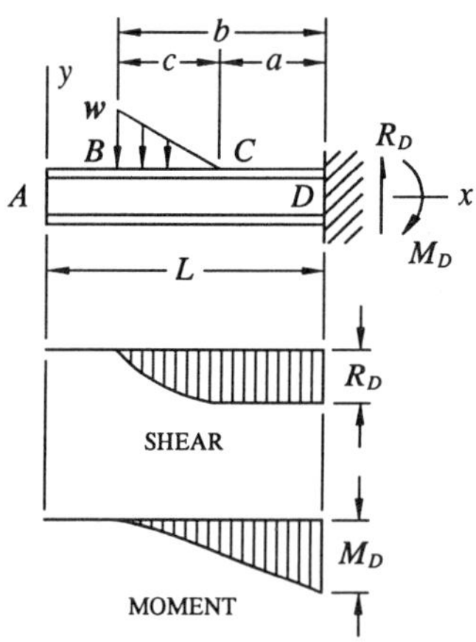

REACTIONS

$$R_D = \frac{1}{2}wc \qquad M_D = \frac{1}{6}wc(a+2b)$$

SHEARS

$$V = 0 \qquad (A \text{ to } B)$$

$$V = \frac{1}{2}\frac{w}{c}[c^2 - (L-a-x)^2] \qquad (B \text{ to } C)$$

$$V = \frac{1}{2}wc \qquad (C \text{ to } D)$$

BENDING MOMENTS

$$M = 0 \qquad (A \text{ to } B)$$

$$M = \frac{1}{6}\frac{w}{c}(3c+L-b-x)(x-L+b)^2 \qquad (B \text{ to } C)$$

$$M = \frac{1}{6}wc(3x-3L+a+2b) \qquad (C \text{ to } D)$$

DEFLECTIONS

$$y = -\frac{1}{120}\frac{wc}{EI}[(5a^2+10ab+15b^2)(L-x) - a^3 - 2a^2b - 3ab^2 - 4b^3] \qquad (A \text{ to } B)$$

$$y = -\frac{1}{120}\frac{wc}{EI}\left[\frac{(L-x-a)^5}{c^2} - 10(L-x)^3 + (10a+20b)(L-x)^2\right] \qquad (B \text{ to } C)$$

$$y = -\frac{1}{12}\frac{wc}{EI}(a+2b-L+x)(L-x)^2 \qquad (C \text{ to } D)$$

$$y_{\max} = -\frac{1}{120}\frac{wc}{EI}(5a^2L + 10abL + 15b^2L - a^3 - 2a^2b - 3ab^2 - 4b^3) \quad \text{at } A$$

TABLE A-1 REFERENCE BEAM FORMULA SOLUTIONS (continued)

Case 9 BEAM SIMPLY-SUPPORTED AT BOTH ENDS—Concentrated load at center span.

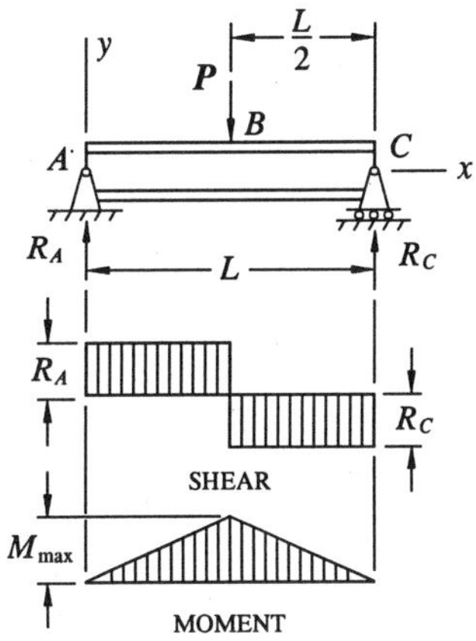

REACTIONS

$$R_A = \frac{P}{2} \qquad R_c = \frac{P}{2}$$

SHEARS

$$V = -\frac{P}{2} \qquad (A \text{ to } B)$$
$$V = \frac{P}{2} \qquad (B \text{ to } C)$$

BENDING MOMENTS

$$M = -\frac{1}{2}Px \qquad (A \text{ to } B)$$
$$M = -\frac{1}{2}P(L-x) \qquad (B \text{ to } C)$$
$$M_{max} = -\frac{PL}{4} \quad \text{at } B$$

DEFLECTIONS

$$y = -\frac{1}{48}\frac{P}{EI}(3L^2x - 4x^3) \qquad (A \text{ to } B)$$
$$y_{max} = -\frac{1}{48}\frac{PL^3}{EI} \quad \text{at } B$$

Case 10 BEAM SIMPLY-SUPPORTED AT BOTH ENDS—Concentrated load at any point.

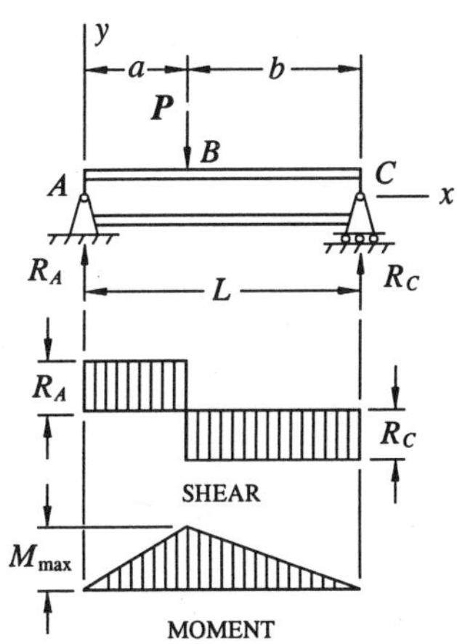

REACTIONS

$$R_A = \frac{Pb}{L} \qquad R_C = \frac{Pa}{L}$$

SHEARS

$$V = -\frac{Pb}{L} \qquad (A \text{ to } B)$$
$$V = \frac{Pa}{L} \qquad (B \text{ to } C)$$

BENDING MOMENTS

$$M = -\frac{Pbx}{L} \qquad (A \text{ to } B)$$
$$M = -\frac{Pa}{L}(L-x) \qquad (B \text{ to } C)$$
$$M_{max} = -\frac{Pab}{L} \quad \text{at } B$$

DEFLECTIONS

$$y = -\frac{Pbx}{6EIL}(L^2 - b^2 - x^2) \qquad (A \text{ to } B)$$
$$y = -\frac{Pa(L-x)}{6EIL}[2Lb - b^2 - (L-x)^2] \qquad (B \text{ to } C)$$
$$y_{max} = -\frac{Pab}{27EIL}(a+2b)\sqrt{3a^2+6ab} \quad \text{at } x = \sqrt{\frac{1}{3}a^2 + \frac{2}{3}ab} \quad \text{when } a > b.$$

TABLE A-1 REFERENCE BEAM FORMULA SOLUTIONS (continued)

Case 11 BEAM SIMPLY-SUPPORTED AT BOTH ENDS—Uniform load over entire span.

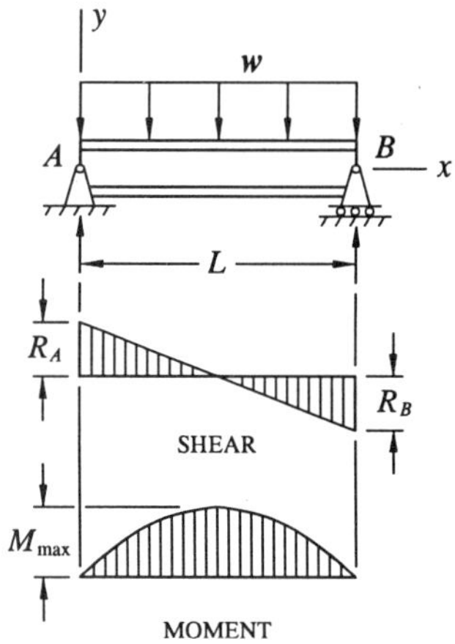

REACTIONS

$$R_A = \frac{wL}{2} \qquad R_B = \frac{wL}{2}$$

SHEARS

$$V = -\frac{1}{2}w(L-2x)$$

BENDING MOMENTS

$$M = -\frac{1}{2}w(Lx - x^2)$$

$$M_{max} = -\frac{wL^2}{8} \quad \text{at } x = \frac{L}{2}$$

DEFLECTIONS

$$y = -\frac{1}{24}\frac{wx}{EI}(L^3 - 2Lx^2 + x^3)$$

$$y_{max} = -\frac{5}{384}\frac{wL^4}{EI} \quad \text{at } x = \frac{L}{2}$$

Case 12 BEAM SIMPLY-SUPPORTED AT BOTH ENDS—Uniform load partially distributed over span.

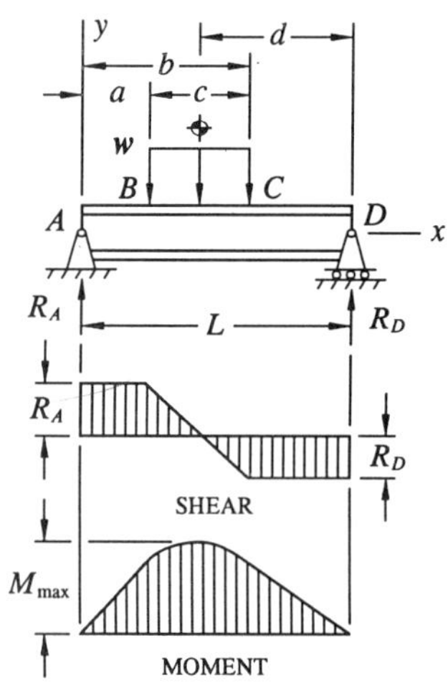

REACTIONS

$$R_A = \frac{wcd}{L} \qquad R_D = \frac{1}{2}\frac{wc}{L}(2a+c)$$

SHEARS

$$V = -R_A \qquad (A \text{ to } B)$$

$$V = -\frac{w}{L}(cd - Lx + aL) \qquad (B \text{ to } C)$$

$$V = R_D \qquad (C \text{ to } D)$$

BENDING MOMENTS

$$M = -R_A x \qquad (A \text{ to } B)$$

$$M = -R_A x + \frac{1}{2}w(x-a)^2 \qquad (B \text{ to } C)$$

$$M = -R_A x + \frac{1}{2}wc(2x - a - b) \qquad (C \text{ to } D)$$

$$M_{max} = -R_A\left(a + \frac{R_A}{2w}\right) \quad \text{at } x = a + \frac{R_A}{w}$$

DEFLECTIONS

$$y = -\frac{1}{48EI}\left[-8R_A(x^3 - L^2x) - \frac{wcx}{L}(8d^3 - 2bc^2 + c^3 + 2c^2L)\right] \qquad (A \text{ to } B)$$

$$y = -\frac{1}{48EI}\left[-8R_A(x^3 - L^2x) - \frac{wcx}{L}(8d^3 - 2bc^2 + c^3 + 2c^2L) + 2w(x-a)^4\right] \qquad (B \text{ to } C)$$

$$y = -\frac{1}{48EI}\left[-8R_A(x^3 - L^2x) - \frac{wcx}{L}(8d^3 - 2bc^2 + c^3) + wc(2x-a-b)^3 - wc(2bc^2 - c^3)\right] \qquad (C \text{ to } D)$$

TABLE A-1 REFERENCE BEAM FORMULA SOLUTIONS (continued)

Case 13 BEAM SIMPLY-SUPPORTED AT BOTH ENDS—Uniformly varying distributed load.

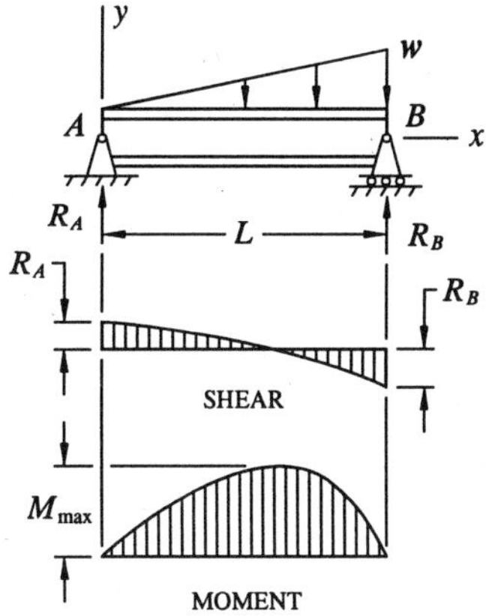

REACTIONS

$$R_A = \frac{1}{6}wL \qquad R_B = \frac{1}{3}wL$$

SHEARS

$$V = -\frac{1}{6}wL + \frac{1}{2}\frac{wx^2}{L}$$

BENDING MOMENTS

$$M = -\frac{wx}{6L}(L^2 - x^2)$$

$$M_{max} = -\frac{wL^2}{9\sqrt{3}} \quad \text{at } x = \frac{L}{\sqrt{3}}$$

DEFLECTIONS

$$y = -\frac{wx}{360EIL}(3x^4 - 10L^2x^2 + 7L^4)$$

$$y_{max} = -.00652\frac{wL^4}{EI} \quad \text{at } x = .5193L$$

Case 14 BEAM SIMPLY-SUPPORTED AT BOTH ENDS—Uniform load partially distributed over span.

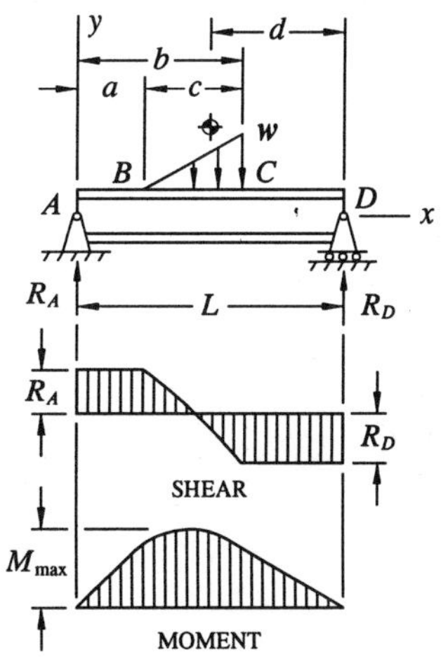

REACTIONS

$$R_A = \frac{1}{2}\frac{wcd}{L} \qquad R_D = \frac{1}{2}\frac{wc}{L}(L-d)$$

SHEARS

$$V = -R_A \qquad (A \text{ to } B)$$

$$V = -R_A + \frac{1}{2}\frac{w}{c}(x-a)^2 \qquad (B \text{ to } C)$$

$$V = R_D \qquad (C \text{ to } D)$$

BENDING MOMENTS

$$M = -R_A x \qquad (A \text{ to } B)$$

$$M = -R_A x + \frac{w(x-a)^3}{6c} \qquad (B \text{ to } C)$$

$$M = -R_A x + \frac{1}{6}wc(3x - a - 2b) \qquad (C \text{ to } D)$$

$$M_{max} = -R_A\left[a + \frac{2}{3}c\sqrt{\frac{d}{L}}\right] \quad \text{at } x = a + c\sqrt{\frac{d}{L}}$$

DEFLECTIONS

$$y = -\frac{1}{6EI}\left[-R_A(x^3 - L^2x) - \frac{1}{2}wcx\left(\frac{d^3}{L} + \frac{c^2}{6} - \frac{c^2b}{6L} + \frac{17}{270}\frac{c^3}{L}\right)\right] \qquad (A \text{ to } B)$$

$$y = -\frac{1}{6EI}\left[-R_A(x^3 - L^2x) + \frac{w(x-a)^5}{20c} - \frac{1}{2}wcx\left(\frac{d^3}{L} + \frac{c^2}{6} - \frac{1}{6}\frac{bc^2}{L} + \frac{17}{270}\frac{c^3}{L}\right)\right] \qquad (B \text{ to } C)$$

$$y = -\frac{1}{6EI}\left[-R_A(x^3 - L^2x) + \frac{1}{2}wc\left(\frac{(3x-a-2b)^3}{27} - d^3\frac{x}{L} - \left(\frac{L-x}{L}\right)\left(\frac{1}{6}bc^2 - \frac{17}{270}c^3\right)\right)\right] \qquad (C \text{ to } D)$$

TABLE A-1 REFERENCE BEAM FORMULA SOLUTIONS (continued)

Case 15 BEAM FIXED AT ONE END, SIMPLY-SUPPORTED AT THE OTHER—Concentrated load at center span.

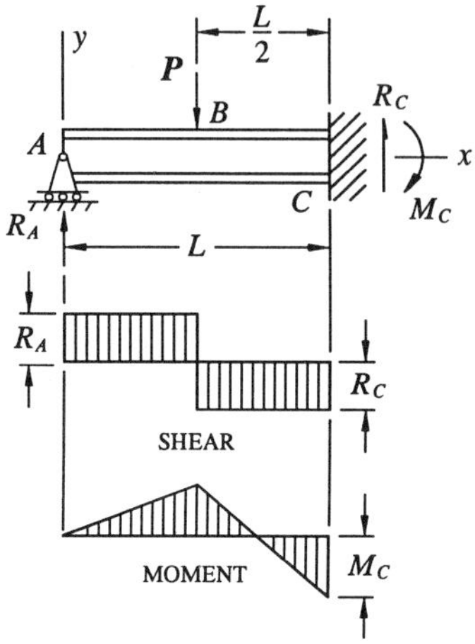

REACTIONS

$$R_A = \frac{5P}{16} \qquad R_C = \frac{11P}{16} \qquad M_C = \frac{3PL}{16}$$

SHEARS

$$V = -\frac{5P}{16} \qquad (A \text{ to } B)$$

$$V = \frac{11P}{16} \qquad (B \text{ to } C)$$

BENDING MOMENTS

$$M = -\frac{5P}{16}x \qquad (A \text{ to } B)$$

$$M = -\frac{P}{16}(8L - 11x) \qquad (B \text{ to } C)$$

DEFLECTIONS

$$y = -\frac{1}{96}\frac{P}{EI}(-5x^3 + 3L^2x) \qquad (A \text{ to } B)$$

$$y = -\frac{1}{96}\frac{P}{EI}\left[-5x^3 + 16\left(x - \frac{L}{2}\right)^3 + 3L^2x\right] \qquad (B \text{ to } C)$$

$$y_{\max} = -.00932\frac{PL^3}{EI} \quad \text{at } x = .4472L$$

Case 16 BEAM FIXED AT ONE END, SIMPLY-SUPPORTED AT THE OTHER—Concentrated load at any point.

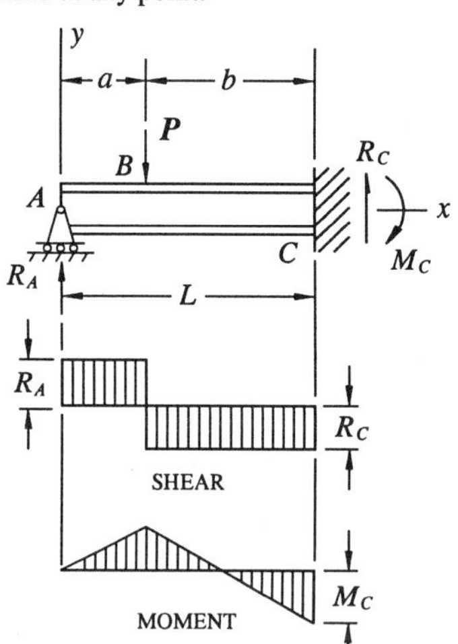

REACTIONS

$$R_A = \frac{1}{2}\frac{P}{L^3}(3b^2L - b^3)$$

$$R_C = P - R_A$$

$$M_C = \frac{1}{2}\frac{P}{L^2}(b^3 + 2bL^2 - 3b^2L)$$

SHEARS

$$V = -R_A \qquad (A \text{ to } B)$$

$$V = R_C \qquad (B \text{ to } C)$$

BENDING MOMENTS

$$M = -R_Ax \qquad (A \text{ to } B)$$

$$M = -R_Ax + P(x - L + b) \qquad (B \text{ to } C)$$

DEFLECTIONS

$$y = -\frac{1}{6EI}[-R_A(x^3 - 3L^2x) - 3Pb^2x] \qquad (A \text{ to } B)$$

$$y = -\frac{1}{6EI}[-R_A(x^3 - 3L^2x) - P(3b^2x - (x-a)^3)] \qquad (B \text{ to } C)$$

TABLE A-1 REFERENCE BEAM FORMULA SOLUTIONS (continued)

Case 17 BEAM FIXED AT ONE END, SIMPLY-SUPPORTED AT THE OTHER—Uniform load over entire span.

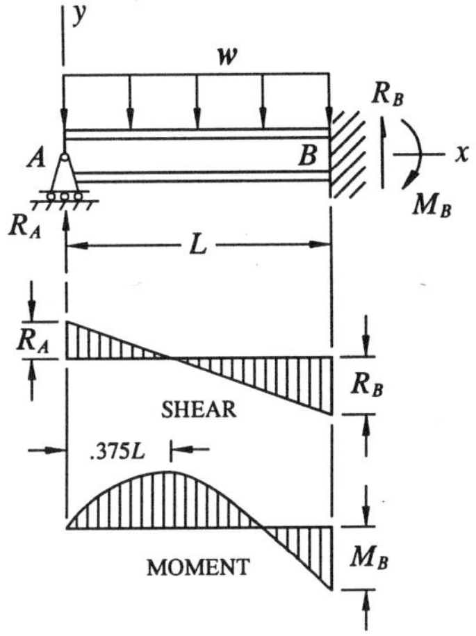

REACTIONS

$$R_A = \frac{3wL}{8} \qquad R_B = \frac{5wL}{8} \qquad M_B = \frac{wL^2}{8}$$

SHEARS

$$V = -\frac{w}{8}(3L - 8x)$$

BENDING MOMENTS

$$M = -\frac{w}{8}(3xL - 4x^2)$$

DEFLECTIONS

$$y = -\frac{1}{48}\frac{w}{EI}(-3Lx^3 + 2x^4 + L^3x)$$

$$y_{max} = -.0054\frac{wL^4}{EI} \quad \text{at } x = .4215L$$

Case 18 BEAM FIXED AT ONE END, SIMPLY-SUPPORTED AT THE OTHER—Uniform load partially distributed over span.

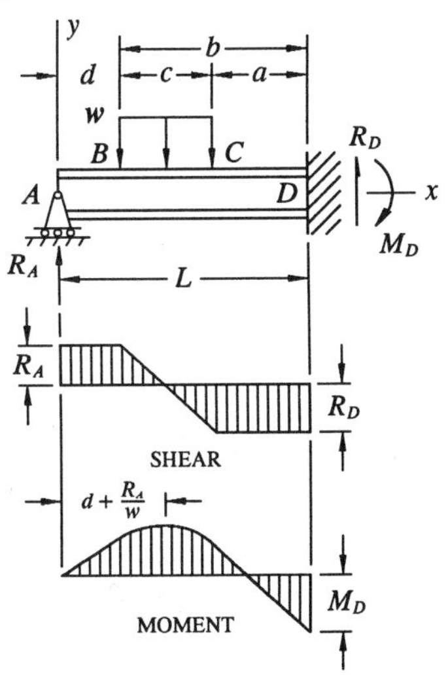

REACTIONS

$$R_A = \frac{1}{8}\frac{wc}{L^3}[4L(a^2 + ab + b^2) - a^3 - ab^2 - a^2b - b^3]$$

$$R_D = wc - R_A$$

$$M_D = \frac{wc}{2}(c + 2a) - R_AL$$

SHEARS

$$V = -R_A \qquad (A \text{ to } B)$$

$$V = -R_A + w(x - d) \qquad (B \text{ to } C)$$

$$V = wc - R_A \qquad (C \text{ to } D)$$

BENDING MOMENTS

$$M = -R_Ax \qquad (A \text{ to } B)$$

$$M = -R_Ax + \frac{w}{2}(x - d)^2 \qquad (B \text{ to } C)$$

$$M = -R_Ax + \frac{wc}{2}(2x - 2d - c) \qquad (C \text{ to } D)$$

DEFLECTIONS

$$y = -\frac{1}{EI}\left[-\frac{R_A}{6}(x^3 - 3L^2x) - \frac{wcx}{6}(3a^2 + 3ac + c^2)\right] \qquad (A \text{ to } B)$$

$$y = -\frac{1}{EI}\left[-\frac{R_A}{6}(x^3 - 3L^2x) - \frac{wcx}{6}(3a^2 + 3ac + c^2) + \frac{w}{24}(x - d)^4\right] \qquad (B \text{ to } C)$$

$$y = -\frac{1}{EI}\left[-\frac{R_A}{6}(x^3 - 3L^2x + 2L^3) - \frac{wc}{6}(2a + c)^2\left(\frac{2a + c}{8} - \frac{3L}{4} - \frac{(2x - 2d - c)^3}{8(2a + c)^2} + \frac{3x}{4}\right)\right] \qquad (C \text{ to } D)$$

TABLE A-1 REFERENCE BEAM FORMULA SOLUTIONS (continued)

Case 19 BEAM FIXED AT ONE END, SIMPLY-SUPPORTED AT THE OTHER—Uniformly varying distributed load.

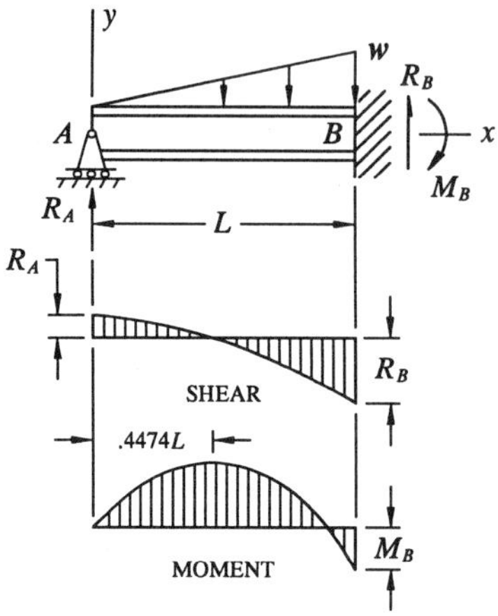

REACTIONS

$$R_A = \frac{1}{10}wL \qquad R_B = \frac{4}{10}wL \qquad M_B = \frac{1}{15}wL^2$$

SHEARS

$$V = -\frac{1}{10}\frac{w}{L}(L^2 - 5x^2)$$

BENDING MOMENTS

$$M = -\frac{1}{30}\frac{w}{L}(3L^2x - 5x^3)$$

DEFLECTIONS

$$y = -\frac{1}{120}\frac{w}{EIL}(-2L^2x^3 + L^4x + x^5)$$

$$y_{max} = -.00238\frac{wL^4}{EI} \quad \text{at } x = L\sqrt{\frac{1}{5}}$$

Case 20 BEAM FIXED AT ONE END, SIMPLY-SUPPORTED AT THE OTHER—Uniformly varying distributed load.

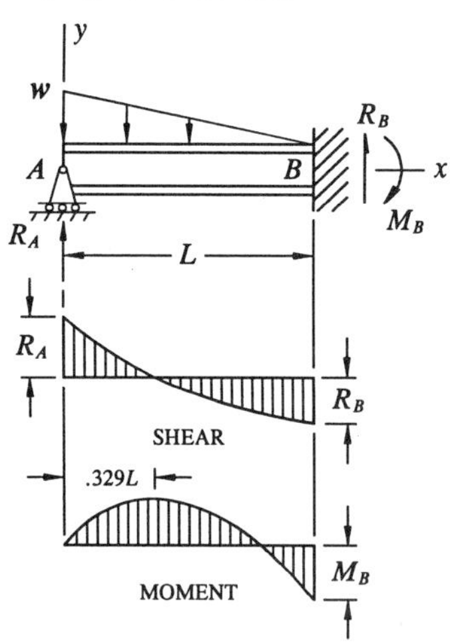

REACTIONS

$$R_A = \frac{11}{40}wL \qquad R_B = \frac{9}{40}wL \qquad M_B = \frac{7}{120}wL^2$$

SHEARS

$$V = -\frac{1}{40}\frac{w}{L}(11L^2 - 40Lx + 20x^2)$$

BENDING MOMENTS

$$M = -\frac{1}{120}\frac{w}{L}(33L^2x - 60Lx^2 + 20x^3)$$

DEFLECTIONS

$$y = -\frac{1}{240}\frac{w}{EIL}(-11L^2x^3 + 3L^4x + 10Lx^4 - 2x^5)$$

$$y_{max} = -.00304\frac{wL^4}{EI} \quad \text{at } x = .402L$$

TABLE A-1 REFERENCE BEAM FORMULA SOLUTIONS (continued)

Case 21 BEAM FIXED AT BOTH ENDS—Concentrated load at center span.

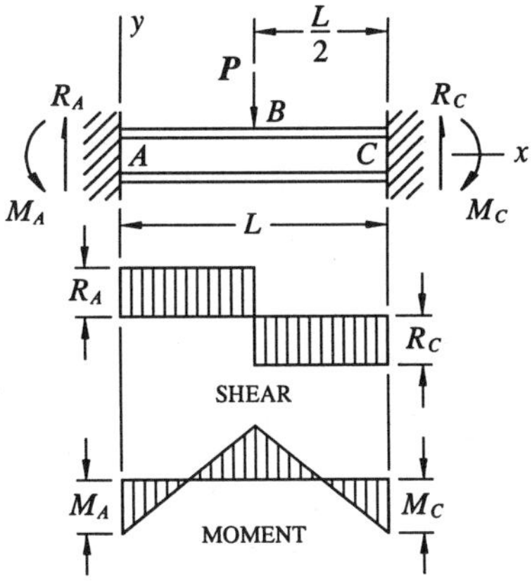

REACTIONS

$$R_A = \frac{P}{2} \qquad R_C = \frac{P}{2}$$
$$M_A = \frac{PL}{8} \qquad M_C = \frac{PL}{8}$$

SHEARS

$$V = -\frac{P}{2} \quad (A \text{ to } B)$$
$$V = \frac{P}{2} \quad (B \text{ to } C)$$

BENDING MOMENTS

$$M = -\frac{P}{8}(4x - L) \quad (A \text{ to } B)$$
$$M = -\frac{P}{8}(3L - 4x) \quad (B \text{ to } C)$$

DEFLECTIONS

$$y = -\frac{P}{48EI}(3Lx^2 - 4x^3)$$
$$y_{\max} = -\frac{PL^3}{192EI} \quad \text{at } B$$

Case 22 BEAM FIXED AT BOTH ENDS—Concentrated load at any point.

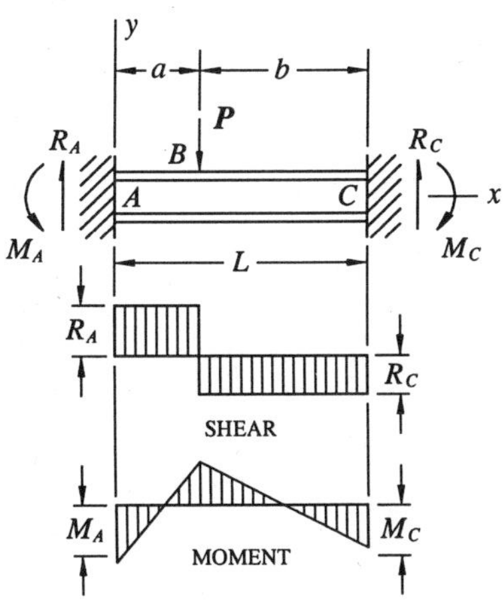

REACTIONS

$$R_A = \frac{Pb^2}{L^3}(3a + b) \qquad R_C = \frac{Pa^2}{L^3}(3b + a)$$
$$M_A = \frac{Pab^2}{L^2} \qquad M_C = \frac{Pa^2b}{L^2}$$

SHEARS

$$V = -R_A \quad (A \text{ to } B)$$
$$V = R_C \quad (B \text{ to } C)$$

BENDING MOMENTS

$$M = -R_Ax + \frac{Pab^2}{L^2} \quad (A \text{ to } B)$$
$$M = -R_Ax + \frac{Pab^2}{L^2} + P(x - a) \quad (B \text{ to } C)$$

DEFLECTIONS

$$y = -\frac{1}{6}\frac{Pb^2x^2}{EIL^3}(3aL - 3ax - bx) \quad (A \text{ to } B)$$
$$y = -\frac{1}{6}\frac{Pa^2(L-x)^2}{EIL^3}[3bL - (3b + a)(L - x)] \quad (B \text{ to } C)$$

TABLE A-1 REFERENCE BEAM FORMULA SOLUTIONS (continued)

Case 23 BEAM FIXED AT BOTH ENDS—Uniform load over entire span.

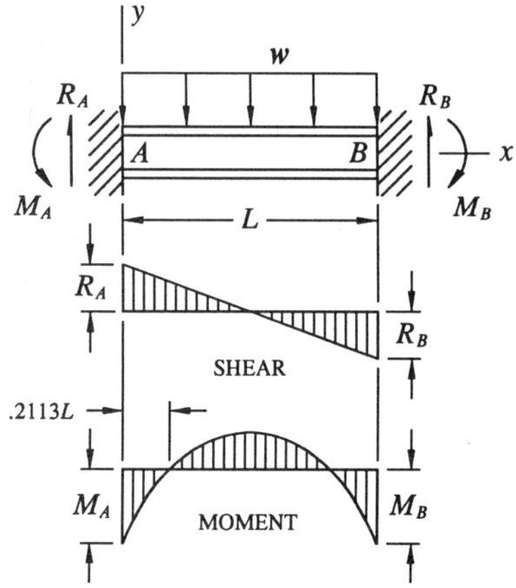

REACTIONS

$$R_A = \frac{wL}{2} \qquad R_B = \frac{wL}{2}$$

$$M_A = \frac{wL^2}{12} \qquad M_B = \frac{wL^2}{12}$$

SHEARS

$$V = -\frac{w}{2}(L-2x)$$

BENDING MOMENTS

$$M = -\frac{w}{12}(6Lx-6x^2-L^2)$$

DEFLECTIONS

$$y = -\frac{wx^2}{24EI}(L^2-2Lx+x^2)$$

$$y_{\max} = -\frac{wL^4}{384EI} \quad \text{at } x = \frac{L}{2}$$

Case 24 BEAM FIXED AT BOTH ENDS—Uniformly varying distributed load.

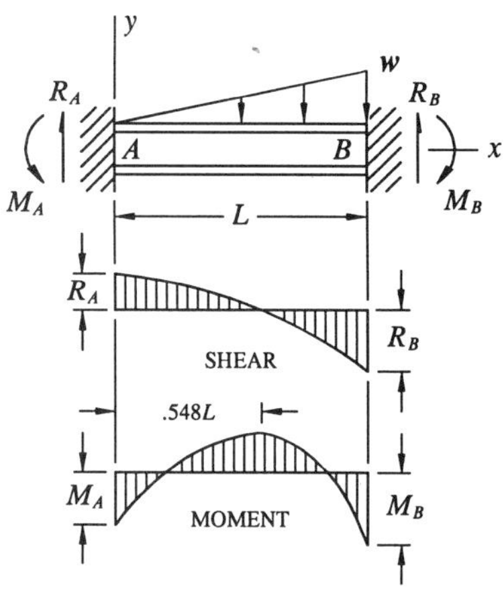

REACTIONS

$$R_A = \frac{3}{20}wL \qquad R_B = \frac{7}{20}wL$$

$$M_A = \frac{1}{30}wL^2 \qquad M_B = \frac{1}{20}wL^2$$

SHEARS

$$V = -\frac{w}{20L}(3L^2-10x^2)$$

BENDING MOMENTS

$$M = -\frac{w}{300L}(45L^2x-10L^3-50x^3)$$

DEFLECTIONS

$$y = -\frac{w}{120EIL}(2L^3x^2-3L^2x^3+x^5)$$

$$y_{\max} = -.001308\frac{wL^4}{EI} \quad \text{at } x = .525L$$

APPENDIX E

Design Mechanical and Physical Properties of Metallic Materials for Aerospace Vehicle Structures

In this appendix, the mechanical and physical properties of different materials that are used in some of the problem solutions of this book are presented. Their published values are taken from the Military Standardization Handbook, *Metallic Materials and Elements for Aerospace Vehicle Structures,* more commonly known as "MIL-HDBK-5F." The following selection of materials are taken from this handbook:

(1) 2024 aluminum alloy extrusions, QQ-A-200/3, p. 647
(2) 2024 aluminum alloy sheet and plate, QQ-A-250/4, p. 648
(3) clad 2024 aluminum alloy sheet and plate, QQ-A-250/5, p. 649.

The mechanical and physical properties associated with these materials are determined from static testing of numerous test specimens at room-temperature,[1] and their values expressed as minimum guaranteed allowables using statistical analysis of the test results. Their tabulated values will provide the means by which an engineer can reliably predict the structural behavior or adequacy of his engineering designs.

All of the information and data contained within MIL-HDBK-5F have been reviewed by the Department of Defense and the Federal Aviation Administration to insure their accuracy prior to publication. The design mechanical and physical properties of commonly used materials (steels, aluminum alloys, magnesium alloys, titanium alloys, heat-resistant alloys, beryllium, and special purpose metals and alloys) are provided in this handbook for both commercial and military aircraft designs; since, in general, the strength requirements of most materials are very often the same for different conventional aircraft designs. Those engineers who are actively pursuing a professional career in structural design engineering should become familiar with the general usage of this document.

Most aerospace companies will furnish their own prescribed structural engineering manuals. These manuals should only be used by the company for whom these documents were originally issued. For instance, the methods, procedures, and material data contained within a company's structures manual should not be interchanged, substituted for, or used to substantiate the aircraft structure of another company. An exception to this rule would be if Company A was to subcontract part of their own aircraft structure to Company B. In this case, Company B would use Company A's manual for the actual subcontract work, not its own in-house version. Of course, the fundamental equations of stress analysis that are given and used throughout this book, so basic to our understanding and study of strength of materials, can always be fully utilized on any type, sort, or category of aircraft vehicle structure.

The engineer is referred to Tables A-2 through A-4, where the design mechanical and physical properties of different materials are presented. The mechanical-property values F_{tu}, F_{ty}, F_{cy}, F_{su}, F_{bru}, and F_{bry} listed in each table are established in accordance with general aviation requirements from various federal and military procuring or certificating agencies on an A-, B-, or S-basis. Certain values in these tables also include the specific orientations of the grain directions (L, LT, or ST) of the material. In Fig. A-13, a simple plate element is shown defined by its established grain directions in accordance with the specific material processing methods indicated.

---

[1] The effect of different temperatures on the properties of a material can also be evaluated by using the graphical solutions provided in this handbook.

TABLE A-2 Design Mechanical and Physical Properties of 2024 Aluminum Alloy Extrusion

Specification	QQ-A-200/3																
Form	Extruded Bar, Rod, and Shapes																
Temper	T3,T3510, and T3511													T81,T8510, and T8511			
Thickness, in	≤ 0.249		0.250-0.499		0.500-0.749		0.750-1.499		1.500-2.999		3.000-4.499		1.500-2.999	3.000-4.499	0.050-0.249	0.250-1.499	1.500-4.500
Cross-section area, in^2	≤ 20								≤ 25				> 25, ≤ 32		≤ 20		≤ 32
Basis	A	B	A	B	A	B	A	B	A	B	A	B	S	S	S	S	S
Mechanical Properties:																	
F_{tu}, ksi:																	
L	57	61	60	62	60	62	65	70	70	74	70	74	68	68	64	66	66
LT	54	58	56	57	54	56	56	60	55	58	54	57	53	52	64	64	61
F_{ty}, ksi:																	
L	42	47	44	47	44	47	46	54	52	54	52	54	48	48	56	58	58
LT	37	41	38	40	37	39	37	43	39	41	39	41	36	36	55	57	57
F_{cy}, ksi:																	
L	34	38	37	39	38	40	41	48	49	50	49	51	45	45	57	59	59
LT	41	45	41	44	40	43	40	47	42	44	41	43	39	38	57	59	59
F_{su}, ksi:	29	31	31	32	30	31	33	35	34	36	33	35	33	32	35	36	39
F_{bru}[a], ksi:																	
(e/D = 1.5)	84	90	78	81	78	80	84	90	88	93	86	91	86	84	94	96	92
(e/D = 2.0)	108	114	98	101	97	101	105	113	111	118	109	115	108	106	123	123	117
F_{bry}[a], ksi:																	
(e/D = 1.5)	61	68	55	59	55	59	57	67	63	66	62	65	59	57	79	82	82
(e/D = 2.0)	71	79	67	71	67	71	69	81	77	80	75	78	71	69	93	96	96
e, percent (S-basis):																	
LT	12	...	12	...	12	...	10	...	10	...	10	...	8	8	4	5	5
E, 10^3 ksi	10.8																
E_c, 10^3 ksi	11.0																
G, 10^3 ksi	4.1																
μ	0.33																
Physical Properties:																	
ω, lb/in^3	0.101																
C, K, and α	See Figure 3.2.3.0 of MIL-HDBK-5F.																

[a]Bearing values are "dry pin" values per Section 1.4.7.1 of MIL-HDBK-5F.

TABLE A-3 Design Mechanical and Physical Properties of 2024 Aluminum Alloy Sheet and Plate

Specification	QQ-A-250/4																
Form	Coiled Sheet		Flat Sheet and Plate												Sheet		Plate
Temper	T4		T42[a]				T62[a]		T81		T851[b]				T861[b]		
Thickness, in	0.010-0.249		0.010-0.499	0.500-1.000	1.001-2.000	2.001-3.000	0.010-0.499	0.500-3.000	0.010-0.249		0.250-0.499		0.500-1.000	1.001-1.499	0.020-0.062	0.063-0.249	0.250-0.500
Basis	A	B	S	S	S	S	S	S	A	B	A	B	S	S	S	S	S
Mechanical Properties:																	
F_{tu}, ksi:																	
L	62	64	62	61	60	58	64	63	67	68	67	68	66	66	71	72	70
LT	62	64	62	61	60	58	64	63	67	68	67	68	66	66	70	71	70
F_{ty}, ksi:																	
L	40	42	38	38	38	38	50	50	59	61	58	60	58	57	63	67	64
LT	40	42	38	38	38	38	50	50	58	60	58	60	58	57	62	66	64
F_{cy}, ksi:																	
L	40	42	38	38	38	38	...	...	59	61	58	60	58	56	63	67	64
LT	40	42	38	38	38	38	...	...	58	60	59	61	58	57	65	69	67
F_{su}, ksi:	37	38	37	37	36	35	...	...	40	41	38	39	37	37	40	40	40
F_{bru}[c], ksi:																	
(e/D = 1.5)	93	96	93	92	90	87	...	...	100	102	102	103	100	100	108	110	108
(e/D = 2.0)	118	122	118	116	114	110	...	...	127	129	131	133	129	129	140	142	140
F_{bry}[c], ksi:																	
(e/D = 1.5)	56	59	53	53	53	53	...	...	83	86	86	89	86	85	90	96	93
(e/D = 2.0)	64	67	61	61	61	61	...	...	94	97	101	105	101	99	105	112	109
e, percent (S-basis):																	
LT	d		d	8	d	4	5	5	5	...	5	...	5	5	3	4	4
E, 10^3 ksi	See Table 3.2.3.0(d) of MIL-HDBK-5F.																
E_c, 10^3 ksi																	
G, 10^3 ksi																	
μ																	
Physical Properties:																	
ω, lb/in^3	0.101																
C, K, and α	See Figure 3.2.3.0 of MIL-HDBK-5F.																

[a] These allowables apply when samples of material supplied in the O or F temper are heat treated to demonstrate response to heat treatment. Properties obtained by the user however, may be lower than those listed if the material has been formed or otherwise cold or hot worked, particularly in the annealed temper, prior to solution heat treatment.
[b] Bearing values are "dry pin" values per Section 1.4.7.1 of MIL-HDBK-5F.
[c] See Table 3.1.2.1.1 of MIL-HDBK-5F.
[d] See Table 3.2.3.0(c) of MIL-HDBK-5F.

TABLE A-4 Design Mechanical and Physical Properties of Clad 2024 Aluminum Alloy Sheet and Plate

Specification	QQ-A-250/5																			
Form	Flat Sheet and Plate																			
Temper	T3								T351											
Thickness, in	0.008-0.009		0.010-0.062		0.063-0.128		0.129-0.249		0.250-0.499		0.500-1.000[a]		1.001-1.500[a]		1.501-2.000[a]		2.001-3.000[a]		3.001-4.000[a]	
Basis	A	B	A	B	A	B	A	B	A	B	A	B	A	B	A	B	A	B	A	B
Mechanical Properties:																				
F_{tu}, ksi:																				
L	59	60	60	61	62	63	63	64	62	64	61	63	60	62	60	62	58	60	55	57
LT	58	59	59	60	61	62	62	63	62	64	61	63	60	62	60	62	58	60	55	57
ST	...	...	...	...	...	...	...	...	...	...	...	...	...	...	...	...	52	54	49	51
F_{ty}, ksi:																				
L	44	45	44	45	45	47	45	47	46	48	45	48	45	48	45	47	44	46	39	41
LT	39	40	39	40	40	42	40	42	40	42	40	42	40	42	40	42	40	42	39	41
ST	...	...	...	...	...	...	...	...	...	...	...	...	...	...	...	...	38	40	38	39
F_{cy}, ksi:																				
L	36	37	36	37	37	39	37	39	37	39	37	39	37	39	36	38	35	37	33	35
LT	42	43	42	43	43	45	43	45	43	45	42	45	42	44	42	44	41	43	39	41
ST	...	...	...	...	...	...	...	...	...	...	...	...	...	...	...	...	46	48	44	47
F_{su}, ksi:	37	37	37	38	38	39	39	40	37	38	36	37	35	37	35	37	34	35	32	34
F_{bru}[b], ksi:																				
(e/D = 1.5)	96	97	97	99	101	102	102	104	94	97	92	95	91	94	91	94	88	91	83	86
(e/D = 2.0)	119	121	121	123	125	127	127	129	115	119	113	117	111	115	111	115	107	111	102	106
F_{bry}[a], ksi:																				
(e/D = 1.5)	68	70	68	70	70	73	70	73	69	72	69	72	69	72	69	72	69	72	67	70
(e/D = 2.0)	82	84	82	84	84	88	84	88	82	86	82	86	82	86	82	86	82	86	80	84
e, percent (S-basis):																				
LT	10	...	c	...	15	...	15	...	12	...	8	...	7	...	6	...	4	...	4	...
E, 10^3 ksi																				
Primary	10.5								10.7											
Secondary	9.5				10.0				10.2											
E_c, 10^3 ksi																				
Primary	10.7								10.9											
Secondary	9.7				10.2				10.4											
G, 10^3 ksi	...																			
μ	0.33																			
Physical Properties:																				
ω, lb/in^3	0.101																			
C, K, and α	...																			

[a] These values have been adjusted to represent the average properties across the whole section, including the 2-1/2 percent nominal cladding thickness.
[b] See Table 3.1.2.1.1 of MIL-HDBK-5F. Bearing values are "dry pin" values per Section 1.4.7.1 of MIL-HDBK-5F.
[c] See Table 3.2.3.0(f) of MIL-HDBK-5F.

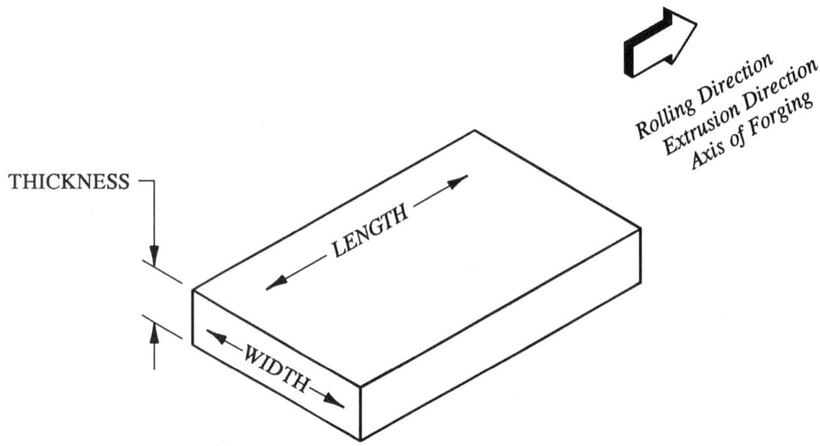

LENGTH (L) Longitudinal Grain Direction.
WIDTH (LT) Longitudinal Transverse Grain Direction.
THICKNESS (ST) Short Transverse Grain Direction.

FIGURE A-13 Grain directions for specific material processing methods of a plate.

In many aircraft design cases, whether they pertain to commercial or military aircraft structures, the A-basis values in the mechanical-property tables are ordinarily used. Under certain design limitations, however, B-values are permitted, as specified by the approving agency. The S-basis values are acceptable where A-basis values are neither available nor specifically indicated in a table. To insure a high degree of reliability for the mechanical properties specified in MIL-HDBK-5F, statistical analysis requirements have been imposed on the tested data.

The mechanical and physical properties listed in each table are applicable to static loading conditions only. Static loading is applied gradually to a structure; whereas, dynamic loading is characterized by its impact loading (that is, loading which is applied rapidly to a structure). The mechanical-property tables in MIL-HDBK-5F will provide the necessary strength characteristics of different materials for the aeronautical engineer to use in his selection of reliable material alternatives for a well-designed aircraft structure.

When a structural member is tested in tension or compression, it is customary to plot the stress and strain relationships of its tested data. To help illustrate this, a typical tension stress-strain diagram is drawn in Fig. A-14. The stress is computed on the basis of the applied load of the structure divided by its "original" cross-sectional area ($f_n = P/A$). Strains are measured by the change in length between two fixed points on the test structure divided by the "original" length of the structure between the fixed points ($\varepsilon = \Delta L/L$).

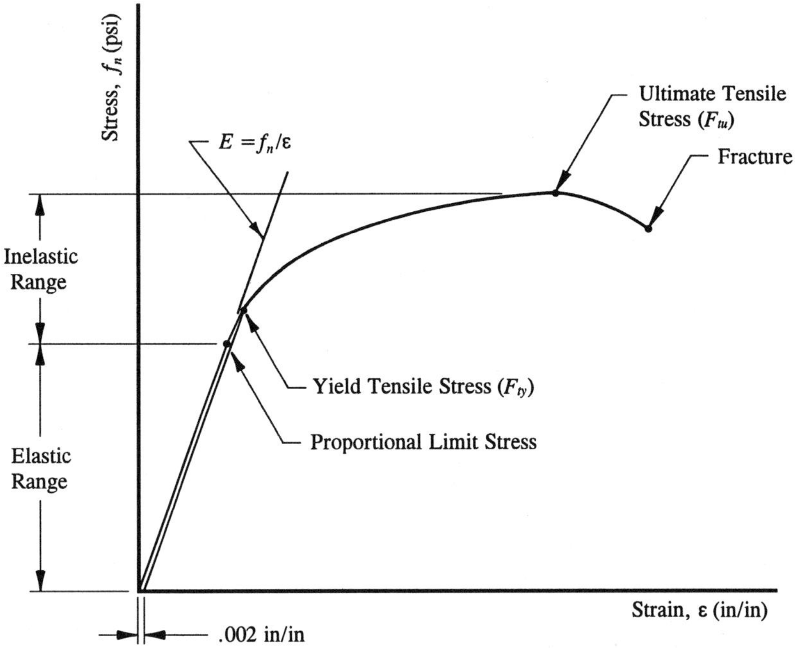

Inelastic range = stresses that occur above the proportional limit stress.
Elastic range = stresses that occur below the proportional limit stress.

FIGURE A-14 Typical stress-strain diagram in tension.

The modulus of elasticity E is defined as the straight-line portion of the stress-strain curve in that same figure. Mathematically, the modulus of elasticity can be written using the definition for the slope of a line. Thus, we have

$$E = \frac{\text{rise}}{\text{run}} = \frac{f_n}{\varepsilon}. \tag{A-9}$$

Equation A-9 should be familiar to most practicing engineers. It is known as Hooke's law, and is only valid in the elastic range of stresses of a material. Where this line just begins to deviate from a straight line establishes what is called the proportional limit stress of the material. All stresses which exceed this value are termed "inelastic" or "plastic." This means that when a structure is subjected to inelastic stress design, it will not return to its original design shape when the applied loads are removed. However, if stresses are held below the proportional limit of the material, no permanent deformation of the structure will occur.

The highest stress point of a tension stress-strain curve determines the ultimate tension stress allowable F_{tu} of the material. In compression, however, the ultimate compression stress allowable F_{cu} (for most metallic materials) is physically impossible to measure accurately. In essence, under compression loading the material tested begins to expand as it continues to support the increasing compression load. If the test specimen is made very short, thereby preventing the member from column action, the compression member theoretically will not fail. Under normal design conditions, the value of the ultimate tensile stress F_{tu} is used as the criterion or basis for limiting the ultimate strength of a material in compression. That is, the value of F_{cu} is set equal to the value of F_{tu} for that material. Of course, higher stress allowables in compression may sometimes be used if their values can be verified from actual test data. Good engineering judgment is the prime prerequisite in establishing the ultimate compression stress allowable of a particular design. For this reason, the values of F_{cu} are not listed in the mechanical-property tables furnished in MIL-HDBK-5F.

In conclusion, discretion must always be used when applying allowable stress data in structural designs because of other design conditions that might actually override their use, such as fatigue, plastic deformation, instability requirements, creep considerations, resistance to stress-corrosion and dynamic effects. These may be more sensitive design parameters than the general strength requirements of the particular design.

For most commonly used aircraft metallic materials used by the aeronautical engineer, the yield stress of the material (F_{cy} or F_{ty}) will not usually exhibit a clear and well-defined stress point on a stress-strain curve. To establish such a point for practical design use, it is usually permissible to determine the yield stress at a strain value of .002 in/in. That is, a line is drawn parallel to the elastic portion of the stress-strain curve at .002 in/in of strain, and where this line intersects the curve will determine the yield stress of the material.[1] If a tension stress-strain curve is used, the yield stress is tension; whereas, if a compression stress-strain curve is used, the yield stress is compression.

To safeguard an aircraft against premature structural failure of its component parts, a good design should achieve adequate strength requirements of its basic structure while still attaining the lightest possible weight overall. In this way, the general performance characteristics of the aircraft are not appreciably altered nor does it jeopardize the structural safety of the aircraft design. The bearing ultimate and yield stress allowables (F_{bru} and F_{bry}) mentioned earlier in this appendix will be specifically covered in Chapter 3 when our attention will focus on the design and analysis of structural joints and connections.

---

[1] Since this value is above the proportional limit stress of the material, it also represents "*some degree of acceptable yielding*" of the material.

APPENDIX F

Calculation of Moment of Inertia

The moment of inertia I_{na} of the cross-sectional area of a beam around its neutral axis is a measure of the resistance to bending of that beam. This value is used in the well-known flexure formula (Eq. 2-5, $f_b = \pm Mc/I_{na}$) to determine the elastic bending stresses at any point on the cross-sectional area. There are several known calculation methods that can be employed in the computation of this quantity. The method most widely used in the aerospace industry today is to set up the solution in tabular form. This will be the method presented in this section.

The moment of inertia of a cross-sectional area is dependent upon its geometric shape and size. Its value is a constant for each particular shaped area about a prescribed or designated axis of bending. The moment of inertia for some standard shapes are tabulated in Table A-5. The values of I_o given in this table are measured around the horizontal axes o-o passing through the centroids of these standard shaped areas. To verify the geometric properties of these standard shapes, the engineer is referred to an integral calculus textbook on this subject.

In general, most beam cross-sectional areas can be partitioned into combinations of these simple cross-sectional shapes. The main emphasis of this appendix will be to determine the moment of inertia of different combinations of these standard shapes. The first of these equations necessary to calculate this quantity is presented here.

TABLE A-5 SECTION PROPERTIES OF STANDARD SHAPES

Rectangle

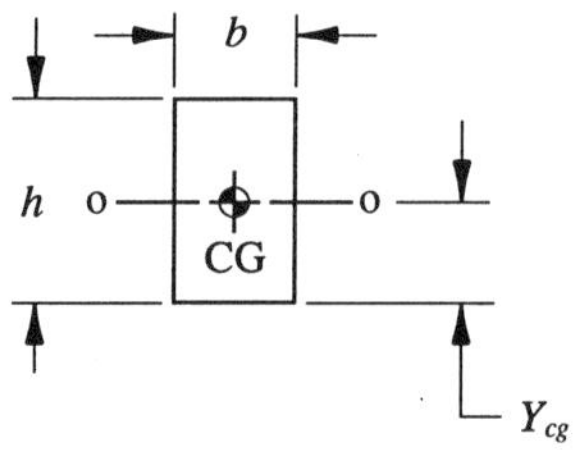

$I_o = bh^3/12$
$Y_{cg} = h/2$
$A = bh$

Triangle

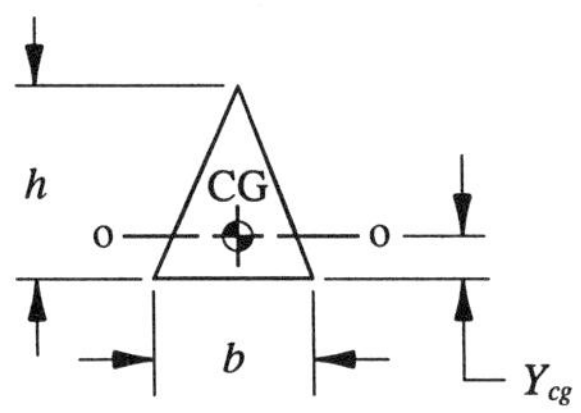

$I_o = bh^3/36$
$Y_{cg} = h/3$
$A = bh/2$

Circle

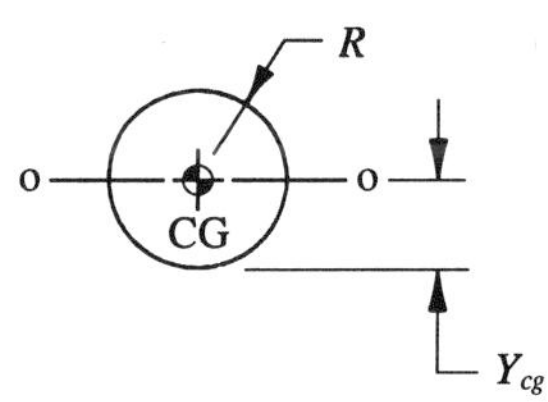

$I_o = \pi R^4/4$
$Y_{cg} = R$
$A = \pi R^2$

Fillet

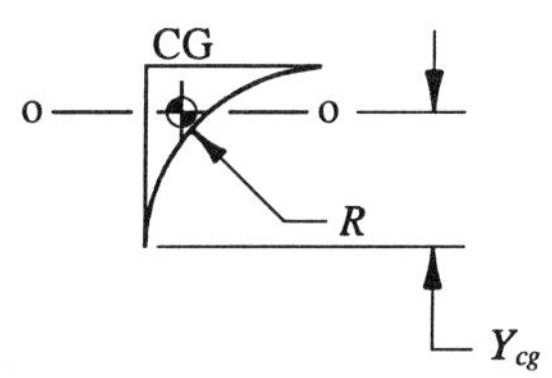

$I_o = .007545R^4$
$Y_{cg} = .7766R$
$A = .2146R^2$

$$Y_{cg} = \frac{\Sigma\, Ay}{\Sigma\, A} \qquad \text{(A-10)}$$

where: $\Sigma\, A = A_1 + A_2 + A_3 + \ldots + A_n$

$\Sigma\, Ay = A_1y_1 + A_2y_2 + A_3y_3 + \ldots + A_ny_n$

A = area of a standard shaped section

y = distance measured from the centroid (center of gravity) of a standard shaped section to an arbitrary established reference axis.

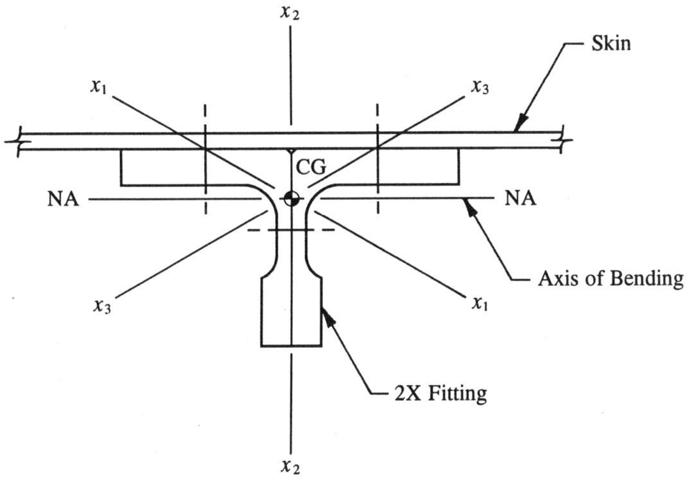

FIGURE A-15 Moment of inertia of the section area about the axis of bending of the beam.

Simply put in words, this equation locates the center of gravity of an entire cross-sectional area by taking a weighted average of all its standard shaped areas with respect to their centroid locations from an arbitrary established reference axis. It is also very useful in solving general centroid location problems, that is, of the beam cap centroid variety.

The second equation calculates the moment of inertia I_{cg} of the total cross-sectional area around the centroidal axis of the total section. Note in particular that this equation also incorporates the distance Y_{cg} found by Eq. A-10. Hence this quantity must be found first.

$$I_{cg} = \Sigma I_o + \Sigma Ay^2 - Y_{cg}(\Sigma Ay) \tag{A-11}$$

where: $\Sigma I_o = (I_o)_1 + (I_o)_2 + (I_o)_3 + \dots + (I_o)_n$

$\Sigma Ay^2 = A_1 y_1^2 + A_2 y_2^2 + A_3 y_3^2 + \dots + A_n y_n^2$

I_o = moment of inertia of a standard shaped section around its own centroidal axis.

For any particular cross-sectional area there can exist an infinite number of values of moment of inertia passing through the center of gravity of the section (see Fig. A-15). However, the required moment of inertia to be used in the flexure formula must be compatible with the axis of bending of the beam. This occurs at the neutral axis of the section area. For example, if a beam physically bends about a horizontal axis, the moment of inertia of the cross-section must also be calculated around that horizontal axis but coincident with the neutral axis of the cross-section.[1] The neutral axis is based on the equilibrium of internal forces across a section area; whereas, the centroidal axis is solely a function of the geometric shape of the section area. The centroidal axis always passes through the centroid or center of gravity of a cross-sectional area.

To find the neutral axis for inelastic stress design, the engineer is referred to an advanced textbook on this subject, where the study of plasticity of inelastic stress designs can more aptly be treated (those stresses which occur above the proportional limit of the material). Specifically, it can be shown that stresses are no longer linear in the plastic range of a stress-strain curve, and the neutral axis of a section will shift slightly in a direction to balance the net axial loads across the section to zero. In the paragraph which subsequently follows, the location of the neutral axis in conjunction with the elastic behavior of a structural design will be fully developed.

In elastic stress design, so long as the material properties of a cross-section behave elastically (that is, stresses which occur below the proportional limit of the material), and the compression and tension stress-strain curves are identical, the neutral axis will remain coincident with the centroidal axis. Mathematically, the following equations are directly formulated from these general limitations made on the structural behavior of the material:

$$Y_{na} = Y_{cg} \qquad \textbf{(A-12)}$$

and therefore

$$I_{na} = I_{cg}\,. \qquad \textbf{(A-13)}$$

In this form, the moment of inertia can now be directly substituted into the flexure formula (Eq. 2-5) since its value is in general agreement with the basic definitions used to apply this expression. Note further that even if calculated bending stresses by this equation do result in the inelastic stress range, their values, if used for a particular design, should nonetheless be slightly conservative. Therefore, so long as a conservative approach to the analysis is deemed acceptable, the engineer should have absolutely no reservations as to the general applicability of Eqs. A-12 and A-13 to conservative solutions of inelastic bending design. The specific criteria established by a company's structural engineering department will govern whether a structure requires the additional fine-tuning of its structural members for inelastic stress design. Such a decision may of course be based upon other design considerations, such as fatigue, crack growth propagation, deformation requirements, etc. These parameters must not be overlooked if the structure is to be properly designed.

---

[1] The beam described in Fig. A-15 will bend around the neutral axis of the composite section parallel to the plane of the attached sheet (as indicated by the skin in this figure).

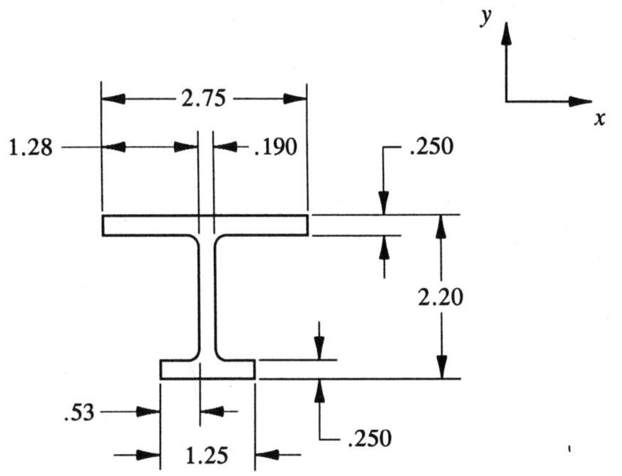

FIGURE A-16 Extrusion drawing. (Net area to minimum tolerance. Nominals used for simplicity. Specific type of material omitted.)

Example A-2 Find the moments of inertia through the centroid of the longeron extrusion shown in Fig. A-16 parallel to the rectangular coordinate axes x and y. In solving such problems correctly, it is highly recommended that the calculations be performed in tabular form.

SOLUTION: In the analysis of most aircraft designs, it is common practice for hand calculations to neglect the contributions of the moments of inertia of the fillets of a cross-sectional area. For this reason, the fillet areas are shown shaded in

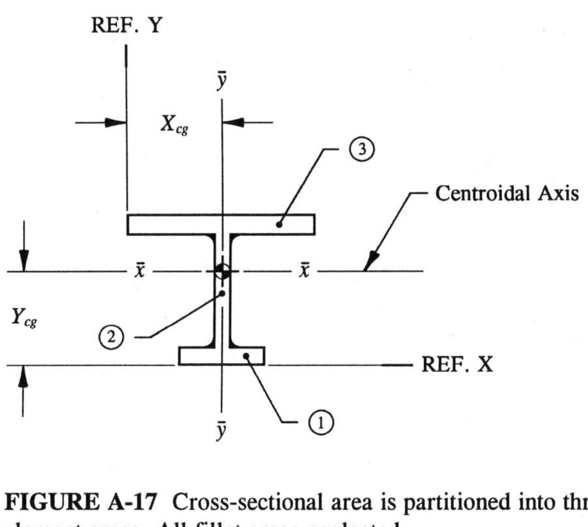

FIGURE A-17 Cross-sectional area is partitioned into three rectangular element areas. All fillet areas neglected.

Fig. A-17—to distinguish them from those areas considered effective in the actual computation of moment of inertia. However, if the moments of inertia of these fillets are believed to be significant quantities for weight reduction, their values can easily be accounted for in the computational tables that follow using the section properties given in Table A-5 for that particular standard shaped area.

For this example, the cross-sectional area given in Fig. A-17 is conveniently partitioned into three rectangular-shaped areas to represent the total moment of inertia of the section in tabular form. Each element area is shown numerically symbolized in that same figure. Next, the most remote distances from the total cross-sectional area are chosen to establish the reference axes X and Y. In this way, for each element area the distances x and y measured from these axes will be positive values in Tables A-6 and A-7. The values of b and h are also filled out in each table. The b dimensions are always taken parallel to the reference axis; while the h dimensions are perpendicular to this axis. It then remains to evaluate the remaining values indicated across the tables (use $A = bh$ and $I_o = bh^3/12$ for a rectangular-shaped area). In the final step, Eqs. A-10 and A-11 are applied using the appropriate column totals of each table.

TABLE A-6 MOMENT OF INERTIA AROUND THE $\bar{x}$-AXIS

Element	b	h	y	A	Ay	Ay^2	I_o
1	1.250	0.250	0.125	0.312	0.039	0.005	0.002
2	0.190	1.700	1.100	0.323	0.355	0.391	0.078
3	2.750	0.250	2.075	0.687	1.427	2.960	0.004
			Total	1.322	1.821	3.356	0.084

$$Y_{cg} = \frac{\Sigma Ay}{\Sigma A} = \frac{1.821}{1.322} = 1.377 \text{ in}$$

$$I_{cg} = \Sigma I_o + \Sigma Ay^2 - Y_{cg}(\Sigma Ay)$$

$$I_{cg} = .084 + 3.356 - 1.377(1.821) = .932 \text{ in}^4.$$

To distinguish I_{cg} from those values which could theoretically be calculated around other axes of this cross-sectional area, the subscript $\bar{x}$ is more appropriately used. Its designation is used to indicate the particular axis about which the moment of inertia is computed. For the value just obtained in this example, this corresponds to the $\bar{x}$-axis, or

$$I_{\bar{x}} = I_{cg} = .932 \text{ in}^4.$$

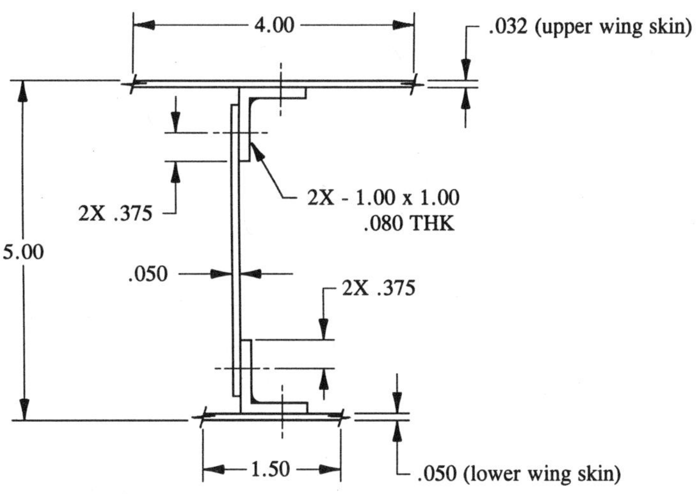

FIGURE A-18 Wing spar section.

TABLE A-7 MOMENT OF INERTIA AROUND THE $\bar{y}$-AXIS

Element	b	h	x	A	Ax	Ax^2	I_o
1	0.250	1.250	1.375	0.312	0.430	0.591	0.041
2	1.700	0.190	1.375	0.323	0.444	0.611	0.001
3	0.250	2.750	1.375	0.687	0.945	1.300	0.433
			Total	1.322	1.819	2.502	0.475

$$X_{cg} = \frac{\Sigma Ax}{\Sigma A} = \frac{1.819}{1.322} = 1.376 \text{ in}$$

$$I_{cg} = \Sigma I_o + \Sigma Ax^2 - X_{cg}(\Sigma Ax)$$

$$I_{cg} = .475 + 2.502 - 1.376(1.819) = .474 \text{ in}^4.$$

In a similar manner, the preferred designation for this moment of inertia corresponds to the $\bar{y}$-axis, or

$$I_{\bar{y}} = I_{cg} = .474 \text{ in}^4.$$

Additional example problems will be presented throughout this book to cover a greater variety of possible solutions to different cross-sectional shapes that might be encountered in actual engineering design. One of these possible structural configurations is described in the following example problem:

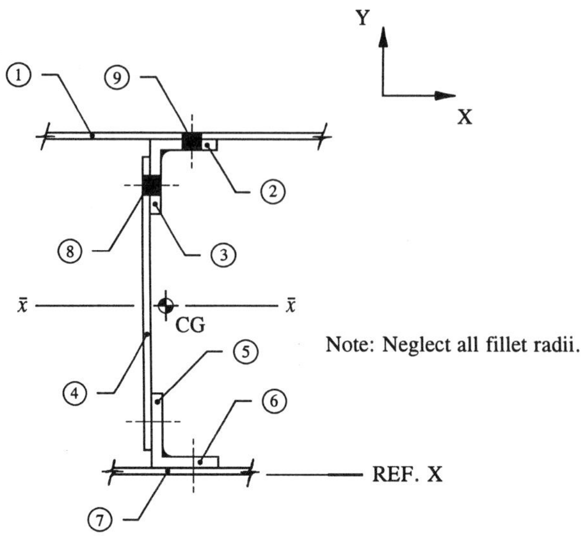

FIGURE A-19 Wing spar net cross-sectional area through the holes.

Example A-3 A built-up wing spar whose cross-sectional dimensions are shown in Fig. A-18 is subjected to a bending moment about a horizontal axis. If the moment produces tension in the upper wing skin and compression in the lower skin, what is the moment of inertia of the total cross-sectional area for elastic stress design? All rivets are 6/32 in diameter (this corresponds to a nominal hole diameter of .191 in, see Table 3-1). Assume that the effectivity of the upper wing skin in tension is 4.0 in.

SOLUTION: In accordance with the development and application of the flexure formula for elastic stress design, the moment of inertia is found around the neutral axis of the built-up section. It will be recalled from previous discussions presented in this appendix that if calculated bending stresses are below the proportional limit of the material, the neutral axis must pass through the centroid of the section area. The axes are said to be coincident (i.e., $Y_{na} = Y_{cg}$). And for elastic stress design, $I_{na} = I_{cg}$ (see Eq. A-13). Even so, for most practical design applications, the bending stresses computed by the flexure formula are the quantities desired. That is, even though the flexure formula is not valid in the inelastic range of stresses, its practical application is nevertheless very important in inelastic stress design—the calculated values yield at most only slightly conservative results anyway. If the amount of conservatism, however, is not acceptable for practical design, the techniques of plastic (inelastic) stress design should then be employed.

The bending moment described in this example will produce tension stresses above the neutral axis of the section area. The rivet holes there are considered ineffective (see the shaded areas in Fig. A-19), and therefore, their areas should not be included in the computation of moment of inertia (for a brief review of net tension stresses, see discussion in Sec. 2.2). A simple way to accomplish the actual computation of moment of inertia when rivet holes are present in a tension member is to subtract the contribution of each rivet hole from the total moment of inertia of the cross-sectional area. Consider Table A-8, where the rivet holes (elements #8 and #9) are subtracted from the total moment of inertia of the section area (elements #1 through #7) for this example.

After the values of *b*, *h*, and *y* have been completely filled in for each element area represented in Table A-8, the indicated operations across the table are performed. The appropriate column totals are then substituted into Eqs. A-10 and A-11 to find the required moment of inertia of the total section area around the centroidal axis. Lastly, Eqs. A-12 and A-13 are each applied to the wing spar section for elastic stress design.

TABLE A-8 MOMENT OF INERTIA AROUND THE $\bar{x}$-AXIS

Element	b	h	y	A	Ay	Ay^2	I_o
1	4.000	0.032	4.984	0.128	0.638	3.180	0.000
2	1.000	0.080	4.928	0.080	0.394	1.943	0.000
3	0.080	0.920	4.428	0.074	0.326	1.443	0.005
4	0.050	4.418	2.509	0.221	0.554	1.391	0.359
5	0.080	0.920	0.590	0.074	0.043	0.026	0.005
6	1.000	0.080	0.090	0.080	0.007	0.001	0.000
7	1.500*	0.050	0.025	0.075	0.002	0.000	0.000
8	0.130	0.191	4.343	– 0.025	– 0.108	– 0.468	– 0.000
9	0.191	0.112	4.944	– 0.021	– 0.106	– 0.523	– 0.000
			Total	0.686	1.750	6.993	0.369

* Assumed effective sheet width in compression (approximately 30*t* for 2024 aluminum alloy materials).

$$Y_{cg} = \frac{\Sigma\, Ay}{\Sigma\, A} = \frac{1.750}{.686} = 2.551 \text{ in}$$

$$I_{cg} = \Sigma\, I_o + \Sigma\, Ay^2 - Y_{cg}(\Sigma\, Ay)$$

$$I_{cg} = .369 + 6.993 - 2.551(1.750) = 2.898 \text{ in}^4.$$

And then, for elastic stress design, we obtain:

$$I_{na} = I_{cg} = 2.898 \text{ in}^4.$$

The tabulation method of this appendix is also recommended for use when structural members are added to the basic cross-sectional area, as when a

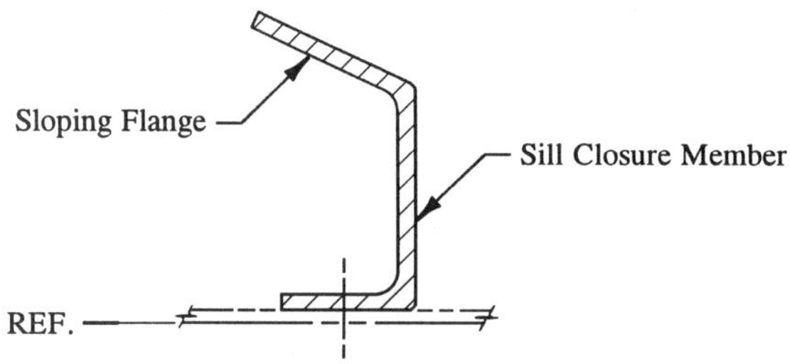

FIGURE A-20 Irregular shaped cross-sectional area.

reinforcement strap is added to a structure for additional strength. The procedure is done without changing or disrupting the previous figures in the table. Here, the values for the reinforcement are added to the table and new totals calculated. However, if the reinforcement is added below the reference baseline, the distance y of the member would be listed as a negative quantity in this table.

Example A-4 For the sill closure member shown in Fig. A-20, describe a method of partitioning that would simplify the computation of moment of inertia? Neglect the fillet and chamfer areas of the section.

SOLUTION: For an irregular shaped section, the tabulation method of this appendix is again employed. This remains the most straightforward method to determine the moment of inertia for this section. For this example, cleaver sectioning of the cross-sectional area will greatly simplify the actual computations of this quantity. To accomplish this, it was decided to completely encase the upper flange of the cross-sectional area by the heavy, bold lines of element #1, as shown in Fig. A-21. Within this enclosure, elements #2, #3, and #4 are partitioned into three triangular areas. Their negative contributions to the moment of inertia are then subtracted from element #1 which encased them. This technique will correctly define the

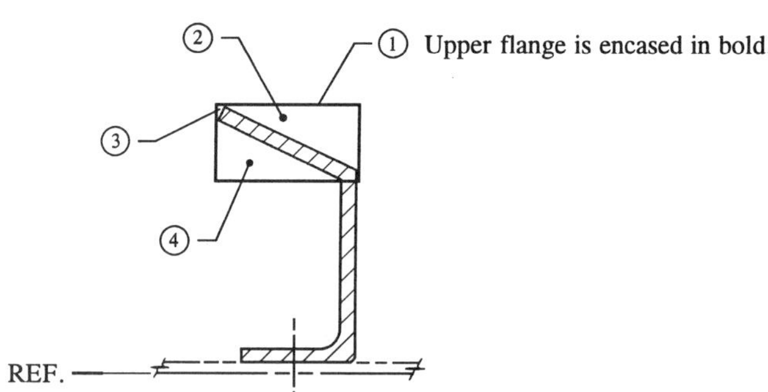

FIGURE A-21 Upper flange is shown partitioned into standard element areas.

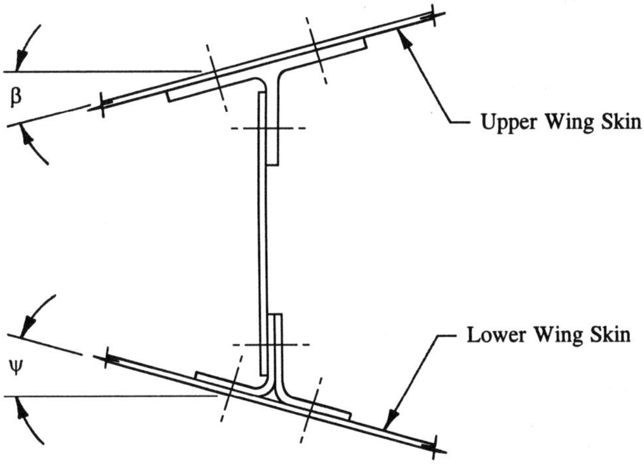

FIGURE A-22 Actual front wing spar cross-section.

sloping flange of the sill closure member. Of course, the skin, web, and lower flange areas are also partitioned and included in the final tabulation.

For most cross-sectional areas used in actual design cases, the foregoing method of partitioning is unnecessary and should be avoided. Such a case is shown in Fig. A-22, where the slope of the wing skins are considered small. Here, the engineer should base his moment of inertia computation on the wing skins being actually horizontal, as shown in Fig. A-23. Whether a particular section area requires the extra fine-tuning or not of its cross-sectional area is strictly up to the judgment of the design engineer in charge to decide. If his decision justifies the additional cost in man-hours, the more detailed method of partitioning should of course be used.

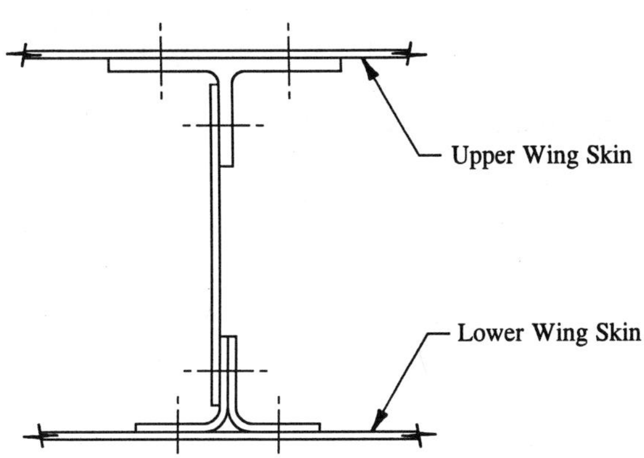

FIGURE A-23 Simplified front wing spar cross-section.

APPENDIX G

Calculation of Principal Moments of Inertia

The principal moments of inertia of a cross-sectional area are fully described and evaluated in this appendix. Their numerical values are used in the well-known flexure formula (Eq. 2-5, $f_b = \pm Mc/I_{na}$) to compute the bending stresses at any point on the exposed cross-sectional area of a member. The physical property which they represent is an indication or measure of the inherent resistance of a member to bending around its principal bending axes.

Before the formulas and procedures of this appendix are presented, it is suggested that the tabulation method of analysis of Appendix F, "Calculation of Moment of Inertia," be completely and thoroughly reviewed. If, however, these principles are clearly understood now, the engineer is encouraged to continue reading through the rest of the material contained in this appendix. The supplementary material which follows is merely an extension of these principles.

The particular method used in this appendix is quite simple, it consists of computing the conventional moments of inertia around a set of horizontal and vertical axes, and then using these results to determine the principal moments of inertia I_{x_p} and I_{y_p} around the principal bending axes x_p and y_p, respectively. By definition, the principal bending axes are those axes about which the maximum and minimum moments of inertia are said to occur. These axes are always mutually perpendicular and must pass through the centroid of area of the beam. Only then can the true representation of internal stress distribution of the member be accurately described. A good understanding of these concepts now will help the engineer recognize the basic relationships of these principles as they apply to actual engineering solutions.

It was shown in Sec. 2.3 that when a cross-sectional area has no axis of symmetry, like an L-section or Z-section, the applied or internal bending moments must be resolved into bending components which act in planes parallel and perpendicular to the principal bending axes which pass through the centroid of the cross-sectional area. In this form, the bending components are compatible with their corresponding principal bending planes, and, as such, should properly indicate the true stress distribution of the member. Clearly, the effects of bending on a structure are such as to cause the beam to bend around either principal bending axes of the cross-sectional area, or both.[1] Unless, of course, to prevent this beam action the structure is physically constrained from doing so by other external structures.

The following list of equations are required to locate the principal bending axes x_p and y_p and compute the corresponding minimum and maximum principal moments of inertia I_{x_p} and I_{y_p} from which these values are based:

$$I_{xy} = \Sigma Axy - AX_{cg}Y_{cg} \qquad \textbf{(A-14)}$$

$$\tan 2\alpha = \frac{2I_{xy}}{I_y - I_x} \qquad \textbf{(A-15)}$$

$$I_{x_p} = I_x \cos^2\alpha + I_y \sin^2\alpha - I_{xy} \sin 2\alpha \qquad \textbf{(A-16)}$$

$$I_{y_p} = I_x \sin^2\alpha + I_y \cos^2\alpha + I_{xy} \sin 2\alpha \qquad \textbf{(A-17)}$$

where: $\Sigma Axy = A_1x_1y_1 + A_2x_2y_2 + A_3x_3y_3 + \ldots + A_nx_ny_n$

A = total cross-sectional area

x = distance measured perpendicular from the rectangular coordinate axis Y to the centroid of an element area

y = distance measured perpendicular from the rectangular coordinate axis X to the centroid of an element area

α = angle measured between the centroidal and principal axes (a positive angle is measured counterclockwise)

I_{xy} = product of inertia with respect to a set of parallel centroidal axes

I_y = moment of inertia around the conventional rectangular coordinate axis y passing through the centroid of the total area

[1] A column, however, will physically bend about the minimum principal axis of the member (see Chapter 7, "Column Members," for the analysis and design of these particular members).

I_x = moment of inertia around the conventional rectangular coordinate axis x passing through the centroid of the total area

I_{x_p} = moment of inertia around the principal axis x_p passing through the centroid of the total area

I_{y_p} = moment of inertia around the principal axis y_p passing through the centroid of the total area

X_{cg} = distance measured perpendicular from the rectangular coordinate axis Y to the centroid of the total cross-sectional area

Y_{cg} = distance measured perpendicular from the rectangular coordinate axis X to the centroid of the total cross-sectional area.

These equations can also be used in finding the moments of inertia about any axis lying at an angle α between the principal axes and the conventional rectangular coordinate axes. However, their practical applications to actual engineering problems are rather doubtful.

The necessary formulas and procedures to determine the principal moments of inertia of a cross-sectional area are summarized below:

(1) From an arbitrary chosen reference axes system (this usually refers to a horizontal and vertical coordinate system in x and y), locate the centroid of the cross-sectional area:

$$X_{cg} = \frac{\Sigma\, Ax}{\Sigma\, A} \quad \text{and} \quad Y_{cg} = \frac{\Sigma\, Ay}{\Sigma\, A}.$$

(2) The conventional moments of inertia I_x and I_y parallel to the reference axes chosen in step 1 are computed. The following equations will produce values which will pass through the centroid of the cross-sectional area:

$$I_x = I_{cg} = \Sigma\, I_o + \Sigma\, Ay^2 - Y_{cg}\,(\Sigma\, Ay)$$
$$I_y = I_{cg} = \Sigma\, I_o + \Sigma Ax^2 - X_{cg}\,(\Sigma\, Ax).$$

(3) In this last step, the principal moments of inertia I_{x_p} and I_{y_p} are evaluated. This is accomplished by applying Eqs. A-14 through A-17 of this appendix.

APPENDIX H

Bending Stress Relationship Between a Built-up Beam and an Integral Beam

In this appendix, we will show how important the requirements of size and spacing of fasteners are to a well-designed, efficient structure. Let us begin by developing an example showing the differences in bending stresses that can occur for (1) two separate members attached together by a system of fasteners and (2) two separate members not attached together by any external means or system of fasteners. To simplify our solution, rectangular section areas are chosen for these members. This in no way implies that other cross-sectional shapes could not be used. On the contrary, the results here are presented to facilitate our solution and to show the most dramatic differences in stresses possible: this occurs for a beam composed of rectangular cross-sectional members.

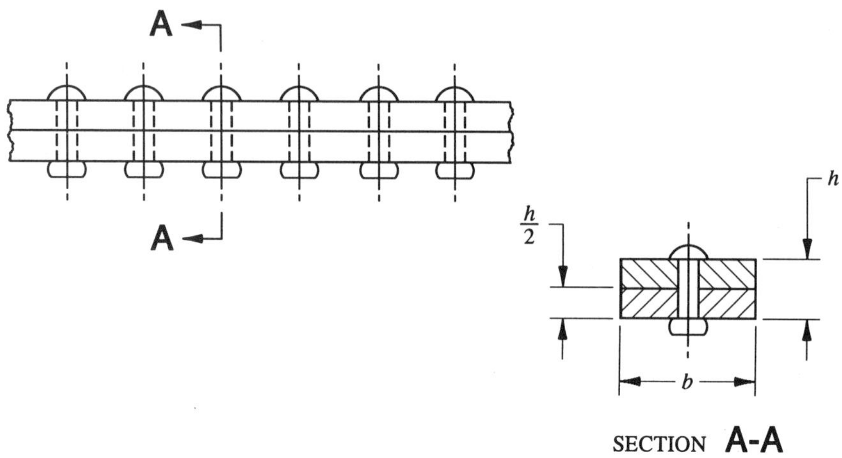

FIGURE A-24 Beam composed of rectangular cross-sectional members riveted together along their lengths.

Let us begin: If two rectangular members are attached together by a system of fasteners along their lengths, what bending stresses will develop at sections along the beam? Such a beam is shown in Fig. A-24. The size and spacing of fasteners are assumed to be structurally adequate to make these rectangular sections act together as a unit—thereby physically duplicating the behavior of an integral beam. In Sec. 4-4, the actual shear flow computations required to accomplish this structural arrangement of members are presented. For now, let us make this general statement or assumption: When the beam is vertically loaded, bending moments will develop along its length. Further, let us assume that a maximum bending moment M_{max} develops somewhere between the supported ends of the beam. The bending stresses caused by such a moment are determined by the flexure formula. Thus

$$f_b = \pm \frac{Mc}{I_{na}} \quad \text{(from Eq. 2-5)}$$

where: M = internal bending moment
c = distance to the extreme fibers of the cross-sectional area
I_{na} = moment of inertia of the total cross-sectional area.

Substituting the appropriate values into this expression gives:

$$f_b = \pm \frac{M_{max}\left[\frac{h}{2}\right]}{\frac{bh^3}{12}} = \pm \frac{6M_{max}}{bh^2}$$

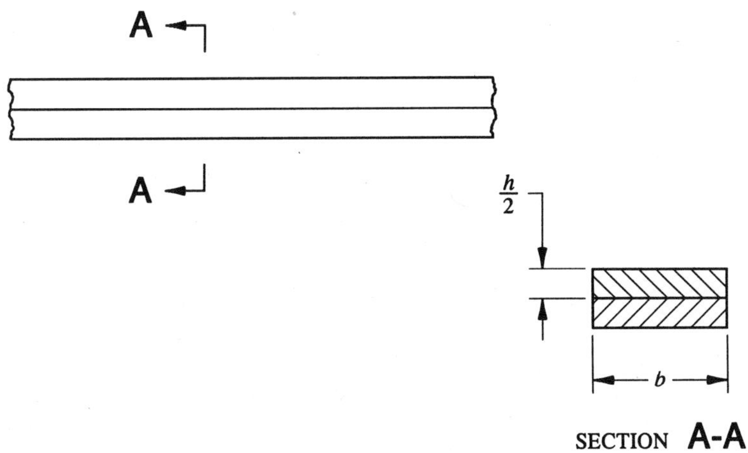

FIGURE A-25 Beam composed of rectangular cross-sectional members (no riveting along their lengths).

where: $M = M_{\max}$
$c = h/2$
$I_{na} = bh^3/12$ (standard equation for a rectangular section, from Appendix F, Table A-5, page 654).

This bending stress corresponds to the value for which the structure would simulate the structure of an integral beam if its members making up the total section area were properly fastened together.

Now, what stresses will develop if the same rectangular sections are used, but the members are not fastened together structurally (see Fig. A-25)? The following reasoning is described for such a case: To be consistent with the loads applied, the same bending moment $M_{\max}$ across the section is assumed. However, in this case, since the members are not attached together, each will physically act as a separate beam. Theoretically, this means that ½ of the bending moment will be carried by each separate member. And, if ½ of the bending moment is applied to ½ of the beam section, isn't that the same as our previous solution to simulate the structure of an integral beam? The answer to this question is "no." Let us see just why this is so. Follow along now for the computation of bending stresses if the members acted separately:

$$f_b = \pm \frac{Mc}{I_{na}}$$

where: $M = M_{\max}/2$
$c = h/4$

$$I_{na} = \frac{b\left[\frac{h}{2}\right]^3}{12} = \frac{bh^3}{96}.$$

Substituting these values into the flexure formula, we obtain:

$$f_b = \pm \frac{\frac{M_{\max}}{2}\left[\frac{h}{4}\right]}{\frac{bh^3}{96}} = \pm \frac{12M_{\max}}{bh^2}.$$

The stress here is twice that computed for the structure of an integral beam section, even though the total combined cross-sectional area was the same as that used for our former solution. This clearly shows how important the proper sizing and spacing of fasteners are to an overall design—bending stresses are dramatically reduced—which in turn can significantly reduce structural weight.

The engineer must always strive to optimize his fastener designs: anything less is structurally unacceptable. Conclusion: A built-up beam structure can physically be considered structurally as good as an integral beam if the individual members of the built-up section are properly attached to the main structure by an adequate size and spacing of fasteners. The shear flow equation, Eq. 4-3, is the basis of this optimization. If this equation is not followed explicitly, a built-up structure is designed for less than its fullest strength or capacity, and must therefore require a reduction in moment of inertia—a rather poor design alternative. In fact, no known method, other than through some form of structural testing, has been devised to determine intermediate cases of moment of inertia: that is, where structural members of a built-up section are less than fully fastened or secured to their primary structures. To avoid this unnecessary complication, the engineer should always make sure that fasteners of separately attached members of a built-up beam are properly sized and spaced according to shear flow design.

APPENDIX I

Inter-Rivet Buckling Using the Equation for the Inelastic Instability of a Flat Sheet in Compression

An alternative method of analysis that is sometimes used by aerospace companies to determine the inter-rivet buckling stress of a riveted member is given by the equation below:

$$F_{ir} = \frac{c\pi^2 E_t}{12(1 - \mu^2)}\left[\frac{t}{s}\right]^2$$

where: F_{ir} = allowable inter-rivet buckling stress

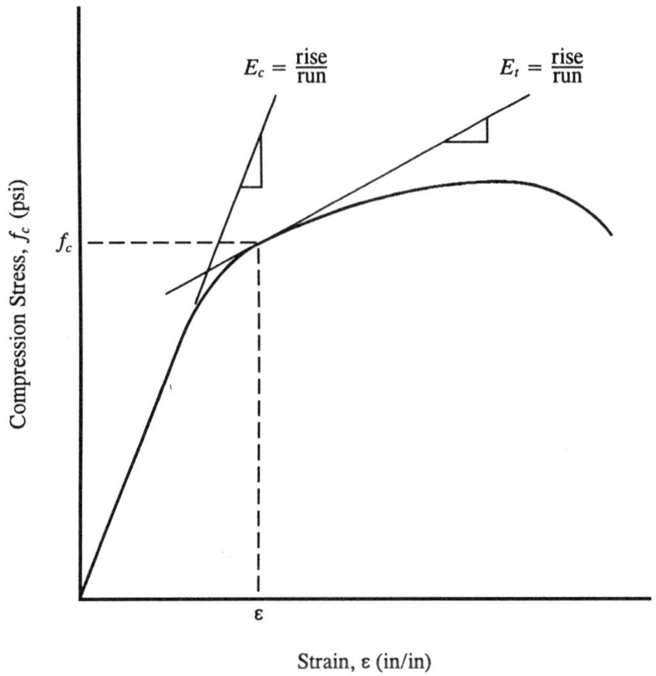

FIGURE A-26 Typical stress-strain diagram for compression.

E_t = compression tangent-modulus
μ = Poisson's ratio (see mechanical-property tables for specific materials in MIL-HDBK-5)
t = skin thickness
s = fastener spacing
c = end-fixity coefficient (refer to Table 6-1, page 363).

This equation is based on sheet or plate stability of members in compression, and is only presented here for general discussion (or for general reference use) for those engineers currently using this method of analysis.

The compression tangent-modulus E_t is defined as the slope (or rise/run) of a tangent line drawn on a stress-strain diagram at a point on the curve corresponding to either a stress or a strain. See Fig. A-26. In the elastic range, the compression tangent-modulus E_t is the same value as the compression modulus of elasticity E_c or Young's modulus. The tangent modulus E_t is a measure of the bending stiffness of a member in the inelastic range of stresses, while Young's modulus E_c is a measure of bending stiffness of a member in the elastic range of stresses.

When a sheet or plate buckles at a stress above the proportional limit of the material, a reduction in plate bending stiffness occurs. The effects of exceeding this limit on the buckled member are incorporated into a plasticity correction factor η. Or,

$$\eta = \frac{E_t}{E_c}.$$

However, if column curves are used, the effects of exceeding the proportional limit of the material are inherently included in their graphical solutions. For this reason, the preferred method of analysis in Sec. 6.2 will be used to determine the solution of inter-rivet buckling of compression-loaded members.

APPENDIX J

Inelastic Bending

In Chapter 2, the flexure formula ($f_b = \pm Mc/I_{na}$, Eq. 2-5) was used to determine internal stresses in a structure caused by bending moments in the elastic range of a stress-strain curve. However, once the structure has exceeded the proportional limit of the material, this equation is no longer valid. That is, its solution will predict maximum fiber stresses that are sometimes too high for practical design use. Although this equation depicts a linear variation of stress with applied bending moment, "real structure" does not behave so simply at higher loads. Its

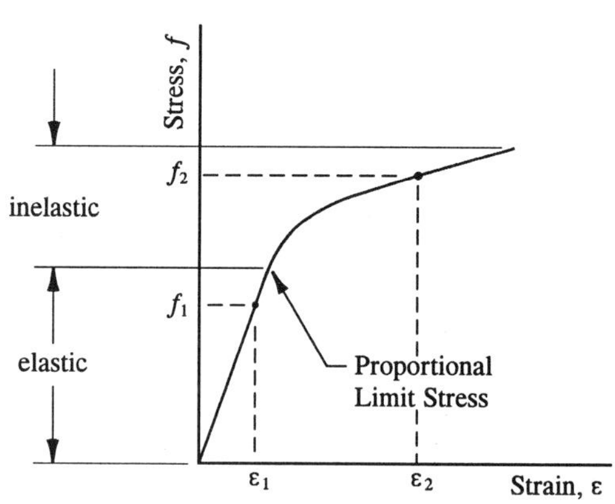

FIGURE A-27 Typical stress-strain diagram showing stresses below and above the proportional limit stress of the material.

solution to problems of inelastic stress design is however acceptable where some conservatism of the overall design of the structure is desirable.

In those cases which preclude local instability, failure of a member in bending will occur above the proportional limit of the material or inelastic range of stresses. The extreme fiber stresses of an actual structure in bending will begin to yield, while interior points of that structure, operating at lower stress levels, will experience increases in stress. The natural tendency of the structure to behave in this way describes what is commonly referred to as "a redistribution of load." The resulting effect is a nonlinear variation of stress.

Using a typical stress-strain curve, Fig. A-27, the theory of inelastic bending is explained in the following way: As the internal bending moment of the structure is increased, internal strains at the extreme fibers will increase to the values ε_1 and ε_2, as shown in Fig. A-28(a). The stress distributions f_1 and f_2 corresponding to these internal strains are shown in Fig. A-28(b). Note, in particular, that the internal stress distribution in the inelastic range is nonlinear for f_2. Now, if the stress distribution given by the flexure formula is superimposed in Fig. A-28(b), notice that the extreme fiber stress f_b exceeds that given by inelastic theory.

Thus, to avoid a weight penalty as a result of computing stresses by the simplified elastic stress distribution method (i.e., $\pm Mc/I_{na}$), a simple procedure for determining the ultimate allowable bending stress F_{bu} of a member in the inelastic range will be presented. The equation is written as follows:

$$F_{bu} = f_m + f_0(K - 1) \qquad \textbf{(A-18)}$$

where: $f_m = F_{tu}$

f_0 = this value is determined from design curves for specific material types (approximate this value by using the lower value of F_{ty} or F_{cy})

K = beam section shape factor[1] (for a rectangular section, $K = 1.5$).

To predict the ultimate failure of a member in bending in the inelastic range of stresses, the following expression is written:

$$\text{Margin of Safety} = \text{M.S.} = \frac{F_{bu}}{f_b k} - 1$$

where: F_{bu} = ultimate allowable bending stress[2]

f_b = ultimate internal bending stress (calculated from Mc/I_{na} for beam sections symmetrical about the neutral axis)

k = fitting factor for commercial aircraft design.

---

[1] The determination of this value for complex shapes, the engineer is referred to an advanced textbook on this subject.

[2] This term is also referred to as the "bending modulus of rupture."

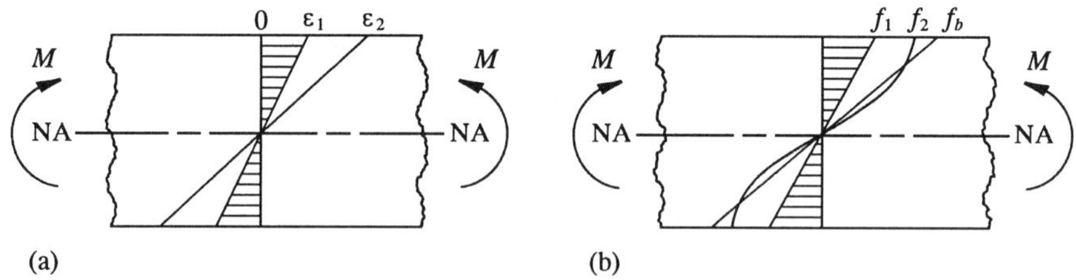

FIGURE A-28 (a) Internal strains due to an increased bending moment (b) Stress distributions corresponding to these internal strains.

A further comment: Since the tension and compression stress-strain curves of most materials are not identical, the neutral axis for inelastic bending is not coincident with the centroidal axis of the cross-sectional area. To account for this condition, it is generally accepted-practice by experienced engineers to use the smaller value of the yield tension or compression stress of the material in Eq. A-18. In so doing, it is assumed that the stress-strain curve of the other is identical. This assumption will greatly simplify the solution for ultimate bending strength, while only introducing a slightly conservative result to the designed structure.[1]

Additionally, a member that is limited by design to a prescribed stress level—for example, fatigue, crippling, or permanent set—can actually preclude the inelastic stress design of that member. In such cases, the value of f_m in Eq. A-18 would then become the limiting stress level. Of course, to solve this equation, the corresponding value of f_0 must also be known.

[1] For a more detailed discussion of this subject, the engineer is referred specifically to an aerospace company structures manual.

INDEX

— NOTES —

— NOTES —

— NOTES —

— NOTES —

— NOTES —

ISBN 0-9647014-0-5

59500

9 780964 701403